ESTROGENS AND HUMAN DISEASES

ANNALS OF THE NEW YORK ACADEMY OF SCIENCES
Volume 1089

ESTROGENS AND HUMAN DISEASES

Edited by H. Leon Bradlow and Giuseppe Carruba

Published by Blackwell Publishing on behalf of the New York Academy of Sciences
Boston, Massachusetts
2006

Library of Congress Cataloging-in-Publication Data

Estrogens and human diseases / edited by H. Leon Bradlow and
Giuseppe Carruba.
  p. ; cm. – (Annals of the New York Academy of Sciences,
ISSN 0077-8923 ; v. 1089)
  Includes bibliographical references and index.
  ISBN-13: 978-1-57331-669-9 (alk. paper)
  ISBN-10: 1-57331-669-5 (alk. paper)
  1. Estrogen–Physiological effect–Congresses. 2. Estrogen–
Pathophysiology–Congresses. 3. Nervous system–Degeneration–
Endocrine aspects–Congresses. I. Bradlow, H. Leon. II. New York
Academy of Sciences. III. Series.
  [DNLM: 1. Neoplasms–drug therapy–Congresses.
2. Estrogens–physiology–Congresses. 3. Estrogens–therapeutic
use–Congresses. 4. Neurodegenerative Diseases–drug
therapy–Congresses. W1 AN626YL v.1089 2006 / QZ 267 E82 2006]

  QP572.E85E836 2006
  616.8'0461–dc22

                                                    2006033052

The *Annals of the New York Academy of Sciences* (ISSN: 0077-8923 [print]; ISSN: 1749-
6632 [online]) is published 28 times a year on behalf of the New York Academy of Sciences
by Blackwell Publishing, with offices located at 350 Main Street, Malden, Massachusetts
02148 USA, PO Box 1354, Garsington Road, Oxford OX4 2DQ UK, and PO Box 378
Carlton South, 3053 Victoria Australia.

Information for subscribers: Subscription prices for 2006 are: Premium Institutional:
$3850.00 (US) and £2139.00 (Europe and Rest of World).
Customers in the UK should add VAT at 5%. Customers in the EU should also add VAT
at 5% or provide a VAT registration number or evidence of entitlement to exemption.
Customers in Canada should add 7% GST or provide evidence of entitlement to exemption.
The Premium Institutional price also includes online access to full-text articles from 1997 to
present, where available. For other pricing options or more information about online access
to Blackwell Publishing journals, including access information and terms and conditions,
please visit www.blackwellpublishing.com/nyas.

Membership information: Members may order copies of the *Annals* volumes directly
from the Academy by visiting www.nyas.org/annals, emailing membership@nyas.org,
faxing 212-298-3650, or calling 800-843-6927 (US only), or +1 212-298-8640 (International). For more information on becoming a member of the New York Academy of Sciences,
please visit www.nyas.org/membership.

Journal Customer Services: For ordering information, claims, and any inquiry concerning
your institutional subscription, please contact your nearest office:
UK: Email: customerservices@blackwellpublishing.com; Tel: +44 (0) 1865 778315;
Fax +44 (0) 1865 471775
US: Email: customerservices@blackwellpublishing.com; Tel: +1 781 388 8599 or
1 800 835 6770 (Toll free in the USA); Fax: +1 781 388 8232
Asia: Email: customerservices@blackwellpublishing.com; Tel: +65 6511 8000;
Fax: +61 3 8359 1120
Members: Claims and inquiries on member orders should be directed to the Academy at
email: membership@nyas.org or Tel: +1 212 838 0230 (International) or 800-843-6927
(US only).

Printed in the USA.
Printed on acid-free paper.

Mailing: The *Annals of the New York Academy of Sciences* are mailed Standard Rate. **Postmaster:** Send all address changes to *Annals of the New York Academy of Sciences*, Blackwell Publishing, Inc., Journals Subscription Department, 350 Main Street, Malden, MA 01248-5020. Mailing to rest of world by DHL Smart and Global Mail.

Disclaimer: The Publisher, the New York Academy of Sciences, and the Editors cannot be held responsible for errors or any consequences arising from the use of information contained in this publication; the views and opinions expressed do not necessarily reflect those of the Publisher, the New York Academy of Sciences, or the Editors.

Annals are available to subscribers online at the New York Academy of Sciences and also at Blackwell Synergy. Visit www.annalsnyas.org or www.blackwell-synergy.com to search the articles and register for table of contents e-mail alerts. Access to full text and PDF downloads of *Annals* articles are available to nonmembers and subscribers on a pay-per-view basis at www.annalsnyas.org.

The paper used in this publication meets the minimum requirements of the National Standard for Information Sciences Permanence of Paper for Printed Library Materials, ANSI Z39.48-1984.

ISSN: 0077-8923 (print); 1749-6632 (online)
ISBN-10: 1-57331-669-5 (paper); ISBN-13: 978-1-57331-669-9 (paper)

A catalogue record for this title is available from the British Library.

Digitization of the *Annals of the New York Academy of Sciences*

An agreement has recently been reached between Blackwell Publishing and the New York Academy of Sciences to digitize the entire run of the *Annals of the New York Academy of Sciences* back to volume one.

The back files, which have been defined as all of those issues published before 1997, will be sold to libraries as part of Blackwell Publishing's Legacy Sales Program and hosted on the Blackwell Synergy website.

Copyright of all material will remain with the rights holder. Contributors: Please contact Blackwell Publishing if you do not wish an article or picture from the *Annals of the New York Academy of Sciences* to be included in this digitization project.

Sponsors and Organizers for the Conference

Ettore Majorana Foundation and Centre for Scientific Culture
Prof. Antonino Zichichi, President and Director International School of Medical Sciences

Biagio Agostara, M. Ascoli Cancer Hospital Centre, Palermo, Italy

H. Leon Bradlow, Hackensack University Medical Center, Jurist Institute for Biomedical Research, Hackensack, New Jersey, USA

Giuseppe Carruba, Department of Experimental Oncology and Clinical Applications, University Medical School, University of Palermo, Italy

Louisa Massimo, Director Emeritus, Department of Pediatric Hematology and Oncology, "G. Gaslini" Scientific Children's Hospital, Genoa, Italy

ANNALS OF THE NEW YORK ACADEMY OF SCIENCES

Volume 1089
November 2006

ESTROGENS AND HUMAN DISEASES

Editors
H. LEON BRADLOW AND GIUSEPPE CARRUBA

This volume is the result of a meeting entitled **Estrogens and Human Diseases**, sponsored by the Ettore Majorana Foundation and Centre for Scientific Culture, and held on May 15–21, 2006, in Erice, Italy.

CONTENTS

Minisymposium

The Puzzle of Myelodysplastic Syndrome: Focusing on Immunophenotyping,
Cytogenetics, and Molecular Genetics

Part VII. Estrogens and Cardiovascular Diseases

Part VIII. Estrogens and Immune Diseases

Financial assistance was received from:

- Regione Siciliana
- Provincia Regionale di Palermo
- AIRC – Associazione Italiana per la Ricerca sul Cancro
- AMGEN
- CELBIO
- Schering-Plough Oncology
- Unionfarma

Preface

Around 30 years ago, Professor Luigi Castagnetta initiated a series of conferences at the Ettore Majorana Foundation and Centre for Scientific Culture in Erice, Sicily, each offering a particular perspective on the subject of hormones and cancer. Sadly, because of his untimely death on September 16, 2004, we did not have the benefit of his participation in the conference that has led to the present volume. Nevertheless the conference held in the same Erice site on May 15–22, 2006, unmistakably bore the imprint of his personality and scientific insight. It was Professor Castagnetta who, very shortly before his death, originally broached the idea of a conference on the subject of Estrogens and Human Disease, and with his customary exuberance, gave momentum to the project. We, along with Luisa Massimo and Biagio Agostara, co-directors of the course, enthusiastically began planning the project. Although it was difficult for us to imagine one of our meetings in Erice without "Gigi," as we used to call him, we were determined to carry his concept to completion, out of our admiration and love for him and hope to hold future meetings.

We continue to share his appreciation of the Ettore Majorana Centre, a remarkable venue for scientific meetings. It comprises a group of former monasteries and convents nestled among the winding, cobblestone streets of Erice—an ancient mountaintop settlement. This ancient ambience is a striking counterpoint to the very modern scientific meetings.

This eighth advanced course of the series on Experimental Oncology and its Clinical Application was mainly focused on the potential role that estrogens may play not only in classical endocrine-related tumors, such as those of the breast or prostate, but also in several other human nosological entities, including neurodegenerative disorders and cardiovascular and immune-related diseases. Topics ranged from the impact of endogenous and exogenous estrogens on human development and cancer risk, to novel aspects in the mechanisms of estrogen action, to estrogen implication in human malignancies (breast, prostate, liver), to the emerging role of estrogen in neurodegenerative disorders (Alzheimer's disease, multiple sclerosis, Parkinson's disease), to estrogen action in the cardiovascular system (including both genomic and nongenomic), to estrogen effects on cells of the immune system and their relevance to immune response and autoimmune diseases. The resulting inferences for clinics, diagnosis, prognosis, and treatment were also presented and extensively discussed. A large room was allocated for interactive discussion, aiming to favor the cross-fertilization process between the faculty and the audience. Furthermore, younger scientists were allowed to present their own experimental data orally

Ann. N.Y. Acad. Sci. 1089: xiii–xiv (2006). © 2006 New York Academy of Sciences.
doi: 10.1196/annals.1386.038

in specifically designed sessions, to provide a close interaction with major experts in the field and to discuss, also informally, technical and methodological aspects.

The articles in this volume are arranged, with a few exceptions, in the same sequence as they were presented, and are grouped into the main topics of the conference. After some brief tributes to Professor Castagnetta, the meeting began with a plenary talk on May 15 by Luisa Massimo on children's art and cancer. The body of the Course Sessions (8 overall) began on May 16 with Session I on Estrogens, Development, and Cancer, followed by Session II on New Insights into Estrogen Action, and the day ended by a first series of poster papers by younger presenters. During the following two days (May 17 and 18), Sessions III, IV, and V were dedicated to Estrogens and Cancer and focused, respectively, on breast cancer, prostate cancer, and liver cancer, the latter being followed by a second series of poster presentations. The fifth day (May 19) began with a keynote lecture by Professor Cavalieri on Catechol Quinones and Cancer; Session VI introduced a new area by dealing with Estrogens and Neurodegenerative Disorders. This was followed by a minisymposium on Myelodysplastic Syndromes. On May 20, two additional Sessions VII and VIII were dedicated to Estrogens and Cardiovascular Diseases and to Estrogens and Immune Diseases, respectively, with a final poster session in between the two. The course ended with closing remarks by the directors.

We wish to express our gratitude to all the coworkers of Prof. Castagnetta and to all the invited speakers and attendees of the course for their significant contributions. Last, but not least, we owe special thanks to Dr. Lucia Polito for providing us with the same generous support that she gave to Professor Castagnetta during her many years of loyal collaboration with him.

This is with our hope to keep this series of conferences going in the years to come.

H. LEON BRADLOW
Hackensack University Medical Center
Hackensack, New Jersey, USA

GIUSEPPE CARRUBA
University of Palermo, Italy

Inside Cancer Complexity

After two successful Advanced Courses held in Erice in 2001 and 2003 with Professor Luigi Castagnetta and Professor H. Leon Bradlow, published in the *Annals of the New York Academy of Sciences*, we have decided to honor Dr. Castagnetta's memory by organizing this course entitled "Estrogens and Human Diseases" together with his former students Professor Giuseppe Carruba and Dr. Lucia Polito. We feel that this meeting is especially important in order to continue an open-minded dialogue, this time in another field of cancer research.

Scientists from several countries are here and will present their outstanding work. I wish to thank them for their contributions and for their generosity.

Moving quickly from the experimental stage to biological significance is the promise of improving both survival rates and quality of life of cancer patients at all ages, including childhood. If we understand the biological mechanisms of carcinogenesis we certainly will be able to improve the treatment strategies, and open up a wide range of future prospects. Thanks to ongoing new discoveries, it is now possible to study cancer from several viewpoints. Currently, the most important areas include specific genetic signature identification by microarray technology, angiogenesis inhibition, immunoliposomes based upon the development of liposomes carrying antibody molecules charged with cytotoxic drugs on their surface, antisense oligonucleotides, and radioactive compounds. Translational research and innovation are the linkage from basic to clinical research.

What about children with cancer? I would like to shift this introductory lecture to a completely different area related to my daily activity, how children with cancer express themselves through drawings.

Before describing this work, I wish to take a moment to remember Professor Luigi Castagnetta, to whom this course is dedicated, and to add that he was an extremely generous person and scientist; he had a great humanistic culture, as most outstanding Sicilian people do, and a natural communicative ability. His collaborators and students considered him a beloved teacher, an older brother, a "maestro" always ready to help them. He will always remain a great example to the investigators involved in the study of the biology of cancer, and not only in Italy. Working with him meant, for me, building something good together. He was a true and faithful friend, and an excellent scientific partner.

LUISA M. MASSIMO
*Department of Pediatric Hematology
and Oncology "G. Gaslini" Scientific
Children's Hospital, Genova, Italy*

Ann. N.Y. Acad. Sci. 1089: xv (2006). © 2006 New York Academy of Sciences.
doi: 10.1196/annals.1386.019

In Tribute to Luigi Castagnetta—Drawings

A Narrative Approach for Children with Cancer

LUISA M. MASSIMO AND DANIELA A. ZARRI

Department of Pediatric Hematology and Oncology, G. Gaslini Children's Research Hospital, Genova, Italy

ABSTRACT: In troublesome situations, each of us uses verbal communication carefully, at times diminishing our meaning with words of little significance. However, since the need to communicate remains a part of us, body language or other forms of expression are put into use. Inside a hospital a child is always a stranger with regards to the uneasiness that accompanies his/her experience. Because diagnostic and therapeutic ends are the primary concern of the health care professionals, there is often little sign of affection in their impersonal gestures, glances, and body language. Graphic and pictorial communication, therefore, holds great importance for sick children since this is an area they have easier access to, and that they cultivate at school and through play. This activity fulfills their innate need to communicate with themselves and with others. Children express themselves through drawings, using them as a stage to dramatize their needs, wishes, anxieties, and joys. When in hospital, children are afraid, and they feel embarrassed around strangers and even parents, especially when the parents are speaking with their children's caregivers. The children are afraid of making a poor impression and of being rejected by adults, of being considered inadequate and untruthful. Their need for truth and for communication unfolds through artistic expression, and this is the basis of art therapy. The opportunity to express themselves through drawings is what makes the ill child his/her own therapeutic agent through a self-healing mechanism. This may be further guided so as to lead to an increase in self-esteem, which in turn will lead to both enhancement of their full expressive possibilities and to positive feedback of their self-image. In addition to verbal language itself, art therapy is the preferred and ideal means to communicate following the rules of "narrative-based medicine," and to understand children. In this study spontaneous drawings of 50 Italian children affected by leukemia or cancer in different stages were evaluated during 2003 at the

Address for correspondence: Prof. Luisa M. Massimo, M.D., Department of Pediatric Hematology and Oncology, G. Gaslini Children's Research Hospital, Largo G, Gaslini 5, 16147 Genova, Italy. Voice: +39-010-591788; fax: +39-010-593129.

e-mail: luisamassimo@ospedale-gaslini.ge.it.

Ann. N.Y. Acad. Sci. 1089: xvi-xxiii (2006). © 2006 New York Academy of Sciences.
doi: 10.1196/annals.1386.020

outpatient clinic of the G.Gaslini Children's Hospital. Ages ranged from 4 to 14 years (median 8 years); 27 were males and 23 females. They drew in three situations: spontaneously when they were alone; with play workers; and with the psychologist. Pictures emerging from these settings have proven to be significant and denote the children's perception of the disease, and of their fears and hopes. The children's drawings allowed them to depict their present and future relationship with the disease, with the hospital, and with the environment in general. Their pictures reflected not only their current state of mind, but also past experiences and future prospects. Art therapy proved to be a vitally important means of "narrative" communication for severely sick children in hospital. Thus, collecting and evaluating drawings in an attempt to establish the intellectual, cultural, and emotional status of each child is of paramount importance. To this end, play workers have been trained to carefully observe each child while drawing. Such extremely important collaboration prevents the loss of relevant and vital details. This research confirms our theory that art therapy has to be included in the total care of a severely ill child while in hospital. Drawings accompanied by comments certainly provide a broader approach to better understanding the child's anxiety and feelings.

KEYWORDS: art therapy for sick children; children's communication through drawings; drawings in hospital care

INTRODUCTION

Inside a hospital a child feels like a stranger because of the uneasiness that accompanies his new experience. He/she usually does not receive suitable explanations, although good communication is essential in order to establish any type of alliance. This includes the therapeutic alliance and the agreement between the patient and the professional caregivers that lead to mutual fulfillment. Diagnostic and therapeutic ends are always kept in mind when dealing with these children. In troublesome situations each of us uses verbal communication carefully, at times diminishing our meaning with a wealth of words that have little significance. However, since the need to communicate remains, body language or other forms of expression are put into use. Often there is a lack of affection in the impersonal gestures, glances, and body language of the health care professionals. Children are thus deprived of the opportunity to communicate on the two simplest levels, but they still have the option of graphic and pictorial communication. This is an area to which they have easy access. It is cultivated at school and through play, and it satisfies their natural need to communicate. They express themselves through drawings, using them as a stage to dramatize their requests, needs, wishes, anxieties, and joys. When in hospital, children are afraid, and they are embarrassed around strangers, and around their parents, especially when the parents are speaking with the health care professionals. Children are afraid of making a poor impression and of being rejected by adults, of being considered inadequate and untruthful. Their need for truth and for communication unfolds through artistic expression. The opportunity to express themselves through drawings makes the sick children their own therapeutic agents through a self-healing mechanism. This may be further guided so as to lead to an increase in self-esteem, to help them achieve their full expressive possibilities and to get positive feedback of their self-image. Art therapy is the preferred and ideal means of communication with a child.

MATERIALS AND METHODS

In the Department of Pediatric Hematology and Oncology, a multistep method was developed in an effort both to investigate the emotional status of sick children and to reduce stressful response to hospitalization and the dramatic changes in their lives. In this study the spontaneous drawings of 50 Italian children affected by leukemia or cancer in different stages were evaluated during 2003 at the outpatient clinic of the G. Gaslini Children's Hospital. Their ages ranged from 4 to 14 years (median 8 years); 27 were males and 23 were females. They came from different Italian geographic areas, social classes, and cultural backgrounds, thus enabling us to evaluate multiple experiences. They were cared for by three trained play workers and one psychologist (D.A.Z.).

We decided to use drawings for our investigation since they are easy to propose and to collect, and because specific protocols for collection and interpretation already exist. In order to establish the rules, we discussed our project with the play workers in an attempt to identify the most appropriate moment for collection and to choose the best approach in order to avoid distorting the communication. We evaluated whether it was appropriate to pressure children to produce drawings and when and whether this request might elicit refusal or tension. We decided that each drawing had to be accompanied by an interview and a written description by the child or, if this was not possible, the written description would be provided by the play worker or by the psychologist. We also decided to collect both spontaneous and solicited drawings, even by simply asking "Can you draw me a picture?" In case of reticence, the subsequent suggestion was "Can you make up a story from your drawing?" The child was free to choose both the topic and the technique, and was given time to start drawing. The teacher stood beside him/her with a neutral encouraging attitude, avoiding any comments or suggestions concerning aesthetic aspects. If the child asked for approval, the answer was "Interesting; tell me what / who that is," thus rewarding the child and even evaluating the subconscious contents.

RESULTS

The drawings that emerged from these settings denote the perception of the disease and of the child's fears and hopes. The comment written by each adolescent and school-age child or by the play worker allowed us to acquire a better understanding of the painter's meaning and feelings. Some very interesting data emerged from the longitudinal study because each child made several paintings over the course of the year while in different health and emotional states, including disease onset, remission, off-treatment, and relapse. In most cases the drawings helped us to understand and appreciate the improvement in the child's feelings that resulted from the environment, from the psychosocial support tightly linked to the achieved results, and from the overall helping strategy developed within the department for the whole family.

DISCUSSION

Although psychological research and therapy in children is usually dependent upon drawings, the scientific literature on this topic is surprisingly scarce. The only general statement that can be made is that the drawings cannot be the sole indicator of the child's status, but must be assessed within a more global study. We agree with this conclusion and believe that interviewing and surveying the children, their siblings, and their parents, as well as carefully studying the children's spontaneous drawings are among the simplest techniques for evaluating the existence, nature, and extent of the patients' feelings (including fantasies and misunderstandings). This knowledge might help us to modify possible distortions both of perception and behavior. Drawing is a spontaneous act for any child. His/her signs have a precise meaning, but they are not always related to their actual experience. Children often merely want to draw or to comment upon a fiction, a reality that is not related to their life and/or feelings. Nevertheless, their drawings always have a meaning that allows us to understand whether there are disturbances in their psychological development or in their feelings. As patients, children have impaired verbal communication channels; yet good communication is very important in order to establish a positive therapeutic alliance with the caregivers. This result can be achieved with the help of nonverbal tools, such as play, drawings, and other handicraft activities. Drawing is an accepted, indeed, preferred activity in hospitals since it is a simple, easy game for children, the drawings can be collected and preserved, and it does not disturb life in the ward. However, a verbal comment is essential to help us understand the child's meaning and feelings. We followed an interview protocol as well as modalities for collection and feedback. Since our activity was not aimed at making a diagnosis or psychotherapy, we have chosen the large setting of playrooms in which team activities could be carried out. This choice was advantageous since the children enjoyed the great freedom they were given to express themselves.

As a result of the large immigration of families from poor countries all over the world to European nations, over the last few years several children who do not speak Italian have been admitted to our department. Drawing is a great opportunity to provide them with entertainment in the playroom and a good quality of life. However, our experience teaches us that we can never be sure of our interpretation of their drawings, since they lack both comments, and the answers to several important questions that we usually get from our little painters.

Among the scarce medical literature on art therapy for sick children, which mostly concerns drawings, we would like to mention a few important articles. Pope-Grattan et al.[1] were among the first investigators who considered children's drawings to be an important indicator in the evaluation of stress and anxiety. They examined 72 human figure drawings made by 43 patients affected by Duchenne's muscular dystrophy, accompanied by a description according to 11 emotional indicators and according to directionality quadrants. They were able to assess physical inadequacy, immaturity, body anxiety, and insecurity. A few years later, Light and Simmons[2] studied a group of healthy children aged 5 to 8 years by a "communication game" using drawings. The results showed the maturity of the older children as compared to the younger ones. Harrison et al.[3] carried out a controlled study of children's drawings as a means of distinguishing 48 children with chronic asthma from 52 healthy controls. The study involved three observers using different methods of investigation. The observer with a knowledge of "drawings per se" was clearly much better ($P < 0.001$) at detecting children with asthma, while the results obtained by the other two observers were no better than random chance. One of them used a scoring method, while the other used a direct assessment technique based on his experience of children with chronic disease. Drawings by kindergarten children were analyzed by Mumcuoglu[4] in order to study the emotional reaction of children to head lice. He found that the choice of color was significant (black was used by 43% of the children, indicating that the subject of lice is associated with anxiety and fear) as were the unhappy faces and omissions of mouths in the drawings. Mares[5] proposed his own method of verbal–graphic diagnostics of children's experience with painful interventions in hospital. The children's drawings were analyzed by means of quantitative and qualitative indicators. He realized that the painful intervention itself is not as stressful for the ill child as the circumstances under which it is performed, which include inadequate preparation, impersonal environment, and absence of social support. That same year, we reported our observations on children drawing their ideas of the central venous catheter. Sometimes it was seen as a dangerous and invasive "foreign body," but mostly it created a psychological state of dependency and became the only means of salvation.[6] Few studies have examined the reliability and validity of the indicators of emotional distress in children's projective drawings, that is, detail, line heaviness even as a way to measure childhood depression and anxiety.[7–9] The reliability and validity of children's art work in clinical investigation were studied by Thomas and Jolley,[10] who realized that children's drawings taken on their own are too complex and inherently ambiguous to be the sole indicator of the emotional experiences of the children who drew them. Research on very young children, carried out by Thomas *et al.*, came to the same conclusion,[11] Cox and Rowlands used three different school methods—Steiner, Montessori, and traditional—to study the effect of art education on healthy children. They concluded that the approach to art education in Steiner method schools is not only conducive to more highly rated imaginative drawings in terms of general drawing ability and use of color, but also to more accurate and detailed observational drawings.[12] Many other authors have investigated the meaning of drawings made by normal, healthy children, mostly to study the affection within their families.[13]

In our research, the method we chose yielded very good results since the attention the children received made them more willing to cooperate. We noticed that they often started by drawing apparently impersonal, conventional situations to test the attitude of the adult toward them, especially when their thoughts were "improper." Cartoon characters or the classic incomplete small houses are structured defenses against an intrusion into intimacy or are drawn when they fear an unpleasant reaction. The discreet attention they receive in the subsequent interviews is the key to opening the closed doors and windows of those small houses. Children frequently produce a significant soliloquy while they draw, and spy on the reaction of adults to their verbal production, thus testing the listener's degree of interest. Therefore, it is necessary to pay careful attention to the words, gestures, and behavior of the children, and to display this attention very clearly. Through this approach, we collected a great deal of data from our Italian patients. We then used these data as the basis for our evaluation of foreign children's drawings, at least initially, since we could not interview them. In childhood, any type of danger is seen as something bringing about physical destruction, and regardless of its severity, a disease is as frightening as other events.

We observed that sick children give different types of messages using different personal techniques. We placed the drawings into two main categories. The first category includes drawings related to their past, covering a long time span, and a wide range of situations that were not influenced by the disease. In these drawings, they often represent themselves as being physically normal, without the existing alopecia, scars, mutilations. They interpret their relationships with parents, friends, animals, and objects in their everyday lives in the same way. They maintain a similar attitude even with regards to their comments. The second category includes drawings showing their perception of the disease and of themselves as sick children. In their paintings they are either absent protagonists in often painful stories, or they are present and the representation of their physical aspect is more realistic. Drawings also show the child's fear of loneliness, which is closely related to their fear of physical destruction, as the child is always aware of his/her vulnerability and dependence on adults. Hunters, witches, predators, monsters, sharks, wolves remind them of the fairy tales as an anthropomorphic representation. The dark side of caregivers and parents, such as Cinderella's and Snow White's stepmothers, is what is often seen.

Doctors and nurses are not represented together with relatives in scenes of daily life, whereas relatives are sometimes present in scenes of hospital life. This is especially common in the illustration of moments spent with those devoted to their health care, for instance, parties in the ward or activities in playrooms. Among the drawings of the second category, teachers and school rooms are often represented as reassuring people and environments that maintain, even in hospital, the characteristics of attention and listening, as well as of interaction that is devoid of any prejudice, which is often shown in daily life. Finally, all the drawings produced during follow-up visits, months or even years after therapy was ended, show how much children and adolescents feel threatened by disease, physicians, nurses, and other health care professionals, sometimes beyond their own conscious perception.

In conclusion, we strongly suggest taking art therapy into consideration and including it in the total care of children affected either by cancer or by other severe diseases that require long periods of hospital treatment. In these circumstances, drawings accompanied by comments would certainly help provide a broader approach to better understanding the child's anxieties and feelings.[14]

REFERENCES

1. POPE-GRATTAN, M.M., C.N. BURNETT & C.V. WOLFE. 1976. Human figure drawings by children with Duchenne's muscular dystrophy. Phys. Ther. **56:** 168–176.
2. LIGHT, P. & B. SIMMONS. 1983. The effects of a communication task upon the representation of depth relationships in young children's drawings. J. Exp. Child Psychol. **35:** 81–92.
3. HARRISON, J.A., N.B. MOGRIDGE & K.P. DAWSON. 1990. Can the study of spontaneous drawings indicate those children with chronic illness? N.Z. Med. J. **103:** 219–221.
4. MUMCUOGLU, K.Y. 1991. Head lice in drawings of kindergarten children. Isr. J. Psychiatry Relat. Sci. **28:** 25–32.
5. MARES, J. 1996. The use of kinetic children's drawings to explore the pain experiences of children in hospital. Acta Medica **39:** 73–80.
6. ZARRI, D., F. MONTALCINI & L. MASSIMO. 1996. The central venous catheter for young patients: an "umbilical cord" fantasy. Bone Marrow Transplant. **2**(Suppl.): 129–133.
7. JOINER, T.E. JR, K.L. SCHMIDT & J. BARNETT. 1996. Size, detail, and line heaviness in children's drawings as correlates of emotional distress: (more) negative evidence. J. Pers. Assess. **67:** 127–141.
8. ZAHR, L.K. 1998. Therapeutic play for hospitalized preschoolers in Lebanon. Pediatr. Nurs. **24:** 449–454.
9. THOMAS, G.V. & R.P. JOLLEY. 1998. Drawing conclusions: a re-examination of empirical and conceptual bases for psychological evaluation of children from their drawings. Br. J. Clin. Psychol. **37:** 127–139.
10. CLATWORTHY, S., K. SIMON & M.E. TIEDEMAN 1999. Child drawing: hospital – an instrument designed to measure the emotional status of hospitalized school-aged children. J. Pediatr. Nurs. **14:** 2–9.

11. THOMAS, G.V., R.P. JOLLEY, E.J. ROBINSON & H. CHAMPION. 1999. Realist errors in children's responses to pictures and words as representations. J. Exp. Child Psychol. **74:** 1–20.
12. ROWLANDS COX, M.V. 2000. The effect of three different educational approaches on children's drawing ability: Steiner, Montessori and traditional. Br. J. Clin. Psychol. **70:** 485–503.
13. MADIGAN, S., M. LADD & S. GOLDBERG. 2003. A picture is worth a thousand words: children's representations of family as indicators of early attachment. Attach. Hum. Dev. **5:** 19–37.
14. MASSIMO, L. 1997. L'assistenza integrata in onco-ematologia pediatrica. Minerva Pediatr. **49:** 507–511.

The Role of Estrogens in Normal and Abnormal Development of the Prostate Gland

GAIL S. PRINS, LIWEI HUANG, LYNN BIRCH, AND YONGBING PU

Department of Urology, University of Illinois at Chicago, Chicago, Illinois, USA

ABSTRACT: Estrogens play a physiologic role during prostate development with regard to programming stromal cells and directing early morphogenic events. However, if estrogenic exposures are abnormally high during the critical developmental period, permanent alterations in prostate branching morphogenesis and cellular differentiation will result, a process referred to as neonatal imprinting or developmental estrogenization. These perturbations are associated with an increased incidence of prostatic lesions with aging, which include hyperplasia, inflammation, and dysplasia. To understand how early estrogenic exposures can permanently alter the prostate and predispose it to neoplasia, we examined the effects of estrogens on prostatic steroid receptors and key developmental genes. Transient and permanent alterations in prostatic AR, ERα, ERβ, and RARs are observed. We propose that estrogen-induced alterations in these critical transcription factors play a fundamental role in initiating prostatic growth and differentiation defects by shifting the prostate from an androgen-dominated gland to one whose development is regulated by estrogens and retinoids. This in turn leads to specific disruptions in the expression patterns of key prostatic developmental genes that normally dictate morphogenesis and differentiation. Specifically, we find transient reductions in *Nkx*3.1 and permanent reductions in *Hox*b-13, which lead to differentiation defects particularly within the ventral lobe. Prolonged developmental expression of *Bmp*-4 contributes to hypomorphic growth throughout the prostatic complex. Reduced expression of *Fgf*10 and *Shh* and their cognate receptors in the dorsolateral lobes leads to branching defects in those specific regions in response to neonatal estrogens. We hypothesize that these molecular changes initiated early in life predispose the prostate to the neoplastic state upon aging.

KEYWORDS: prostate; estradiol; estrogen; steroid receptors; *Hox*b-13; *Nkx*3.1; sonic hedgehog; fibroblast growth factor-10

Address for correspondence: Gail S. Prins, P.h.D., Department of Urology, M/C 955, University of Illinois at Chicago, 820 South Wood, Chicago, IL 60612, USA. Voice: 312-413-9766; fax: 312-996-1291.
e-mail: gprins@uic.edu

Ann. N.Y. Acad. Sci. 1089: 1–13 (2006). © 2006 New York Academy of Sciences.
doi: 10.1196/annals.1386.009

INTRODUCTION

Prostate gland development is under hormonal regulation, primarily mediated by androgens that dictate its growth and differentiation.[1,2] In addition, the developing prostate is sensitive to other protein and steroid hormones including estrogens.[2] In humans, under the continuous influence of maternal and placental estrogens during fetal development, extensive squamous metaplasia arises within the prostatic epithelium, which sloughs at birth after maternal estrogen levels fall.[3] These effects are mediated through estrogen receptors α and β (ERα and ERβ), which are expressed at high levels in the developing prostate stroma and epithelium, respectively.[4] The natural role, if any, for estrogens during human prostatic development is unknown; however, it is possible that estrogens normally program the prostate gland in a manner that affects their growth and function throughout life.

Studies with various rodent models support a physiologic role for estrogens in prostate development, particularly with regard to programming of prostatic stromal cells.[5,6] In contrast to humans, in whom prostate development is completed *in utero,* the rodent prostate gland is rudimentary at birth and undergoes extensive branching morphogenesis followed by functional differentiation during the first 15 days of life.[7] Thus the neonatal rodent prostate has emerged as a useful model for evaluating the role of endogenous and exogenous estrogens during prostate development. With this rodent model, it has been shown that elevated perinatal levels of endogenous estrogens (maternal or excess local production) or exogenous estrogens (diethylstilbesterol or, potentially, environmental estrogens) lead to permanent disturbances in prostate growth and predispose to precancerous lesions, a process referred to as developmental estrogenization or estrogen imprinting.[8] The specific model used in our laboratory to study developmental estrogenization of the prostate gland is the Sprague–Dawley rat given injections of 25 μg estradiol on neonatal days 1, 3, and 5. While considered a "high-dose" exposure, most of this estradiol is bound to the high levels of circulating α-fetoprotein in the neonate, and free circulating estradiol levels are estimated at 1/100th of this amount. This neonatal exposure to estradiol results in a permanent reduction in prostatic growth and activational response to androgens during adulthood, an effect mediated in part through a permanent reduction in androgen receptor (AR) expression.[9–12] Upon aging, prostatic hyperplasia and dysplasia are prominent in neonatally estrogenized rats, and PIN-3 (prostatic intraepithelial neoplasia) lesions are observed when these animals are given exogenous testosterone.[13,14] Although all prostate lobes are permanently imprinted by elevated estrogens, there is some lobe specificity to the response. Thus branching deficiencies are notable in the dorsal and lateral lobes while the ventral prostate, although hypomorphic, shows normal branching patterns.[15] Structural and functional epithelial cytodifferentiation during development is perturbed or, for some end-points, permanently blocked by neonatal estrogens as determined by markers for basal and luminal cytokeratins and secretory proteins (PBP, DLP protein, urokinase, 26 kD protease) [10,16,17] and the greatest differentiation defects are consistently observed in the ventral prostate lobe. The molecular basis for neonatal estrogenization of the prostate gland with lobe-specific responses will be the focus of this review article.

MECHANISM OF ACTION: STEROID RECEPTORS

Estrogen action in the rat prostate gland is mediated through stromal ERα[18] and epithelial ERβ.[19] Importantly, studies with ER knockout mice (αERKO and βERKO) showed that stromal cell ERα is the dominant ER mediating developmental estrogenization of the prostate.[17] During the first 5–10 days of life, ERα is present in the mesenchymal cells of the proximal regions of the growing ducts. Following estrogenic exposure, there is a transient upregulation of this protein within periductal stromal cells along the length of the ducts, which allows for amplification of estrogenic action during this critical period.[18] This, in turn, leads to a transient expression of progesterone receptor (PR) in these stromal cells that are normally negative for PR.[20] In addition, prostatic retinoid receptors (RARs and RXRs) and intraprostatic retinoid levels are immediately and permanently elevated following neonatal estrogenic exposure, which allows for the amplification of retinoid signals during development and with aging.[21,22] It is particularly significant that these increases in ER, PR, and RAR levels occur at the same time that AR is drastically downregulated.[10,12] These changes are summarized in the schematic shown in FIGURE 1. Following a brief exposure to high levels of estrogen during the neonatal critical period, the temporal expression patterns as well as quantitative levels of several key steroid receptors (transcription factors), are drastically altered. Thus, the prostate is no longer under predominant androgen regulation, but is rather driven by estrogenic and retinoid signals through the ERs, PR, RARs, and RXRs. We propose that the net effect of these changes is that the programming and organizational signals that normally dictate and determine prostate development during discrete temporal windows are permanently and irretrievably altered.

DEVELOPMENTAL GENES

Continuous branching morphogenesis of glandular structures is dictated by time-specific and region-specific expression of master regulatory genes.[23] Although common morphogenetic paradigms exist for all branched structures studied to date, the critical difference is that spatial and temporal combinations

(A)

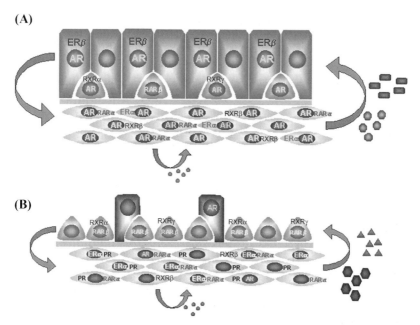

(B)

FIGURE 1. Schematic representation of steroid receptor expression in postnatal day 5–10 developing prostates from oil-treated control rats (**A**) and neonatally estrogenized rats (**B**). In the normal developing prostate (**A**), androgen receptor (AR) is the dominant steroid receptor in both epithelial and stromal cells. Under the influence of androgens, the stromal cells produce and secrete specific paracrine factors that dictate growth and differentiation of the gland. As epithelial cells differentiate, AR levels markedly increase and ERβ expression is induced. Other steroid receptors are expressed in a cell-specific manner and regulate cell-specific gene expression during critical developmental windows. Estrogen receptor α (ERα) is expressed at low levels in periductal stromal cells in the proximal region of the elongating ducts. RARβ is expressed in a subpopulation of basal epithelial cells, whereas RARα and γ are localized to periductal stromal cells along the ductal length. RXRα and RXRγ are expressed by basal cells, while RXRβ localizes to periductal stromal cells. Following a brief exposure to high levels of estrogens during the neonatal critical period, the prostatic steroid receptor profile is drastically altered (**B**). AR is absent in epithelial cells and is present at very low levels in stromal cells, thus dampening the androgen signaling pathway in the developing prostate. ERα is upregulated and expressed at high levels in periductal stromal cells along the length of the ducts, and progesterone receptor (PR) is induced in those same cells under the influence of estrogen. The number of cells expressing RARα and RARβ is markedly increased. Thus, estrogen exposure has switched the developing prostate from an androgen-dominated tissue to one that is regulated by estrogen, progesterone, and retinoids.

of these genes give rise to unique structures. While the "prostatic code" is not well defined at the present time, recent activity in this field has led to an early map.[17,24–31,42] We are currently interested in determining whether neonatal exposure to estrogens can alter prostatic development through changes in the expression of these key developmental genes.

HOMEOBOX GENES: *Nkx* 3.1 AND *Hox*b 13

Several specific homeobox genes have been identified within the developing prostate tissue and are thought to account for prostate determination and to play a role in morphogenesis and cellular differentiation. These include members of the *Hox* gene family,[32] and the NK gene family.[31] Importantly, a growing body of evidence supports a role for estrogens, progesterone, and retinoids in regulating homeobox genes in a variety of structures including the lungs and uterus.[33–35] Furthermore, fetal exposure to diethylstilbestrol (DES) resulted in strong downregulation of uterine *Hoxa*-10 expression.[33] Thus we explored the effects of neonatal estradiol exposure on prostatic *Nkx*3.1 and *Hox*b 13 genes to determine whether these genes may be downstream of estrogen action in the prostate.

*Nkx*3.1 is a member of the NK family of homeobox transcription factors whose expression in the murine male reproductive tract is restricted to UGS-derived prostate and bulbourethral gland epithelium.[25,36] Importantly, this gene is expressed in the fetal mouse UGS epithelium at the sites of bud formation, suggesting a role for *Nkx*3.1 in prostate determination.[24,25] Continued expression of this gene is believed to be important for epithelial cell differentiation. Using qRT-PCR, we measured the ontogeny of *Nkx*3.1 expression in the rat ventral prostate and found peak expression at postnatal day 10 (FIG. 2A) when the epithelial cells undergo cytodifferentiation.[10] Although continued expression

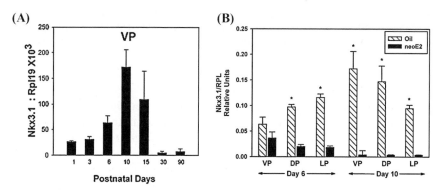

FIGURE 2. Real-time qRT-PCR of *Nkx*3.1 expression in the developing rat prostate lobes. Samples were amplified in duplex using a SYBR-green assay and data were normalized to the ribosomal protein, RPL19 mRNA co-amplified for each tissue. **A:** Ventral lobe (VP) expression levels of days 1, 3, 6, 10, 15, 30, and 90 of life show a peak of expression at postnatal day 10 with low steady-state expression observed in adulthood. **B:** Postnatal days 6 and 10 expression levels in the VP, dorsal (DP), and lateral (LP) prostate lobes of rats exposed to oil (*hatched bars*) or 25 µg estradiol benzoate on days 1, 3, and 5 of life (*solid bars*). N = 4–10 assays/group. *$P < 0.01$ compared to estradiol-treated rats at same time point. (from Pu *et al.* Reprinted by permission.)

in the adult prostate is believed to be important in maintaining differentiation, the relative levels are small compared to the expression on postnatal days 5–15. To determine the effects of early estrogen exposure on *Nkx*3.1 expression, we performed *in situ* hybridization[17] and real-time RT-PCR[42] on developing and adult prostates of control and estrogenized rats. Neonatal estrogens immediately and strongly suppressed *Nkx*3.1 expression in the developing prostate (FIG. 2B). However, this downregulation of *Nkx*3.1 was transient, and similar expression levels were observed between controls and estrogenized prostates by day 30 and thereafter.[17] Nonetheless, it is important to stress that the developmental peak in *Nkx*3.1 expression was abolished by neonatal estrogens. We propose that a transient disruption in *Nkx*3.1 expression at a critical time when epithelial cells normally differentiate into basal and luminal layers[10] may contribute to the perturbed epithelial differentiation seen throughout the prostate lobes of the estrogen-exposed animals.

Prostate specification has been shown to be regulated in part through the most posterior genes of the *Hox* cluster, the *Hox*13 genes.[32] Of the three *Hox*13 genes expressed in the prostate (*Hox*a-13, *Hox*b-13, and *Hox*d-13), *Hox*b-13 is unique in that it is expressed solely by epithelial cells and its increased expression postnatally correlates with epithelial differentiation.[17,30,37] In the rat prostate, we quantitated *Hox*b-13 mRNA by qRT-PCR and *in situ* hybridization throughout development and into adulthood and found an increasing anterior-to-posterior expression gradient with low levels in the dorsal lobe, moderate levels in the lateral lobe, and high expression throughout the epithelium of the ventral prostate lobes.[15] This suggests an increasingly important role for *Hox*b-13 in the rat ventral lobe, which is similar to findings reported for the mouse prostate, where expression was exclusively confined to the ventral prostate and targeted deletion of *Hox*b-13 resulted in ventral lobe-specific defects. When we transfected *Hox*b-13 into cultured rat prostate basal cells, they differentiated into a luminal phenotype suggesting a specific role for *Hox*b-13 in epithelial cell differentiation.[38] Following neonatal exposure to estrogen, *Hoxb*-13 expression was immediately and permanently suppressed in all prostate lobes with the most significant reduction (80%) observed in the ventral prostate gland.[17] Since this loss directly correlated with the loss of epithelial cell differentiation and secretory gene expression, we propose that estrogen-initiated loss of prostatic *Hoxb*-13 may play a critical role in mediating the differentiation defects observed in the developmentally estrogenized prostate gland. Furthermore, since *Hox*b13 was most severely reduced in the ventral lobe, where it plays a more prominent role as compared to the more anterior prostate lobes (unpublished data), its suppression may lead to the marked differentiation defects preferentially seen in the ventral prostate.

SECRETED SIGNALING MOLECULES

In addition to developmental regulation by homeobox genes, branching morphogenesis occurs as a complex interplay between epithelial and mesenchymal cells. While many secreted epithelial–mesenchymal signals have been characterized, a small number of signaling molecules have been found to be critical during embryogenesis.[23] In particular, combinations of *Hedgehogs, Wnts, Bmps*, and *Fgfs* to a large extent control soft tissue development. These positive and negative regulatory molecules are spatially and temporally regulated and communicate signals between cells via their cognate receptors. We have recently examined the ontogeny and localization of *Bmp*-4, sonic hedgehog (*Shh*), and *Fgf*-10 in the normal developing rat prostate lobes and those exposed neonatally to estradiol to determine whether alterations in their signaling pathways are involved in mediating specific aspects of the estrogenized phenotype.

Bmp-4 as a Negative Regulator of Prostate Ductal Outgrowth

Bone morphogenetic proteins (*Bmps*) are members of the Tgfβ superfamily and, in general, act as inhibitors of proliferation during development.[39] *Bmps* initiate cell signaling by activating Type I and Type II transmembrane receptors with intracellular pathways involving Smads 1, 3, and 5. In the mouse prostate, *Bmp*4 mRNA is localized to the mesenchyme and levels decline postnatally.[46] While targeted disruption of *Bmp*4 is embryonically lethal, heterozygotes possessed an increased number of branching tips in the murine ventral prostate implicating *Bmp*4 as a negative regulator of prostate growth.[46] We localized and quantitated *Bmp*4 mRNA expression in the prostate lobes of the developing rat (FIG. 3A) and found that it was initially intense and broad throughout the prostatic mesenchyme (seen in dorsal and lateral lobes at day 1) and subsequently condensed to cells adjacent to the elongating ducts as morphogenesis progressed (seen in the more developed ventral lobe at day 1). Expression levels of *Bmp*4 mRNA rapidly declined in control prostate lobes within 6 days following birth (FIG. 3B, hatched bars). These findings support the concept that broad *Bmp*4 expression in the mesenchyme suppresses ductal outgrowth during early developmental stages and that rapid loss postnatally is permissive for ductal outgrowth and branching morphogenesis. Following neonatal estrogen exposure, *Bmp*4 expression did not decline, but rather remained at relatively high perinatal levels until after day 15 (FIG. 3B, solid bars), which may contribute to prolonged growth suppression in the prostate lobes. To directly test whether elevated *Bmp*4 contributes to growth inhibition following estrogen exposure, we cultured newborn ventral lobes (VPs) as previously described in 10^{-8} M testosterone (T), T + 1.0 μg/mL *noggin* (a specific *Bmp*4 antagonist), T + 20 μM estradiol (E) or T + E + *noggin*. Rudimentary prostates at day 0 grew to fully branched lobes by day 8 in the presence of T and this was further enhanced by the addition of *noggin* (FIG. 4 C). Culture in T + E retarded distal prostate outgrowth ($P < 0.05$) and addition of *noggin* partially reversed (by ~40%) this estrogen-induced growth inhibition (FIG. 3C). Thus we propose that the continued postnatal expression of *Bmp*4

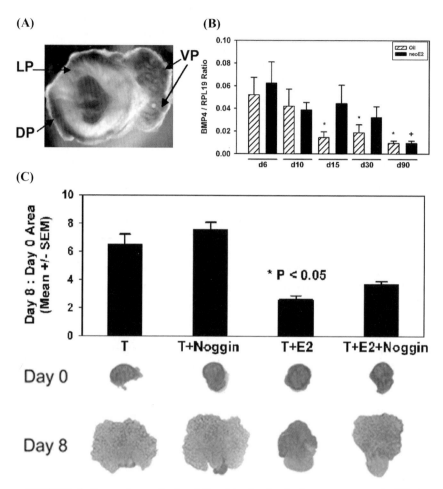

FIGURE 3. Expression and role of *Bmp*4 in the developing rat prostate. **A:** Whole-mount *in situ hybridization* of *Bmp*4 mRNA expression in a day 1 prostate complex shows broad mesenchymal *Bmp*4 expression in dorsal (DP) and lateral (LP) lobes at the early budding stage and signal condensation in periductal mesenchyme as ducts elongate and branch in the more advanced ventral (VP) prostate. **B:** VP *Bmp*4 mRNA levels over time as measured by real time qRT-PCR. Expression declined in control rats (*hatched bar*) as morphogenesis proceeds with significant loss by day 15 (*$P < 0.05$ vs. day 6 oil-treated tissue). Following neonatal estradiol exposure (*solid bars*), *Bmp*4 expression remained at high perinatal levels until after day 30 ($+ P < 0.01$ vs. day 6 estrogen-treated tissue). *Bars* represent mean ± SEM of 4–6 samples. **C:** VP organ culture for 8 days in the presence of 10^{-8} M testosterone (T), T + *noggin* (a *Bmp*4 antagonist), T plus 20 µg estradiol (T + E) and T + E + *noggin*. Contralateral lobes were used for the T-only group and the T + E groups. A *bar graph* shows the area on day 8 normalized to day 0 (bars represent mean ± SEM for 6 experiments), while representative photos from each group at start of culture (day 0) and after 8 days are shown below. *$P < 0.05$ vs. T + E + *noggin*.

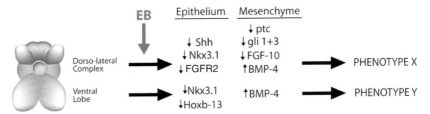

FIGURE 4. A schematic representation of the lobe-specific, estrogen-induced alterations in critical morphoregulatory genes in the rodent prostate. Brief neonatal exposure to high-dose estradiol results in alterations in expression, of key developmental genes in a lobe-specific manner that produces lobe-specific phenotypes. In the dorsoalateral lobes, estrogens suppress *Shh* signaling and *Fgf*10 signaling, transiently reduce *Nkx*3.1 expression, and increase *Bmp*-4 levels. This results in phenotype X, which consists of branching deficiencies, hypomorphic growth, and mild epithelial differentiation defects. In the ventral lobe, estrogens permanently suppress *Hox*b-13, transiently suppress *Nkx*3.1, and increase *Bmp*-4 expression postnatally. This leads to phenotype Y, which consists of severe differentiation defects and hypomorphic growth. In total, both common and unique phenotypes are proposed to result from differential regulation of key morphoregulatory genes by early estrogenic exposures.

in estrogen-exposed rats prolongs the growth-inhibitory actions of this secreted factor, which contributes to the hypomorphic prostate gland phenotype.

Sonic Hedgehog (Shh) and Fibroblast Growth Factor 10 (Fgf 10) as Regulators of Branching Morphogenesis

Shh is a secreted glycoprotein produced by epithelial cells at mesenchymal interfaces in developing tissues, where it plays a critical role in growth and branching morphogenesis.[40] Importantly, *Shh* has been shown to regulate many other developmental genes including *Hox* genes as well as *Nkx*3.1. The murine UGS and prostate epithelial cells produce *Shh* as early as fetal day 17 and the levels decline with development.[28] Secreted *Shh* protein activates target cells through a membrane receptor *patched* (*ptc*) localized in mesenchymal cells. Following a cascade of molecular signals, this ultimately results in increased levels of *gli* transcription factors.[41] We recently characterized the *Shh* expression patterns in the developing rat prostate lobes and localized *Shh* to the distal tip epithelial cells of outgrowing ducts while *ptc* and *glis* were expressed by periductal mesenchymal cells in the distal aspects of the gland.[47] Between days 1–15 of postnatal life, a marked decrease was observed in *Shh* expression with the greatest decrease occurring between days 1–6. Through cross talk with other secreted morphogens including *Bmp*4 and *Fgf*10, a specific role in ductal outgrowth was determined. Importantly, neonatal exposure to estradiol resulted in a significant reduction in *Shh*, *ptc*, *gli*1, and *gli*3 expression in the dorsal and lateral lobes by neonatal day 1, which persisted through development. Interestingly, ventral prostate expression of *Shh, ptc*, and *glis* was unaffected by the estrogenic exposure. This differential effect on *Shh* expression by estrogens may play a role in the previously noted lobe-specific estradiol response where branching was abolished in the dorsolateral region, whereas ventral branching was minimally affected by neonatal estrogen exposure.

Developmental studies have also shown an essential role for $Fgf10$ in stimulating prostatic budding, ductal outgrowth, and branching morphogenesis.[31,43] $Fgf10$ is secreted by prostate mesenchymal cells and interacts with a unique splice variant of the Fgf transmembrane receptor family, the $FgfR2iiib$, which is expressed on prostatic epithelial cells,[44] thus establishing a specific paracrine communication. We recently determined that $Fgf10$ and $FgfR2iii$b localize to the distal periductal mesenchymal cells and distal tip epithelial cells, respectively (distal signaling center), of elongating and branching ducts in the separate rat prostate lobes where they regulate the expression of multiple morphoregulatory genes including increased *Shh*, *ptc*, *Bmp7*, *Hox*b13, and *Nkx*3.1 and decreased *Bmp4* levels.[45] Ventral and lateral lobe organ cultures and mesenchyme-free ductal cultures were used to demonstrate a direct role for $Fgf10/FgfR2iii$b in ductal elongation, branching, epithelial proliferation, and differentiation. On the basis of these findings, we propose that localized expression and feedback loops between several morphoregulatory factors in the developing prostate contribute to tightly regulated branching morphogenesis.[45]

Similar to *Shh-ptc-gli*, neonatal estrogen exposure downregulated $Fgf10$ and $FgfR2iii$b expression in the dorsolateral prostate specifically, whereas ventral lobe expression of these genes was unaffected.[43] Furthermore, lateral prostate organ culture studies demonstrated that growth and branching inhibition as well as $Fgf10/FgfR2iii$b suppression are mediated directly at the prostatic level. Finally, exogenous $Fgf10$ added to lateral lobe cultures in the presence of T + E fully rescued the growth and branching deficits due to estrogen exposure.[45] Together with the *Shh-ptc-gli* experiments, our findings demonstrate that reductions in $Fgf10$ signaling are a proximate cause of *Shh-ptc-gli* down-regulation, which together results in branching inhibition of the dorsolateral prostate following neonatal estrogen exposure.

CONCLUSIONS

In summary, we have shown that early exposure to high levels of estrogens initiates permanent structural and functional alterations in the prostate gland which last throughout life. We propose that this effect is initiated through upregulated levels of stromal ERα, which in turn results in altered steroid receptor expression throughout the developing gland. Rather than being an androgen-dominated process, prostatic development becomes regulated by alternate steroids including estrogens and retinoids. This, in turn, leads to disruptions in the coordinated expression of several critical developmental genes including the homeobox genes *Hox*b13 and *Nkx*3.1 as well as secreted ligands *Shh*, Fgf-10, and *Bmp4* (schematized in FIG. 4). Since a precise temporal expression pattern of these and other molecules is normally required for appropriate growth and differentiation of the prostatic epithelium and stroma, the estrogen-initiated disruption in this pattern would lead to permanent growth as well as branching and differentiation defects of the prostate gland. The ultimate consequences of this developmental estrogenization are a prostate predisposed to hyperplasia and dysplasia in adulthood and sensitized to more severe lesions, including cancer, as the animals age.

ACKNOWLEDGMENTS

We gratefully acknowledge Oliver Putz for the graphic representation of our data. This work has been supported by NIH Grant DK 40890.

REFERENCES

1. LASNITZKI, I. & T. MIZUNO. 1980. Antagonistic effects of cyproterone acetate and oestradiol on the development of the fetal rat prostate gland induced by androgens in organ culture. Prostate **1:** 147–156.
2. PRICE D. 1936. Normal development of the prostate and seminal vesicles of the rat with a study of experimental postnatal modifications. Am. J. Anat. **60:** 79–127.
3. ZONDEK, L.H. & T. ZONDEK. 1980. Congenital malformations of the male accessory sex glands in the fetus and neonate. *In* Male Accessory Sex Glands. E. Spring-Mills and E.S.E. Hafez, Eds : 17–37. Elsevier–North Holland. New York.
4. ADAMS, J.Y., I. LEAV, K.M. LAU, *et al.* 2002. Expression of estrogen receptor beta in the fetal, neonatal, and prepubertal human prostate. Prostate **52:** 69–81.
5. JARRED, R.A., S.J. MCPHERSON, J.J. BIANCO, *et al.* 2002. Prostate phenotypes in estrogen-modulated transgenic mice. Trends Endocrinol. Metab. **13:** 163–168.
6. TILLEY, W., D. HORSFALL, E. MCK. CANT & V. MARSHALL. 1985. Specific binding of oestradiol to guinea-pig prostate cytosol and nuclear fractions. J. Steroid Biochem. **22:** 705–711.
7. HAYASHI, N., Y. SUGIMURA, J. KAWAMURA, *et al.* 1991. Morphological and functional heterogeneity in the rat prostatic gland. Biol. Reprod. **45:** 308–321.
8. SANTTI, R., R.R. NEWBOLD, S. MAKELA, *et al.* 1994. Developmental estrogenization and prostatic neoplasia. Prostate **24:** 67–78.
9. PRINS, G.S.. 1992. Neonatal estrogen exposure induces lobe-specific alterations in adult rat prostate androgen receptor expression. Endocrinology **130:** 3703–3714.
10. PRINS, G.S. & L. BIRCH. 1995. The developmental pattern of androgen receptor expression in rat prostate lobes is altered after neonatal exposure to estrogen. Endocrinology **136:** 1303–1314.
11. PRINS, G.S., C. WOODHAM, M. LEPINSKE & L. BIRCH. 1993. Effects of neonatal estrogen exposure on prostatic secretory genes and their correlation with androgen receptor expression in the separate prostate lobes of the adult rat. Endocrinology **132:** 2387–2398.
12. WOODHAM, C., L. BIRCH & G.S. PRINS. 2003. Neonatal estrogens down regulate prostatic androgen receptor levels through a proteosome-mediated protein degradation pathway. Endocrinology **144:** 4841–4850.
13. PRINS, G.S. 1977. Developmental estrogenization of the prostate gland. *In* Prostate: Basic and Clinical Aspects. R.K. NAZ, Ed.: 247–265. CRC Press. Boca Raton, FL.

14. PUTZ, O. & G.S. PRINS. 2002. Prostate gland development and estrogenic imprinting. *In* Steroid Hormones and Cell Cycle Regulation. K.L. BURNSTEIN, Ed.: 73–89. Kluwer. Boston, MA.

15. PU, Y., L. HUANG & G.S. PRINS. 2004. Neonatal estrogen exposure alters epithelial differentiation in rat prostate through down regulation of *Hoxb*-13. J. Androl. **25:** 330–337.

16. CHANG, W.Y., M.J. WILSON, L. BIRCH & G.S. PRINS. 1999. Neonatal estrogen stimulates proliferation of periductal fibroblasts and alters the extracellular matrix composition in the rat prostate. Endocrinology **140:** 405–415.

17. PRINS, G.S., L. BIRCH, H. HABERMANN, *et al*. 2001. Influence of neonatal estrogens on rat prostate development. Reprod. Fertil. Dev. **13:** 241–252.

18. PRINS, G.S. & L. BIRCH. 1997. Neonatal estrogen exposure up-regulates estrogen receptor expression in the developing and adult rat prostate lobes. Endocrinology **138:** 1801–1809.

19. PRINS, G.S., M. MARMER, C. WOODHAM, *et al*. 1998. Estrogen receptor-β messenger ribonucleic acid ontogeny in the prostate of normal and neonatally estrogenized rats. Endocrinology **139:** 874–883.

20. SABHARWAL, V., O. PUTZ & G.S. PRINS. 2003. Neonatal estrogen exposure induces progesterone receptor expression in the developing prostate gland. Presented at the 95th Annual Meeting of the American Urologic Association, Atlanta, GA.: 97

21. PRINS, G.S., W.Y. CHANG, Y. WANG & R.B. VAN BREEMEN. 2002. Retinoic acid receptors and retinoids are up-regulated in the developing and adult rat prostate by neonatal estrogen exposure. Endocrinology **143:** 3628–3640.

22. PU, Y., L. DENG, P.J.P. DAVIES & G.S. PRINS. 2003. Retinoic acid metabolizing enzymes, binding proteins, and RXRs are differentially expressed in the developing and adult rat prostate lobes and are altered by neonatal estrogens in a lobe-specific manner. Presented at the 85th Annual Meeting of the Endocrine Society, Philadelphia, PA. **P3-236:** 530.

23. HOGAN, B.L.M.. 1999. Morphogenesis. Cell **96:** 225–233.

24. BHATIA-GAUR, R., A.A. DONJACOUR, P.J. SCIAVOLINO, *et al*. 1999. Roles for *Nkx*3.1 in prostate development and cancer. Gen. Devel. **13:** 966–977.

25. BIEBERICH, C.J., K. FUJITA, W.W. HE & G. JAY. 1996. Prostate-specific and androgen-dependent expression of a novel homeobox gene. J. Biol. Chem. **271:** 31779–31782.

26. KOPACHIK, W., S.W. HAYWARD & G.R. CUNHA. 1998. Expression of hepatocyte nuclear factor-3a in rat prostate, seminal vesicle, and bladder. Dev. Dyn. **211:** 131–140.

27. LAMM, M.L., W.S. CATBAGAN, R.J. LACIAK, *et al*. 2002. Sonic hedgehog activates mesenchymal Gli1 expression during prostate ductal bud formation. Dev. Biol. **249:** 349–366.

28. PODLASEK, C.A., D.H. BARNETT, J.Q. CLEMENS, *et al*. 1999. Prostate development requires sonic hedgehog expressed by the urogenital sinus epithelium. Dev. Biol. **209:** 28–39.

29. PODLASEK, C.A., J.Q. CLEMENS & W. BUSHMAN. 1999. *Hoxa*-13 gene mutation results in abnormal seminal vesicle and prostate development. J. Urol. **161:** 1655–1661.

30. SREENATH, T., A. OROSZ, K. FUJITA & C.J. BIEBERICH. 1999. Androgen-independent expression of *hoxb*-13 in the mouse prostate. Prostate **41:** 203–207.

31. THOMSON, A.A. & G.R. CUNHA. 1999. Prostatic growth and development are regulated by FGF10. Development **126:** 3693–3701.

32. WAROT, X., C. FROMENTAL-RAMAIN, V. FRAULOB, *et al.* 1997. Gene dosage-dependent effects of the *Hoxa*-13 and *Hoxd*-13 mutations on morphogenesis of the terminal parts of the digestive and urogenital tracts. Development **124:** 4781–4791.

33. MA, L., G.V. BENSON, H. LIM, *et al.* 1998. Abdominal B(AbdB) *hoxa* genes: regulation in adult uterus by estrogen and progesterone and repression in mullerian duct by the synthetic estrogen diethylstilbestrol (DES). Dev. Biol. **197:** 141–154.

34. MARSHALL, H., A. MORRISON, M. STUDER, *et al.* 1996. Retinoids and hox genes. FASEB **9:** 969–978.

35. WOOD, H.B., S.J. WARD & G.M. MORRISS-KAY. 1996. Effects of all-*trans*-retinoic acid on skeletal pattern, 5'HoxD gene expression, and RARb2/b4 promoter activity in embryonic mouse limbs. Dev. Gen. **18:** 74–84.

36. SCHIAVOLINO, P.J., E.W. ABRAMS, L. YANG, *et al.* 1997. Tissue-specific expression of murine *Nkx3.*1 in the male urogenital system. Dev. Dyn. **209:** 127–138.

37. ECONOMIDES, K.D. & M.R. CAPECCHI. 2003. *Hoxb13* is required for normal differentiation and secretory function of the ventral prostate. Development **130:** 2061–2069.

38. HUANG, L., Y. PU, L. BIRCH & G.S. PRINS. 2006. Posterior Hox gene expression and differential androgen regulation in the developing and adult rat prostate lobes. Endocrinology. In press.

39. HOGAN, B.L.M.. 1996. Bone morphogenetic proteins in development. Curr. Opin. Gen. & Dev. **6:** 432–438.

40. BELLUSCI, S., Y. FURUTA, M. RUSH, *et al.* 1997. Involvement of sonic hedgehog (Shh) in mouse embryonic lung growth and morphogenesis. Development **124:** 53–63.

41. WALTERHOUSE, D., J. YOON & P. IANNACCONE. 1999. Developmental pathways: sonic hedgehog-patched-GLI. Environ. Health Persp. **107:** 167–171.

42. HUANG, L., Y. PU, S. ALAM, *et al.* 2004. Estrogenic regulation of signaling pathways and homeobox genes during rat prostate development. J. Androl. **25:** 330–337.

43. DONJACOUR, A.A., A.A. THOMSON & G. CUNHA. 2003. FGF-10 plays an essential role in the growth of the fetal prostate. Dev. Biol. **261:** 39–54.

44. FINCH, P., G. CUNHA, J. RUBIN, *et al.* 1995. Pattern of keratinocyte growth factor and keratinocyte growth factor receptor expression during mouse fetal development suggests a role in mediating morphogenetic mesenchymal-epithelial interactions. Dev. Dynam. **203:** 223–240.

45. HUANG, L., Y. PU, S. ALAM, *et al.* 2005. The role of Fgf10 signaling in branching morphogenesis and gene expression in the rat prostate gland: lobe-specific suppression by neonatal estrogens. Dev. Biol. **278:** 396–414.

46. PODLASEK, J., J.Q. CLEMENS, J. LEE & W. BUSHMAN. 1999. Bone morphogenetic protein-4 is a negative regulator of prostate ductal branching. J. Urol. **161:** 125.

47. PU, Y., L. HUANG & G.S. PRINS. 2004. Sonic hedgehog-patched-gli signaling in the developing rat 44. Prostate gland: lobe-specific suppression by neonatal estrogens reduces ductal growth and branching. Dev. Biol. **273:** 257–275.

Timing of Dietary Estrogenic Exposures and Breast Cancer Risk

SONIA DE ASSIS AND LEENA HILAKIVI-CLARKE

Department of Oncology, Georgetown University, Washington, D.C. 20057, USA

ABSTRACT: The same dietary component, such as fat or phytochemicals in plant foods, can have an opposite effect on breast cancer risk if exposed *in utero* through a pregnant mother or at puberty. Dietary exposures during pregnancy often have similar effects on breast cancer risk among mothers and their female offspring. High fat intake and obesity are illustrative examples: excessive pregnancy weight gain that increases high birth weight is associated with increased breast cancer risk among mothers and daughters. High body weight during childhood is inversely linked to later breast cancer risk. The main reason why the age when dietary exposures occur determines their effect on breast cancer risk likely reflects the extensive programming of the mammary gland during fetal life and subsequent reprogramming at puberty and pregnancy. Programming is a series of epigenetic/transcriptional modifications in gene expression that can be influenced by changes in the hormonal environment induced, for example, by diet. Because epigenetic modifications are inherited by daughter cells, they can persist throughout life if they occur in mammary stem cells or uncommitted mammary myoepithelial or luminal progenitor cells. Our results indicate that the estrogen receptor (ER), mitogen-activated protein kinase (MAPK), and the tumor suppressors BRCA1, p53, and caveolin-1 are among the genes affected by diet-induced alterations in programming/reprogramming. Consequently, mammary gland morphology may be altered in a manner that increases or reduces susceptibility to malignant transformation, including an increase/reduction in cell proliferation, differentiation, and survival, or in the number of terminal end buds (TEBs) or pregnancy-induced mammary epithelial cells (PI-MECs) that are the sites where breast cancer is initiated. Thus, dietary exposures during pregnancy and puberty may play an important role in determining later risk by inducing epigenetic changes that modify vulnerability to breast cancer.

KEYWORDS: breast cancer; estrogens; diet; timing of exposure

Address for correspondence: Leena Hilakivi-Clarke, Ph.D., Department of Oncology, Georgetown University, Research Building E407, 3970 Reservoir Road NW, Washington, D.C. 20057, USA. Voice: +001-202-687-7237; fax: +001-202-687-7505.
e-mail : Clarkel@georgetown.edu

Ann. N.Y. Acad. Sci. 1089: 14–35 (2006). © 2006 New York Academy of Sciences.
doi: 10.1196/annals.1386.039

TIMING OF DIETARY EXPOSURE AFFECTS
BREAST CANCER RISK

Breast cancer risk is determined not only by what a woman eats when she is diagnosed, but more importantly, what her mother ate whilst she was pregnant or nursing her. Furthermore, what a woman ate as a child or when she was pregnant may have an impact on her breast cancer risk later in life. We will review data suggesting that several dietary factors, including dietary fat or genistein in soy foods, may have different effects on breast cancer risk, depending on when during a woman's lifetime she is exposed to them. This likely reflects the fact that many dietary components modify hormonal environment by altering circulating estrogen concentrations or by containing factors that can activate or inhibit steroid receptors; timing of estrogenic exposures determines their effect on breast cancer risk. The studies reviewed below mostly have utilized animal models, reflecting difficulties in obtaining accurate dietary information retrospectively in human populations, particularly regarding maternal and childhood dietary exposures in women diagnosed with breast cancer in adult life.

Estradiol

Although lifetime exposure to elevated levels of estrogens has been proposed to increase breast cancer risk, this dogma is mostly based on observations that earlier menarche and later menopause are both associated with higher breast cancer risk.[1] However, the possibility that the factors that modulate puberty onset, rather than puberty onset itself, may be the ones primarily causing a shift in breast cancer incidence has not been considered. Findings in animal studies indicate that *in utero* exposure to estradiol (E2) or a high fat diet that increases pregnancy E2 levels accelerate puberty onset and increase carcinogen-induced mammary tumorigenesis,[2] while an exposure to E2 before weaning protects the gland from malignant transformation although it also causes an early puberty onset.[3] These studies show that the same hormone—E2—can either increase or reduce mammary tumorigenesis, depending on when during the development the rats are exposed to it. The story becomes even more complicated: an exposure to E2 at the level mimicking pregnancy hormonal environment after carcinogen administration reduces mammary tumorigenesis,[4] but so does a depletion of estrogens by ovariectomy.[5] In ovariectomized rats treated with a carcinogen[6] or in athymic mice inoculated with human (estrogen receptor) ER-positive breast cancer cells,[7] E2 exposure promotes tumor growth.

Studies that have compared blood estrogen levels to breast cancer risk in women indicate that the levels either during pre- or postmenopausal years increase postmenopausal breast cancer risk, but have no effect on premenopausal breast cancer risk.[8,9] Elevated *in utero* estrogenic environment may increase breast cancer risk in humans: daughters of women who were exposed to a synthetic estrogen, diethylstilbestrol (DES), during the fetal period to avoid miscarriage have been reported to be at an increased breast cancer risk.[10,11] However, because of methodologic weaknesses, results of the DES studies need to be interpreted with caution. To our knowledge, no studies have been conducted in humans that have compared circulating hormone levels during fetal development or childhood to later breast cancer risk.

There are several proxy measures of estrogenic exposures, including high fat intake and high body weight. They correlate with elevated circulating estrogen concentrations due to aromatization of androgens to estrogens taking place in the adipose tissue. Some dietary factors include estrogenic components, such as genistein in soy foods. The effects of soy, fat intake, and obesity during fetal period, puberty, and pregnancy on breast cancer risk are summarized below.

Genistein

Studies conducted in animal models of breast cancer show that similarly to E2, the timing of exposure to soy food products has age-dependent effects on breast cancer risk. This may be because soy contains genistein, which is a weak estrogenic compound (for review, see Ref. 12). Thus, an exposure to genistein *in utero* or during prepuberty leads to opposing changes in mammary tumorigenesis: genistein administered to pregnant dams increases the risk of mammary cancer in the female offspring,[13] while prepubertal exposure before weaning decreases the risk.[14,15] Exposure to genistein after a carcinogen exposure does not seem to affect mammary tumorigenesis.[12] Human ER-positive MCF-7 breast cancer cells, inoculated to ovariectomized mice to model postmenopause, begin to grow when exposed to genistein.[16]

In humans, high soy food intake during childhood is linked to reduced mammary tumorigenesis,[17,18] and a recent meta-analysis suggested that an exposure during adult life reduces premenopausal breast cancer risk.[12] Many women consume genistein supplements rather than soy foods, but no studies have been conducted to investigate whether these supplements would have an impact on breast cancer risk in human populations. Findings in mice show that although genistein stimulates the growth of breast tumors, if it is given with soy flour to mimic natural soy intake, no stimulation is seen.[19] Thus, purified isoflavone supplements may have different effects on breast cancer risk than soy foods.

Fat Intake

Epidemiological studies that have addressed dietary fat intake during adult life have generated conflicting data.[20,21] Total fat intake at the time women were diagnosed may not be associated with breast cancer risk, although intake of specific fats, such as saturated,[22] monounsaturated, [23] or n-3 polyunsatured fatty acids,[24,25] might be. Animal studies concur with the human data and show that some dietary fats promote mammary tumorigenesis, some have no effect and some are protective,[26–28] when comparisons are done between high and low fat intake. Animal studies further indicate that high fat (fat source: corn oil high in n-6 polyunsaturated fatty acids [PUFAs]) intake during pregnancy increases both dams' and female offspring's breast cancer risk,[2,29] but an exposure before weaning has no effect.[30] Rats exposed to n-3 PUFAs, derived mainly from fish, either *in utero* or before weaning, exhibit lower mammary tumorigenesis than that in rats fed n-6 PUFA-based fats.[30,31]

Obesity

Similarly to fat intake and estrogen exposures, obesity has timing-of-exposure-dependent effects on breast cancer risk. Among human populations, high birth weight has been shown to confer increased breast cancer risk in several studies.[32–37] This increase may be limited to premenopausal breast cancer. Being overweight or obese during childhood and adolescence appears to be protective against breast cancer.[34,35] Body weight has also been inversely associated with breast cancer in premenopausal women.[38–40] Postmenopausal obesity and weight gain through adult life increases postmenopausal breast cancer risk in case–control and cohort studies.[41] Excessive weight gain during pregnancy, adjusted for body mass index (BMI) at the time of diagnosis, increases the risk of post- but not premenopausal breast cancer.[42,43]

During reproductive years, adipose-derived estrogens suppress the ovarian estrogen production by affecting the pituitary-hypothalamic axis, and thus in premenopausal women BMI does not correlate with circulating estrogen concentrations.[44] Thus, other factors besides changes in E2 levels may explain why obesity reduces premenopausal breast cancer risk. Obesity alters the levels and bioavailability of several hormones and growth factors,[45] including leptin, insulin-like growth factors, adiponectin, tumor necrosis factor, NF-κB, and mitogen-activated protein kinase (MAPK).

WHY DOES TIMING OF ESTROGENIC/DIETARY EXPOSURES DETERMINE THE EFFECT ON BREAST CANCER RISK?

Epigenetic Modifications

The main reason why timing of dietary exposures determines their effect on breast cancer risk is probably related to extensive programming of the mammary gland during fetal life and then reprogramming at puberty and pregnancy.

During fetal development, epigenetic reprogramming interprets the information in the genetic code by means that do no involve a change in DNA sequence.[46] The most common epigenetic alteration is methylation of cytosine in the 5′ position in CpG dinucleotides in a gene's promoter region, resulting in silencing of gene expression. Another common form of epigenetic regulation involves modifications of histones that can result in activation or inactivation of chromatin. The epigenetic modifications are then inherited in somatic daughter cells, so that cell identity is maintained throughout life. The scheduled epigenetic reprogramming can be modified by factors that influence the epigenome, such as steroid hormones, [47–49] maternal intake of folic acid, [50] or genistein.[51] Furthermore, epigenetic changes may program the mammary gland morphology, because methylation of genes in the mammary gland is shown to coordinate mammary epithelial differentiation.[52]

Targets of Epigenetic Modifications: Stem Cells

The most strategic target for epigenetic modifications is the mammary stem cell. All mammary structures originate from somatic stem cells; if a stem cell is implanted to an empty fat pad, it can build an entire epithelial tree.[53,54] There also is convincing evidence that breast cancer is initiated in mammary stem cells.[55] Stem cells have a long life, they are resistant to apoptosis, and they divide asymmetrically to give rise to uncommitted progenitor cells.[56] Progenitor cells can rapidly multiple and give rise to committed luminal and myoepithelial progenitors and further to differentiated luminal and myoepithelial cells. Thus, if events leading to breast cancer—mutations and/or epigenetic modifications—occur in mammary stem cells, these cells give rise to affected daughter cells that may not be able to differentiate and instead keep proliferating. Interestingly, many breast tumors are entirely luminal, whilst some contain both luminal and myoepithelial cells,[57,58] suggesting that luminal lineage is targeted by factors that induce breast cancer. This may be related to the data indicating that myoepithelial cells in a normal mammary gland act as tumor suppressors.[59] Cancer myoepithelial cells may be different from normal myoepithelial cells and induce growth, migration, and invasion of breast cancer cells, undermining the integrity of basement membrane.[59]

Does the number of stem cells that compose less than 1% of mammary epithelial population [56] determine a gland's susceptibility to malignant transformation? Baik *et al.*[60] have proposed that elevated *in utero* hormone and/or growth factor levels increase later breast cancer risk by increasing the total number of replicating immature stem cells and eventually the number of cells at risk for malignant transformation. The group provided indirect evidence to support the hypothesis by showing that cord blood growth factor levels that may be associated with later increase in breast cancer risk were linked to the number of cord blood hemotopoietic stem cells. However, perhaps more important than the number is an increase in the susceptibility of the stem cells to changes that initiate breast cancer. Stem cells are located in a niche, a microenvironment that regulates stem cell behavior [61,62] and that might also protect them from malignant transformation by expressing genes that inhibit DNA adduct accumulation and repair DNA damage. Because myoepithelial cells are part of the mammary niche,[63] alterations in them may be critical in determining risk of breast cancer.

Changes in Gene Expression Following in Utero Hormonal/Dietary Modifications

At present, no studies have been conducted that have examined whether maternal dietary exposures that alter later susceptibility to breast cancer would do so because they epigenetically modify the expression of genes that either increase or reduce the likelihood that breast cancer is initiated upon an exposure to a chemical carcinogen or radiation. Findings obtained in other target organs besides the breast suggest that this might be the case. Maternal exposure to DES during pregnancy, which increases uterine cancer risk in daughters [64] and female mouse pups,[65] induces persistent expression of the proto-oncogene *c-fos*, and *lactoferrin* genes, and permanent repression of *Hoxa-10* and *Hoxa-11* in the female uterine tract.[47–49] Although the changes in *c-fos* and *lactoferrin* expression resulted from hypomethylation of GpC promoters, changes in *Hoxa*s might reflect changes in chromatin structure induced by histone modifications.

Genes Potentially Mediating the Breast Cancer Increasing Effects of Altered in Utero Hormonal Environment

Because E2, genistein, high fat diet and high birth weight all are associated with increased fetal estrogenic environment, we have been focusing on changes in the mammary ER-α levels. *In utero* exposure to E2 or genistein upregulates the expression of this receptor,[13,66] consistent with the observation that ER was found to be hypomethylated in the mammary glands of rats exposed to E2-increasing high fat diet *in utero*.[67] High-birth-weight rats, in contrast, exhibit a significantly reduced mammary ER-α expression.[68] This finding may reflect the lack of effect of the high birth weight–inducing obesity-inducing diet (OID) on maternal E2 levels and an increase in maternal leptin levels instead.[69] Maternal exposure to subcutaneous leptin injections reduces mammary ER-α content (Yu *et al.*, unpublished data), indicating that elevated fetal leptin levels may have caused downregulation of ER-α. These findings suggest that both an increase and a reduction in mammary ER-α expression are linked to an increase in susceptibility to develop mammary tumors.

High birth weight is associated with increased activation of MAPK in an adult mammary gland.[68] MAPK pathway is identified as a key regulator of a group of genes called Polycomb (PcG) that prevent lineage-specific cell differentiation.[70,71] Thus, high birth weight may increase later breast cancer risk by affecting stem cell fate. This is in line with an observation that diet-activated signals influence stem cell proliferation and differentiation in the *Drosophila* ovary.[72]

Changes in Gene Expression after Pubertal Hormonal/Dietary Modifications

Postpubertal dietary exposures may also induce persistent epigenetic changes. Neonatal exposure to leptin normalizes the programmed effects of fetal undernutrition on accelerated weight gain and increased plasma levels of glucose and insulin [73]; however, it is not known whether this is a result of leptin's affecting epigenetic regulation of gene expression. The sensitivity to long-lasting epigenetic modifications is not limited only to fetal and early postnatal development; postweaning exposure to a synthetic methyl-donor-deficient diet induced a persistent loss of imprinting in the insulin-like growth factor 2 (Igf2) locus in the kidney.[74]

Pubertal Hormonal/Dietary Exposures and Changes in Mammary Gland Gene Expression

Alterations in gene expression patterns in the mammary gland of animals prepubertally fed a diet that reduced their later breast cancer risk may provide clues to the pathways linked to susceptibility to develop this disease. Our preliminary data generated in gene microarrays indicate that these genes are probably related to cell proliferation, apoptosis, and differentiation (Shajahan and Hilakivi-Clarke, unpublished data); functional assays have shown that these end points are affected by early life exposure to E2 or genistein.[3] We also have found that an exposure to E2 or genistein during prepuberty exhibits increased expression of BRCA1 mRNA in the rat mammary gland.[3] Furthermore, prepubertal E2 and/or genistein exposures upregulate the gene expression and protein levels of caveolin-1 [66] and Pten,[75] suggesting an increase in tumor suppressor functions.

Changes in Gene Expression after Pregnancy Hormonal/Dietary Modifications

Pregnancy has a dual effect on breast cancer risk. A full-term pregnancy, especially at an early age, provides a long-lasting protection against breast cancer, whereas first pregnancy after age 30 increases the risk.[76,77] Pregnancy has also been shown to increase the risk of developing breast cancer for 3–5 years after parturition, when compared to the risk in age-matched nulliparous women.[78–80] The short-term increase in risk may occur because of the growth-enhancing effects of pregnancy hormones on cells that have already undergone the first steps of neoplastic transformation. In contrast, the long-term protective effects of parity may be because of the pregnancy-induced elimination of mammary cells that are most susceptible for breast cancer, either by altering their gene expression patterns or by differentiation, or by both mechanisms.[81,82] These changes will also take place in the breasts of older women, but if their breast cell(s) have already undergone malignant transformation, the protective alterations are not sufficient to reverse the cancer initiation. Younger women have a lower probability of initiated cells than older women and thus the protective effects of pregnancy are apparent in this group.

The dual effects of pregnancy on breast cancer risk observed in humans have been recapitulated in animal studies. Pregnancy before or soon after an exposure to a mammary carcinogen has been shown to completely block or significantly reduce the development of mammary tumors in rats.[81] If pregnancy takes place a few weeks after a carcinogen exposure (that is, when the carcinogen has induced a formation of microtumors), the protective effect is partially lost.

Altered Hormone Levels during Pregnancy and Breast Cancer Risk

Although age at first pregnancy is a strong determinant of breast cancer risk, several factors are known to modulate the protective effects of parity. A higher risk of breast cancer has been reported for women whose pregnancy estrogen levels were elevated. Most of the evidence comes from indirect measures of estrogenicity. For instance, mothers who suffered from severe nausea or vomiting during pregnancy [83] or gave birth to heavy infants [84] are at increased risk. Direct evidence for the role of pregnancy estrogen levels on breast cancer risk originates from studies of women who were exposed to DES during pregnancy.[85] In addition to DES, other studies have linked pregnancy estrogen levels directly to breast cancer risk: a nested case–control study recently found that women with higher estrone levels during the third trimester of pregnancy had twice the incidence of breast tumors of the controls.[86]

Conversely, lower levels of estrogens during pregnancy seem to decrease breast cancer risk. Maternal levels of circulating alpha-fetoprotein, a glycoprotein that binds to estrogen and suppresses its activity [87,88] during pregnancy, are inversely associated with breast cancer risk.[89,90] Furthermore, women who suffered from pre-eclampsia and pregnancy hypertension are at reduced risk of developing breast cancer.[78,91] This may reflect higher levels of testosterone in these women, which may reflect a reduction in aromatization of testosterone to estrogens or increased testosterone synthesis.

An increase in estrogen levels during pregnancy is clearly not the only change associated with increased breast cancer risk among mothers. Gestational glycosuria or diabetes, another common complication during pregnancy, has been shown to increase breast cancer risk. Women in the highest quartile of glucose intolerance during pregnancy had a tenfold higher risk than women in the lowest quartile.[92] Caution needs to be exercised when interpreting these results because the study contains a low number of subjects. However, another study conducted in the British Women's Heart and Health cohort also found increased breast cancer risk in women who had gestational glycosuria or diabetes mellitus.[93]

Exposure to modifiable risk factors during pregnancy affects the risk of breast cancer. Weight gain of more than 15 kg during pregnancy was associated with 62% increase in breast cancer risk when compared to women who gain the recommend amount (11 to 15 kg).[42] In animal studies, dietary fat intake during pregnancy has been shown to affect dams' mammary tumorigenesis. Rats fed a diet high in n-6 PUFAs during pregnancy had a fourfold higher tumor incidence compared to that of the control group.[29] The increase in mammary tumorigenesis was accompanied by a twofold increase in E2 levels when measured near the end of pregnancy.[29] Another study showed that rat dams who gain an excessive amount of weight during pregnancy exhibit a significantly increased DMBA-induced mammary tumorigenesis. The exposure that results an excessive pregnancy weight gain—an OID—did not increase pregnancy E2 levels, but increased circulating leptin levels.[69] This is consistent with a study showing that an exposure to leptin during pregnancy increases dam's mammary tumorigenesis, while E2 exposure lengthened tumor latency and modestly increased the final tumor incidence (De Assis *et al.*, unpublished data).

Pregnancy-Induced Changes in Gene Expression

Pregnancy induces several changes in the gene signaling patterns in the mammary gland. ER-α, progesterone receptor (PR), and epidermal growth factor receptor (EGFR) are lower in the mammary glands of parous than nulliparous animals.[94,95] Pregnancy hormonal environment can be mimicked by exposing mice or rats to similar levels of estrogens and progesterone than detected during a normal pregnancy.[4] Sivaraman and coworkers[96] did not detect any differences in the mRNA expression of ER, PR, cyclins D1, and D2, the cell cycle inhibitors p16, p21, and p27, and the tumor suppressor p53, but found that protein levels of p53, p21, and mdm2 levels were higher in the mice exposed to pregnancy-mimicking hormonal manipulation. In addition to upregulating p53, pregnancy increases the levels of another tumor suppressor gene, BRCA1.[97] An increase in the expression of tumor suppressor genes might be part of the mechanism that prevents high pregnancy estrogen levels from inducing DNA damage and genetic alterations.[98] The function of both

BRCA1 and p53 has been linked to DNA damage repair and maintenance of genetic stability.[99–101]

D'Cruz et al.[82] compared gene expression patterns between parous and nulliparous animals using cDNA microarrays. Several different strains of mice and rats were included in the study. The investigators identified a panel of 38 genes that were differentially expressed in the parous animals. On the basis of expression pattern of these genes, it was possible to reproducibly distinguish between parous and nulliparous states of the mammary gland of both rats and mice. The differentially expressed genes fell into three categories: growth factors that stimulate proliferation, growth factors that stimulate differentiation, and genes related to immune responses. Cell proliferation-linked growth factors, such as amphiregulin, leptin, and IGF-1 were expressed at lower levels in the parous than nulliparous gland. In contrast, differentiation-inducing transforming growth factor (TGF)-β3 and several of its transcriptional targets were upregulated. These findings suggest that pregnancy might reduce breast cancer risk by reducing the expression of genes that participate in inducing cell proliferation and by increasing expression of genes that induce differentiation.

Genes Potentially Mediating the Breast Cancer Increasing Effects of Altered Pregnancy Hormonal Environment

To determine whether alterations in the pregnancy hormonal environment that increase dams' mammary tumorigenesis affect gene expression in the mammary gland, we studied gene expression profiles in the mammary tissues of rats which had been treated with leptin or E2 during pregnancy. Both exposures increase the dam's mammary tumorigenesis (de Assis *et al.*, unpublished data). Affymetrix Rat RG-U34A GeneChip® arrays were used, and data were analyzed by applying several new algorithms for gene selection and neural network construction. Using the algorithms, 54 genes were found to be upregulated and 52 downregulated in the fully involuted mammary glands of rats exposed to either leptin or E2 during pregnancy. Among the genes that were upregulated were those related to MAPK signaling, while genes that were downregulated in rats exposed to E2 or leptin during pregnancy included those linked to TGF-β signaling. The present findings suggest that excessive levels of E2 or leptin during pregnancy may counteract molecular changes linked to pregnancy's ability to reduce breast cancer risk.

CHANGES IN MAMMARY GLAND MORPHOLOGY AS A RESULT OF FETAL, PUBERTAL, OR PREGNANCY HORMONAL/DIETARY EXPOSURES

Hormonal and dietary exposures at the times when the mammary gland is undergoing programming/reprogramming should change mammary gland morphology, particularly if the changes occur in stem cells. These morphological changes could then contribute to altered susceptibility to breast cancer initiation, for example, by offering more targets for malignant transformation or fewer (myoepithelial) cells that suppress tumorigenesis. Therefore, we briefly review the sequence of events from fetal period to involution that occur in the rodent mammary gland. Several previous reviews have described these events in detail.[102–104]

Fetal Development

The mammary fat pad in mice and rats appears at midgestation when the primary mammary rudiment penetrates the underlying mesenchyma.[105,106] Signaling molecules important for epithelial–mesenchymal interactions participate in the development of the fetal mammary gland.[107] Although steroid hormones, growth hormone (GH) or prolactin are not required for the fetal mammary development, experimental manipulations taking place *in utero,* that, for example, increase maternal estrogenic activity, alter the mammary gland morphology at the time of exposure and long term.[2,108–113]

Effects of in Utero Exposures on Mammary Gland Development in Experimental Models

Neonatal treatment of mice with E2, DES, or tamoxifen, a selective ER modulator, changes mammary gland morphology [113] and cell proliferation and differentiation [108] within mammary epithelial tree. Our studies show [2,110] that *in utero*/neonatal E2 exposure increases the number of terminal end buds (TEBs) and delays their differentiation to alveolar buds and lobules. Furthermore, TEBs themselves are altered; they contain fewer apoptotic cells and the number of proliferating cells is increased in the *in utero*-E2-exposed rats.[66] Maternal dietary exposures during pregnancy that have been shown to increase female offspring's mammary tumorigenesis—genistein, high-fat diet or OID which leads to high birth weight—all induce an increase in the number of TEBs.[114] These findings suggest that developmental patterns of TEBs, including their number and the level of cell proliferation/apoptosis occurring in the TEBs, may be programmed *in utero*. Furthermore, maternal diet during pregnancy appears to influence the programming.

Because TEBs are the targets of malignant transformation in the rodent mammary gland,[115] an increase in the number of TEBs by fetal estrogenic manipulations is likely to increase the gland's susceptibility to carcinogen-induced mammary tumorigenesis.

Pubertal Development

The mammary rudiment containing a primitive ductal tree is quiescent until at about 3 weeks of postnatal age, when ovarian hormone production starts and large club-shaped TEBs appear at the tips of growing epithelial ducts. They consist of a mass of body cells that give rise to luminal cells and a top layer of cap cells that give rise to myoepithelial cells.[56] Luminal and myoepithelial cells form the two layers of mammary epithelium: luminal cells are the inner layer, and myoepithelial cells are the outer layer in ducts and alveolar structures. Because cap cells have been found among body cells,[116] they might be the origins of body cells and thus also of luminal cells. Cap cells have been postulated to be multipotent mammary stem cells,[56] although these cells may as well just be the cells that regulate motility of TEBs.[117]

Estrogens and ER are necessary for pubertal mammary epithelial growth.[118] In addition, GH and insulin-like growth factor 1 (IGF-1) are required.[119] TGF-β and epidermal growth factor (EGF) appear to be important, but lack of progesterone or prolactin signaling has no apparent effect on mammary gland development.[116,120,121] Because many of these hormones and growth factors are either secreted from stroma and have an epithelial receptor, or their receptors are located in the stroma and they are secreted from the epithelium,[122] similarly to the fetal period, the stromal–epithelial interactions are essential in regulating the pubertal mammary gland development.

Effects of Pubertal Exposures on Mammary Gland Development in Experimental Models

Administration of E2 to prepubertal rats has an opposite effect on mammary gland development compared to *in utero* E2 exposure. Thus, it reduces the number of TEBs [3] and reduces cell proliferation and increases apoptosis with the TEBs.[66] Prepubertal exposure to genistein has a similar effect than prepubertal E2 exposure.[14,15] Furthermore, prepubertal exposure to the OID increases body weight at weaning and reduces the number of TEBs (Khan and Hilakivi-Clarke, unpublished data). These findings suggest a link between the reduced number of TEBs induced by prepubertal estrogenic manipulations and the reduced risk for malignant transformation.

Pregnancy

Pregnancy is characterized by extensive epithelial proliferation and formation of highly differentiated alveolar structures that produce milk.[123,124] Early in pregnancy, the terminal ductules branch and elongate, while later during pregnancy, their differentiation to alveoli predominates. The stromal compartment shrinks as the glandular components of the breast enlarge. These changes

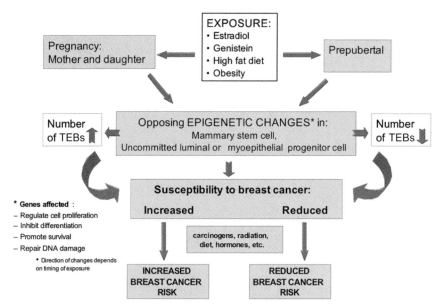

FIGURE 1. A hypothetical model that explains how timing of exposure to hormones or dietary factors modifies later breast cancer risk by inducing epigenetic changes in mammary stem cells, or uncommitted luminal or myoepithelial cells that then determine an individual's susceptibility to malignant transformation. The epigenetic changes in gene expression induced by exposures during pregnancy in the mother and her female offspring may be opposite to the changes induced by exposures during puberty, and be reflected by an increase or reduction in the number of terminal end buds (TEBs), respectively. TEBs are the structures where malignant tumors are initiated in the rat mammary gland, and corresponding structures in the human breast, terminal ductal lobular units, are the sites where most human breast cancers occur.

occur mainly in response to estrogen, progesterone, and prolactin that are required for a successful completion of all pregnancy-related events. However, additional regulators, including TGFβ and signal transducer and activator of transcription (STAT) also affect mammary gland development during pregnancy, lactation, and involution.[124]

Although circulating estrogen and progesterone levels are dramatically reduced at parturition, the functional gland architecture is maintained by prolactin[109] in mothers who nurse their infant. The secretory luminal cells produce large volumes of milk, and contraction of the myoepithelial cells eject the milk through the nipple. When lactation ceases, most epithelial cells undergo apoptosis and those remaining shrink and become inactive. As a result, the alveoli and ducts regress back to a resting state, and the stroma including adipose cells reappears. The architecture of the postlactational mammary gland and the composition of the supporting tissues are not identical to the nulliparous gland. For example, in humans, the number of the least-differentiated terminal ductal lobular unit (TDLU) (called TDLU1) is significantly reduced during pregnancy, and the number of differentiated TDLU2 and TDLU3 is increased.[4,125] In rats and mice, TEBs terminally differentiate to lobulo-alveolar structures during pregnancy,[115] and they do not reappear post partum. Furthermore, resting mammary glands of parous individuals have a slower growth rate and lower binding of carcinogen than the glands of nulliparous individuals.[115]

Effects of Pregnancy Exposures on Mammary Gland Development in Experimental Models

We have investigated whether maternal exposure to E2, leptin, or OID during pregnancy has persistent effects on cell proliferation in rat dams.[69] Results indicated that they all increased the number of proliferating cells in the rat mammary gland, when determined 3 months after the pregnancy; that is, the increase was permanent. These findings are consistent with Siverman *et al.*'s "cell fate hypothesis," which states that pregnancy hormones induce a molecular switch in mammary stem cells that leads to changes in cell proliferation and response to DNA damage.[96] The molecular changes then inhibit cell proliferation in response to subsequent exposures to hormones or carcinogens.[96,126] Wagner and Smith[127] might have identified in mice the cells that serve as targets of pregnancy-related alterations, that is, the pregnancy-induced mammary epithelial cells (PI-MECs). These cells originate from cells that differentiate during pregnancy and fail to undergo apoptosis during postlactational remodeling. PI-MECs have been shown to be cellular targets for pregnancy-enhanced mammary tumorigenesis, and therefore these cells are uniquely suitable for studying the mechanisms mediating the effects of pregnancy dietary manipulations on breast cancer risk.

CONCLUSIONS

Emerging evidence suggests that the developmental stage when hormonal and dietary exposures that elevate hormone levels occur determines whether they increase, reduce or have no effect on breast cancer risk. Exposures to elevated hormonal environment during pregnancy seem to increase both the mother's and her female offspring's breast cancer risk, while pubertal exposures to the same hormone/dietary components are protective. The key mediators of these exposures during periods when the mammary gland is undergoing extensive modeling/remodeling are probably epigenetic changes that may occur in undifferentiated mammary luminal and myoepithelial cell lineages in the developing mammary gland and PI-MECs in the pregnant mammary gland. As a consequence of the epigenetic changes, unopposed cell proliferation, perhaps linked to impaired DNA repair, increased cell survival, and reduced differentiation are anticipated to take place. Breast cancer, however, is initiated only when the epigenetically altered cells are exposed to cancer-initiating factors, such as radiation, carcinogens, and high levels of hormones. In normally functioning mammary cells in individuals not exposed to elevated hormonal environment *in utero* or during pregnancy, cancer initiators do not necessarily cause any harm, because the cells can either repair the damage or undergo apoptosis. Cells in individuals exposed to high estrogenic environment at puberty appear to exhibit a further increase in their ability to undergo apoptosis and repair DNA damage.[3,66,128] Consequently, the most likely targets of epigenetic changes induced by *in utero*, pubertal, or pregnancy hormonal/dietary exposures are genes that repair DNA damage or induce apoptosis. It may not be a coincidence that the majority of inherited breast cancers are caused by mutations in genes that have these two functions, such as BRCA1, BRCA2, and p53. Epigenetic changes in genes that induce cell proliferation and inhibit cell lineage–specific differentiation are probably also targeted by timing of hormonal/dietary exposures, because their excessive activation could overpower cell repair mechanisms.

In summary, we propose that interindividual differences in susceptibility to cancer initiation result from exposures to altered hormonal environment—induced by maternal and childhood diet—during pregnancy or childhood (FIG. 1). Gene polymorphisms were initially believed to explain the differences in cancer susceptibility, but thus far none of the known polymorphisms appears to be strongly linked to susceptibility to develop breast cancer.[129,130] If epigenetic changes determine who is likely to develop breast cancer and who is not, dietary factors that reverse these change may be useful in preventing breast cancer. At present time, several dietary factors have been identified that modify the epigenome,[131] including folic acid in green leafy vegetables and epigallocatechin gallate (EGCG) in green tea.

ACKNOWLEDGMENT

This work was supported by grants from the NCI (U54 CA00100971, RO1 CA89950 and R21 ES013858), American Institute for Cancer Research, and Breast Cancer Research Foundation.

REFERENCES

1. KELSEY, J.L., M.D. GAMMON & E.M. JOHN. 1993. Reproductive factors and breast cancer. Epidemiol. Rev. **15:** 36–47.
2. HILAKIVI-CLARKE L., R. CLARKE, I. ONOJAFE, *et al.* 1997. A maternal diet high in n-6 polyunsaturated fats alters mammary gland development, puberty onset, and breast cancer risk among female rat offspring. Proc. Natl. Acad. Sci. USA **94:** 9372–9377.

3. CABANES, A., M. WANG, S. OLIVO, *et al.* 2004. Prepubertal estradiol and genistein exposures up-regulate BRCA1 mRNA and reduce mammary tumorigenesis. Carcinogenesis **25:** 741–748.
4. RAJKUMAR, L., R. C. GUZMAN, J. YANG, *et al.* 2001. Short-term exposure to pregnancy levels of estrogen prevents mammary carcinogenesis. Proc. Natl. Acad. Sci. USA **98:** 11755–11759.
5. GANDILHON, P., R. MELANCON, J. DJIANE & P.A. KELLY. 1982. Comparison of ovariectomy and retinyl acetate on the growth of established 7,12-dimethylbenz[a]anthracene-induced mammary tumors in the rat. J. Natl. Cancer Inst. **69:** 447–451.
6. KERDELHUE, B. & J. JOLETTE. 2002. The influence of the route of administration of 17beta-estradiol, intravenous (pulsed) versus oral, upon DMBA-induced mammary tumour development in ovariectomised rats. Breast Cancer. Res. Treat. **73:** 13–22.
7. CLARKE, R., R.B. DICKSON & M.E. LIPPMAN. 1992. Hormonal aspects of breast cancer. Growth factors, drugs and stromal interactions. Crit. Rev. Oncol. Hematol. **12:** 1–23.
8. VERKASALO, P.K., H.V. THOMAS, P.N. APPLEBY, *et al.* 2001. Circulating levels of sex hormones and their relation to risk factors for breast cancer: a cross-sectional study in 1092 pre- and postmenopausal women (United Kingdom). Cancer Causes Control **12:** 47–59.
9. KEY, T.J. 1999. Serum oestradiol and breast cancer risk. Endocr. Relat. Cancer **6:** 175–180.
10. PALMER, J.R., E.E. HATCH, C.L. ROSENBERG, *et al.* 2002. Risk of breast cancer in women exposed to diethylstilbestrol in utero: preliminary results (United States). Cancer Causes Control **13:** 753–758.
11. SANDERSON, M., M.A. WILLIAMS, J.R. DALING, *et al.* 1998. Maternal factors and breast cancer risk among young women. Paediatr. Perinat. Epidemiol. **12:** 397–407.
12. TROCK, B.J., L. HILAKIVI-CLARKE & R. CLARKE. 2006. Meta-analysis of soy intake and breast cancer risk. J. Natl. Cancer Inst. **98:** 459–471.
13. HILAKIVI-CLARKE, L., E. CHO, I. ONOJAFE, *et al.* 1999. Maternal exposure to genistein during pregnancy increases carcinogen-induced mammary tumorigenesis in female rat offspring. Oncol. Rep. **6:** 1089–1095.
14. FRITZ, W.A., L. COWARD, J. WANG & C.A. LAMARTINIERE. 1998. Dietary genistein: perinatal mammary cancer prevention, bioavailability and toxicity testing in the rat. Carcinogenesis **19:** 2151–2158.
15. HILAKIVI-CLARKE, L., I. ONOJAFE, M. RAYGADA, *et al.* 1999. Prepubertal exposure to zearalenone or genistein reduces mammary tumorigenesis. Br. J. Cancer **80:** 1682–1688.
16. ALLRED, C.D., K.F. ALLRED, Y.H. JU, *et al.* 2001. Soy diets containing varying amounts of genistein stimulate growth of estrogen-dependent (MCF-7) tumors in a dose-dependent manner. Cancer Res. **61:** 5045–5050.
17. WU, A.H., P. WAN, J. HANKIN, *et al.* 2002. Adolescent and adult soy intake and risk of breast cancer in Asian-Americans. Carcinogenesis **23:** 1491–1496.
18. SHU, X.O., F. JIN, Q. DAI, *et al.* 2001. Soyfood intake during adolescence and subsequent risk of breast cancer among Chinese women. Cancer Epidemiol. Biomarkers Prev. **10:** 483–488.
19. ALLRED, C.D., K.F. ALLRED, Y.H. JU, *et al.* 2004. Soy processing influences growth of estrogen-dependent breast cancer tumors. Carcinogenesis **25:** 1649–1657.

20. BOYD, N.F., J. STONE, K.N. VOGT, *et al.* 2003. Dietary fat and breast cancer risk revisited: a meta-analysis of the published literature. Br. J. Cancer **89:** 1672–1685.
21. SMITH-WARNER, S.A., D. SPIEGELMAN, H.-O. ADAMI, *et al.* 2001. Types of dietary fat and breast cancer: a pooled analysis of cohort studies. Int. J. Cancer **92:** 767–774.
22. CHO, E., D. SPIEGELMAN, D.J. HUNTER, *et al.* 2003. Premenopausal fat intake and risk of breast cancer. J. Natl. Cancer Inst. **95:** 1079–1085.
23. WOLK, A., R. BERGSTROM, D. HUNTER, *et al.* 1998. A prospective study of association of monounsaturated fat and other types of fat with risk of breast cancer. Arch. Intern. Med. **158:** 41–45.
24. CAYGILL, C.P.J. & M.J. HILL. 1995. Fish n-3 fatty acids and human colorectal and breast cancer. Eur. J. Cancer Prev. **4:** 329–332.
25. GOODSTINE, S.L., T. ZHENG, T.R. HOLFORD, *et al.* 2003. Dietary $(n\text{-}3)/(n\text{-}6)$ fatty acid ratio: possible relationship to premenopausal but not postmenopausal breast cancer risk in U.S. women. J. Nutr. **133:** 1409–1414.
26. WELSCH, C.W. 1992. Relationship between dietary fat and experimental mammary tumorigenesis: a review and critique. Cancer Res. **52:** 2040–2048.
27. ROGERS, A.E. 1997. Diet and breast cancer: studies in laboratory animals. J. Nutr. **127:** 933S–935S.
28. CAVE, W.T. 1991. Dietary n-3 (omega-3) polyunsaturated fatty acid effects on animal tumorigenesis. FASEB J. **5:** 2160–2166.
29. HILAKIVI-CLARKE, L., I. ONOJAFE, M. RAYGADA, *et al.* 1996. Breast cancer risk in rats fed a diet high in n-6 polyunsaturated fatty acids during pregnancy. J. Natl. Cancer Inst. **88:** 1821–1827.
30. OLIVO, S.E. & L. HILAKIVI-CLARKE. 2005. Opposing effects of prepubertal low and high fat n-3 polyunsaturated fatty acid diets on rat mammary tumorigenesis. Carcinogenesis **26:** 1563–1572.
31. HILAKIVI-CLARKE, L., E. CHO, A. CABANES, *et al.* 2002. Dietary modulation of pregnancy estrogen levels and breast cancer risk among female rat offspring. Clin. Cancer Res. **8:** 3601–3610.
32. MICHELS, K.B. & F. XUE. 2006. Role of birthweight in the etiology of breast cancer. Int. J. Cancer **119:** 2007–2025.
33. STAVOLA, B.L., R. HARDY, D. KUH, *et al.* 2000. Birthweight, childhood growth and risk of breast cancer in a British cohort. Br. J. Cancer **83:** 964–968.
34. HILAKIVI-CLARKE, L., T. FORSEN, J.G. ERIKSSON, *et al.* 2001. Tallness and overweight during childhood have opposing effects on breast cancer risk. Br. J. Cancer **85:** 1680–1684.
35. AHLGREN, M., M. MELBYE, J. WOHLFAHRT & T.I. SORENSEN 2004. Growth patterns and the risk of breast cancer in women. N. Engl. J. Med. **351:** 1619–1626.
36. MCCORMACK, V.A., S.S. DOS I, I. KOUPIL, *et al.* 2005. Birth characteristics and adult cancer incidence: Swedish cohort of over 11000 men and women. Int. J. Cancer **115:** 611–617.
37. VATTEN, L.J., T.I. NILSEN, S. TRETLI, *et al.* 2005. Size at birth and risk of breast cancer: prospective population-based study. Int. J. Cancer **114:** 461–464.
38. HUANG, Z., S.E. HANKINSON, G.A. COLDITZ, *et al.* 1997. Dual effects of weight and weight gain on breast cancer risk. JAMA **278:** 1407–1411.
39. TRENTHAM-DIETZ, A., P.A. NEWCOMB, B.E. STORER, *et al.* 1997. Body size and risk of breast cancer. Am. J. Epidemiol. **145:** 1011–1019.

40. POTISCHMAN, N., C.A. SWANSON, P. SIITERI & R.N. HOOVER. 1996. Reversal of relation between body mass and endogenous estrogen concentrations with menopausal status. J. Natl. Cancer Inst. **88:** 756–758.
41. KABUTO, M., S. AKIBA, R. STEVENS, *et al.* 2000. A prospective study of estradiol and breast cancer in Japanese women. Cancer Epidemiol. Biomarkers Prev. **9:** 575–579.
42. KINNUNEN, T.I., R. LUOTO, M. GISSLER, *et al.* 2004. Pregnancy weight gain and breast cancer risk. BMC Womens Health **4:** 7–17.
43. HILAKIVI-CLARKE, L., R. LUOTO, T. HUTTUNEN & M. KOSKENVUO. 2005. Pregnancy weight gain and premenopausal breast cancer risk. J. Reprod. Med. **50:** 811–816.
44. TRICHOPOULOS, D., A. POLYCHRONOPOULOU, J. BROWN & B. MACMAHON. 1983. Obesity, serum cholesterol, and estrogens in premenopausal women. Oncology **40:** 227–231.
45. LORINCZ, A.M. & S. SUKUMAR. 2006. Molecular links between obesity and breast cancer. Endocr. Relat. Cancer. **13:** 279–292.
46. SANTOS, F. & W. DEAN. 2004. Epigenetic reprogramming during early development in mammals. Reproduction. **127:** 643–651.
47. BLOCK, K., A. KARDANA, P. IGARASHI & H.S. TAYLOR. 2000. *In utero* diethylstilbestrol (DES) exposure alters Hox gene expression in the developing mullerian system. FASEB J. **14:** 1101–1108.
48. LI, S., L. MA, T. CHIANG, *et al.* 2001. Promoter CpG methylation of Hox-a10 and Hox-a11 in mouse uterus not altered upon neonatal diethylstilbestrol exposure. Mol. Carcinog. **32:** 213–219.
49. LI, S., R. HANSMAN, R. NEWBOLD, *et al.* 2003. Neonatal diethylstilbestrol exposure induces persistent elevation of *c-fos* expression and hypomethylation in its exon-4 in mouse uterus. Mol. Carcinogen. **38:** 78–84.
50. COONEY, C.A., A.A. DAVE & G.L. WOLFF. 2002. Maternal methyl supplements in mice affect epigenetic variation and DNA methylation of offspring. J. Nutr. **132:** 2393S–2400S.
51. DOLINOY, D.C., J. R. WEIDMAN, R.A. WATERLAND & R.L. JIRTLE. 2006. Maternal genistein alters coat color and protects Avy mouse offspring from obesity by modifying the fetal epigenome. Environ. Health Perspect. **114:** 567–572.
52. PLACHOT, C. & S.A. LELIEVRE. 2004. DNA methylation control of tissue polarity and cellular differentiation in the mammary epithelium. Exp. Cell Res. **298:** 122–132.
53. KORDON, E.C. & G.H. SMITH. 1998. An entire functional mammary gland may comprise the progeny from a single cell. Development. **125:** 1921–1930.
54. SHACKLETON, M., F. VAILLANT, K.J. SIMPSON, *et al.* 2006. Generation of a functional mammary gland from a single stem cell. Nature **439:** 84–88.
55. AL-HAJJ, M., M.S. WICHA, A. ITO-HERNANDEZ, *et al.* 2003. Prospective identification of tumorigenic breast cancer cells. Proc. Natl. Acad. Sci. USA **100:** 3983–3988.
56. SMALLEY, M. & A. ASHWORTH. 2003. Stem cells and breast cancer: a field in transit. Nat. Rev. Cancer **3:** 832–844.
57. SORLIE, T., C.M. PEROU, R. TIBSHIRANI, *et al.* 2001. Gene expression patterns of breast carcinomas distinguish tumor subclasses with clinical implications. Proc. Natl. Acad. Sci. USA **98:** 10869–10874.
58. PEROU, C.M., T. SORLIE, M.B. EISEN, *et al.* 2000. Molecular portraits of human breast tumours. Nature **406:** 747–752.

59. ADRIANCE, M.C., J.L. INMAN , O.W. PETERSEN & M.J. BISSELL. 2005. Myoepithe-lial cells: good fences make good neighbors. Breast Cancer Res. **7:** 190–197.
60. BAIK, I., W.J. DEVITO, K. BALLEN, *et al.* 2005. Association of fetal hormone levels with stem cell potential: evidence for early life roots of human cancer. Cancer Res. **65:** 358–363.
61. XI, R. & T. XIE. 2005. Stem cell self-renewal controlled by chromatin remodeling factors. Science **310:** 1487–1489.
62. BUSZCZAK, M. & A.C. SPRADLING. 2006. Searching chromatin for stem cell identity. Cell **125:** 233–236.
63. POLYAK, K. & M. HU. 2005. Do myoepithelial cells hold the key for breast tumor progression? J. Mammary Gland Biol. Neoplasia **10:** 231–247.
64. GIUSTI, R.M., K. IWAMOTO & E.E. HATCH. 1995. Diethylstilbestrol revisited: a review of the long-term health effects. Ann. Intern. Med. **122:** 778–788.
65. MCLACHLAN, J.A., R.R. NEWBOLD & B.C. BULLOCK. 1980. Long-term effects on the female mouse genital tract associated with prenatal exposure to diethyl-stilbestrol. Cancer Res. **40:** 3988–3999.
66. HILAKIVI-CLARKE, L., A. SHAJAHAN, B. YU & A.S. DE. 2006. Differentiation of mammary gland as a mechanism to reduce breast cancer risk. J. Nutr. **136:** 2697S–2699S.
67. YENBUTR, P., L. HILAKIVI-CLARKE & A. PASSANITI. 1998. Hypomethylation of an exon I estrogen receptor CpG island in spontaneous and carcinogen-induced mammary tumorigenesis in the rat. Mech. Ageing Dev. **106:** 93–102.
68. DE ASSIS, S., K. GALAM & L. HILAKIVI-CLARKE. 2006. High birth weight increases mammary tumorigenesis in rats. Int. J. Cancer **119:** 1537–1546.
69. DE ASSIS, S., M. WANG, S. GOEL, *et al.* 2005. Excessive weight gain during pregnancy increases carcinogen-induced mammary tumorigenesis in Sprague-Dawley and lean and obese Zucker rats. J. Nutr. **136:** 998–1004.
70. NYSTUL, T.G. & A.C. SPRADLING. 2006. Breaking out of the mold: diversity within adult stem cells and their niches. Curr. Opin. Genet. Dev. **16:** 463–468.
71. VONCKEN, J.W., H. NIESSEN, B. NEUFELD, *et al.* 2005. MAPKAP kinase 3pK phosphorylates and regulates chromatin association of the polycomb group protein Bmi1. J. Biol. Chem. **280:** 5178–5187.
72. LAFEVER, L. & D. DRUMMOND-BARBOSA. 2005. Direct control of germline stem cell division and cyst growth by neural insulin in *Drosophila*. Science **309:** 1071–1073.
73. VICKERS, M.H., P.D. GLUCKMAN, A.H. COVENY, *et al.* 2005. Neonatal leptin treatment reverses developmental programming. Endocrinology **146:** 4211–4216.
74. WATERLAND, R.A., J.R. LIN, C.A. SMITH & R.L. JIRTLE. 2006. Post-weaning diet affects genomic imprinting at the insulin-like growth factor 2 (Igf2) locus. Hum. Mol. Genet. **15:** 705–716.
75. DAVE, B., R.R. EASON, S.R. TILL, *et al.* 2005. The soy isoflavone genistein pro-motes apoptosis in mammary epithelial cells by inducing the tumor suppressor PTEN. Carcinogenesis **26:** 1793–1803.
76. MACMAHON, B., P. COLE, T.M. LIN, *et al.*1970. Age at first birth and breast cancer. Bull. World Health Organ. **43:** 209–221.
77. MERRILL, R.M., S. FUGAL, L.B. NOVILLA & M.C. RAPHAEL. 2005. Cancer risk associated with early and late maternal age at first birth. Gynecol. Oncol. **96:** 583–593.

78. HSIEH, C., M. PAVIA, M. LAMBE, *et al.* 1994. Dual effect of parity on breast cancer risk. Eur. J. Cancer **30A:** 969–973.
79. BRUZZI, P., E. NEGRI & C. LA VECCHIA.1988. Short term increase in risk of breast cancer after full term pregnancy. Br. Med. J. **297:** 1096–1098.
80. WILLIAMS, E.M.I., L. JONES, M.P. VESSEY & K. MCPHERSON. 1990. Short term increase in risk of breast cancer associated with full pregnancy. Br. Med. J. **300:** 578–579.
81. RUSSO, J., G.A. BALOGH, R. HEULINGS, *et al.* 2006. Molecular basis of pregnancy-induced breast cancer protection. Eur. J. Cancer Prev. **15:** 306–342.
82. D'CRUZ, C.M., S.E. MOODY, S.R. MASTER, *et al.* 2002. Persistent parity-induced changes in growth factors, TGF-beta3, and differentiation in the rodent mammary gland. Mol. Endocrinol. **16:** 2034–2051.
83. ENGER, S.M., R.K. ROSS, B. HENDERSON & L. BERNSTEIN. 1997. Breastfeeding history, pregnancy experience and risk of breast cancer. Br. J. Cancer **76:** 118–123.
84. WOHLFAHRT, J. & M. MELBYE. 1999. Maternal risk of breast cancer and birth characteristics of offspring by time since birth. Epidemiology **10:** 441–444.
85. COLTON, T., R. GREENBERG, K. NOLLER, *et al.* 1993. Breast cancer in mothers prescribed diethylstilbestrol in pregnancy. JAMA **269:** 2096–2100.
86. PECK, J.D., B.S. HULKA, C. POOLE, *et al.* 2002. Steroid hormone levels during pregnancy and incidence of maternal breast cancer. Cancer Epidemiol. Biomarkers Prev. **11:** 361–368.
87. ALLEN, S.H., J.A. BENNETT, G.J. MIZEJEWSKI, *et al.* 1993. Purification of alpha-fetoprotein from human cord serum with demonstration of its antiestrogenic activity. Biochim. Biophys. Acta **1202:** 135–142.
88. VAKHARIA, D. & G.J. MIZEJEWSKI. 2000. Human alpha-fetoprotein peptides bind estrogen receptor and estradiol, and suppress breast cancer. Breast Cancer Res. Treat. **63:** 41–52.
89. MELBYE, M., J. WOHLFAHRT, U. LEI, *et al.* 2000. Alpha-fetoprotein levels in maternal serum during pregnancy and maternal breast cancer incidence. J. Natl. Cancer Inst. **92:** 1001–1005.
90. RICHARDSON, B.E., B.S. HULKA, J.L. PECK, *et al.* 1998. Levels of maternal serum alpha-fetoprotein (AFP) in pregnant women and subsequent breast cancer risk. Am. J. Epidemiol **148:** 719–727.
91. RICHARDSON, B.E., J.D. PECK & J.K. WORMUTH. 2000. Mean arterial pressure, pregnancy-induced hypertension, and preeclampsia: evaluation as independent risk factors and surrogates for high maternal serum alpha-fetoprotein in estimating breast cancer risk. Cancer Epidemiol. Biomarkers Prev. **9:** 1349–1355.
92. DAWSON, S.I. 2004. Long-term risk of malignant neoplasm associated with gestational glucose intolerance. Cancer **100:** 149–155.
93. LAWLOR, D.A., G.D. SMITH & S. EBRAHIM. 2004. Hyperinsulinaemia and increased risk of breast cancer: findings from the British Women's Heart and Health Study. Cancer Causes Control **15:** 267–275.
94. THORDARSON, G., E. JIN, R.C. GUZMAN, *et al.* 1995. Refractoriness to mammary tumorigenesis in parous rats: is it caused by persistent changes in the hormonal environment or permanent biochemical alterations in the mammary epithelia? Carcinogenesis **16:** 2847–2853.
95. YANG, J., K. YOSHIZAWA, S. NANDI & A. TSUBURA. 1999. Protective effects of pregnancy and lactation against N-methyl-N-nitrosourea-induced mammary carcinomas in female Lewis rats. Carcinogenesis **20:** 623–628.

96. SIVARAMAN, L., L.C. STEPHENS, B.M. MARKAVERICH, et al. 1998. Hormone-induced refractoriness to mammary carcinogenesis in Wistar-Furth rats. Carcinogenesis **19:** 1573–1581.
97. MARQUIS, S.T., J.V. RAJAN, A. WYNSHAW-BORIS, et al. 1995. The developmental pattern of BRCA1 expression implies a role in differentiation of the breast and other tissues. Nat. Genet. **11:** 17–26.
98. HILAKIVI-CLARKE, L. 2000. Estrogens, BRCA1 and breast cancer risk. Cancer Res. **60:** 4993–5001.
99. GOWEN, L.C., A.V. AVRUTSKAYA, A.M. LATOUR, et al.1998. BRCA1 required for transcription-coupled repair of oxidative DNA damage. Science **281:** 1009–1012.
100. WELCSH, P.L., M.K. LEE , R. M. GONZALEZ-HERNANDEZ, et al. 2002. BRCA1 transcriptionally regulates genes involved in breast tumorigenesis. Proc. Natl Acad. Sci. USA **99:** 7560–7565.
101. OREN, M. 1992. p53: the ultimate tumor suppressor gene. FASEB **6:** 3169–3176.
102. VILLADSEN, R. 2005. In search of a stem cell hierarchy in the human breast and its relevance to breast cancer evolution. APMIS **113:** 903–921.
103. MEDINA, D. 2005. Mammary developmental fate and breast cancer risk. Endocr. Relat. Cancer **12:** 483–495.
104. STERNLICHT, M.D. 2006. Key stages in mammary gland development: the cues that regulate ductal branching morphogenesis. Breast Cancer Res. **8:** 201.
105. RUSSO, J., B.A. GUSTERSON, A.E. ROGERS, et al. 1990. Comparative study of human and rat mammary tumorigenesis. Lab. Invest. **62:** 244–278.
106. ROSEN, J.M., R. HUMPHREYS, S. KRNACIK, et al.1994. The regulation of mammary gland development by hormones, growth factors, and oncogenes. Prog. Clin. Biol. Res. **387:** 95–111.
107. HENNIGHAUSEN, L. & G.W. ROBINSON. 2001. Signaling pathways in mammary gland development. Dev. Cell **1:** 467–475.
108. HOVEY, R.C., M. SAI-SATO, A. WARRI, et al. 2005. Effects of neonatal exposure to diethylstilbestrol, tamoxifen, and toremifene on the BALB//c mouse mammary gland. Biol. Reprod. **72:** 423–435.
109. HOVEY, R.C., J.F. TROTT & B.K. VONDERHAAR. 2002. Establishing a framework for the functional mammary gland: from endocrinology to morphology. J. Mammary Gland Biol. Neoplasia **7:** 17–38.
110. HILAKIVI-CLARKE, L., E. CHO, M. RAYGADA & N. KENNEY. 1997. Alterations in mammary gland development following neonatal exposure to estradiol, transforming growth factor alpha, and estrogen receptor antagonist ICI 182780. J. Cell Physiol. **170:** 279–289.
111. WARNER, M.R. 1976. Effect of various doses of estrogen to BALB/cCrgl neonatal female mice on mammary growth and branching at 5 weeks of age. Cell Tissue Kinet. **9:** 429–438.
112. TAMOOKA, T. & H.A. BERN. 1982. Growth of mouse mammary glands after neonatal sex hormone treatment. J. Natl. Cancer Inst. **69:** 1347–1352.
113. JONES, L.A. & H.A. BERN. 1979. Cervicovaginal and mammary gland abnormalities in BALB/cCrgl mice treated neonatally with progesterone and estrogen, alone or in combination. Cancer Res. **39:** 2560–2567.
114. HILAKIVI-CLARKE, L. 2006. Nutritional modulation of terminal end bud: its relevance to breast cancer prevention. Curr. Cancer Drug Targets. In press.
115. RUSSO, J. & I.H. RUSSO. 1987. Biological and molecular bases of mammary carcinogenesis. Lab. Invest. **57:** 112–137.

116. WOODWARD, W.A., M.S. CHEN, F. BEHBOD & J.M. ROSEN. 2005. On mammary stem cells. J. Cell Sci. **118:** 3585–3594.

117. SAPINO, A., L. MACRI, P. GUGLIOTTA, *et al.* 1993. Immunophenotypic properties and estrogen dependency of budding cell structures in the developing mouse mammary gland. Differentiation **55:** 13–18.

118. DANIEL, C.W. & G.B. SILBERSTEIN. 1987. Postnatal development of the rodent mammary gland. *In* The Mammary Gland: Development, Regulation, and Function. G.B. Silberstein & C.W. Daniel, Eds.: 3–36. Plenum Press. New York.

119. KLEINBERG, D.L., M. FELDMAN & W. RUAN. 2000. IGF-I: an essential factor in terminal end bud formation and ductal morhogenesis. J. Mammary Gland Biol. Neoplasia. **5:** 7–17.

120. COLEMAN, S., G.B. SILBERSTEIN & C.W. DANIEL. 1988. Ductal morphogenesis in the mouse mammary gland: evidence supporting a role for epidermal growth factor. Dev. Biol. **127:** 304–315.

121. EWAN, K.B., G. SHYAMALA, S.A. RAVANI, *et al.* 2002. Latent transforming growth factor-beta activation in mammary gland: regulation by ovarian hormones affects ductal and alveolar proliferation. Am. J. Pathol. **160:** 2081–2093.

122. STERNLICHT, M.D., H. KOUROS-MEHR, P. LU & Z. WERB. 2006. Hormonal and local control of mammary branching morphogenesis. Differentiation **74:** 365–381.

123. RUSSO, J., D. MAILO, Y.F. HU, *et al.* 2005. Breast differentiation and its implication in cancer prevention. Clin. Cancer Res. **11:** 931s–936s.

124. OAKES, S.R., H.N. HILTON & C. J. ORMANDY. 2006. The alveolar switch: coordinating the proliferative cues and cell fate decisions that drive the formation of lobuloalveoli from ductal epithelium. Breast Cancer Res. **8:** 207.

125. RUSSO, I.H. & J. RUSSO. 2000. Hormonal approach to breast cancer prevention. J. Cell Biochem. **77:** 1–6.

126. SIVARAMAN, L., S.G. HILSENBECK, L. ZHONG, *et al.* 2001. Early exposure of the rat mammary gland to estrogen and progesterone blocks co-localization of estrogen receptor expression and proliferation. J. Endocrinol. **171:** 75–83.

127. WAGNER, K.U. & G.H. SMITH. 2005. Pregnancy and stem cell behavior. J. Mammary Gland Biol. Neoplasia **10:** 25–36.

128. HILAKIVI-CLARKE, L., S.E. OLIVO, A. SHAJAHAN, *et al.* 2005. Mechanisms mediating the effects of prepubertal (*n*-3) polyunsaturated fatty acid diet on breast cancer risk in rats. J. Nutr. **135:** 2946S–2952S.

129. YE, Z. & J.M PARRY. 2002. The CYP17 MspA1 polymorphism and breast cancer risk: a meta-analysis. Mutagenesis **17:** 119–126.

130. MONTGOMERY, K.G., J.H. CHANG, D.M. GERTIG, *et al.* 2005. The AIB1 glutamine repeat polymorphism is not associated with risk of breast cancer before age 40 years in Australian women. Breast Cancer Res. **7:** R353–R356.

131. DAVIS, C.D. & E.O. UTHUS. 2004. DNA methylation, cancer susceptibility, and nutrient interactions. Exp. Biol. Med. (Maywood) **229:** 988–995.

From Adult Stem Cells to Cancer Stem Cells

Oct-4 Gene, Cell–Cell Communication, and Hormones during Tumor Promotion

JAMES E. TROSKO

Pediatrics and Human Development, Michigan State University, East Lansing, Michigan 48824, USA

ABSTRACT: Carcinogenesis is characterized by "initiation," "promotion," and "progression" phases. The "stem cell theory" and "dedifferentiation" theories are used to explain the origin of cancer. Growth control for stem cells, which lack functional gap junctional intercellular communication (GJIC), involves negative soluble or niche factors, while for progenitor cells, it involves GJIC. Tumor promoters, *hormones*, and growth factors inhibit GJIC reversibly. Oncogenes stably inhibit GJIC. Cancer cells, which lack growth control and the ability to terminally differentiate and to apoptose, lack GJIC. The Oct3/4 gene, a POU (Pit-Oct-Unc) family of transcription factors was thought to be expressed only in embryonic stem cells and in tumor cells. With the availability of normal adult human stem cells, tests for the expression of Oct3/4 gene and the stem cell theory in human carcinogenesis became possible. Human breast, liver, pancreas, kidney, mesenchyme, and gastric stem cells, HeLa and MCF-7 cells, and canine tumors were tested with antibodies and polymerase chain reaction (PCR) primers for Oct3/4. Adult human breast stem cells, immortalized nontumorigenic and tumor cell lines, but not the normal differentiated cells, expressed Oct3/4. Adult human differentiated cells lose their Oct-4 expression. Oct3/4 is expressed in a few cells found in the basal layer of human skin epidermis. The data demonstrate that normal adult stem cells and cancer stem cells maintain expression of Oct3/4, consistent with the stem cell hypothesis of carcinogenesis. These Oct-4 positive cells might represent the "cancer stem cells." A strategy to target "cancer stem cells" is to suppress the Oct-4 gene in order to cause the cells to differentiate.

Address for correspondence: James E. Trosko, Ph.D., Pediatrics and Human Development, Michigan State University, 246 Food Safety and Toxicology. Voice: 517-432-3100, ext. 188; fax: 517-432-6340.
e-mail: james.trosko@ht.msu.edu

Ann. N.Y. Acad. Sci. 1089: 36–58 (2006). © 2006 New York Academy of Sciences.
doi: 10.1196/annals.1386.018

KEYWORDS: Oct3/4 gene; gap junctional intercellular communication; adult stem cells; tumor promoter; cancer stem cells

Some would argue that the search for the origin and treatment of this disease will continue over the next quarter century in much the same manner as it has in the recent past, by adding further layers of complexity to the scientific literature that is already complex almost beyond measure. But we anticipate otherwise: those researching the cancer problem will be practicing a dramatically different type of science than we have experienced over the past 25 years. Surely much of this change will be apparent at the technical level. But ultimately, the more fundamental change will be conceptual.[1]

—D. HANAHAN AND R.A WEINBERG

DROWNING IN MOLECULAR CANCER FACTS WITHOUT THE LIFE VEST OF CONCEPTS

One needs only to pick up the latest cancer journals to find articles about supported research to generate mountains of data with sophisticated modern technologies by skilled specialists in search of molecular details of expressed genes or activated/deactivated oncogenes or tumor suppressor genes, respectively, in one type of cancer cell or another. Yet, one asks what these facts tell us about the cause of carcinogenesis of any or all cancers, let alone the development of efficacious cancer preventive or treatment strategy. Some might argue that there are a few current conceptual paradigms to drive and interpret these experiments. For example, the "oncogene" and "tumor suppressor" gene paradigms are perfect examples of useful paradigms. Yet, when one views diagrams in articles and commercial advertisements that illustrate the genes, their coded protein structures, signal pathways, and DNA structures, one notes they always are shown in a single cell. Well, cancer is a disease of the whole body. As V.R. Potter has stated to make us more sensitive to this fact, "The cancer problem is not merely a cell problem, it is a problem of cell interaction, not only within tissues, but also with distal cells in other tissues. But in stressing the whole organism, we must also remember that the integration of normal cells with the welfare of the whole organism is brought about by molecular messages acting on molecular receptors."[2]

The goal of this report is simple. It is to respond positively to Hanahan and Weinberg's challenge to re-conceptualize the nature of the carcinogenic process and to offer an integrated series of concepts about carcinogenesis, in general, as it might bear on understanding and preventing human breast cancer, while recognizing that the solution will not be simple. As a story of Albert Einstein is told when he gave a public lecture to lay persons about his recent theory of relativity, a young reporter came up to him and asked, "Professor Einstein, now that you physicists understand the makings of the universe, don't you think it is *complicated*?" "Young man," Einstein replied, "If you know nothing of the makings of the universe, it is, indeed, *complicated*; however, when you begin to understand, it is merely *complex!*"

It will be asserted that understanding the concepts of the "stem cell" origin of cancer,[3–5] the multistage, multimechanism process of "initiation," "promotion," and "progression" phases of carcinogenesis,[6] the mutation/epigenetic theory of carcinogenesis, oncogene/tumor suppressor genes of oncogenesis, gap junctional intercellular communication and cancer, and the "cancer stem cell" hypothesis will assist in achieving what Hanahan and Weinberg have stated in there guste. In brief, this new integrative way of viewing the general carcinogenic process should be applicable to all forms of cancer, solid tumors as well as "soft" tumors. Specifically, it should also be applicable to human breast cancer.

FACTS ARE, AT BEST, INCOMPLETE; AT WORSE, DEAD WRONG!

From experimental *in vitro* work on human breast cancer cells (i.e., MCF-7; mutagenesis and cytotoxicity assays), experimental carcinogenesis studies on rodents (bioassays to test carcinogens; initiators/promoters of breast carcinogenesis; clinical chemoprevention and therapeutic trials), analysis of breast cancer genetic predispositions, molecular genetic animal models, and epidemiological studies have already proved that our understanding of breast carcinogenesis is "complicated." Genetic factors, gender factors, developmental stage factors, dietary factors, exogenous chemicals and hormones, cultural and behavior factors contribute to either increasing of decreasing the risk of breast cancer (as with other cancers). Contributions by others to this symposium will delineate known genes (oncogenes; tumor suppressor genes), hormones (i.e., estrogens, their metabolites) and chemicals (dietary; pollutants) and postulated mechanisms (mutagenesis; epigenetic) by which they might contribute to breast carcinogesis. Others will demonstrate many altered gene expression patterns seen in different kinds of breast cancer thought to be predictors of potential intervention therapeutic strategies.

A fact generally assumed to hold true for all cancers is that each cancer cell within the tumor, while it might be genotypically and phenotypically unique from the other tumor cells, has been derived from a single normal cell.[7] Further, an assumption that has taken on the façade of a fact has grown into a powerful paradigm, namely, the idea that the normal target cell that gives rise, ultimately, to an invasive, malignant tumor cell is a "mortal" cell that must be "immortalized" first, in order to survive long enough to acquire the so-called "hallmarks" of cancer.[1] In other words, it is now generally accepted that all forms of cancer, including human breast cancer, must exhibit these six phenotypes: (*a*) self-sufficiency in growth control; (*b*) insensitivity to growth-inhibitory signals; (*c*) evasion of programmed cell death; (*d*) limited (less replicative) potential; (*e*) sustained angiogenesis; and (*f*) tissue invasion and metastasis. More will be said about these "hallmarks" later.

In addition, it is also generally accepted that "no one thing" causes cancer and that those aforementioned factors do in fact contribute in some manner to carcinogenesis, although at present there is no universal acceptance of the mechanisms or the phase of carcinogenesis by which they work. Today, most agree that mutations in genes, as well as epigenetic alterations in the expression of genes without mutations, can contribute to the carcinogenic process. However, exactly where in the process, and whether the mutation or epigenetic alteration of a gene(s) is (are) the "cause" or consequence of the carcinogenic process, has to be determined. To really muddy the understanding of how each factor might contribute to the mechanisms of carcinogenesis, particularly if the agent can mutate a gene, the relative weakness of assays to determine whether chemical agents cause mutations has been a real stumbling block.[8]

MULTISTAGE, MULTIMECHANISM NATURE OF CARCINOGENESIS

Probably, the experimental demonstration of the fact that to produce a cancer in an animal, one had to sequentially expose the animal to a unique set of agents/conditions before a tumor appeared. When exposed to a "carcinogen" at a dose/concentration that was below a threshold to produce a cancer during the lifetime of an animal (mouse, rat, rabbit), but followed by sustained, chronic exposure to a noncarcinogen that finally allowed tumors (skin, liver, mammary) to appear, the concepts of "initiation," "promotion," and "progression" were conceived.[9] The interpretation of these whole-animal tumor studies generated these "operationally" distinct phases of the carcinogenic process. Currently, it is observed that the initiation phase requires an agent that can induce an "irreversible" change in one single cell. It is further assumed that the "initiation" agent must be a mutagen and the process of mutagenesis, which produces, for all practical purposes, an irreversible change in DNA, is the mechanism of "initiation." This interpretation is supported by observations that many physical (UV, X rays) and chemical agents can be "initiators" in animal systems. In addition, mutations (gene and chromosomal) are found in most cancer cells (exception might be teratoma—see later). One cannot deny that human genetic syndromes (xeroderma pigmentosum, Down's, retinoblastoma, etc.), which can predispose the affected individuals to a variety of cancers inherit mutations (gene and chromosomal), that are associated with those particular cancers. The relatively recent discoveries of "oncogenes" and "tumor suppressor genes" have also provided strong evidence of a role of mutations in the initiation/promotion/progression process of carcinogenesis.

To provide a bit of support for a nonmutagenic (i.e., "epigenetic") mechanism for the initiation phase of carcinogenesis might be the production of teratomas.

If an irreversible mutation was responsible for teratomas, it would be very difficult to explain how a single cell from a teratoma when transplanted back to the blastocyst of a genetically marked mouse could contribute to a normal mosaic mouse.[10] In other words, if this teratoma cell had an irreversible mutation in some critical gene that blocked normal development to produce a teratoma, then how could that cell, when placed back into the microenvironment of a normal blastocyst, contribute to the production of normal tissues in the normal mosiac mouse? The alterative explanation is that in the original pregnant animal, if the developing embryo is exposed to some abnormal microenvironment, altered gene transcription could have occurred without mutating the gene(s), such that the normal careful orchestration of gene expression patterns needed for embryonic/fetal development does not occur. Rather, the stem cells are not organized or induced to differentiate in an organized sequence, even though differentiation can occur in a grossly disorganized fashion to form hair, bone, teeth, etc. in the teratoma mass.

In addition, one must not forget that some epigenetic changes could be "irreversible," which appears to be the case during normal development and differentiation, when a stem cell commits to a specific lineage progenitor cell that gives rise to specific cell types, not all the potential cell types existing in the genome of that stem cell or progenitor cell. This does not exclude the possibility of "transdifferentiation" of a committed adult stem cell.[11]

Many agents or conditions that do not induce DNA damage, inhibit repair of DNA damage, or directly cause mutations *do* contribute to the promotion phase of carcinogenesis; these observations lead to the interpretation that "epigenetic" mechanisms contribute to the promotion phase of carcinogenesis (FIG. 1). Chemicals, such as DDT, phorbol ester, saccharin, polybrominated biphenyls, pthalates, perfluoro-sulfanated compounds, and phenobarbital, which are not mutagenic and which do not "initiate" carcinogenesis, are good tumor promoters.[12] The fact that the tumor promotion process occurs after exposure to an initiator, means that a promoter must be present at or above "threshold" levels,[13] and that promoters must be given to an animal (or human being) in a regular, sustained fashion for a long period of time. Experimental observations show that the interruption of the regular, sustained exposure can stop or even reverse the promotion process.[14] Re-establishment of an interrupted promotion process can lead to the restoration of the promotion of the initiated cells. This demonstrated that a cell that was previously initiated "remembers" it was previously irreversibly changed and can resume the promotion process. Physical irritation, wound healing, or intrinsic growth stimuli (such as in a growing fetus, neonate, or adolescent) can act as a tumor promoter. Now there is evidence that chronic inflammation by various cytokines and other inflammatory agents (including toxins from bacteria, fungi, viruses, as well as several external chemicals) can act as promoters.[15]

These epigenetic agents and conditions that can act as tumor promoters seem to work by causing the single initiated cell to clonally expand to form

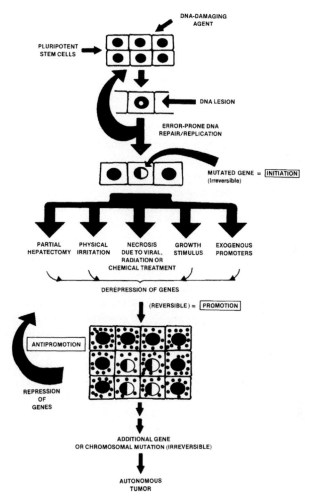

FIGURE 1. A diagrammatic heuristic scheme to depict the postulated mechanisms of the initiation and promotion phase of carcinogenesis. DNA lesions, induced by physical or chemical mutagens, are substrates that can be fixed if they are not removed in an error-free manner prior to DNA replication. Promotion includes those conditions (i.e., wounding, cytotoxicity, exogenous promoters) in which a pluripotent, but surviving, initiated cell can escape the nonproliferative state. The buildup of initiated cells allows them to "resist" the antimitotic influence of neighboring noninitiated cells. This, together with a second mutation, might allow a given cell to have autonomous, invasive properties of a malignant cell. (From Trosko and Tai.[15] Reprinted, by permission from Springer-Verlag).

sectors in tissues of embryonic-like or partially differentiated cells, such as a papilloma in the skin, polyps in the colon, nodes in the breast or foci in the liver. Experimentally, then, promoters act as "mitogens" rather than "mutagens." In addition, experimentally, they also appear to block apoptosis.[16] Therefore, operationally, promotion involves the clonal expansion of initiated cells by stimulating mitogenesis in these initiated cells (which, by virtue of the initiation process, blocks terminal differentiation), as well as blocking the apoptosis of these cells. The two promotion processes lead to the selective accumulation of these initiated cells, whereas any normal cell stimulated to proliferate and to differentiate can, in time, die by apoptosis or senescence. Interruption of the promotion process not only stops the increase in cell growth of the initiated cell, but also allows initiated cells to die by apoptosis (explaining the regression or shrinkage of papillomas or focus after stoppage of phorbol ester treatment of skin and phenobarbital of liver-initiated cells).[14]

The speculated mechanism to explain the epigenetic molecular/biochemical mechanisms of tumor promotion is the alteration of the expression of genes, either at the transcriptional, translational, or posttranslational levels. At the cell level it is the stimulation of cell proliferation and the inhibition of apoptosis. What has been largely ignored is that this process of promotion is a whole-animal phenomenon, not an *in vitro* cellular or molecular response. It occurs in tissues and organs. It has been hypothesized that the operational phenomenon of tumor promotion involves oxidative stress-induced intracellular signaling,[17] which sends signals (*a*) to the nuclei to cause transcriptional alterations of gene expression and (*b*) to modulate extracellular communication either by secreted factors for soft tissue cells (lymphoreticular cells) and gap junctional intercellular communication, which controls cell proliferation,[18] differentiation,[19] and apoptosis.[20] Most, if not all, known tumor promoters have been shown to reversibly inhibit cell–cell communication at threshold levels (characteristics of tumor promoters *in vivo*).[21]

In addition, many of the tumor-promoting agents/conditions can induce oxidative stress. While, traditionally, oxidative stress has been interpreted as causing "oxidative" damage, which translated into meaning DNA damage and mutations, oxidative stress leading to redox changes in cells can and does lead to intracellular signaling. Classic examples are phorbol ester (TPA), perchlorophenol (PC), and estrogen.[22–24] Early on it was shown that TPA seemed to induce DNA damage and chromosomal damage.[25] Yet it induced both cell growth and induced differentiation in both cells in culture and *in vivo*. A mutagen (initiator) works by random DNA damage and can lead to inhibited cell growth and necrotic cell death. It could not explain wholesale differentiation of a population of cells that it worked on by random DNA damage and mutagenesis. Promoters actually stimulate cell growth and block cell death by apoptosis. The signaling needed for cell proliferation often is associated by the activation of the MAPK pathway, which is associated with promoters.

Because of the gross numbers of artifacts intrinsic in all *in vitro* assays to measure mutations, as well as the misinterpretation of the data generated by these "indirect" surrogate measures of mutations, there have been far too many agents classified as mutagenic or "genotoxic."[26,27] In addition, just because a tumor appears in an animal after long-term exposures to high levels of a chemical, which has an identified a mutation in an oncogene or tumor suppressor gene, does not necessarily mean that a chemical caused the mutation found in that tumor.[28] In fact, a more likely interpretation is that the high level and chronic exposure to the "carcinogen" actually promoted preexisting, spontaneously "initiated" or mutated cells.[8]

Lastly, what does "initiation" actually do to prevent a normal cell from senescing or terminally differentiating? To answer that question, more will have to be examined related to the original normal cell that is "initiated."

THE STEM CELL THEORY OF CARCINOGENESIS

Two of the earliest theories of carcinogenesis are the "stem cell theory"[3-5] and the "de-differentiation" theory.[29] These theories, for the most part, were generated independent of the "initiation," "promotion," and "progression" concept. The monoclonal origin of cells within a tumor contributed indirectly to the stem cell theory. On the other hand, those believing in the de-differentiation theory posit that any of the 100 trillion cells of the body (except those real terminally differentiated cells such as red blood cells; or lens cells, those that have lost their nuclei) could re-program to the embryonic state and then start on the multistage, multimechanism process with a diploid cell. (Remember, any polyploid normal cell, such as the tetra- and octoploid human hepatocytes, would have to activate/inactivate multiple oncogenes or tumor suppressor genes before it could get started to be initiated and be seen as premalignant liver foci, which are primarily diploid.)

Although these theories of carcinogenesis were generated before— (*a*) the isolation or partial characterization of embryonic or adult stem cells; (*b*) the generation of experimental data on the initiation/promotion/progression model of carcinogenesis; or (*c*) the relatively recent demonstration of "re-programming" of genes during somatic nuclear transfer into oocytes,[30]—there are some observations that allow us to integrate these new facts into one hypothesis or concept. The current paradigm driving most thinking in the carcinogenesis process is the idea that a normal, "mortal" cell must first be "immortalized" and then neoplastically transformed. This idea clearly conforms to the multistep, multimechanism hypothesis of carcinogenesis. This paradigm would then necessitate the concept of "re-programming" of a normal, "mortal" cell, since these normal, mortal cells are thought to have a finite life time (i.e., the "Hayflick" lifespan),[31] while a population of cancer cells (at least *in vitro* up until recently) were thought to be immortal, such as HeLa and MCF-7 cell lines. The classic publication of Land *et al.*[32] provided the experimental observations that supported this paradigm. In that experiment when the myc oncogene was transfected into a population of primary rodent cells *in vitro* (recall that this population would be heterogeneous, with a few adult stem cells, progenitor cells with a finite life span, and terminally differentiated cells) only a few cells survived, which were probably the orginal normal immortal stem cells that have been blocked from terminally differentiating or senescing. Of the few cells that survived the "crises," these were "immortal" but not yet tumorigenic. Only then were these immortalized cells capable of accruing other changes to become neoplastically transformed because they could proliferate for a long time, which is needed to accumulate the necessary mutational/epigenetic changes required for the cell to exhibit all the hallmarks of cancer.

THE CHALLENGE TO THE MORTAL-TO-IMMORTAL PARADIGM SEQUENCE FOR CARCINOGENESIS

With the recent ability to isolate and characterize stem cells, and assuming the accepted definition of a stem cell as one that has the ability to both self-renew and to differentiate into many different cell types, it is normally assumed that the normal state of a stem cell is that of unlimited capacity to proliferate. In other words, *stem cells are naturally "immortal" until they are induced to terminally differentiate or senesce.* Therefore, if the stem cell is the target cell for the "initiation" of the carcinogenic process, *then the new paradigm that would challenge the current paradigm would be that the first step of carcinogenesis would be to inhibit the stem cell from terminal differentiation.* Another way to state this is that the "initiation" step prevents the "mortalization" of a naturally "immortal" stem cell. It is exactly the opposite concept of the current paradigm.

Since normal stem cells can divide either symmetrically or asymmetrically, what the initiation event actually does to these normal stem cells is to block cell division irreversibly and asymmetrically, but permit symmetrical cell division (FIG. 2). The scientific challenge, then, would be to determine what intrinsic (genes) and extrinsic (external) factors control whether a cell divides one way or another. It seems that stem cells exist in a unique, protected microenvironment ("niche") by which they interact directly with a signaling extracellular matrix, as well as with secreted negative growth factors. Possibly by mutating, the genes involved in the cell–matrix interaction and the signaling mechanism linking that interaction with the genes for determining asymmetrical division would lead to uncontrolled symetrical cell division.[33]

While one might argue that this change in concept about the paradigm for the sequence and target for the carcinogenic process is but "semantics," one should see that it now gives new direction to understanding the mechanism for the start of the carcinogenic process. The new paradigm states that one should start to see whether adult normal stem cells can be neoplastically transformed more easily than normal progenitor cells. In addition, this paradigm states that one should look for genes that regulate cell–matrix interactions and the signaling in stem cell proliferation leading to symmetrical or asymmetrical cell divisions.

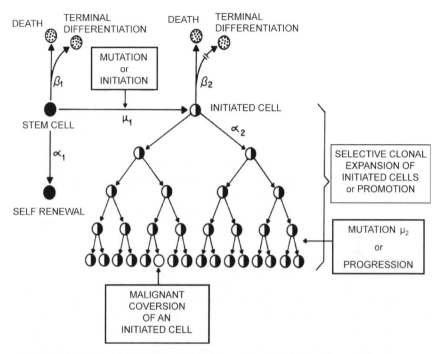

FIGURE 2. The initiation/promotion/progression model of carcinogenesis showing (1) rate of terminal differentiation and death of stem cell; (2) rate of death, but not of terminal differentiation of the initiated cell; (3) rate of cell division of initiated cells; (4) rate of the molecular event leading to initiation (i.e. mutation); and (5) rate at which the second event occurs within an initiated cell (from Trosko et al.[68] Reprinted by permission.)

STEM CELLS, PROGENITOR CELLS, CELL–CELL COMMUNICATION, AND TISSUE HOMEOSTASIS

In multicellular organisms, such as a human being, the 100 trillion cells consists of a few adult stem cells, their lineage-derived, limited-life-span daughter progenitor cells, and the n-stage terminally differentiated cells. To regulate the careful concatenation of gene expression to bring about the correct expression needed for normal embryonic, fetal, neonatal, adolescent, mature, and aging development, a delicately integrated communication network must be maintained. This was beautifully described by Markert.[34]

> Cells interact and communicate during embryonic development and through inductive stimuli mutually direct the divergent courses of their differentiation. Very little cell differentiation is truly autonomous in vertebrate organisms. The myriad cell phenotypes present in mammals, for example, must reflect a corresponding complexity in the timing, nature, and amount of inductive interactions. Whatever the nature of inductive stimuli may be, they emerge as

a consequence of specific sequential interactions of cells during embryonic development.

The first embryonic cells, blastomeres, of mice and other mammals are all totipotent. During cleavage and early morphologenesis these cells come to occupy different positions in the three-dimensional embryo. Some cells are on the outside, some inside. The different environments of these cells cause them to express different patterns of metabolism in accordance with their own developing programs of gene function. These patterns of metabolism create new chemical environments for nearby cells and these changed environments induce yet new programs of gene function in responding cells. Thus a progressive series of reciprocal interactions is established between the cellular environment and the genome of each cell. These interactions drive the cell along a specific path of differentiation until a stable equilibrium is reached in the adult. Thereafter little change occurs in the specialized cells and they become remarkably refractory to changes in the environment. They seem stably locked into the terminal patterns of gene function characteristic of adult cells. The genome seems no longer responsible to the signals that were effective earlier in development.

Of course, changes can occur in adult cells that lead to renewed cell proliferation and altered differentiation as seen in neoplasms, both benign and malignant, but such changes are very rare indeed when one considers the number of cells potentially available for neoplastic transformation. Possibly, mutations in regulatory DNA of dividing adult cells can occasionally lead to new and highly effective programs of gene function that we recognize as neoplastic or malignant. However, most genetic changes in adult cells can probably lead to cell death since random changes in patterns of gene activity are not likely to be beneficial.

Extracellular communication between cells and the matrix must be accomplished by stationary or secreted factors (e.g., collagen, laminin, hormones, cytokines, and growth factors). These stationary and secreted factors then trigger intracellular signals within the affected cells having receptors to these factors that transfer these signals to (*a*) the nuclei of the affected cells and (*b*) membrane organelles such as gap junctions or receptors[35] (FIG. 3).

It appears that initial characterization of several embryonic and adult stem cells is that they lack functional gap junctional intercellular communication (GJIC).[33] Given that GJIC has been hypothesized to play a role in the growth control or contact inhibition for progenitor cells (epithelial, endothelial, fibroblast) and that stem cells also have growth control without GJIC, one could argue that GJIC plays no or little role in growth control. However, growth control for stem cells could be by negative secreted growth regulators from the differentiated cells of their lineage (see Ref. 36). In mature tissues, such as those of liver or kidney, few cells (stem or progenitor) are proliferating. Only during massive tissue injury will there be compensatory replacement of those cells (in many mature tissues, the replaced cells are "scar" cells, not the originally differentiated cells of that tissue). In some organs, such as the skin,

Gap Junctions in Cellular Homeostasis

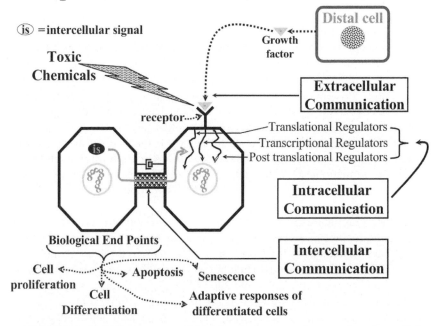

FIGURE 3. Endogenous extracellular signals that can trigger various intracellular signal-transducing mechanisms can either increase or decrease gap junctional intercellular communication between the cells in a multicellular organism. Growth, wound healing tissue repair, pattern formation or tissue differentiation, programmed cell death, and adaptive responses of tissues occur when either there is an up- or downregulation of gap junction function. (From Trosko and Inoue.[69] Reprinted by permission.)

blood system, or intestinal tract, there is constant cell replacement. In some organs, such as those that must also maintain internal volume size, but must have constant replacement, such as the lung or testes, there is also a homeostatic balance of birth and loss of cells. In summary, extracellular communication triggers intracellular signaling, which, in turn, affects intercellular signaling either by secreted factors or through gap junctions.

CANCER AS THE RESULT OF DYSFUNCTIONAL HOMEOSTATIC CONTROL OF CELL PROLIFERATION, CELL DIFFERENTIATION, AND APOPTOSIS

Characteristics of cancer cells are the so-call "hallmarks" of cancer.[1] The loss of growth control or loss of contact inhibition,[37] the inability to terminally differentiate, or to apoptose properly seem to be just the opposite of normal cells (either stem or progenitor). Cancer has been classically viewed as a "disease of differentiation,"[3] as well as a "stem cell disease,"[4] or oncogeny as partially blocked ontogeny.[5]

Another interesting observation in cancer is that, while all the cells within the tumor are clonally derived from one cell, they are very heterogeneous in terms of both genotype and phenotype. Often they are characterized as "genomically unstable," leading to the diversity of both genotypes and phenotypes. Some investigators have speculated that one of the early steps of carcinogenesis is the induction of genomic instability.[38] Yet, it must be determined whether genomic stability is the cause or consequence of carcinogenesis.

One of the very early hypotheses to suggest a mechanistic basis for the loss of growth control or inability to regulate differentiation was the rendering of GJIC nonfunctional.[39] Without functional GJIC, assuming that GJIC is a necessary process for growth control and differentiation for progenitor cells, then these cancer phenotypes would result.

Another very interesting observation that is constantly overlooked is the fact that there appears to be only two classes of cancer cells, both of which do not have functional GJIC. Upon close examination, there are two classes of dysfunctional GJIC. One is where a cell does not express its connexin or gap junction genes (e.g., HeLa and MCF-7 cancer cell lines) and the other is where the cancer cell expresses its connexin genes, but the protein is not transported, assembled, or functional, such as those with activated scr, ras, neu, raf, because the connexin protein is postranslationally modified.[40] It is interesting to note that the tumorigenicity of the HeLa and MCF-7 cells can be ameliorated by transcriptional activation of the connexin genes.[41,42] This leads to a new strategy for both chemoprevention and chemotherapy of cancer (FIG. 4)

CANCER STEM CELLS: A RE-DISCOVERY OF AN OLD IDEA

A relatively recent article had described the isolation from human breast cancer tissues of a unique subset of cancer cells within the tumor that was capable of repopulating the tumor, whereas most of the breast cancer cells were not capable of perpetuating the tumor.[43] The emergence of the "cancer stem" concept has taken the cancer field by storm as though this was never anticipated. Indeed, to some extent it is true because most have generalized that all cancer cells were "immortal." Now it seems, especially with more rigorous extension of the original findings,[44] that several other types of "cancer stem" cells have been reported.[45]

Now the experimental scientific question to be answered is: "Where did this cancer stem cell come from?" Two possible explanations come to mind: first, they were derived from adult normal stem cells. Alternatively, they were derived from normal differentiated progenitor cells that "de-differentiated" or

Origin of Two Types of GJIC Deficient Tumor Cells: Hypothesis"

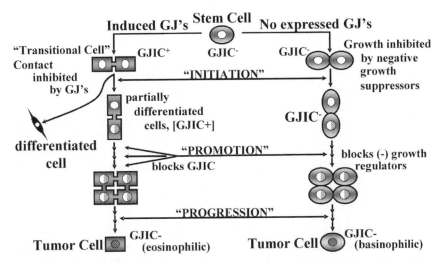

FIGURE 4. The figure illustrates how two types of cancer cells could arise from either pluripotent stem cells (lacking expressed connexin genes and having no GJIC) or from very early transit cells, which express connexin genes and have functional GJIC after exposure to an initiator. Initiation is that process which would prevent the stem or transit cell from terminal differentiation (loss of telomerase activity). These initiated stem or initiated transit cells would be growth-suppressed either by secreted negative growth regulators or by gap junction–dependent "contact inhibition," respectively. If these initiated stem or initiated transit cells are exposed chronically to agents that either inhibit the secreted negative growth regulator or its receptor-dependent signaling (initiated stem cell) or downregulate gap junctional intercellular communication (initiated transit cell), these initiated cells would proliferate, accumulate, and accrue sufficient genetic/epigenetic changes sufficient to become "promoter independent" and invasive and metastatic. In the end, both tumor types lack functional GJIC, one because of the transcriptional suppression of the connexin genes (stem cells); the other because various mutations/activated oncogenes/deactivated/loss of tumor suppressor genes cause downregulation of the expressed connexins and gap junctions (transit cells). Strategically and tactically, based on this hypothesis, the approach to chemoprevention and chemotherapy would be very different.

"re-programmed" to a more "embryonic "state. To address this question, our lab isolated many different normal adult human stem cells (kidney, breast, pancreas, liver, mesenchyme). In addition, the lab had previously shown that these normal adult stem cells were characterized by the lack of functional GJIC and being able to differentiate with various inducers. This differentiation was accompanied by the induction of connexin genes and functional GJIC. Also a wholesale conversion of markers occurred during this differentiation process.[46] Later, we showed that the normal human breast epithelial stem cell could be kept in the immortal state by transfection with SV40,[47] and then later induced to become weakly tumorigenic with repeated X-ray exposures. These clones could then be converted to highly tumorigenic cells by transfection with the activated ERB 2/neu oncogene.[48] The interpretation of our result, using Occam's razor, was that, since we could not induce "immortalization" in the normal differentiated daughter cells of the adult breast epithelial cells, we could prevent mortalization in the adult stem cells with SV40 and later neoplastically transform them; the original normal, immortal, adult stem cell was the "target" cell for the transformation process. The neoplastically derived breast tumor cell resembled many of the original phenotypes of the normal adult breast stem cell. Several of the markers that remained were the nonexpression of $C \times 43$ and no functional GJIC and the expression of estrogen receptor.[49] The normal differentiated daughter expressed $C \times 43$ and maspin gene. The normal adult breast cell that was classified as an adult stem cell was demonstrated when the cells were induced to form a three-dimensional, budding, ductal "organoid" very similar, morphologically and biochemically, to *in vivo* human breast tissue structures.[50]

However, the strongest evidence for the stem cell's being the target cell for carcinogenesis and being the potential origin of the "cancer" stem cells came when papers stated that the transcription factor needed for maintaining "stemness," Oct3/4 or from hence, Oct4, was found in embryonic stem cells but not in normal tissues.[51] Later, Oct4 was observed in a few tumors that were examined. It was concluded by these authors that Oct4 expression in tumor cells was "restored" by the transformation process.[52,53] This was the stimulus for our lab to test whether it was the adult stem cell or the differentiated adult cells that might be the "target" cell to initiate the cancer process. Since our lab had at hand cultures of isolated human adult kidney, breast, pancreas, liver, and mesenchyme stem cells, we tested for the expression of Oct4 in these cells, their differentiated daughters, and tumor cells from these organs, as well as a few tumor cell lines (HeLa and MCF-7), in addition to normal human and canine skin.[43] The results indicated that Oct4 was expressed in all the adult normal stem cells, but not in their differentiated daughter cells. It was also expressed, rarely, in normal tissue, but was expressed in a heterologous fashion in the HeLa and MCF-7 cell lines.[43] This can be seen in the human breast stem cell and normal, immortalized, weakly and highly tumorigenic derivatives (FIG. 5).

Moreover, even more evidence supported the hypothesis that the "cancer stem cell" was derived from the adult normal stem cell when our lab examined 83 canine tumors for the expression of Oct4 in the tumors. The results showed that 100% of the tumors had expressed Oct4; however, the frequency within each tumor was variable, in that some tumors expressed a small frequency, while others expressed a larger frequency.[54]

This is now consistent with the idea that within tumors one can find cells that have a biomarker for stem cells (Oct4), suggesting that it came from the normal adult stem cells. It has yet to be shown that these are the actual cells that can maintain the tumor growth or are the true "cancer stem cells." To explain the non-Oct4-expressing cells within the tumor, one could speculate that as the tumor grows, its microenvironment changes. This could alter the expression of genes, including repressing the gene for maintaining "stemness." This would cause partial differentiation of the cancer stem cell, as was described by Potter.[5] In addition, in each organism in which a tumor is found, the frequency of Oct4-expressing cells could be influenced by physiological factors influencing the microenvironment of the cancer stem cells, either favoring symmetrical cell division to increase the frequency of cancer stem cells with expressed Oct4 or by altering cell division to be asymmetrical to force "partial differentiation" of these "cancer stem" cells. It has yet to be determined whether the frequency of these Oct4 cancer stem cells might be correlated with the clinical outcomes of treatment of each tumor.

GENERIC CONCEPTS OF CARCINOGENESIS TO SPECIFIC HYPOTHESIS OF HUMAN BREAST CARCINOGENESIS

Assuming that (a) the adult stem cells are the target cells for the "initiation" of the multistage, multimechanism process of carcinogenesis, and (b) that these cells are promoted to accrue the phenotypic changes needed for the "hallmarks of cancer," then what experimental evidence might exist to support or reject this hypothesis? Since normal human breast epithelial stem cells have been isolated and partially characterized, as well as shown to be blocked from terminal differentiation by SV40 and then neoplastically transformed by treatment with X rays and transfected ErB2/Neu oncogene, the first direct evidence showed that normal adult stem cells could be neoplastically transformed *in vitro*, a very difficult task for normal human cells. Moreover, these normal human breast stem cells expressed the estrogen receptor gene that was maintained during SV40 immortalization (and actually blocked mortalization) and during neoplastic transformation.[55] This represents the majority of estrogen receptor phenotypes in actual human cancers.

Another important piece of experimental evidence that supports the human breast stem cell as targets for breast carcinogenesis is the demonstration that the "stemness-requiring" gene, Oct4, has been shown to be expressed in normal human breast stem cells, repressed during the differentiation of the breast stem cell, maintained when the normal breast stem cell was blocked from mortalization by SV40, and subsequently neoplastically transformed by X-rays and the ErB2/Neu oncogene (FIG. 5).

In this experimental case, the Oct4 gene expression was not first repressed and then "re-programmed" or "restored" by integration of SV40, as would be required by the opposing paradigm, stating that the breast differentiated progenitor cell (which does not express the Oct4 gene) reactivate the Oct4 gene. In fact, in the experiment,[47] the differentiated breast epithelial cell, which expressed the estrogen receptor and connexin 43 gene, was never "immortalized" by SV40.

In effect, the phenotype of the human breast neoplastic cell derived from this study was very similar to the classic MCF-7 breast carcinoma cell line (e.g., no expression of $C \times 43$; estrogen receptor expression; telomerase-positive; Oct4 expression–positive, tumorigenic). However, a significant number of human breast cancers are estrogen receptor–negative. Are these cells derived from the normal differentiated epithelial cells with no Oct4, expressed $C \times 43$, reduced telomerase, and no expressed estrogen receptor? Do these cells represent normal, "mortal" cells that have their Oct4 gene "re-programmed" or restored by the "initiation" event?

HUMAN BREAST TUMOR PROMOTION: EPIGENETIC PROCESS INVOLVING REDOX SIGNALING–INDUCED OXIDATIVE STRESS, ALTERED GENE EXPRESSION CONTROLLING MITOGENESIS AND APOPTOSIS, AS WELL AS REVERSIBLE INHIBITION OF GJIC

If the normal human breast stem cell is the cell that is "initiated," what then promotes these cancers? A general concept about promotion is that chemical promoters reversibly block GJIC. However, if "cancer stem cells" are derived from normal adult stem cells and if these "cancer stem cells" share many of the phenotypes, such as Oct4 expression and estrogen receptor, but no expression or functional gap junctions, then tumor promoters of "cancer stem cells" must be different from the cancer non-stem cells.[40] Promoters of these breast cancer stem cells might include estrogen and other agents that act as mitogens and inhibitors of apoptosis for initiated cancer stem cells that do not have functional GJIC. If the breast cancer non-stem cells do not express the estrogen receptor, then estrogens would not act as a promoter by modulating connexin expression or inhibiting functional GJIC by receptor–dependent mechanisms. This, of course, does not exclude estrogen receptor-independent mechanisms.

While hormones, such as 17 beta-estradiol, can either increase or decrease the expression of connexins and the function of gap junctions in various hormone-regulated tissues,[56,57] the exact cellular mechanism, regulation of genes and signal cascades that influence the tumor promotion process are both complex and not yet systematically examined in human breast tissue. However, early studies have shown in one system that the effect of estrogen on uterine epithelium requires interaction with the surrounding stromal cells. In other words, the direct cell contact between the stromal cells and breast epithelium, which might not involve gap junctions between the two cell types (although gap junctions do exist between the homogenous stromal and epithelial cells) could result in a secreted factor from the stromal cells stimulated by estrogens, which inhibits GJIC in the breast epithelial cells.[58] This could lead to mitogenetic hyperplasia.

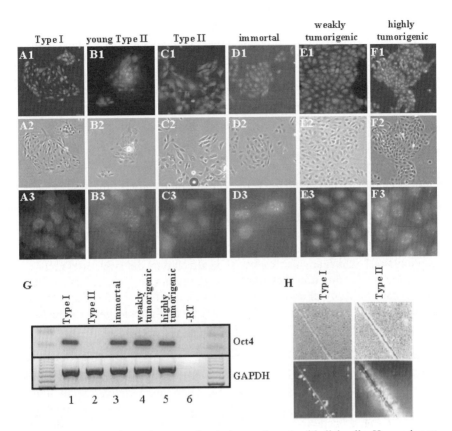

FIGURE 5. Oct4 protein expression in human breast epithelial cells. Human breast stem cells (type I) (A), differentiated daughter cells (young and mature type II) (B and C), an immortal cell line (SV40-transfected type I cells) (D), a weakly tumorigenic cell line (X-ray-transformed) (E), and a highly tumorigenic cell line (neu oncogene-transduced) (F) were immunostained, with Oct4 showing in red or green (A1–F1). (A2)–(F2) are phase-contrast images showing the morphology of the cells. (A3)–(F3) are higher magnification images of A1–F1 superimposed on 40,60-diamidino-2-phenylindole dihydrochloride (DAPI) blue nuclear stain. Punctate staining of Oct4 was seen in most cell types, located in the nucleus, except for mature type II cells (C3). In (B) Oct4 staining was heterogeneously distributed in young type II cells, only the cells in the center of the colony staining positive. Scale bars: (A1)–(F2) 60 mm; (A3)–(F3) 20 mm. (G) RT-PCR analysis of Oct4 expression in type I human breast stem cells (lane 1) and human breast immortal (lane 3), weakly tumorigenic (lane 4) and highly tumorigenic cell lines (lane 5). No expression of Oct4 was seen in type II differentiated cells (lane 2). Monkey ES cells were used as a positive control (lane 6). Lane 7 is a no-template control. (H) Scrape loading dye transfer assay (SL/DT) was used to examine GJIC in human breast epithelial cells. Type I cells were deficient in GJIC. Young and mature type II cells were efficient in GJIC.

Another approach to understanding the role of estrogens in breast carcino-genesis is to view the role of endogenous/exogenous agents in induction of oxidative stress. While the normal view is to ascribe oxidative stress leading to oxidative damage (as it could lead to macromolecular damage to nucleic acids, proteins, and lipids), a rapidly growing of body of evidence suggests that many chronic diseases associated with oxidative stress are not always associated with necrosis, DNA or protein damage, but rather altered gene expression through oxidative signaling.[59] Of course, oxidative damage by es-trogens to DNA has been postulated to play a role in the induction of genomic mutations.[60]

A systematic study, both *in vitro* with normal human breast stem cells, normal human differentiated breast epithelium and breast stromal cells, human breast cancer stem cells, and breast cancer non-stem cells and *in vivo*, will have to be done to determine how estrogen might affect proliferation, apoptosis (measures of tumor promotion) of these cell types, in addition to the status of gap junctions, which are also known to be affected by oxidative stress.[61]

Yet, the normal function of estrogens and hormones, in general, is epigenetic, that is, they work by altering cell proliferation, differentiation, and adaptive responses of differentiated cells via signaling and altered gene expression. Specifically, gene expression is highly regulated by the coordination of extra-, intra- and gap junctional intercellular communication systems that maintain tissue homeostasis.

Oxidative stress has been postulated to play a significant role in tumor promotion.[62] Indeed, TPA and organic and hydrogen peroxides act as tumor promoters and not as initiators, [63] suggesting that these oxidants are not muta-gens but rather epigenetic effectors. Hydrogen peroxide has also been demon-strated to be a promoter but not an initiator using two-stage *in vivo* carcino-genesis model systems and transformation in *in vitro* systems.[63,64] In addition, recent research has started a shift in the understanding of how ROS (reac-tive oxygen species) can reversibly control the expression of genes at non-cytotoxic levels.[65] In one study, over 100 genes and signaling proteins have been reported to be sensitive to reductive and oxidative (redox) states in a cell.[66]

Bringing this general series of observations to the concept that estrogens might be a tumor promoter by generating oxidative stress is the report that, indeed, oxidative stress has been demonstrated in estrogen-induced renal car-cinogenesis.[24] In addition, oxidative stress has been shown to effect the expres-sion of both ER-alpha and ER-beta.[67] In summary, the weight of the evidence seems to be consistent with the idea that estrogen can be a tumor promoter of initiated breast stem cells, which have the estrogen receptor, by its ability to induce oxidative stress–induced signaling. Within the microenvironment of these tumors, partial differentiation might occur, leading to the initiated estro-gen receptor–positive cancer "stem cells" forming estrogen receptor–negative cells.

REFERENCES

1. HANAHAN, D. & R.A. WEINBERG. 2000. The hallmarks of cancer. Cell **100:** 57–70.
2. POTTER, V.R. 1978. Biochemistry of Cancer. *In* Cancer Research. J. Holland & E. Frei, Eds.: 178–192. Lea and Febiger. Philadelphia, PA.
3. MARKERT, C. 1968. Neoplasia: a disease of cell differentiation. Cancer Res. **28:** 1908–1914.
4. PIERCE, G.P. 1974. Neoplasm differentiation and mutations. Am. J. Pathol. **77:** 103–118.
5. POTTER, V.R. 1978. Phenotypic diversity in experimental hepatomas: the concept of partially blocked ontogeny. Br. J. Cancer **38:** 1–23.
6. WEINSTEIN, I.B., C.S. GATTANI, P. KIRSCHMEIER, *et al.* 1984. Multistage carcinogenesis involves multiple genes and multiple mechanisms. J. Cell Physiol. Suppl. **3:** 127–137.
7. FIALKOW, P.J. 1979. Clonal origin of human tumor. Am. Rev. Med. **30:** 135–176.
8. TROSKO, J.E. & B.L. UPHAM. 2005. The emperor wears no clothes in the field of carcinogen risk assessment: ignored concepts in cancer risk assessment. Mutagenesis **20:** 81–90.
9. BEREBLUM, P.M. 1954. A speculative review: the probable nature of promoting action and its significance in the understanding of the mechanism of carcinogenesis. Cancer Res. **14:** 471–477.
10. MINSK, B. & K. ILLMENSI. 1976. Totipotency and normal differentiation of single teratocarcinoma cells cloned by injecting into blastocysts. Proc. Natl. Acad. Sci. USA **73:** 549–553.
11. DI GIOACCHINO, G., C. DI CAMPLI, M.A. ZOCCA, *et al.* 2005. Transdifferentiation of stem cells in pancreatic cells: state of the art. Transplant. Proc. **37:** 2662–2663.
12. TROSKO, J.E. & C.C. CHANG. 1988. Nongenotoxic mechanisms in mechanisms in carcinogenesis: role of inhibited intercellular communication. *In* Banbury Report 31: Carcinogen Risk Assessment: New Directions in the Quantitative and Qualitative Aspects. R.W. Hart & F.D. Hoerger. Eds.: 139–170. Cold Spring Harbor Laboratory. Cold Spring Harbor, NY.
13. TROSKO, J.E. & R.J. RUCH. 1998. Cell-cell communication in carcinogenesis. Front. Biosci. **3:** 208–236.
14. GOODMAN, J.A. 2001. Operational reversibility is a key aspect of carcinogenesis. Toxicol. Sci. **64:** 147–148.
15. TROSKO, J.E. & M.-H. TAI. 2006. Adult stem cell theory of the multistage, multi-mechanism theory of carcinogenesis: role of inflammation on the promotion of initiated stem cells. *In* Infection and Inflammation: Impacts on Oncogenesis. T. Dittmar, Ed.: 45–65. S. Karger AG. Amsterdam.
16. BURSCH, F., F. OBERHAMMER & R. SCHULTE-HERMANN. 1992. Cell death by apoptosis and its protective role against disease. Trends Pharmacol. Sci. **13:** 245–251.
17. UPHAM, B.L. & J. WAGNER. 2001. Toxicant-induced oxidative stress in cancer. Toxicol. Sci. **64:** 1–3.
18. LOEWENSTEIN, W.R. 1966. Permeability of membrane junctions. Ann. N.Y. Acad. Sci. **137:** 441–472.
19. WEI, C.-J., X. XU & C.W. LO. 2004. Connexins and cell signaling in development and disease. Annu. Rev. Cell Dev. Biol. **20:** 811–838.
20. WILSON, M.R., T.W. CLOSE & J.E. TROSKO. 2000. Cell population dynamics (apoptosis, mitosis, and cell-cell communication) during disruption of homeostasis. Exp. Cell Res. **254:** 257–268.

21. TROSKO, J.E. 2001. Is the concept of "tumor promotion" a useful paradigm? Mol. Carcinogen. **30:** 131–137.
22. CERUTTI, P.A. 1985. Prooxidant states and tumor promotion. Science **227:** 375–381.
23. UMEMURA, T., S. KAI, R. HASEGAWA, et al. 1999. Pentachlorophenol (PCP) produces liver oxidative stress and promoters but does not initiate hepatocarcinogenesis in B6C3F1 mice. Carcinogenesis **20:** 1115–1120.
24. BHAT, H.K., G. CALAF, T. HEI, et al. 2003. Critical role of oxidative stress in estrogen-induced carcinogenesis. Proc. Natl. Acad. Sci. USA **100:** 3913–3918.
25. BIRBOIM, H.C. 1982. DNA strand breakage in human leukocytes exposed to a tumor promoter, phorbol myristate acetate. Science **215:** 1247–1249.
26. TROSKO, J.E. 1997. Challenge to the simple paradigm that "carcinogens" are "mutagens" and to the *in vitro* and *in vivo* assays used to test the paradigm. Mutat. Res. **373:** 245–249.
27. TROSKO, J.E. 1988. A failed paradigm: carcinogenesis is more than mutagenesis. Mutagenesis **3:** 363–366.
28. THILLY, W.G. 2003. Have environmental mutagens caused oncomutations in people? Nat. Genet. 255–259.
29. SELL, S. 1993. Cellular origin of cancer: dedifferentiation or stem cell maturation arrest? Environ. Health Perspect. **101:** 15–26.
30. COWAN, C., J. ATIENZA, D. MELTON, et al. 2005. Nuclear reprogramming of somatic cells after fusion with human embryonic stem cells. Science **309:** 1369–1373.
31. HAYFLICK, L. 1965. The limited *in vitro* lifetime of human diploid cell strains. Exp. Cell Res. **37:** 614–636.
32. LAND, H., L.F. PARADA & R.A. WEINBERG. 1983. Tumorigenic conversion of primary embryo fibroblast requires at least at least two cooperating oncogenes. Nature **304:** 596–602.
33. TROSKO, J.E., C.C. CHANG, M.R. WILSON, et al. 2000. Gap junctions and the regulation of cellular functions of stem cells during development and differentiation. Methods **20:** 245–264.
34. MARKERT, C.L. 1984. Genetic control of cell interactions in chimeras. Develop. Genet. **4:** 267–279.
35. TROSKO, J.E., C.C. CHANG, B.L. UPHAM, et al. 1998. Epigenetic toxicology as toxicant-induced changes in intracellular signaling leading to altered gap junctional intercellular communication. Toxicol. Lett. 102–103: 71–78.
36. TROSKO, J.E., C.C. CHANG, B.V. MADHUKAR, et al. 1996. Intercellular communication: a paradigm for the interpretation of the initiation/ promotion/progression model of carcinogenesis. In: Chemical Induction of Cancer: Modulation and Combination Effects. 205–225. Birkhauser, Boston.
37. BOREK, C. & L. SACHS. 1966. The difference in contact inhibition of cell replication between normal cells and cells transformed by different carcinogens. Proc. Natl. Acad. Sci. USA **56:** 1705–1711.
38. TLSY, T.D., A. BRIOT, A. GUALBERTO, et al. 1995. Genomic instability and cancer. Mutation Res. **337:** 1–7.
39. LOEWENSTEIN, W.R. 1966. Permeability of membrane junctions. Ann. N.Y. Acad. Sci., **137:** 441–472.
40. TROSKO, J.E. 2003. The role of stem cells and gap junctional communication in carcinogenesis. J. Biochem Molec. Biol. **36:** 43–48.

41. KING, T.J., L.H. FUKUSHIMA, T.A. DONLON, *et al*. 2000. Correlation between growth control, neoplastic potential and endogenous connexin43 expression in HeLa cell lines: implications tumor progression. Carcinogenesis **21:** 311–315.

42. MOMIYAMA, M., Y. OMORI, Y. ISHIZAKA, *et al*. 2003. Connexin26-mediated gap junctional communication reverses the malignant phenotype of MCF-7 breast cancer cells. Cancer Sci. **94:** 501–507.

43. AL HAJJ, M., M.S. WICHA, A. BENITO-HERNANDEZ, *et al*. 2003. Prospective identification of tumorigenic breast cancer cells. Proc. Natl. Acad. Sci. USA **100:** 3983–3988.

44. PONTI, D., A. COSTA, N. ZAFFARONI, *et al*. 2005. Isolation and *in vitro* propagation of tumorigenic breast cancer cells with stem/progenitor cell properties. Cancer Res. **65:** 5506–551.

45. TAI, M.H., C.C. CHANG, M. KIUPEL, *et al*. 2005. Oct-4 expression in adult stem cells: evidence in support of the stem cell theory of carcinogenesis. Carcinogenesis **26:** 495–502.

46. CHANG, C.C. 2006. Recent translational research: stem cells as the roots of breast cancer. Breast Cancer Res. **8:** 103–105.

47. KAO, C.Y., K. NOMATA, C.S. OAKLEY, *et al*. 1995. Two types of normal human breast epithelial cells derived from reduction mammoplasty: phenotypic characteristization and response to SV40 transfection. Carcinogenesis **16:** 531–538.

48. KANG, K.S., W. SUN, K. NOMATA, *et al*. 1998. Involvement of tyrosine phosphorylation of p185 c-erB2/neu in tumorigenicity induced by X-rays and neu-oncogene in human breast epithelial epithelial cells. Mol. Carcinogen. **21:** 225–233.

49. CHANG, C.C., W. SUN, A. CRUZ, *et al*. 2001. A human breast epithelial cell type with stem cell characteristics to telomerase activation and immortalization. Cancer Res. **59:** 6118–6123.

50. CHANG, C.C., W. SUN, A. CRUZ, *et al*. 2001. A human breast epithelial cell type with stem cell characteristics as target cells for carcinogenesis. Radiat. Res. **155:** 201–207.

51. PESCE, M. & H.R. SCHOLER. 2001. Oct-4: gatekeeper in the beginnings of mammalian development. Stem Cells **19:** 71–278.

52. MONK, M. & C. HOLDING. 2001. Human embryonic genes re-expressed in cancer cells. Oncogenes **20:** 8085–8091

53. GIDEKEL, S., G. PIZOV, Y. BERGMAN, *et al*. 2003. Oct-3/4 is a dose-dependent oncogenic fate determinant. Cancer Cell **4:** 361–370.

54. WEBSTER, J.D., V. YUSBASIYAN-GURKAN, C.C. CHANG, *et al*. 2005. Oct-4 expression in canine neoplasms: a potential role for embryonic genes in cancer progression. Vet. Pathol. **42:** 5.

55. KANG, K.S., I. MORITA, A. CRUZ, *et al*. 1997. Expression of estrogen receptors in a normal human breast epithelial cell type with luminal and stem cell characteristics and its neoplastically transformation cell lines. Carcinogenesis **18:** 251–257.

56. GRUMMER, R., O. TRAUB & E. WINTERHAGER. 1999. Gap junction connexin genes cx26 and cx43 are differentially regulated by ovarian steroid hormones in rat endometrium. Endocrinology **140:** 2509–2516.

57. SAITO, T., R. TANAKA, K. WATABA, *et al*. 2004. Overexpression of estrogen receptor-alpha gene suppresses gap junctional intercellular communication in endometrial carcinoma cells. Oncogene **23:** 1109–1116.

58. ASTRAHANTSEFF, K.N. & J.E. MORRIS. 1994. Estradiol-17 beta stimulates prolif-eration of uterine epithelial cells cultured with stromal cells but not cultured separately. In Vitro Cell Dev. Biol. **30:** 769–776.

59. UPHAM, B.L. & J.E. TROSKO. 2005. A paradigm shift in the understanding of oxidative stress and its implications to exposure of low-level ionizing radiation. Acta Med. Nagasaki **50:** 63–68.

60. CAVALIERI, E.L., D.E. STACK, P.D. DEVANESAN, et al. 1997. Molecular origin of cancer: Catechol estrogen-3,4-quinones as endogenous tumor initiators. Proc. Natl. Acad. Sci. USA **94:** 10937–10942.

61. KLAUNIG, J.E. & L.M. KAMENDULIS. 2004. The role of oxidative stress in carcino-genesis. Annu. Rev. Pharmacol. Toxicol. **44:** 239–267.

62. SLAGA, T.J., A.J. KLEIN-SZANTO, L.L. TRIPLETT, et al. 1981. Skin tumor-promoting activity of benzoyl peroxide, a widely used free radical-generating compound. Science **213:** 1023–1025.

63. KLEIN-SZANTO, A.J. & T.J. SLAGA. 1982. Effects of peroxides on rodent skin epi-dermal hyperplasia and tumor promotion. J. Invest. Dermatol. **79:** 30–34.

64. NAKAMURA, Y., T.D. GINHART, D. WINTERSTEIN, et al. 1988. Early superoxide dismutase-sensitive event promotes neoplastic transformation in mouse epider-mal JB6 cells. Carcinogenesis **9:** 203–207.

65. KOIKE, T., N. KIMURA, K. MIYAZAKI, et al. 2004. Hypoxia induces adhesion molecules in cancer cells: a missing link between Warburg effect and induction of selectin-ligand carbohydrates. Proc. Natl. Acad. Sci USA **101:** 8132–8137.

66. ALLEN, R.G. 2000. Oxidative stress and gene regulation. Free Radic. Biol. Med. **28:** 463–499.

67. TAMIR, S., S. IZRAEL & J. VAYA. 2002. The effect of oxidative stress on ER alpha and ER beta expression. J. Steroid Biochem. Molec. Biol. **81:** 327–332.

68. TROSKO, J. et al. 1998. In Modern Cell Biology. Vol. 7: Gap Junctions. E.L. Hertberg and R.G. Johnson, Eds.: 435–488. Alan R. Liss. New York.

67. TROSKO, J.E. & T. INOUE. 1997. Oxidative stress, signal transduction, and inter-cellular communication in radiation carcinogenesis. In Radiation Injury and the Chernobyl Catastrophe. N. Daniak et al. Eds.: Alpha Med Press. Ohio; published as a supplement to Stem Cells **15**(Suppl. 2): 59–67.

Chromatin Remodeling and Control of Cell Proliferation by Progestins via Cross Talk of Progesterone Receptor with the Estrogen Receptors and Kinase Signaling Pathways

GUILLERMO P. VICENT,[a] CECILIA BALLARÉ,[a] ROSER ZAURIN,[a] PATRICIA SARAGÜETA,[b] AND MIGUEL BEATO[a]

[a]Centre de Regulació Genòmica (CRG), Universitat Pompeu Fabra (UPF), PRBB, Dr Aiguader 88, 08003 Barcelona, Spain

[b]Instituto de Biología y Medicina Experimental, CONICET, Facultad de Ciencias Exactas y Naturales, Universidad de Buenos Aires, 1428 Buenos Aires, Argentina

ABSTRACT: Transcription from the mouse mammary tumor virus (MMTV) promoter can be induced by glucocorticoids or progestins. Progesterone treatment of cultured cells carrying an integrated single copy of an MMTV transgene leads to recruitment of progesterone receptor (PR), SWI/SNF, and SNF2h-related complexes to MMTV promoter. Recruitment is accompanied by selective displacement of histones H2A and H2B from the nucleosome B. In nucleosomes assembled on promoter sequences, SWI/SNF displaces histones H2A and H2B from MMTV nucleosome B, but not from other MMTV nucleosomes or from an rDNA promoter nucleosome. Thus, the outcome of nucleosome remodeling by purified SWI/SNF depends on the DNA sequence. On the other hand, 5 min after hormone treatment, the cytoplasmic signaling cascade Src/Ras/Erk is activated via an interaction of PR with the estrogen receptor, which activates Src. As a consequence of Erk activation PR is phosphorylated, Msk1 is activated, and a ternary complex PR-Erk-Msk1 is recruited to MMTV nucleosome B. Msk1 phosphorylates H3 at serine 10, which is followed by acetylation at lysine 14, displacement of HP1γ, and recruitment of Brg1, PCAF, and RNA polymerase II. Blocking Erk activation or Msk1 activity prevents induction of the MMTV transgene. Thus, the rapid nongenomic effects of progestins are essential for their transcriptional effects on certain progestin target genes. In rat endometrial stromal cells, picomolar concentrations of progestins trigger the cross talk of PR with ERβ that activates the Erk and Akt kinase pathways leading to cell proliferation in the absence of direct transcriptional

Address for correspondence: Dr. Miguel Beato, Center for Genomic Regulation (C.R.G.), PRBB, Dr Aiguader 88, E-08003 Barcelona, Spain. Voice: +34-93-224-0901; fax: +34-93-224-08-99.
e-mail: miguel.beato@crg.es

Ann. N.Y. Acad. Sci. 1089: 59–72 (2006). © 2006 New York Academy of Sciences.
doi: 10.1196/annals.1386.025

effects of the ligand-activated PR. Thus, depending on the cellular context rapid kinase activation and transcriptional effect play different roles in the physiological response to progestins.

KEYWORDS: mouse mammary tumor virus; progesterone receptor; chromatin; transcriptional regulation; histone H1; kinases

The basic unit of chromatin is the nucleosome, which contains a core of histones around which DNA is wrapped in 1.65 left-handed superhelical turns. This core contains two molecules of each of four core histone proteins: H2A, H2B, H3, and H4. Eukaryotic cells contain a fifth class of histones, called linker histones, which bind to the nucleosome and to the linker DNA and alter the stability with which DNA within the nucleosome is associated. The prototype of the linker histones is histone H1, of which there are six somatic isoforms and a testis-specific form. Modulation of the structure and dynamics of the nucleosome is an important regulatory mechanism of all DNA-based processes in eukaryotic cells, such as transcription, DNA replication and repair. Changes in chromatin structure affect the binding of nonhistone proteins, such as transcription factors and the replication machinery, by restricting access to the binding sites within the DNA.

The cell has developed multiple strategies for the optimal use of chromatin as the substrate for DNA-directed processes. The two more important remodeling mechanisms are ATP-dependent chromatin remodeling enzymatic complexes and enzymes that modify the histones posttranslationally. In addition, the cells can incorporate core histone variants to alter the structure and dynamics of specific chromatin regions. ATP-dependent chromatin remodeling complexes utilize the energy from ATP hydrolysis to rearrange both histone–DNA and histone–histone interactions. Most ATP-dependent chromatin remodeling factors are multisubunit complexes with an ATPase as the catalytic center. These ATPase subunits can be classified into three families on the basis of the presence of functional domains: the SWI2/SNF2-, the Mi-2/CHD-, and the ISWI-ATPases.[1] The SWI/SNF family comprises yeast Snf2 and Sth2, *Drosophila melanogaster* brahma (BRM), and mammalian BRM and brahma-like 1 (BRG1). These proteins are characterized by the presence of a bromo domain, which binds acetylated histones.[2] The imitation SWI (ISWI) family of enzymes have a SANT domain, which is thought to act as a histone-binding domain,[3] and may recognize specifically modified histones. There are two ISWI homologues in yeast (Isw1 and Isw2) and mammals (SNF2H and SNF2L). A third class, the chromodomain and helicase-like domain (CHD) family, is characterized by the presence of two amino-terminal chromodomains, which interact with methylated histone tails.[4]

Posttranslational modifications, primarily of the histone-tail domains, such as acetylation of lysines, methylation of lysines or arginines, and phosphorylation of serines and threonines, alter the properties of chromatin, influencing accessibility of the DNA, and in addition, act as signals for the recruitment of nuclear factors.[5,6] Functional cooperation between histone-modifying and ATP-dependent chromatin-remodeling enzymes can mediate positive and negative output on gene regulation. For example, the bromodomain of Brg1 binds the H4 tail when acetylated at K8,[7] and TAFII250 binds the H3 tail when acetylated at both K9 and K14.[8]

Nuclear receptors (NRs) are one of the most abundant classes of transcriptional regulators in animals (metazoans). They regulate diverse functions, such as homeostasis, reproduction, development, and metabolism. NRs share structurally conserved domains and can be regulated through steroids, thyroid hormone, retinoic acid, vitamins, or other proteins. They function as transcription factors, often in complex with other coregulators, and govern transcription of target genes involved in such varied processes as homeostasis, reproduction, development, and metabolism.[9] The steroid/thyroid hormone receptors are members of a very large family of nuclear ligand-activated transcription factors that includes the steroid receptors (those for progesterone [PRs], androgen [ARs], estrogen [ERs], glucocorticoids [GRs], and mineralocorticoids) and receptors for thyroid hormone, retinoids, and vitamin D, as well as an even larger group of proteins termed orphan receptors, whose ligands and/or functions are as yet unknown.[10,11] These receptors play key roles both as transcriptional activators and as repressors in all aspects of biological function, including regulation of development, metabolism, and reproduction.

Control of transcription by steroid hormones often involves binding of the ligand-activated hormone receptors to promoter/enhancer regions of regulated genes followed by recruitment of coregulators, remodeling of chromatin, and formation of the transcription initiation complex. In some cases, regulation of transcription is based on an interaction of the hormone receptors with other sequence-specific transcription factors. But many regulatory regions of hormone-responsive genes contain binding sites for the hormone receptors (hormone-responsive elements [HREs]) and are organized in positioned nucleosomes, which are remodeled in the context of hormone induction. To elucidate these processes, we have studied the induction of the mouse mammary tumor virus (MMTV) promoter by the steroid hormone progesterone.

INTRODUCTION TO THE HORMONAL REGULATION OF THE MMTV PROMOTER

The organization of eukaryotic promoter and enhancer regions in chromatin also plays an essential role in modulating interactions of regulatory proteins and transcription factors with their DNA target sequences. The participation of chromatin dynamics in gene regulation has been studied in great detail. One of the more extensively characterized model systems is the hormonal regulation of the expression of the MMTV. During hormone induction of the MMTV promoter, there are rapid changes in chromatin structure as evidenced by the appearance of a DNase I hypersensitive site in a region containing the HREs.[12] The MMTV HREs were the first to be identified in experiments with the glucocorticoid receptor (GR),[13-15] although they were later shown to bind the progesterone receptor (PR) with high affinity[16,17] and to mediate progesterone activation of transcription.[18]

The MMTV promoter is organized into positioned nucleosomes, with a nucleosome covering the HREs and the binding site for NF1[19] (FIG 1). A full hormonal activation of the promoter requires not only the HREs but also the NF1 binding site, indicating that both factors synergize *in vivo*.[16,20] However, in cell-free transcription experiments with MMTV promoter DNA, the hormone receptors activate transcription,[21] but no synergism with NF1 is detected. Instead NF1 competes with hormone receptors for binding and transactivation of naked DNA templates.[20] In intact cells, however, both hormone receptors and NF1 occupy their binding sites simultaneously after hormone induction on the surface of a nucleosome-like particle[22] (FIG 1). These results suggested an important role of the nucleosomal organization of the promoter for efficient induction.

In addition to PR and NF1, the octamer transcription factor 1 (Oct1) participates in MMTV regulation. In fact, a transcriptional synergism has been described between PR and Oct1 *in vitro* and in transient transfection experiments.[23] However, because these results have not been confirmed in studies with chromatin-organized MMTV promoter sequences, we will not further mention the role of Oct1 in this review.

When the MMTV promoter DNA is assembled into nucleosomes *in vitro*, it adopts a precise rotational orientation on the surface of the histone octamer that exposes the external HREs 1 and 4 but leaves inaccessible the central HREs 2, 3, and 5, which are essential for hormone induction.[24] Moreover, NF1 cannot bind to MMTV promoter sequences assembled into regular nucleosomes because it encircles the DNA double helix completely.[24,25] Therefore, we concluded that the nucleosome must experience changes during induction in order to enable the simultaneous binding of receptors and NF1 and to facilitate their functional synergism.

A few minutes after progesterone treatment of breast cancer cells carrying a single copy of the MMTV promoter integrated in their chromosomes, a characteristic and sharp DNase I hypersensitive site appears near the symmetry axis of the nucleosome encompassing the HREs.[22] The same hypersensitive site can be induced by treatment with moderate concentrations of inhibitors of histone deacetylases, such as sodium butyrate or trichostatin A,[26] suggesting that it reflected an "opening" of the chromatin that can be initiated by a moderate increase in histone acetylation. We have devoted our attention during the last years to understanding the nature of this hormone-induced change in chromatin structure and how it is brought about.

MMTV promoter structure

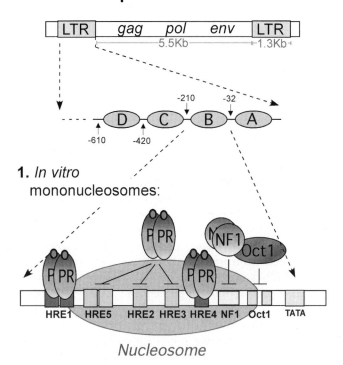

1. *In vitro* mononucleosomes:

Nucleosome

2. *In vivo* after hormone induction:

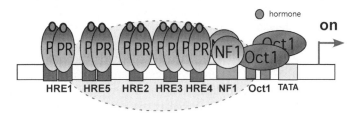

Remodeled nucleosome

FIGURE 1. Schematic representation of the main *cis* elements in the MMTV promoter and their occupancy in nucleosomes assembled *in vitro* (1) and in intact cells after hormone induction (2). The positions covered by the main population of histone octamers are indicated by the oval labeled nucleosome or nucleosome-like particle. The various HREs, the NF1 binding site, the octamer factor 1 binding sites (Oct1), and the TATA box are indicated. The numbers refer to the distance in nucleotides from the transcription start site. The hormone receptor (PR) dimers are represented by violet ovals, the NF1 dimer by green circles, and Oct1 by red ovals. Colors appear in on-line version.

THE LESSONS FROM *IN VITRO* ASSEMBLED DYNAMIC MINICHROMOSOMES

To study the biochemistry of the interaction between hormone receptors and chromatin-organized MMTV promoter sequences, we made use of chromatin assembly systems that generate arrays of nucleosomes mimicking the behavior of natural chromatin. In our hands the best results were obtained with extracts from preblastodermic *Drosophila* embryos, which contain abundant core histones and the machinery needed for efficient chromatin assembly.[27] Minichromosomes assembled in these extracts exhibit the same translational and rotational positioning of nucleosomes over the MMTV promoter as detected in the chromatin of intact breast cancer cells, with a nucleosome occupying the HREs and the NF1 binding sites. In the absence of PR and NF1, these MMTV minichromosomes are transcriptionally silent when assayed in a cell-free transcription system. Addition of the factors individually results in a weak stimulation of transcription by PR and little or no activation by NF1. However, addition of both factors together causes a strong synergistic transcriptional activation, which is dependent on preincubation of the minichromosomes with PR in the presence of ATP, suggesting that an ATP-dependent chromatin remodeling process is needed.[28] Preliminary experiments indicated that the complex responsible for this remodeling event in embryonic extracts is NURF,[29] which is recruited to the minichromosomes by PR.[28]

In DNA footprinting experiments at high concentrations of PR, we detect ATP-dependent binding of the receptors to the HREs, while NF1 is unable to bind to the MMTV promoter in minichromosomes. However, preincubation of the minichromosomes with PR and ATP facilitates binding of NF1 to the promoter, generating a continuous footprint over the HREs and the NF1 site,[28] as reported *in vivo*.[22] Thus, in extracts that assemble dynamic chromatin, one can reproduce the physiological behavior of the MMTV promoter.

At lower, more physiological concentrations of PR, no DNA footprint is observed even in the presence of ATP, but the low levels of receptor are sufficient to synergize with NF1 and to generate a continuous footprint over the HREs and the NF1. These results indicate that under physiological conditions not only does PR help NF1 to bind, but NF1 is needed for optimal PR binding.[28] Intriguingly, the transactivation domain of NF1 is not needed for this reciprocal synergism with PR, suggesting that the only function of NF1 is to stabilize the "open" conformation of the nucleosome and thus to facilitate access of PR to the hidden HREs.

H2A/H2B DIMER DISPLACEMENT *IN VIVO* AND *IN VITRO*

To identify the ATP-dependent remodeling activity involved in opening the MMTV chromatin and to define the nature of the "open" nucleosomal

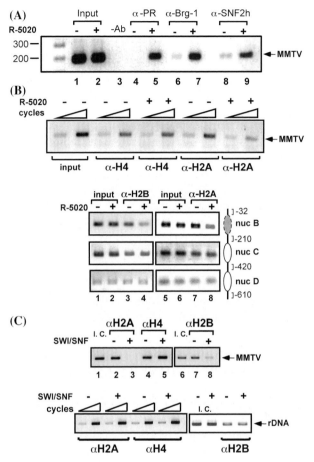

FIGURE 2. Binding of factors and histone stoichiometry on the MMTV promoter. (**A**) Chromatin immunoprecipitation (ChIp) experiments in T47D-ML cells, carrying a single copy of the MMTV promoter integrated in chromatin: recruitment of PR and ATP-dependent chromatin remodeling complexes. Cells were treated with the synthetic progestin R5020 or with vehicle (−) for 30 min and submitted to ChIp experiments using antibodies to PR, the Brg1 ATPase, or the hSnf2h ATPase. The input (1%) and the precipitated DNA were amplified by PCR using oligos specific for nucleosome B of the MMTV promoter.[30] (**B**) ChIp experiments in T47D-ML cells: displacement of H2A and H2B from the MMTV promoter following hormone induction. Cells were treated as described in (**A**) and submitted to ChIp experiments using antibodies against histones H2A, H4 (*upper panel*), and H2B (*lower panel*). The input and the precipitated DNA were amplified using probes specific for MMTV nucleosome B (*upper row*), nucleosome C (*middle row*), and nucleosome D (*bottom row*). (**C**) Displacement of histones H2A and H2B from MMTV but not from rDNA nucleosomes. Recombinant histone octamers were used to assemble nucleosomes by salt dialysis on DNA fragments of equal length derived from the MMTV promoter or from the mouse rDNA promoter. Both sequence position nucleosomes in two main translational frames are seen. On incubation with purified ySWI/SNF in the presence of ATP, ChIp experiments using antibodies against histones H2A, H2B, and H4 were performed.

conformation, we performed chromatin immunoprecipitation (ChIP) experiments in T47D breast cancer cells carrying a single copy of the MMTV
promoter.[22] Thirty minutes after treatment with the synthetic progesterone
analogue R5020, we could detect PR bound to the MMTV promoter, along
with the coactivator Src-1 and the chromatin remodeling complexes Brg1 and
SNF2h (FIG. 2 A).[30] Thus, these two remodeling ATPases could be part of the
complexes responsible for the ATP-dependent changes in chromatin sensitivity
to nucleases detected 30 min after hormone exposure.[22] Simultaneously, there
is a selective loss of histones H2A and H2B from the promoter nucleosome B,
but not from the adjacent nucleosomes C or D (FIG. 2 B).[30]

To test whether ATP-dependent remodeling complexes can displace histones H2A and H2B from MMTV nucleosomes, we performed experiments
with *in vitro* assembled nucleosomes and purified ySWI/SNF complex isolated
from *Saccharomyces cerevisiae*. To our surprise we found that in the presence
of ATP, ySWI/SNF could displace H2A and H2B from MMTV promoter nucleosomes, but not from a mouse ribosomal promoter nucleosome assembled
on DNA fragments of the same length (FIG. 2 C).[30] Since the proteins used
for this assay were highly purified or recombinant, we conclude that the nucleotide sequence contains topological information that determines not only
nucleosome positioning, but also the outcome of the remodeling process.

HORMONE RECEPTORS AND NF1 CAN BIND TO THE MMTV PROMOTER IN POSITIONED H3/H4 TETRAMERS

Is the displacement of both H2A/H2B dimers a reasonable model for explaining the binding of PR and NF1 to MMTV promoter chromatin on hormone
induction? We know that a tetramer of histones H3 and H4 positions MMTV-
promoter sequences in a very similar way as a histone octamer, and that NF1
can bind to a H3/H4 tetramer particle with relatively high affinity.[31] The question is whether PR can access the central HREs in MMTV sequences organized
around an H3/H4 tetramer. To answer this question, we performed band shift
experiments with free DNA as well as with DNA assembled around a histone
octamer or around an H3/H4 tetramer. The results show that whereas PR could
only bind to the exposed HREs on the octamer particle, it could clearly access
the central HREs in the tetramer particle. Thus, a tetramer of histones H3 and
H4 represents a plausible model for the structure of the "open" nucleosome
conformation detected on hormone induction.

HISTONE H1 PARTICIPATES IN OPTIMIZING HORMONE INDUCTION

The experiments described so far do not take into account the linker histones,
an important structural component of metazoan chromatin. Linker histones

form a large family of proteins that share a common globular domain and exhibit variable C-terminal and N-terminal extensions, with basic residues and sites for phosphorylation by various kinases. The globular domain binds DNA at the entry site and at the pseudo dyad, whereas the C-terminal domain contacts the DNA at the exit site and imposes a change on its direction. The structure of the bound N-terminal extension has not been solved. Given these interactions linker histones are considered to seal the nucleosomal DNA and therefore to limit the dynamics of the nucleosome. In fact it has been shown that in the presence of bound histone H1, the ySWI/SNF complex cannot remodel nucleosomes.[32] We therefore investigated the role of histone H1 in the hormonal induction of the MMTV promoter.

Using mononucleosomes assembled by salt dialysis, we found that histone H1 binds asymmetrically to MMTV nucleosomes, with a clear preference for the distal 5′ end of nucleosomal DNA.[33] In agreement with the accepted model, we found that incorporation of H1 into MMTV minichromosomes increases nucleosome spacing and reduces access of general transcription factors to the promoter, thus inhibiting basal transcription.[34] However, the absolute values of transcription and induction by a combination of PR and NF1 were enhanced in H1 containing minichromosomes.[34] This unexpected effect was due to the better positioning of nucleosomes in the presence of H1,[33] and, as a consequence, a better binding of PR[33,34] and a higher proportion of promoters participating in transcription.[34]

But how is the H1 obstacle overcome by the ATP-dependent remodeling activities involved in hormone induction? We found that in the presence of bound PR, H1 is phosphorylated and subsequently removed from the promoter on transcription initiation.[34] Phosphorylation of H1 allows nucleosome remodeling by ATP-dependent complexes.[32] Thus, H1, a structural component of chromatin that functions as a general repressor of transcription, contributes to a better regulation of a hormone-inducible promoter by reducing basal transcription and improving induced transcription.

NONGENOMIC EFFECTS OF PROGESTINS

Apart from their direct transcriptional effects, steroid hormones also exhibit rapid cytoplasmic effects, such as the transient activation of several kinase cascades. The ultimate targets of the activated kinase cascades are not well defined, but likely include transcription factors and factors involved in cell cycle control.[35] Traditionally the nongenomic and genomic actions of steroid hormones have been considered as two independent pathways, but we have tested the possibility that the two pathways converge in the modification of structural components of chromatin.

Five minutes after progesterone administration to breast cancer cells, there is an increase in activity of the components of the Src/Ras/Erk cascade, which

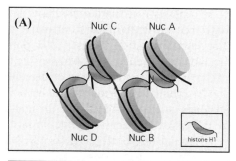

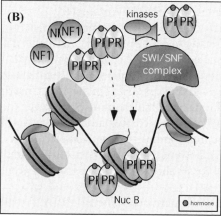

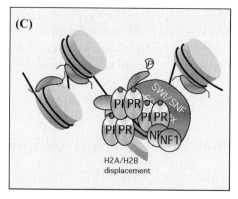

FIGURE 3. Hypothetical model for the initial steps of MMTV promoter induction. Histone H1 is associated with chromatin and improving nucleosome positioning and tightening nucleosome structure. In this way H1 contributes to a further silencing of the gene in the absence of hormone-activated PR, but improves PR binding to the exposed HRE1.[33,34] Nucleosome-bound PR recruits kinases that phosphorylate H1 and H3. Subsequently an ATP-dependent chromatin-remodeling complex is recruited to the promoter and catalyzes displacement of H2A/H2B dimers and NF1 binding. NF1 binds to its cognate site and maintains the open conformation of the nucleosome, permitting additional PR molecules to bind to the previously inaccessible HREs, enhancing recruitment of coactivators and the general transcriptional machinery. It is around this time that H1 is displaced from the promoter.

is essential for progestin-induced cell proliferation.[36] This effect is mediated by a specific interaction between two domains of the N-terminal half of PR and the ligand-binding-domain of ERα, which is activated in the absence of estrogens.[37] Activated ERα interacts directly with c-Src and activates its tyrosine kinase activity and consequently the whole MAP kinase cascade. Because some of the kinases that phosphorylate core histones (Msk1 and 2) and histone H1 (Cdk2) are downstream substrates of Erk, it is conceivable that the rapid cytoplasmic effects of steroid hormones are in some way related to their chromatin targets. Indeed, selective inhibition of Erk or Msk activation in breast cancer cells interferes with chromatin remodeling and blocks transcriptional activation of the promoter. Activated Msk is recruited to the MMTV promoter in a complex with activated PR and Erk and phosphorylates histone H3 at serine 10, leading to displacement of HP1γ and activation of chromatin remodeling.[38] Inhibiting the activation of the kinases compromises progestin activation of classical progesterone target promoter. Our results point to a hitherto unsuspected link between rapid kinase activation and gene induction by steroid hormones.

A hypothetical model of how all the processes described in this review could take place on the MMTV promoter is proposed in FIGURE 3.

In rat endometrial stromal cells, which have no ERα but only minute amounts of ERβ, progestins activate the Src/Ras/Erk pathway and the PI3K/Akt pathway via an interaction of PR with ERβ leading to induction of cell proliferation.[39] The low amount of PR in these cells precludes transcriptional activation of progesterone target genes. Moreover, picomolar concentrations of progestins unable to trigger transcriptional gene regulation are sufficient for activating cell proliferation.[39] Thus, in these cells the effects of progestins on cell proliferation are physiologically uncoupled from their genomic effects. These results indicate that the nature of the cross talk between various signaling pathways used by steroid hormones are cell type–specific and probably specified in the course of cell differentiation.

ACKNOWLEDGMENTS

We wish to thank Jofre Font, CRG, for PR preparation. G.P.V. was a recipient of a fellowship of the Ramón y Cajal Programme. The experimental work was supported by grants from the Departament d´Universitats Recerca i Societat de la Informació (DURSI), Ministerio de Educación y Ciencia (MEC) BMC 2003-02902 and Fondo de Investigación Sanitaria (FIS) PI0411605 and CP04/00087.

REFERENCES

1. EISEN, J.A., K.S. SWEDER & P.C. HANAWALT. 1995. Evolution of the SNF2 family of proteins: subfamilies with distinct sequences and functions. Nucleic Acids Res. **23:** 2715–2723.

2. HASSAN, A.H., P. PROCHASSON, K.E. NEELY, *et al.* 2002. Function and selectivity of bromodomains in anchoring chromatin-modifying complexes to promoter nucleosomes. Cell **111**: 369–379.

3. BOYER, L.A., R.R. LATEK & C.L. PETERSON. 2004. The SANT domain: a unique histone-tail-binding module? Nat. Rev. Mol. Cell. Biol. **5**: 158–163.

4. FLANAGAN, J.F., L.Z. MI, M. CHRUSZCZ, *et al.* 2005. Double chromodomains cooperate to recognize the methylated histone H3 tail. Nature **438**: 1181–1185.

5. JENUWEIN, T. & C.D. ALLIS. 2001. Translating the histone code. Science **293**: 1074–1080.

6. STRAHL, B.D. & C.D. ALLIS. 2000. The language of covalent histone modifications. Nature **403**: 41–45.

7. AGALIOTI, T., G. CHEN & D. THANOS. 2002. Deciphering the transcriptional histone acetylation code for a human gene. Cell **111**: 381–392.

8. JACOBSON, R.H., A.G. LADURNER, D.S. KING & R. TJIAN. 2000. Structure and function of a human TAFII250 double bromodomain module. Science **288**: 1422–1425.

9. ROBINSON-RECHAVI, M., H. ESCRIVA GARCIA & V. LAUDET. 2003. The nuclear receptor superfamily. J. Cell. Sci. **116**: 585–586.

10. EVANS, R.M. 1988. The steroid and thyroid hormone receptor superfamily. Science **240**: 889–895.

11. O'MALLEY, B.W. & O.M. CONNEELY. 1992. Orphan receptors: in search of a unifying hypothesis for activation. Mol. Endocrinol. **6**: 1359–1361.

12. ZARET, K.S. & K.R. YAMAMOTO. 1984. Reversible and persistent changes in chromatin structure accompany activation of a glucocorticoid-dependent enhancer element. Cell **38**: 29–38.

13. CHANDLER, V.L., B.A. MALER & K.R. YAMAMOTO. 1983. DNA sequences bound specifically by glucocorticoid receptor *in vitro* render a heterologous promoter hormone responsive *in vivo*. Cell **33**: 489–499.

14. PAYVAR, F., D. DEFRANCO, G.L. FIRESTONE, *et al.* 1983. Sequence-specific binding of glucocorticoid receptor to MTV DNA at sites within and upstream of the transcribed region. Cell **35**: 381–392.

15. SCHEIDEREIT, C., S. GEISSE, H.M. WESTPHAL & M. BEATO. 1983. The glucocorticoid receptor binds to defined nucleotide sequences near the promoter of mouse mammary tumour virus. Nature **304**: 749–752.

16. CHALEPAKIS, G., J. ARNEMANN, E. SLATER, *et al.* 1988. Differential gene activation by glucocorticoids and progestins through the hormone regulatory element of mouse mammary tumor virus. Cell **53**: 371–382.

17. VON DER AHE, D., S. JANICH, C. SCHEIDEREIT, *et al.* 1985. Glucocorticoid and progesterone receptors bind to the same sites in two hormonally regulated promoters. Nature **313**: 706–709.

18. CATO, A.C., D. HENDERSON & H. PONTA. 1987. The hormone response element of the mouse mammary tumour virus DNA mediates the progestin and androgen induction of transcription in the proviral long terminal repeat region. EMBO J. **6**: 363–368.

19. RICHARD-FOY, H. & G.L. HAGER. 1987. Sequence-specific positioning of nucleosomes over the steroid-inducible MMTV promoter. EMBO J. **6**: 2321–2328.

20. BRUGGEMEIER, U., L. ROGGE, E.L. WINNACKER & M. BEATO. 1990. Nuclear factor I acts as a transcription factor on the MMTV promoter but competes with steroid hormone receptors for DNA binding. EMBO J. **9**: 2233–2239.

21. KALFF, M., B. GROSS & M. BEATO. 1990. Progesterone receptor stimulates transcription of mouse mammary tumour virus in a cell-free system. Nature **344:** 360–362.

22. TRUSS, M., J. BARTSCH, A. SCHELBERT, *et al.* 1995. Hormone induces binding of receptors and transcription factors to a rearranged nucleosome on the MMTV promoter *in vivo*. EMBO J. **14:** 1737–1751.

23. BRÜGGEMEIER, U., M. KALFF, S. FRANKE, *et al.* 1991. Ubiquitous transcription factor OTF-1 mediates induction of the mouse mammary tumour virus promoter through synergistic interaction with hormone receptors. Cell **64:** 565–572.

24. PINA, B., U. BRUGGEMEIER & M. BEATO. 1990. Nucleosome positioning modulates accessibility of regulatory proteins to the mouse mammary tumor virus promoter. Cell **60:** 719–731.

25. EISFELD, K., R. CANDAU, M. TRUSS & M. BEATO. 1997. Binding of NF1 to the MMTV promoter in nucleosomes: influence of rotational phasing, translational positioning and histone H1. Nucleic Acids Res. **25:** 3733–3742.

26. BARTSCH, J., M. TRUSS, J. BODE & M. BEATO. 1996. Moderate increase in histone acetylation activates the mouse mammary tumor virus promoter and remodels its nucleosome structure. Proc. Natl. Acad. Sci. USA **93:** 10741–10746.

27. VENDITTI, P., L. DI CROCE, M. KAUER, *et al.* 1998. Assembly of MMTV promoter minichromosomes with positioned nucleosomes precludes NF1 access but not restriction enzyme cleavage. Nucleic Acids Res. **26:** 3657–3666.

28. DI CROCE, L., R. KOOP, P. VENDITTI, *et al.* 1999. Two-step synergism between the progesterone receptor and the DNA-binding domain of nuclear factor 1 on MMTV minichromosomes. Mol. Cell. **4:** 45–54.

29. TSUKIYAMA, T. & C. WU. 1995. Purification and properties of an ATP-dependent nucleosome remodeling factor. Cell **83:** 1011–1020.

30. VICENT, G.P., A.S. NACHT, C.L. SMITH, *et al.* 2004. DNA instructed displacement of histones H2A and H2B at an inducible promoter. Mol. Cell. **16:** 439–452.

31. SPANGENBERG, C., K. EISFELD, W. STUNKEL, *et al.* 1998. The mouse mammary tumour virus promoter positioned on a tetramer of histones H3 and H4 binds nuclear factor 1 and OTF1. J. Mol. Biol. **278:** 725–739.

32. HORN, P.J., L.M. CARRUTHERS, C. LOGIE, *et al.* 2002. Phosphorylation of linker histones regulates ATP-dependent chromatin remodeling enzymes. Nat. Struct. Biol. **9:** 263–267.

33. VICENT, G.P., M.J. MELIA & M. BEATO. 2002. Asymmetric binding of histone H1 stabilizes MMTV nucleosomes and the interaction of progesterone receptor with the exposed HRE. J. Mol. Biol. **324:** 501–517.

34. KOOP, R., L. DI CROCE & M. BEATO. 2003. Histone H1 enhances synergistic activation of the MMTV promoter in chromatin. EMBO J. **22:** 588–599.

35. BJORNSTROM, L. & M. SJOBERG. 2005. Mechanisms of estrogen receptor signaling: convergence of genomic and nongenomic actions on target genes. Mol. Endocrinol. **19:** 833–842.

36. MIGLIACCIO, A., D. PICCOLO, G. CASTORIA, *et al.* 1998. Activation of the Src/p21ras/Erk pathway by progesterone receptor via cross-talk with estrogen receptor. EMBO J. **17:** 2008–2018.

37. BALLARE, C., M. UHRIG, T. BECHTOLD, *et al.* 2003. Two domains of the progesterone receptor interact with the estrogen receptor and are required for progesterone activation of the c-Src/Erk pathway in mammalian cells. Mol. Cell. Biol. **23:** 1994–2008.

38. VICENT, G.P., C. BALLARE, A.S. NACHT, *et al.* 2006. Induction of progesterone target genes requires activation of Erk and Msk kinases and phosphorylation of histone H3. Mol. Cell. In press.

39. VALLEJO, G., C. BALLARE, J.L. BARANAO, *et al.* 2005. Progestin activation of nongenomic pathways via cross talk of progesterone receptor with estrogen receptor beta induces proliferation of endometrial stromal cells. Mol. Endocrinol. **19:** 3023–3037.

Epigenetics and the Estrogen Receptor

JENNIFER E. LEADER,[a,b] CHENGUANG WANG,[a] VLADIMIR M. POPOV,[a] MAOFU FU,[a] AND RICHARD G. PESTELL[a]

[a]Kimmel Cancer Center, Departments of Cancer Biology and Medical Oncology, Thomas Jefferson University, Philadelphia, Pennsylvania 19107, USA

[b]Interdisciplinary Program in Tumor Biology, Georgetown University, Washington, D.C. 20057, USA

ABSTRACT: The position effect variegation in *Drosophila* and *Schizosaccharomyces pombe,* and higher-order chromatin structure regulation in yeast, is orchestrated by modifier genes of the Su(var) group, (e.g., histone deacetylases ([HDACs]), protein phosphatases) and enhancer E(Var) group (e.g., ATP [adenosine 5′-triphosphate]-dependent nucleosome remodeling proteins). Higher-order chromatin structure is regulated in part by covalent modification of the N-terminal histone tails of chromatin, and histone tails in turn serve as platforms for recruitment of signaling modules that include nonhistone proteins such as heterochromatin protein (HP1) and NuRD. Because the enzymes governing chromatin structure through covalent modifications of histones (acetylation, methylation, phosphorylation, ubiquitination) can also target nonhistone substrates, a mechanism is in place by which epigenetic regulatory processes can affect the function of these alternate substrates. The posttranslational modification of histones, through phosphorylation and acetylation at specific residues, alters chromatin structure in an orchestrated manner in response to specific signals and is considered the basis of a "histone code." In an analogous manner, specific residues within transcription factors form a signaling module within the transcription factor to determine genetic target specificity and cellular fate. The architecture of these signaling cascades in transcription factors (SCITs) are poorly understood. The regulation of estrogen receptor (ERα) by enzymes that convey epigenetic signals is carefully orchestrated and is reviewed here.

KEYWORDS: estrogen receptor; cyclin D1; epigenetics; histone; chromatin

EPIGENETICS

Epigenomics refers to the study of heritable changes in gene expression that occur without a change in DNA sequence. Through the silencing of

Address for correspondence: Richard G. Pestell, Kimmel Cancer Center, Departments of Cancer Biology and Medical Oncology, Thomas Jefferson University, 233 South 10th Street, Philadelphia, PA 19107, USA. Voice: 215-503-5649; fax: 215-503-9334.

e-mail: Dawn.Scardino@mail.jci.tju.edu

Ann. N.Y. Acad. Sci. 1089: 73–87 (2006). © 2006 New York Academy of Sciences.
doi: 10.1196/annals.1386.047

tumor suppressor genes, epigenetic gene regulation frequently plays a critical role in the pathogenesis of cancer. Epigenomic modifications include covalent modifications of DNA and histones as well as noncovalent changes regulating nucleosome positioning. The enzymes regulating epigenetic change have been characterized in a number of animal systems including *Drosophila* and transgenic mice. Recent studies have characterized the mammalian enzymes that regulate epigenetic change. Environmental factors including hormones in turn regulate activities of several enzymes, altering DNA methylation and histone acetylation patterns.

Histone Methylation

Several recent studies have demonstrated the importance of histone methylases and histone demethylases in regulating estrogen receptor (ERα) activity and expression. Posttranslational modification that does not alter DNA sequence requiring methylation occurs both on DNA and on proteins. Methylation of chromatin is often linked to methylation of DNA. A number of histone methylating enzymes directly interact with DNA methylating enzymes (DNA methyltransferases (DNMTs) and methyl-binding proteins).[1] Modification by methylation of DNA is generally targeted to cytosine residues in CpG dinucleotide pairs. Methylation governs genomic stability, retroelement suppression, and gene promoter regulation. Regions of CpG in the mammalian genome include large CpG islands (>500 bp), small CpG islands (200–500 bp) associated with transposons, and nonisland CpGs. DNA methyltransferases are associated with the replication complex in mammalian cells. This finding is consistent with a model in which the signals for methylating sequences in the genome are provided by a pre-existing hemimethylation. Thus, replication of the sequence to daughter chromatids temporarily results in hemimethylated DNA, which is recognized by DNMTs, ensures restoration of the symmetrical methylation of both DNA strands. The other major signal for methylation in mammalian cells is the presence of SINE elements.[36]

Methylation of histones occurs on either lysine or alanine residues, resulting in either condensation or relaxation of the chromatin architecture. Methylation likely provides binding sites for regulatory proteins with specialized binding domains. The main sites of methylation of histones occur on either heterochromatin or euchromatin. Heterochromatin is condensed and considered transcriptionally silent, whereas euchromatin is less densely packed and transcriptionally active. Methylated lysine residues are located characteristically within heterochromatin and demarcate subdomains.[1] Methylated histone residues serve as docking sites for repressive proteins, including the polycomb protein (PC) and heterochromatin protein (HP1), which recognize histone H3, K27 or H3, K9, respectively. HP1 and PC recognize methylated lysine residues through their chromo domain. Other proteins recognize methylated lysine residues though two other motifs, known as the Tudor domain and the WD40 repeat domain.

Histone methylation by protein arginine methyltransferases represents a relatively prevalent modification of proteins. The protein arginine methyl transferases (PRMTs) consist of two types, differing in the asymmetry of the dimethylarginine, product. The Type 1 PRMT forms monomethylarginine and asymmetric dimethylarginine, whereas Type 2 PRMT forms monomethylarginine and symmetric dimethylarginine. The PRMTs, 1, 2, 3, 4, and 6 are Type 1 PRMTs. The Type 2 PRMT is represented by PRMT5, also known as CARM1 (coactivator-associated arginine methyltransferase). Stallcup and coworkers[4] demonstrated that CARM1 encodes both an arginine methyltransferase and a nuclear receptor coactivator, linking posttranslational modification by methylation to ERα receptor signaling.

The histone lysine methylases share a common SET (Su/var, Enhancer of Zeste, Trithorax) domain. The SET domain conveys the *S*-adenosyl-L-methionine cofactor to the epsilon amino group of the lysine residues. The histone H3 lysine 9 methyltransferase group catalyzes H3, lysine 9 methylation and includes *Suv39h1, Suv39 h2, G9a, G9a-related protein* and the *SET DB1* gene products.

Enzymatic demethylation of histone was first described in 1973 by Paik and Kim.[37] The identification of specific proteins regulating this activity took many years to be identified, however. Recently several lysine specific demethylases have been described, including lysine specific demethylase 1 (LSD1), JHDM1, JHDM2A, and JMJD2.[32]

In addition to removal of arginine methylation by lysine demethylases, the methyl group can be removed from the arginine by the conversion of the methylarginine residue into citrulline, referred to as deimination. Deimination is conducted by arginine peptidyl arginine deiminase 4 (PADI4), which converts unmodified arginine and monomethylated arginine to citrulline at specific sites on the tails of H3 and H4.[6] Importantly, for the purpose of this review, PADI4 repressed the estrogen-regulated gene, *pS2*, linking arginine demethylation to ERα signaling.

Histone Acetyltransferases and Deacetylases

ERα function can be regulated by histone acetylases and histone deacetylases (HDACs). Euchromatic DNA is packaged by histones into nucleosomes composed of 147 base pairs of DNA and the core histone proteins (H2A, H2B, H3, and H4). Dramatic alterations in chromatin structure are modulated through posttranslational modification of lysine tails.[9] Conserved lysine residues are present in the amino terminal tails of all four core histones. Acetylation of lysine residues is thought to both neutralize the basic charge of histone tails and to serve as epigenetic markers which provide recognition motifs for docking of proteins that recruit transcriptional activators or repressors. The histone acetyl-transferase (HAT) enzymes were historically described as Type A, located in the nucleus, and Type B, located in the cytoplasm. Type B typically have a housekeeping role, acetylating newly synthesized free histones, whereas Type A HAT acetylate nucleosomal histones within chromatin in the nucleus. The Type A nuclear HATs include five families, the Gcn5-related acetyltransferases (GNATs), the MYST (MOZ, Ybf2/Sas3, Sas2, and Tip60)-related HATs, the HATs regulating general transcription (TAFII250), the CBP/p300 cointegrator HATs; and the p160 coactivator HATs, (SRC-1 and SRC3).[9]

The dynamic remodeling of acetylated lysine residues is mediated through two distinct types of HDACs: trichostatin A (TSA)-sensitive and NAD- regulated. TSA-sensitive HDACs include the class 1 HDACs (HDACs 1, 2, 3, and 8) which are related to the *Saccharomyces cerevisiae* transcriptional regulator RPD3. The class II HDACs are related to the yeast HDA1 protein and include HDACs 4, 5, 6, 7, 9, and 10. HDAC 11 is more related to the Type 1 HDACs and contains a catalytic domain at the N-terminus with HDAC activity.

NUCLEAR RECEPTORS

Nuclear receptors function as transcription factors that govern transcription of genes. Their activity can be regulated by steroids, thyroid hormone, retinoic acids, or vitamins, and they coordinate diverse processes such as homeostasis, reproduction, development, metabolism, and disease.[40] There are four main conserved domains of all nuclear receptors. These domains include the activation function domain (AF), the DNA-binding domain (DBD), the hinge region, and the ligand-binding domain (LBD), the latter being the site of many protein–protein and hormone interactions.

Coregulator proteins, both coactivators and corepressors, work with nuclear receptors in complexes that govern gene expression. Nuclear receptors and the transcriptional apparatus are often linked together through coactivator recruitment of protein complexes. These complexes then can use their histone-modifying abilities to alter the local chromatin structure. Several coactivators that bind to nuclear receptors include steroid receptor coactivator-1 (SRC-1), amplified in breast cancer1/thyroid and RA receptor/SRC-2 (AIB1/ACTR/SRC-2), glucocorticoid receptor interacting protein 1/transcriptional intermediary factor 2/SRC-3 (GRIP1/TIF-2/SRC-3), menin, and p300/CBP and p300/CBP-associated factor (p/CAF).[17,18,51] Corepressors function with unliganded nuclear receptors to silence gene expression. These corepressors include proteins like nuclear receptor corepressor (N-CoR), silencing mediator of retinoid and thyroid hormone receptor (SMRT), Sin3, HDACs, thyroid hormone receptor uncoupling protein (TRUP), BRCA1, NuRD, Suv39h1, DNMT1, pRB2/p130, and E2F4/5.[17,18,51]

THE ESTROGEN RECEPTOR

The last two decades have seen an evolving body of literature providing a compelling case for dynamic regulation of ERα function through both post-translational modification by acetylation and through epigenetic signaling cascades. The nuclear receptor, ERα, is activated by, and controls the activity of, the steroid hormone, estrogen. Together estrogen and its receptor are vitally important in normal development, reproduction, and various diseases. ERα is distributed at the cellular membrane, the cytoplasm, the nucleus, and the mitochondria. The membrane-bound form of ERα regulates nongenomic function through interactions with SHC and caveolin-1, inducing acute activation of PI3 kinase and Akt signaling pathway. The nuclear form provides DNA-dependent regulation of gene expression. Epigenetic regulation has been well characterized for the nuclear located ERα. The role of epigenetic signals of ERα located in other compartments of the cell remains to be better understood.

ERα binds DNA either directly or through other transcription factors (AP-1, Sp1) in order to regulate transcription of target genes. The ERα functional activity in the nucleus is mediated through binding of coactivator and corepressors, which encode enzymes with HAT-modulating activity. The cointegrators CBP/p300 (CREB-binding factor) encode intrinsic HAT activity. The binding of HATs to the ERα provides a docking function leading to acetylation of local histones with consequent nucleosomal destabilization facilitating transcription factor binding to local DNA sequences at promoter regions of estrogen-responsive genes. Some proteins that are already known to bind the ER include members of the p160 family (SRC-1, TIF2/GRIP1/SRC-2, AIB1/ACTR/SRC-3), cyclin D1, menin, and many HATs (CBP, p300, p/CAF).[21,29,30] The p160 coactivator family (SRC1/amplified in breast cancer/activator of the thyroid and RA receptor/ SRC-2 to [AIB1/ACTR/SRC3]) and the related group 1 (GRIP-1/TIP-2/SRC-2) facilitate the interaction between the p300 coactivator and the nuclear receptor. In addition, nuclear receptor repressors of the N-CoR and SMRT complex physically associate with the ERα particularly in the presence of the ERα ligand antagonists such as tamoxifen. The ERα has been shown to physically associate with several corepressors which encode intrinsic HDAC activities including BRCA1 and MTA1.[8] BRCA1 binds the ERα to repress ligand-induced gene expression. BRCA1 repression of ERα is opposed by endogenous cyclin D1 through physical association within local chromatin[45] (FIG. 1). It is plausible that BRCA1 association with ERα may play a role in the recently described finding that transient double-stranded DNA break formation occurs during ERα ligand-dependent gene transcription.[24]

Epigenetic Modifiers Silence the ERα Gene

In breast cancer ERα gene expression is an important prognostic factor.[52] Altered expression and function of ERα coregulators with epigenetic function have been demonstrated to play a role in hormone signaling. The AIB1 protein is frequently amplified in breast cancer correlating with the ER-positive status.[2] The expression levels of TIP2, CBP, and ER are strongly correlated in intraductal breast carcinomas.[31] Furthermore, tamoxifen-resistant tumors show a shorter relapse of survival in samples with low expression of NCoR.[20]

Unfortunately though, 30% of breast cancers are ERα-negative upon diagnosis[22] and many breast cancers can lose ERα expression during progression of the cancer. In many patients epigenetic modification plays a role in the loss of ERα gene expression. Yang et al.[54] demonstrate reduced ERα expression due to increased DNA methylation and/or histone deacetylation.[54] The demethylase PADI4 has been linked to the repression of the estrogen-responsive gene pS2.[6] HDACs bind ERα and HDAC overexpression silences expression of the ER gene.[25] siRNA-mediated reduction of DNMT1 induced ERα expression.[39,53] Two commonly used inhibitors of this silencing mechanism are the DNMT inhibitor, 5-aza-2′-deoxycytidine (5-aza-dC), and the HDAC inhibitor, TSA. Treatment with either inhibitor individually enhanced ERα gene expression.[25,54,55] Use of both 5-aza-dC and TSA enhanced re-expression of both ERα mRNA and protein in human breast cancer cells. The re-expressed ERα was functional and it induced expression of known ERα target genes. Collectively these studies suggest how inhibitors of HDACs and DNMTs may be used to reinduce ERα expression and thereby restore therapeutic response to ERα antagonists.

Macaluso et al.[34] examined further the mechanisms silencing the ERα gene and identified several multimolecular ERα repression complexes. pRb2/p130-E2F4/5-HDAC1-SUV39H1-p300 or pRB2/p130-E3F4/5-HDAC1-DNMT1-SUV39H1 proteins were found on the ERα promoter. These complexes included HDACs, DNMTs, the histone methyltransferase, SUV39H1, and the cell cycle regulatory protein, pRb2/p130. It was hypothesized that protein complexes recruited by pRb2/p130 modulate acetylation or methylation to the ERα promoter, regulating its expression by altering the local chromatin structure through the histone methyltransferases, like SUV39H1. Sharma et al.[42] examined the multimolecular protein complexes upon treatment of cells with 5-aza-dC and TSA. Cells with silenced ERα demonstrated DNA hypermethylation, histone hypoacetylation, H3K9 methylation, and an increased abundance of methyl-binding proteins, DNMTs, and HDACs. Treatment of these cells with the HDAC and DNMT inhibitors led to ERα re-expression, release of the repressor complexes, enrichment of histone acetylation, and decreased H3K9 methylation.

The ERα Works in Regulating Target Gene Transcription with Coregulators

In addition to the HATs and HDAC-containing complexes, ERα forms protein complexes with other coregulatory proteins to govern expression of genes.

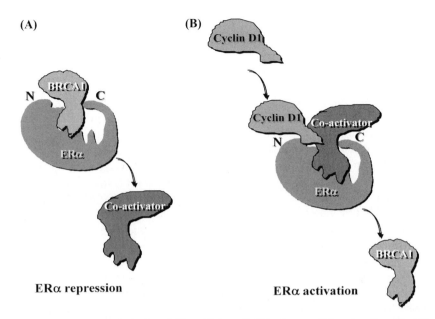

FIGURE 1. Hypothetical model by which cyclin D1 augments ER α signaling. The ER α activity is repressed by BRCA1,[8] Endogenous cyclin D1 opposes the action of BRCA1 at an ERE. Cyclin D1 associates directly with the ERα The prevailing view in cancer biology is that two general classes of cancer genes exist, those that regulate genomic stability including antimutators and DNA repair genes, and a second class of genes regulating cell cycle control. Cyclin D1 shares both properties, promoting DNA synthesis and regulating the function of BRCA1.[43] Estradiol induces BRCA1 to the pS2 ERE in ChIP assays, an effect antagonized by cyclin D1,[43] and E2 induces transient double-strand breaks with the recruitment of DNA repair complexes to the ERE of the pS2 gene. Collectively these studies support a model in which cyclin D1 regulates both cell proliferation and DNA repair function.

A component of a histone methyltransferase complex regulates the ERα to further regulate target genes.[7] Menin is the protein product of the multiple endocrine neoplasia 1 (MEN1) tumor suppressor gene. It is a component of the MLL1/MLL2 H3K4 histone methyltransferase complex, which is typically linked to gene activation. Menin physically associates with the ERα and works as a coactivator to activate the expression of the ERα target gene, pS2 (TFF1).[7] Importantly, MEN1 mutations associated with disease disrupted any ERα-menin interaction and the ERα activity.

Acetylation of the ERα Regulates its Activity

In the first studies demonstrating direct acetylation, the ERα was shown to be acetylated in MCF7 human breast cancer cells by immunoprecipitation Western blotting.[44] GST-fusion proteins of the ERα were then shown to serve as *in vitro* substrates for acetylation in the presence of p300, produced in baculovirus. Deletion analysis identified a minimal region of ERα acetylated by p300. Edman degradation assays and MALDI-TOF mass spectrometry identified the acetylated residues as preferentially lysine K302 and K303 with some minimal acetylation of lysine 299. A minimal ERα peptide was acetylated by p300 with similar efficiency as histone H3. Point mutations of the lysine residues in ERα resulted in ERα mutants that were activated at lower concentrations of E2 than the wild-type ERα. Glutamine or alanine substitutions of the acetylated lysine residues enhanced transactivation; in particular, ERα activation by p300 was enhanced. The alteration in transactivation by the acetylation site was distinct and did not affect activation by other kinases, including mitogen-activated protein kinase or activation by the p68 RNA helicase A.[44] The ERα K303R mutation conferred enhanced activation of ERα activity at low subphysiological levels of hormone. The ERα lysine motif that was acetylated directly by p300 was shown to be conserved across species and the motif was identified in many other phylogenetically related receptors, including the androgen receptor and PPARγ[44] (FIG. 2). Analysis of the related lysine motif in the AR demonstrated a similar biochemical function and growth-regulatory properties.[11,14–16]

Independently of these findings another laboratory had identified a point mutation of the ERα at K303 occurring as a somatic mutation in human breast cancer.[19] The mutation of K303 occurred with high frequency (30%) of early breast cancer lesions, referred to as ductal carcinoma *in situ*. The ERαK303R mutant conveyed a growth advantage to breast carcinoma cells in culture.[19] Growth assays demonstrated that the acetylation site ERαK303R mutation enhanced cellular proliferation in response to low concentrations of estradiol, suggesting the ERα K303R mutation provides a "gain of function" mutation in human breast cancer.

Analysis of other nonhistone substrates for acetylation, such as p53, provides evidence that the acetylation of transcription factors may in turn regulate their phosphorylation[28] by distinct kinases.[28] Thus, acetylation of lysine 320 prevents phosphorylation of serine in the NH2-terminal region of p53. The ERα is phosphorylated by protein kinase A at residue 305. The generation of a kinase-active mutant of the ERα through the introduction of an aspartic acid residue blocked acetylation of the ERα.[5] Studies by Cui *et al.* demonstrating ERα acetylation is linked to phosphorylation of the ERα at residue serine 305 may be of importance to therapy resistance in breast cancer, as PKA activation of ERα has been linked to tamoxifen resistance.[35] These studies suggesting that acetylation and phosphorylation within the ERα are coupled are consistent with prior studies coupling acetylation and phosporylation of the androgen receptor.[11,50]

p53 is known to be acetylated at distinct sites coordinating distinct signaling pathways.[28] It is known that p300/CBP acetylates carboxyl-terminal lysine residues of p53 (lysines 372, 373, 382). P/CAF acetylates a residue within

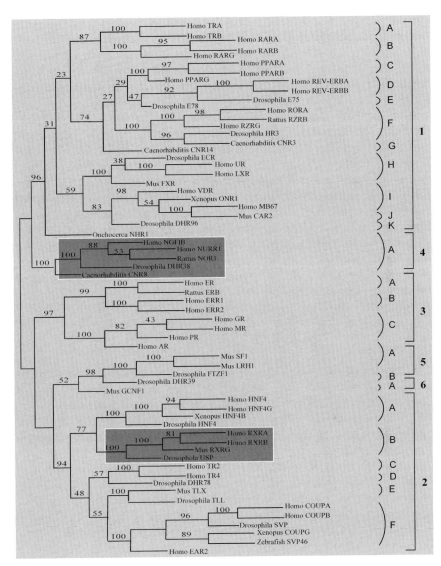

FIGURE 2. Phylogenetic conservation of the acetylation motif. The phylogenetic tree linking nuclear receptors in vertebrate arthropods and nematodes is shown. Nuclear receptors containing the acetylation motif are shown in yellow, whereas nuclear receptors lacking the motif are shown in pink.[49]

the flexible linker region of p53 (lysine 320). In response to genotoxic stress, DNA damage induces acetylation of lysine 320 and lysine 373 with distinguishable kinetics. These two distinct acetylation sites regulate distinct clusters of genes with high-affinity p53-binding sites, promoting cell survival.[28] In contrast K373 regulates interactions with affinity DNA-binding sites found in proapoptotic genes leading to cell death. In keeping with the finding of multiple modular acetylation sites in p53, additional acetylation sites were identified in the ERα at lysine K266 and K268.[27] Contrary to K302/303, which were acetylated directly by p300,[44] K266/268 was acetylated in an assay using p300/p160 (SRC1) and the ligand estradiol.

Although the distinguishable biological functions of the ERα lysine residues remains to be determined, the acetylated residues in the androgen receptor (K302/303) promote DNA synthesis and antiapoptotic signals.[11,14–16] The AR acetylated residues regulate access to DNA in chromatin immune precipitation assays[11] and promote binding to promoters of target genes that induce DNA synthesis such as cyclin D1.[11,14–16] The p53 acetylation site also alters access within the local chromatin structure to enhance DNA binding.[28] In electrophoretic mobility shift assays, the ERα acetylation (K266, and K268) was shown to regulate DNA binding, whereas acetylation of the ERαK303 site does not affect binding. The application of an unbiased proteomic approach to examine ERα residues acetylated *in vivo* under physiological conditions and in tumors will be of interest (FIG. 3).

Cyclin D1 Regulates ERα Activity

The cyclin D1 gene product is overexpressed in 30–40% of cancers and is associated with poor prognosis in ER-positive breast cancer patients.[26,38] Initially cloned as part of a breakpoint rearrangement in parathyroid adenoma, the cyclin D1 protein has subsequently been shown to bind HDACs, the pRB protein, and several transcription factors.[13] Cyclin D1 contributes a catalytic subunit function of a kinase that phosphorylates pRb and NRF1.[41,47] Phosphorylation of pRB in the nucleus regulates DNA synthesis, while phosphorylation of NRF1 regulates mitochondrial biosynthesis.[41,47] At the membrane, cyclin D1 promotes cellular migration, and angiogenesis through induction of cytokines and vascular growth regulatory proteins (VEGF, TSP1).[33]

The role of cyclin D1 in regulating the nuclear receptor is complex. *In vivo*, cyclin D1 knockout mice develop a phenotype of enhanced PPARγ activity with hepatic steatosis due to the inhibition of PPARγ activity by cyclin D1.[48] Cyclin D1 has been shown to associate with the ERα and enhance ERα activity, in part through recruiting the SRC1 p160 coactivator in a ligand-independent manner,[56] and also through antagonizing the ERα corepressor BRCA1.[43] Cyclin D1 functions in regulating both ERα and BRCA1 occupancy in the context of local chromatin at an estrogen response element of the *pS2* gene.[43] The finding that cyclin D1 regulates local chromatin occupancy is consistent with the findings that cyclin D1 binds SUV39, HP1α and HDACs and that the abundance of cyclin D1 determines the local acetylation of histones, including histone H3 Lys9.[10,23,46] It is known that mammary-targeted expression of

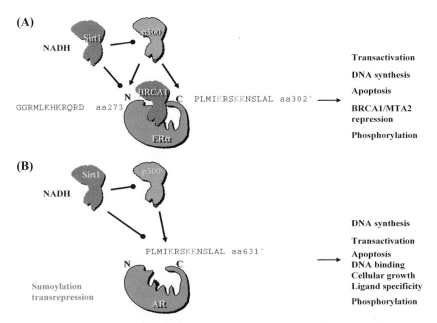

FIGURE 3. The ERα is regulated by TSA and NAD-dependent HDACs. The ERα and the AR are acetylated at conserved lysine residues. Although NAD regulates ERα activity, p300, an essential coactivator of ERα, is also repressed by Sirt1.[3] The AR has been shown to be directly regulated by acetylation in response to physiological stimuli and to be repressed by SIRT1 in a catalytic domain-dependent manner.[12] An acetylated AR substrate functions as an excellent substrate for SIRT1. The nuclear receptor acetylation site governs nuclear receptor function, as indicated to the right, including transactivation DNA synthesis and apoptosis. In the case of the AR, the transrepression and sumoylation of the AR are unaffected by acetylation.

cyclin D1 induces mammary tumorigenesis in transgenic mice. Therefore, it will be of interest to determine the relative importance of these kinase-independent functions of cyclin D1 in inducing mammary tumorigenesis and estrogen responsiveness.

CONCLUSIONS

Over the last decade histone-modifying enzymes have been successfully cloned and characterized. These posttranslational modifications within histone tails provide the basis of signaling modules within the local chromatin, known as the "histone code." Recent studies have demonstrated the presence of similar enzyme complexes associated with the ERα. Similar to histone tails, transcription factors, such as p53 and the nuclear receptors, ERα and the AR, encode signaling modules within the protein, in which one posttranslational modification leads to a sequential commitment to other types of posttranslational modifications. Cascades of acetylation, phosphorylation, and ubiquitination modify the receptors' function, genetic response, and consequent cell fate decisions. Although these signaling cascades in transcription factor or SCITs are poorly understood at this time, the residues for posttranslational modification appear to be well conserved across species. In the same manner that cytoplasmic signaling cascades in the last decades defined kinase modules, so too will the next decade provide important insights into intratranscription factor signaling cascades that may ultimately contribute to the biological specificity of nuclear receptor signaling.

ACKNOWLEDGMENTS

This work was supported in part by R01CA70896, R01CA75503, R01CA86072, and R01CA86071 (to R.G.P.). The Kimmel Cancer Center was supported by the NIH Cancer Center Core Grant P30CA56036 (to R.G.P). This project is funded in part from the Dr. Ralph and Marian C. Falk Medical Research Trust and a grant from the Pennsylvania Department of Health (to R.G.P.). The Department specifically disclaims responsibility for analysis, interpretation, or conclusions.

REFERENCES

1. BANNISTER, A.J. & T. KOUZARIDES. 2005. Reversing histone methylation. Nature **436:** 1103–1106.
2. BAUTISTA, S., H. VALLES, R.L. WALKER, *et al.* 1998. In breast cancer, amplification of the steroid receptor coactivator gene AIB1 is correlated with estrogen and progesterone receptor positivity. Clin. Cancer Res. **4:** 2925–2929.
3. BOURAS, T., M. FU, A.A. SAUVE, *et al.* 2005. SIRT1 deacetylation and repression of P300 involves lysine residues 1020/1024 within the cell-cycle regulatory domain 1. J. Biol. Chem. **280:** 10264–10276.
4. CHEN, D., H. MA, H. HONG, *et al.* 1999. Regulation of transcription by a protein methyltransferase. Science **284:** 2174–2177.
5. CUI, Y., M. ZHANG, R. PESTELL, *et al.* 2004. Phosphorylation of estrogen receptor alpha blocks its acetylation and regulates estrogen sensitivity. Cancer Res. **64:** 9199–9208.
6. CUTHBERT, G.L., S. DAUJAT, A.W. SNOWDEN, *et al.* 2004. Histone deimination antagonizes arginine methylation. Cell **118:** 545–553.
7. DREIJERINK, K.M., K.W. MULDER, G.S. WINKLER, *et al.* 2006. Menin links estrogen receptor activation to histone H3K4 trimethylation. Cancer Res. **66:** 4929–4935.
8. FAN, S., J. WANG, R. YUAN, *et al.* 1999. BRCA1 inhibition of estrogen receptor signaling in transfected cells. Science **284:** 1354–1356.
9. FU, M., C. WANG, Z. LI, *et al.* 2004. Minireview: cyclin D1: normal and abnormal functions. Endocrinology **145:** 5439–5447.
10. FU, M., M. RAO, T. BOURAS, *et al.* 2004. Recruitment of HDACs by cyclin D1 inhibits PPAR-gamma mediated adipogenesis. J. Biol. Chem. **279:** 24745–24756.

11. Fu, M., M. Rao, K. Wu, *et al.* 2004. The androgen receptor acetylation site regulates cAMP and AKT but not ERK-induced activity. J. Biol. Chem. **279:** 29436–29449.

12. Fu, M., A.A. Sauve, M. Liu, *et al.* 2006. The hormonal control of androgen receptor function through SIRT1. Mol. Biol. Cell. **26:** 8122–8135.

13. Fu, M., C. Wang, M. Rao, *et al.* 2005. Cyclin D1 represses p300 transactivation through a CDK-independent mechanism. J. Biol. Chem. **28:** 29728–29742.

14. Fu, M., C. Wang, A.T. Reutens, *et al.* 2000. p300 and p300/cAMP-response element-binding protein-associated factor acetylate the androgen receptor at sites governing hormone-dependent transactivation. J. Biol. Chem. **275:** 20853–20860.

15. Fu, M., C. Wang, J. Wang, *et al.* 2003. Acetylation of the androgen receptor enhances coactivator binding and promotes prostate cancer cell growth. Mol. Cell. Biol. **23:** 8563–8575.

16. Fu, M., C. Wang, J. Wang, *et al.* 2002. The androgen receptor acetylation governs transactivation and MEKK1-induced apoptosis without affecting in vitro sumoylation and transrepression function. Mol. Cell. Biol. **22:** 3373–3388.

17. Fu, M., C. Wang, J. Wang, *et al.* 2002. Acetylation in hormone signaling and the cell-cycle. Cytokine Growth Factor Rev. **13:** 259–276.

18. Fu, M., C. Wang, X. Zhang & R. Pestell. 2003. Nuclear receptor modifications and endocrine cell proliferation. J. Steroid Biochem. Mol. Biol. **85:** 133–138.

19. Fuqua, S.A., C. Wiltschke, Q.X. Zhang, *et al.* 2000. A hypersensitive estrogen receptor-alpha mutation in premalignant breast lesions. Cancer Res. **60:** 4026–4029.

20. Girault, I., S. Tozlu, R. Lidereau & I. Bieche. 2003. Expression analysis of DNA methyltransferases 1, 3A, and 3B in sporadic breast carcinomas. Clin. Cancer Res. **9:** 4415–4422.

21. Hanstein, B., R. Eckner, J. DiRenzo, *et al.* 1996. p300 is a component of an estrogen receptor coactivator complex. Proc. Natl. Acad. Sci. USA **93:** 11540–11545.

22. Hortobagyi, G.N. 1998. Progress in endocrine therapy for breast carcinoma. Cancer **83:** 1–6.

23. Hulit, J., C. Wang, Z. Li, *et al.* 2004. Cyclin D1 genetic heterozygosity regulates colonic epithelial cell differentiation and tumor number in ApcMin mice. Mol. Cell. Biol. **24:** 7598–7611.

24. Ju, B.G., V.V. Lunyak, V. Perissi, *et al.* 2006. A topoisomerase IIbeta-mediated dsDNA break required for regulated transcription. Science **312:** 1798–1802.

25. Kawai, H., H. Li, S. Avraham, *et al.* 2003. Overexpression of histone deacetylase HDAC1 modulates breast cancer progression by negative regulation of estrogen receptor alpha. Int. J. Cancer **107:** 353–358.

26. Kenny, F.S., R. Hui, E.A. Musgrove, *et al.* 1999. Overexpression of cyclin D1 messenger RNA predicts for poor prognosis in estrogen receptor-positive breast cancer. Clin. Cancer Res. **5:** 2069–2076.

27. Kim, M.Y., E.M. Woo, Y.T.E. Chong, *et al.* 2006. Acetylation of estrogen receptor α by p300 at lysines 266 and 268 enhances the deoxyribonucleic acid binding and transactivation activities of the receptor. Mol. Endocrinol. **20:** 1479–1493.

28. Knights, C.D., J. Catania, S.D. Giovanni, *et al.* 2006. Distinct p53 acetylation cassettes differentially influence gene-expression patterns and cell fate. J. Cell. Biol. **173:** 533–544.

29. KRAUS, W.L. & J.T. KADONAGA. 1998. p300 and estrogen receptor cooperatively activate transcription via differential enhancement of initiation and reinitiation. Genes Dev. **12:** 331–342.

30. KRAUS, W.L., E.T. MANNING & J.T. KADONAGA. 1999. Biochemical analysis of distinct activation functions in p300 that enhance transcription initiation with chromatin templates. Mol. Cell. Biol. **19:** 8123–8135.

31. KUREBAYASHI, J., T. OTSUKI, H. KUNISUE, *et al.* 2000. Expression levels of estrogen receptor-alpha, estrogen receptor-beta, coactivators, and corepressors in breast cancer. Clin. Cancer Res. **6:** 512–518.

32. LEADER, J.E., C. WANG, M. FU & R.G. PESTELL. 2006. Epigenetic regulation of nuclear steroid receptors. Biochem. Pharmacol. **72:** 1589–1596.

33. LI, Z., X. JIAO, C. WANG, *et al.* 2006. Cyclin D1 promotes cellular migration through p27^{KIP1}. Cancer Res. **66:** 9986–9994.

34. MACALUSO, M., C. CINTI, G. RUSSO, *et al.* 2003. pRb2/p130-E2F4/5-HDAC1-SUV39H1-p300 and pRb2/p130-E2F4/5-HDAC1-SUV39H1-DNMT1 multimolecular complexes mediate the transcription of estrogen receptor-alpha in breast cancer. Oncogene **22:** 3511–3517.

35. MICHALIDES, R., A. GRIEKSPOOR, A. BALKENENDE, *et al.* 2004. Tamoxifen resistance by a conformational arrest of the estrogen receptor alpha after PKA activation in breast cancer. Cancer Cell **5:** 597–605.

36. NEUMEISTER, P., C. ALBANESE, B. BALENT, *et al.* 2002. Senescence and epigenetic dysregulation in cancer. Int. J. Biochem. Cell. Biol. **34:** 1475.

37. PAIK, W.K. & S. KIM. 1973. Enzymatic demethylation of calf thymus histones. Biochem. Biophys. Res. Commun. **51:** 781–788.

38. PESTELL, R.G., C. ALBANESE, A.T. REUTENS, *et al.* 1999. The cyclins and cyclin-dependent kinase inhibitors in hormonal regulation of proliferation and differentiation. Endocrine Rev. **20:** 501–534.

39. ROBERT, M.F., S. MORIN, N. BEAULIEU, *et al.* 2003. DNMT1 is required to maintain CpG methylation and aberrant gene silencing in human cancer cells. Nat. Genet. **33:** 61–65.

40. ROBINSON-RECHAVI, M., H. ESCRIVA GARCIA & V. LAUDET. 2003. The nuclear receptor superfamily. J. Cell. Sci. **116:** 585–586.

41. SAKAMAKI, T., M.C. CASIMIRO, X. JU, *et al.* 2006. Cyclin d1 determines mitochondrial function in vivo. Mol. Cell. Biol. **26:** 5449–5469.

42. SHARMA, D., J. BLUM, X. YANG, *et al.* 2005. Release of methyl CpG binding proteins and histone deacetylase 1 from the estrogen receptor alpha (ER) promoter upon reactivation in ER-negative human breast cancer cells. Mol. Endocrinol. **19:** 1740–1751.

43. WANG, C., S. FAN, Z. LI, *et al.* 2005. Cyclin D1 antagonizes BRCA1 repression of estrogen receptor alpha activity. Cancer Res. **65:** 6557–6567.

44. WANG, C., M. FU, R.H. ANGELETTI, *et al.* 2001. Direct acetylation of the estrogen receptor alpha hinge region by p300 regulates transactivation and hormone sensitivity. J. Biol. Chem. **276:** 18375–18383.

45. WANG, C., M. FU & R.G. PESTELL. 2005. Estrogen receptor acetylation and phosphorylation in hormone responses. Breast Cancer Online J.

46. WANG, C., M. FU & R.G. PESTELL. 2004. Histone acetylation/deacetylation as a regulator of cell cycle gene expression. Methods Mol. Biol. **241:** 207–216.

47. WANG, C., Z. LI, Y. LU, *et al.* 2006. Cyclin D1 repression of NRF-1 integrates nuclear DNA synthesis and mitochondrial function. Proc. Natl. Acad. Sci. USA. **103:** 11567–11572.

48. WANG, C., N. PATTABIRAMAN, M. FU, *et al.* 2003. Cyclin D1 repression of peroxisome proliferator-activated receptor gamma (PPARgamma) expression and transactivation. Mol. Cell. Biol. **23:** 6159–6173.
49. WANG, X., S.C. MOORE, M. LASZCKZAK & J. AUSIO. 2000. Acetylation increases the alpha-helical content of the histone tails of the nucleosome. J. Biol. Chem. **275:** 35013–35020.
50. WESTWICK, J.K., R.J. LEE, Q.T. LAMBERT, *et al.* 1998. Transforming potential of Dbl family proteins correlates with transcription from the cyclin D1 promoter but not with activation of Jun NH_2-terminal kinase, p38/Mpk2, serum response factor, or c-Jun. J. Biol. Chem. **273:** 16739–16747.
51. XU, L., C.K. GLASS & M.G. ROSENFELD. 1999. Coactivator and corepressor complexes in nuclear receptor function. Curr. Opin. Genet. Dev. **9:** 140–147.
52. YAGER, J.D. & N.E. DAVIDSON. 2006. Estrogen carcinogenesis in breast cancer. N. Engl. J. Med. **354:** 270–282.
53. YAN, P.S., H. SHI, F. RAHMATPANAH, *et al.* 2003. Differential distribution of DNA methylation within the RASSF1A CpG island in breast cancer. Cancer Res. **63:** 6178–6186.
54. YANG, J.B., Z.J. DUAN, W. YAO, *et al.* 2001. Synergistic transcriptional activation of human acyl-coenzyme A: cholesterol acyltransterase-1 gene by interferon-gamma and all-trans-retinoic acid THP-1 cells. J. Biol. Chem. **276:** 20989–20998.
55. YANG, X., A.T. FERGUSON, S.J. NASS, *et al.* 2000. Transcriptional activation of estrogen receptor alpha in human breast cancer cells by histone deacetylase inhibition. Cancer Res. **60:** 6890–6894.
56. ZWIJSEN, R.M.L., R.S. BUCKLE, E.M. HIJMANS, *et al.* 1998. Ligand-independent recruitment of steroid receptor coactivators to estrogen receptor by cyclin D1. Genes Dev. **12:** 3488–3498.

Red Wine Extract Prevents Neuronal Apoptosis *in Vitro* and Reduces Mortality of Transgenic Mice

ROSALBA AMODIO,[a] ENNIO ESPOSITO,[b] CATERINA DE RUVO,[b] VINCENZO BELLAVIA,[a] EMANUELE AMODIO,[a] AND GIUSEPPE CARRUBA[a]

[a]*Experimental Oncology Unit—Department of Oncology, M. Ascoli, ARNAS-Civico, Palermo, Italy*

[b]*Laboratory of Neurophysiology, Istituto di Ricerche Farmacologiche "Mario Negri," Consorzio Mario Negri Sud, Santa Maria Imbaro, Chieti 66030, Italy*

ABSTRACT: In this work, we have investigated the effects of nutritional antioxidants as antidegenerative agents on glutamate-induced apoptosis in primary cultures of cerebellar granule neurons (CGNs). Glutamate-induced apoptosis is also associated with intracellular $[Ca^{2+}]_I$ overload, generation of reactive oxygen species (ROS), depression of cell energy metabolism, cytochrome *c* release, and increase in caspase-3 activity. Pretreatment (3 h) with red wine extract (5 μg/mL) and ascorbic acid (30 μM) blocks glutamate-induced apoptosis in CGNs. *In vivo* experiments carried out on transgenic mice expressing the human mutated Cu, Zn superoxide dismutase (SOD1) G93A ($mSOD1^{G93A}$) show that mice fed with lyophilized red wine have significantly increased survival as compared to control, untreated animals.

KEYWORDS: cerebellar granule cells; apoptosis; lyophilized red wine; ASL; $mSOD1^{G93A}$

INTRODUCTION

Neuronal cell death is a tightly regulated process. It is intimately involved in both normal development of the nervous system and neurological disorders.[1] Developmentally regulated neuron death eliminates the large excess of neurons that are produced, thereby preserving only those neurons needed for proper synaptic connections.[2,3] In contrast, neuron death in the adult brain is common in a variety of disorders including those associated with cerebral ischemia and

Address for correspondence: Dr. Giuseppe Carruba, Experimental Oncology Unit—Department of Oncology, P.O. M. Ascoli, ARNAS-Civico, Palermo, Italy. Voice: +39-091-6664348; fax: +39-091-6664352.

e-mail: lucashbl@unipa.it

Ann. N.Y. Acad. Sci. 1089: 88–97 (2006). © 2006 New York Academy of Sciences.
doi: 10.1196/annals.1386.026

neurodegenerative diseases such as Alzheimer's disease,[4] Huntington's disease,[5] amyotrophic lateral sclerosis,[6] and spinal muscular atrophy.[7] Several studies have shown that extracellular glutamate can be associated with brain injury in many neurodegenerative disorders, although the precise mechanisms are still controversial.[8,9] Glutamate is a major excitatory neurotransmitter in the central nervous system, and, during the postnatal period, glutamate-activated N-methyl-D-aspartate (NMDA) receptors increase $[Ca^{2+}]_I$ influx into cytosol to trigger changes in neuronal metabolism and gene expression, which are necessary for brain development.[10,11] In contrast, overstimulation of NMDA receptors by glutamate induces cell death in a process known as excitotoxicity.[12] Aiming to understand the molecular mechanisms that regulate this process, we have used glutamate to induce neuronal apoptosis on primary cultures of cerebellar granule neurons (CGNs), a suitable *in vitro* model for studying neuronal apoptosis.[13,14] In a recent study, we have showed that excitotoxic death of CGNs induced by glutamate occurs via both necrosis and apoptosis, with apoptosis predominating after exposure to relatively low concentrations of glutamate (50 μM).[15] Many studies have shown that glutamate-induced apoptosis is also consistently associated with intracellular $[Ca^{2+}]_I$ overload, concomitant generation of reactive oxygen species (ROS), and depression of cell energy metabolism.[11,12] This series of biochemical events is associated with cytocrome c release and increase in caspase-3 activity, and production of ROS is thought to represent a central mechanism in the series of biochemical events that ultimately leads to apoptosis.[16,17] Consistent with this hypothesis are the findings that various antioxidants block glutamate-induced apoptosis in CGNs.[18–20] In the present study, we have used a red wine lyophilized extract (a natural antioxidant with potential antiapoptotic activity) to test its antiapoptotic effect on *in vitro* and *in vivo* model systems of neurodegeneration. In addition, the interference of red wine lyophilized extract with ROS formation and caspase-3 activation was investigated *in vitro*. Moreover, we show preliminary results obtained from transgenic mice expressing the human-mutated Cu, Zn superoxide dismutase (SOD1) G93A (mSOD1^{G93A}).[21,22]

EXPERIMENTAL PROCEDURES

Cell Cultures

Primary cultures of cerebellar granule cells were prepared from 8-day-old Wistar rats (Charles River, Italy) according to the procedure described by Levi *et al.*[23] Dissociated cells were suspended in basal Eagle's medium (BME) (Sigma, St Louis, MO, USA) containing 10% heat-inactivated fetal calf serum (Eurobio, Les Ulis Cedex, France), 2-mM glutamine (Sigma), 25-mM KCl (Sigma), 100-mg/mL gentamycin (Sigma), and plated in poly-L-lysine (Sigma)-coated (10 mg/mL) 35-mm petri dishes. Plates used for a single experiment contained equal numbers of cells (2.5×10^6 cells/dish) originating from the same dissociation. Cells were incubated for the desired period at 37°C in humidified 95% air, 5% CO_2. Cytosine-arabinofuranoside (10 mM) (Sigma) was added after 18 h or 20 h to culture medium to prevent replication of non-neuronal cells. All experiments were performed with fully differentiated neurons (8 days in culture). All cultures were fed with 5-mM D-glucose (Sigma) on day 7 *in vitro*.

Measurement of Apoptosis

Apoptosis was measured after application of glutamate (50 mM, final concentration) in the culture medium. Apoptosis was measured by the TUNEL method, conducted using the *in situ* Cell Death Detection kit (Boehringer, Mannheim, Germany), according to the manufacturer's instructions. In brief: cultures were fixed with 4% paraformaldehyde (Sigma) in PBS for 30 min and permeabilized with 0.25% Triton X-100 for 10 min. Cells were rinsed with PBS and covered with labeling reaction mixture containing terminal deoxynucleotidyl transferase (TdT) and fluorescein-deoxyuridine triphosphate (dUTP). Cultures were incubated at 37°C for 1 h. Reactions were terminated by rinsing the cells with PBS. For the correlation of TUNEL with nuclear morphology, cultures were counterstained with PI (5 μg/mL) and observed with an epifluorescent microscope. To confirm the specificity of TUNEL, cultures were treated with 1 μg/mL DNAse I (Sigma) at room temperature for 10 min to create positive controls. TdT was omitted from the labeling reaction mixture in negative controls.

Assay for Caspase-3 Activity

At the appropriate time, treated cells were collected (2 million per sample), washed twice with PBS pH 7.4, and resuspended in 50 μL precooled lysis buffer commercial kit Apo/Alert CPP32 (Clontech Laboratories, Palo Alto, CA, USA). The cells were allowed to swell for 10 min on ice. After incubation, the cellular lysates were centrifuged at 12,000 rpm for 3 min at 4°C to precipitate cellular debris. Protein concentration was determined (Bradford method; Biorad Laboratories, Hercules, CA, USA) in the supernatants. Equal amounts of protein were incubated with 50 μM of the caspase-3 substrate Asp–Glu–Val–Asp-7-amino-4-trifluoromethyl coumarin (DEVD-AFC) (Clontech Laboratories) in a reaction buffer at 37°C for 1 h. The amounts of released 7-amino-4-trifluoromethyl coumarin (Clontech Laboratories) were measured by means of a spectrofluorometer with an excitation wavelength of 380 nm and an emission wavelength of 505 nm. One unit was defined as the amount of enzyme required to release 1 pmol of AFC/h at 37°C.

Measurements of Reactive Oxygen Species

Levels of cellular ROS were measured using the fluorescent probe 2,7-dichlorodihydrofluorescein diacetate (H_2DCFDA; Molecular Probes, OR, USA). In brief: cells were incubated for 30 min at 37°C in the presence of 10 μM H_2DCFDA (added from a 10-mM stock solution in dimethyl sulfoxide) in the original serum-containing medium. H_2DCFDA passively diffuses across the neuronal membranes, where the acetates are cleaved by intracellular esterases. Oxidation of H_2DCFDA occurs almost exclusively in the cytosol and produces a fluorescence response. The amount of intracellular oxidants is proportional to the intensity of fluorescence (measured at excitation wavelength of 488 nm and emission wavelength of 510 nm). After loading with the dye, neurons were washed in Locke's buffer, centrifuged at 1,200 rpm for 5 min, then lysed (Tris–EDTA + Triton 0.2%) for 10 min at 4°C, and centrifuged at 12,000 rpm for 5 min at 4°C. Cytoplasmatic fraction was collected and measured using a spectrofluorimetric assay (CM1T111, Spex Industries, Edison, NJ, USA).

Antioxidants

The following antioxidants were used to test their potential antiapoptotic effect: ascorbic acid (30 mM) (Sigma) and a lyophilized extract of red wine (5 mg/mL), which contains several antioxidant compounds and was provided by Dr D. Rotilio, Consorzio Mario Negri Sud, Italy.

Transgenic Mice

Transgenic mice originally obtained from Jackson Laboratories and expressing a high copy number of mutant human (h) SOD1 with a Gly-93-Ala substitution, or wild-type (WT) hSOD1 mice, were bred and maintained on a C57BL/6 mice strain at the Consorzio Mario Negri Sud, S. Maria Imbaro (CH), Italy. Transgenic mice are identified by PCR.[24] The mice were housed at 21°C ± 1°C with relative humidity 55% ± 10% and 12 h of light. Food (standard pellets) and water were supplied *ad libitum*. Female WT SOD1 were used as controls. Procedures involving animals and their care were conducted in conformity with the institutional guidelines that are in compliance with national (D.L. No. 116, G.U. Suppl. 40, Feb. 18, 1992, Circolare No. 8, G.U., 14 luglio 1994) and international laws and policies (EEC Council Directive 86/609, OJ L 358,1, Dec.12, 1987; NIH Guide for the Care and Use of Laboratory Animals, U.S. National Research Council, 1996). The control mice ($n = 7$) were fed with normal drinking water, whereas the other mice ($n = 8$) were treated with lyophilized red wine dissolved in the drinking water.

Data Analysis

Values from each culture dish represents an $n = 1$ determination and are expressed as mean percentages $\pm$ SEM. The experiments were repeated 3–10 times independently on separate occasion with different cultures. Statistical analysis was performed by one-way analysis of variance (ANOVA) followed by Tukey's test. A P-value of <0.05 was considered significant. Moreover the cumulative probability of survival in mSOD1 mice was followed by Kaplan–Meier survival curve.

RESULTS AND DISCUSSION

The main aim of this study was to investigate the actions of red wine extract in different *in vitro* and *in vivo* models of neuronal apoptosis. A large body of evidence indicates that an unbalanced production of ROS may give rise to oxidative stress, which can induce neuronal damage, ultimately leading to neuronal death by apoptosis or necrosis.[10,16,17] Several studies have shown that nutritional antioxidants can block neuronal death *in vitro* and, hence, may have therapeutic potential in animal models of major neurodegenerative diseases.[15,18,19] We have investigated the effects of nutritional antioxidants as antidegenerative agents on glutamate-induced apoptosis in primary cultures of CGNs. In this study, we have analyzed the pro-apoptotic effect of glutamate by the TUNEL method 24 h after its addition to the culture medium. Interestingly, the effect of glutamate was prevented by a lyophilized extract of red wine (5 mg/mL) and ascorbic acid (30 mM), which were added to the culture medium 3 h before glutamate ($P < 0.01$ glutamate as compared to control, and $P < 0.01$ ascorbic acid and red wine as compared to glutamate) (Fig. 1). Moreover, our results show that red wine extract (5 mg/mL) and ascorbic acid (30 mM) were capable of significantly reducing the rise of ROS production induced by glutamate (50 mM) in this *in vitro* model ($P < 0.01$ glutamate compared with control) (Figs. 2 and 3). Several studies have shown that ascorbic acid could act as a scavenger of OH− and singlet oxygen.[25] Also red wine has been shown to contain compounds that exhibit radical scavenger and antioxidant properties. Thus, it is conceivable that ascorbic acid and red wine extract exert their antiapoptotic effect by reducing ROS formation. Some studies have shown that glutamate-induced ROS formation in CGNs is followed by an increase of cytosolic caspase-3 activity.[26–29] It is therefore conceivable that caspase-3 activation is mediated by intracellular increase in ROS concentration.[27] Thus, another very interesting finding of this study is that both ascorbic acid and red wine extract block the increase of caspase-3 activity induced by glutamate in CGNs ($P < 0.01$ glutamate compared with control and $P < 0.01$ red wine and ascorbic acid compared with glutamate) (Fig. 4). Inasmuch as caspase-3 activation has been shown to play an important role in inappropriate apoptosis,[30] the

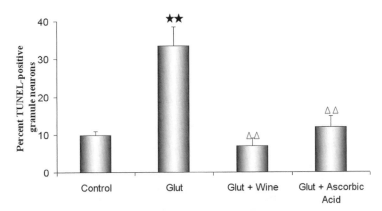

FIGURE 1. Protective effects of lyophilized red wine (5 μg/mL) and ascorbic acid (30 μg/mL) against glutamate-induced apoptosis in cerebellar granule neurons. Apoptotic nuclei were stained by the TUNEL method. Apoptotic nuclei were counted at 1000× in six to seven randomly chosen microscopic fields taken from six different experiments and expressed as the mean (± SEM) percentage of total nuclei stained with PI. **$P < 0.01$ as compared with control; $^{\Delta\Delta}P < 0.01$ as compared with glutamate by one-way ANOVA followed by Tukey's test.

inhibitory effect exerted by ascorbic acid and red wine extract on this enzyme might be relevant for their potential use as antineurodegenerative agents. It is interesting to note that the effects of red wine extract and ascorbic acid were similar to those of DEVD-CHO (50 mM), a specific inhibitor of caspase-3.[27–30]

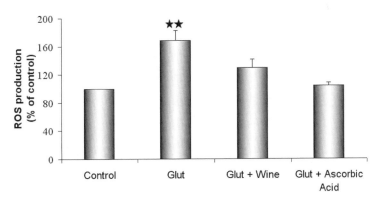

FIGURE 2. Effects of antioxidants on glutamate-induced reactive oxygen species (ROS) production. Data represent the mean (± SEM) percent increase in ROS production measured 6 h after glutamate addition, as compared with control cells. Ascorbic acid and red wine extract were added 3 h before glutamate. Experiments were performed in triplicate. **$P < 0.01$ as compared with control by one-way ANOVA followed by Tukey's test.

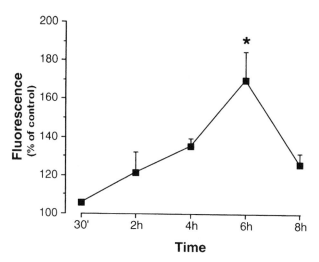

FIGURE 3. Time course of glutamate-induced ROS production. The data represent the mean ± SEM of three independent experiments, and are expressed as the percent change relative to control cells. *$P < 0.05$ as compared with time 0 by one-way ANOVA followed by Tukey's test.

In this respect, we have obtained preliminary results on transgenic mice expressing the human mSOD1^{G93A}, which began to develop amyotrophic lateral sclerosis (ALS) symptoms at the mean age of about 3 months.[31] ASL is a fatal paralytic neurodegenerative disorder mainly characterized by a progressive loss of motoneurons in the cerebral cortex, brainstem, and spinal cord[21] and invariably leading to death within approximately 3–5 years from the onset of symptoms. About 15% of patients with familial ALS (FALS), clinically indistiguishable from the more common sporadic ALS, carry mutations in the gene

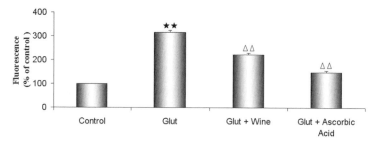

FIGURE 4. Glutamate-induced caspase-3 activity in cerebellar granule neurons: inhibitory effect of lyophilized red wine and ascorbic acid. Caspase-3 activity was expressed as the percentage of fluorescence increase with respect to control. The data represent the mean ±SEM of three independent experiments.**$P < 0.01$ as compared with control; $^{\triangle\triangle}P$ <0.01 as compared with glutamate by one-way ANOVA followed by Tukey's test.

encoding for the free radical scavenging enzyme SOD1.[22,32] The pathogenesis of FALS does not seem to be related to a reduced activity of SOD1, but rather to a novel function of the mutated enzyme which is toxic to motoneurons.[31–33] Support for this hypothesis has come from transgenic mice lines overexpressing the mutated human SOD1 enzyme.[21] Basing our work on the hypothesis that in this strain of animals an increased formation of ROS occurs and on the basis of our *in vitro* experiments, we treated the mice with lyophilized red wine. In this series of experiments red wine was dissolved in the drinking water that was made freely available to the animals. Our results show that mice fed with lyophilized red wine have significantly reduced mortality rates as compared to control, untreated animals (Log-Rank test, $P = 0.017$) (FIG. 5). This could be a consequence of a reduction in the elevated ROS formation that normally occurs in the transgenic mouse. Moreover, we have calculated that the daily intake of polyphenolic compounds expressed as gallic acid equivalent (GAE) was about 20 mg/mouse. These data suggest that red wine extract and ascorbic acid could be used as chemopreventive dietary supplements for neurodegenerative disorders. Further research is necessary to better understand the molecular mechanisms of polyphenolic action and their potential inference in human health.

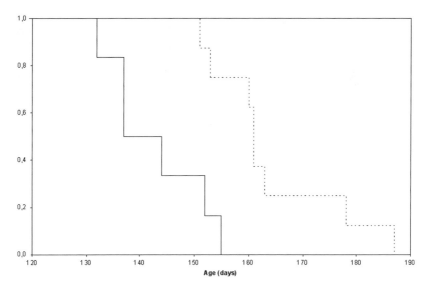

FIGURE 5. Kaplan–Meier survival curve showing cumulative probability of survival in mSOD-1[G93A] mice. Treatment with lyophilized red wine (*dashed line*) significantly prolonged survival when compared with littermates treated with normal drinking water (*solid line*). Log-rank test, $P = 0.017$. The onset of treatment was 30–40 days of age. Mean survival (days): control = 143 ± 4.0; treated = 164 ± 4.5 (+15%).

REFERENCES

1. CONTESTABILE, A. 2002. Cerebellar granule cells as a model to study mechanisms of neuronal apoptosis or survival *in vivo* and *in vitro*. Cerebellum **1**: 41–55. Review.
2. BENN, S.E. & C.J. WOOLF. 2004. Adult neuron survival strategies–slamming on the brakes. Not Rev. Neurosci. **5**: 686–700. Review.
3. OPPENHEIM, R.W. 1991. Cell death during development of the nervous system. Annu. Rev. Neurosci. **14**: 453–501.
4. LOO, D.T. *et al.* 1993. Apoptosis is induced by β-amyloid in cultured central nervous system neurons. Proc. Natl. Acad. Sci. USA **90**: 7951–7955.
5. PORTERA-CAILLIAU, C. *et al.* 1995. Evidence for apoptotic cell death in Huntington disease and excitotoxic animal models. J. Neurosci. **15**: 3775–3787.
6. RABIZADEH, S. *et al.* 1995. Mutations associated with amyotrophic lateral sclerosis convert superoxide dismutase from an apoptotic gene to a proapoptotic gene: studies in yeast and neural cells. Proc. Natl. Acad. Sci. USA **92**: 3024–3028.
7. ROY, N. *et al.* 1995. The gene for neuronal apoptosis inhibitory protein is partially deleted in individuals with spinal muscular atrophy. Cell **80**: 167–178.
8. CHOI, D.W, 1988. Glutamate neurotoxicity and diseases of the nervous system. Neuron **1**: 623–634.
9. DU, Y. *et al.* 1997. Activation of a caspase 3-related cysteine protease is required for glutamate-mediated apoptosis of cultured cerebellar granuleneurons. Proc. Natl. Acad. Sci. USA **94**: 11657–11662.
10. COYLE, J.T. & P. PUTTFARCKEN. 1993. Oxidative stress, glutamate, and neurodegenerative disorders. Science **262**: 689–695.
11. LI, C.Y., T.Y. CHIN, S.H. CHUEH. 2004. Rat cerebellar granule cells are protected from glutamate-induced excitotoxicity by S-nitrosoglutathione but not glutathione. Am. J. Physiol. Cell. Physiol. **286**: C893–C904.
12. GALL, D. *et al.* 2005. Intracellular calcium regulation by burst discharge determines bidirectional long-term synaptic plasticity at the cerebellum input stage. J. Neurosci. **25**: 4813–4822.
13. D'MELLO, S.R. *et al.* 1993. Induction of apoptosis in cerebellar granule neurons by low potassium: inhibition of death by insulin-like growth factor I and cAMP. Proc. Natl. Acad. Sci. USA **90**: 10989–10993.
14. GALLI, C. *et al.* 1995. Apoptosis in cerebellar granule cells is blocked by high KCl, forskolin, and IGF-1 through distinct mechanisms of action: the involvement of intracellular calcium and RNA synthesis. J. Neurosci. **15**: 1172–1179.
15. DE RUVO, C. *et al.* 2000. Nutritional antioxidants as antidegenerative agents. Int. J. Dev. Neurosci. **18**: 359–366.
16. ATABAY, C. *et al.* 1996. Removal of serum from primary cultures of cerebellar granule neurons induces oxidative stress and DNA fragmentation: protection with antioxidants and glutamate. J. Neurosci. Res. **43**: 465–475.
17. HIGUCHI, M. *et al.* 1998. Regulation of reactive oxygen species-induced apoptosis and necrosis by caspase 3-like proteases. Oncogene **17**: 2753–2760.
18. DE GROOT, H. & U. RAUEN. 1998. Tissue injury by reactive oxygen species and the protective effects of flavonoids. Fundam. Clin. Pharmacol. **12**: 249–255.

19. DESCHAMPS, *et al.* 2001. Nutritional factors in cerebral aging and dementia: epidemiological arguments for a role of oxidative stress. Neuroepidemiology **20**: 7–15.

20. ENGELHART, M.J. *et al.* 2002. Dietary intake of antioxidants and risk of Alzheimer's disease. JAMA **287**: 3223–3229.

21. GURNEY, M.E. *et al.* 1994. Motor neuron degeneration in mice that express a human Cu,Zn superoxide dismutase mutation. Science **264**: 1772–1775.

22. DAL, C. & GURNEY. 1995. Neuropathological changes in two lines of mice carrying transgene for mutant human Cu,Zn SOD, and in mice overexpressing wild type human SOD: a model of familial amyotrophic lateral sclerosis. Brain Res. **676**: 25–40.

23. LEVI, G. *et al.* 1984. Autoradiographic localization and depolarization-induced release of acidic amino acids in differentiating cerebellar granule cell cultures. Brain Res. **290**: 77–86.

24. ROSEN, D.R. 1993. Mutations in Cu/Zn superoxide dismutase gene are associated with familial amyotrophic lateral sclerosis. Nature **364**: 362.

25. BODANNES, R.S. & P.C. CHAN. 1979. Ascorbic acid as a scavenger of singlet oxygen. FEBS Lett. **105**: 195–196.

26. DU, Y. *et al.* 1997. Activation of a caspase 3-related cysteine protease is required for glutamate-mediated apoptosis of cultured cerebellar granule neurons. Proc. Natl. Acad. Sci. USA **94**: 11657–11662.

27. HIGUCHI, M. *et al.* 1998. Regulation of reactive oxygen species-induced apoptosis and necrosis by caspase 3-like proteases. Oncogene **17**: 2753–2760.

28. KERRY, N.L. & M. ABBEY. 1997. Red wine and fractioned phenolic compounds prepared from red wine inhibit low density lipoprotein oxidation *in vitro*. Atherosclerosis **135**: 93–102.

29. FAUNONNEAU, B. *et al.* 1997. Comparative study of radical scavenger and antioxidant properties of phenolic compounds from *Vitis vinifera* cell cultures using *in vitro* tests. Life Sci. **61**: 2103–2110.

30. NICHOLSON, D.W. 1999. ICE/CED3-like proteases as therapeutic targets for the control of inappropriate apoptosis. Nat. Biotechnol. **14**: 297–301.

31. WATANABE, M. *et al.* 2001. Histological evidence of protein aggregation in mutant SOD1 transgenic mice and in amyotrophic lateral sclerosis neural tissues. Neurobiol. Dis. **8**: 933–941

32. GREENLUND, L.J.S., T.L. DECKWERTH & E.M. JOHNSON. 1995. Superoxide dismutase delays apoptosis: a role for reactive oxygen species in programmed neuronal death. Neuron **14**: 303–315.

33. DE GROOT, H. & U. RAUEN. 1998. Tissue injury by reactive oxygen species and the protective effects of flavonoids. Fundam. Clin. Pharmacol. **12**: 249–255.

Regulatory Cytokine Gene Polymorphisms and Risk of Colorectal Carcinoma

ANTONINO CRIVELLO,[a,b] ANTONIO GIACALONE,[a,b]
MARINA VAGLICA,[c] LETIZIA SCOLA,[a,b] GIUSI IRMA FORTE,[a,b]
MARIA CATENA MACALUSO,[c] CRISTINA RAIMONDI,[c]
LAURA DI NOTO,[c] ALBERTO BONGIOVANNI,[c] ANGELA ACCARDO,[c]
GIUSEPPINA CANDORE,[b] LAURA PALMERI,[c] ROBERTO VERNA,[d]
CALOGERO CARUSO,[b] DOMENICO LIO,[a,b] AND SERGIO PALMERI[c]

[a]Patologia Clinica, Dipartimento di Biopatologia e Metodologie Biomediche, University of Palermo, Palermo, Italy

[b]Gruppo di Studio sull'Immunosenescenza, Dipartimento di Biopatologia e Metodologie Biomediche, Università di Palermo, Palermo, Italy

[c]U.O Terapie Oncologiche Innovative, Dipartimento di Discipline Chirurgiche e Oncologiche, Università di Palermo, Palermo, Italy

[d]Centro di Ricerca per la Sperimentazione Clinica, Università degli Studidi Roma "La Sapienza," Rome, Italy

ABSTRACT: It is well established that cancer arises in chronically inflamed tissue, and this is particularly notable in the gastrointestinal tract. Classic examples include *Helicobacter pylori*–associated gastric cancer, hepatocellular carcinoma, and inflammatory bowel disease–associated colorectal cancer. Growing evidence suggests that these associations might be not casual findings. Focusing on individual cytokines has generated evidence that anti-inflammatory cytokine interleukin (IL)-10 and transforming growth factor-beta1 (TGF-β1) may have a complex role in gastrointestinal carcinogenesis. As an example, IL-10-deficient mice develop severe atrophic gastritis and a chronic enterocolitis, developing colorectal cancer similar to human inflammatory bowel disease–associated neoplasia. TGF-β1 is a multifunctional signaling molecule with a wide array of roles. Animal experiments suggest that TGF-β1 plays a biphasic role in carcinogenesis by protecting against the early formation of benign epithelial growths, but promoting a significant stimulation of tumor growth invasion and metastasis during tumor progression. We assessed association of functional polymorphisms (−1082G/A;

Address for correspondence: Prof. Domenico Lio, Chair of Clinical Pathology, Immunosenescence Study Group, General Pathology Section, Department of Pathobiology and Biomedical Methodologies, University of Palermo, Corso Tukory 211, 90134 Palermo, Italy. Voice: +39-09-1655-5913; fax: +39-09-1655-5933.
e-mail: dolio@unipa.it

Ann. N.Y. Acad. Sci. 1089: 98–103 (2006). © 2006 New York Academy of Sciences.
doi: 10.1196/annals.1386.002

−592C/A) and TGF-β1 (−509C/T; +869C/T) influencing the IL-10 production to colorectal cancer risk in a case–control study of 62 patients and 124 matched controls. No significant differences were observed among cancer patients and controls for IL-10 −1082G/A; −592C/A genotype frequencies. Evaluation of odds ratios (OR) for the TGF-β1 +869C/T genotypes showed a significant increased risk for individuals bearing +869CC genotype compared to +869CT- and +869TT-positive individuals. These results suggest that the +869C allele, responsible for a Leu→Pro substitution in the signal peptide sequence of the TGF-β1 protein, may have a predisposing role in the development of colorectal cancer.

KEYWORDS: colorectal cancer; gene polymorphisms; TGF-β1; IL-10

INTRODUCTION

Immune response has a significant impact on the potential for malignancy. In particular, it is well established that cancer may arise in chronically inflamed tissue, and this is particularly notable in the gastrointestinal tract.[1-3] The importance of type I inflammatory response, in particular, is also demonstrated by experiments that show that B cell–deficient *Helicobacter*-infected mice are not protected from severe atrophy and metaplasia.[2] In colorectal adenomas and carcinomas, there is a predominance of CD4- and CD3-positive cells.[3] Thus CD4 T lymphocytes and their cytokine products are extremely important in the malignant transformation of chronically inflamed tissue.[4-6] Cytokines play a central role in the regulation of inflammatory response. Focusing on individual cytokines has generated evidence that anti-inflammatory cytokines, such as interleukin (IL)-10 and transforming growth factor-beta1 (TGF-β1), may have a complex role in gastrointestinal carcinogenesis.[5] As an example, IL-10-deficient mice develop severe atrophic gastritis and a chronic enterocolitis, developing colorectal cancer similar to human inflammatory bowel disease–associated neoplasia.[6,7] On the other hand, IL-10 is an immunosuppressive cytokine that may facilitate the development of cancer by supporting tumor escape from the immune response. TGF-β1 is a multifunctional signaling molecule with a wide array of roles.[8,9] Experimental models suggest that TGF-β1 plays a biphasic role in carcinogenesis by not only protecting against the early formation of benign epithelial growths, but also by promoting malignant transformation invasion and metastasis during tumor progression.[10,11]

We typed 62 colorectal cancer cases and 124 age- and sex-matched controls for four main functional polymorphisms of the IL-10 (−1082G/A; −592C/A) and TGF-β1 (−509C/T; +869C/T) genes, influencing level of cytokine production, to assess the association of these SNPs with the susceptibility to colorectal cancer.

MATERIALS AND METHODS

Blood samples from 62 patients were collected at the Department of Oncology and Surgical Disciplines, University of Palermo, where colon cancer diagnosis and grading were clinically assessed. The control group consisted of 124 unrelated age- and sex-matched healthy subjects, recruited in the same geographic area. Written informed consent was obtained from all the subjects according to Italian laws. Genomic DNA was isolated from peripheral blood leukocytes by a standard method using proteinase K digestion followed by standard salting-out technique.[12]

TGF-β1 –509C/T and +869C/T SNPs[13] were investigated by means of the amplification refractory mutation system (ARMS)-PCR technique, using two allele-specific PCR reactions for each SNP per DNA sample.[14] IL-10 –1082G/A and –592C/A SNPs were genotyped as previously described.[14]

Allele and genotype frequencies were analyzed for differences in distribution between patients and healthy controls by means of chi-square exact test with Yates correction. Odds ratio with the 95% confidence interval was obtained using Woolf's approximation method. The obtained P-values were multiplied for the number of possible genotypes of each SNP typed. P-corrected (Pc) < 0.05 was considered the significance limit.

RESULTS AND DISCUSSION

The distribution of genotypes for each polymorphism typed was in agreement with the expected values fitting in the Hardy–Weinberg equation. No significant differences were observed among cancer patients and controls for IL-10 –1082G/A, and –592C/A genotype frequencies (TABLE 1). These data are in agreement with results reported by Macarthur et al.[15] suggesting that investigated IL-10 polymorphisms do not play an important role in susceptibility to colorectal carcinoma. The two SNPs at –1082G→A and –592C→A taken into account are in strong linkage. Thus, the possible haplotypes are: –1082G/–592C, –1082A/–592C, and –1082A/–592A.[16] These haplotypes are associated with differential IL-10 production, as demonstrated by reporter gene assays, although, in some cases, differing results have been described in cells undergoing distinct stimuli.[17] These polymorphisms have been reported in association with development of inflammatory diseases, such as inflammatory bowel diseases,[18] suggesting a role as supporter of inflammation involved in development of colorectal cancer. Thus, larger studies to confirm present data are required.

Similar results were obtained evaluating –509C/T SNP (TABLE 1), which induced a YY1 consensus sequence in a region of the promoter associated with negative transcription regulation,[19] when we analyzed the differences of genotype distribution between cases and healthy controls. On the contrary, the evaluation of +869C/T SNP inducing Leu10pro substitution in TGF-β1 signal

TABLE 1. Percentage of homozygous and heterozygous subjects for the –1082G/A and –592C/A IL-10 and –509C/T TGF-β1 SNPs in 62 patients affected by colorectal carcinoma and in 124 healthy controls

	Genotypes	Patients	Controls	OR (CI 95%)	Pc*
IL-10 1082G/A	–1082GG	12 (19.4)	26 (21.0)	0.90 (0.42–1.94)	ns
	–1082GA	34 (54.8)	60 (48.4)	1.29 (0.70–2.39)	ns
	–1082AA	16 (25.8)	38 (30.6)	0.79 (0.40–1.56)	ns
IL-10 –592C/A	–592CC	31 (50.0)	69 (55.6)	0.80 (0.43–1.47)	ns
	–592CA	28 (45.2)	48 (38.7)	1.30 (0.70–2.42)	ns
	–592AA	3 (4.8)	7 (5.7)	0.85 (0.21–3.41)	ns
TGF-β1 –509C/T	–509CC	19 (30.6)	44 (35.5)	0.80 (0.42–1.54)	ns
	–509CT	29 (46.8)	58 (46.8)	1.00 (0.54–1.84)	ns
	–509TT	14 (22.6)	22 (17.7)	1.35 (0.64–2.87)	ns
TGF-β1 +869C/T	+869CC	35 (56.4)	41 (33.1)	2.62 (1.40–4.91)	0.011
	+869CT	23 (37.1)	61 (49.2)	0.61 (0.33–1.14)	ns
	+869TT	4 (6.5)	22 (17.7)	0.31 (0.11–0.97)	ns

*P-corrected (Pc) value. the obtained P-value was multiplied for the number of the possible genotypes for each SNP.
 TGF-β1 +869C/T genotype distribution was found significantly increased in colorectal cancer patients group compared to the control group 3×2 $Pc = 0.012$.

peptide allowed us to identify a significant increased risk for colon–rectal carcinoma associated with +869CC genotype (TABLE 1). It has been reported that the amount of TGF-β in serum is higher for Pro10 homozygotes than Leu10 homozygotes.[19] So the effect of the Leu10Pro polymorphism on the amount of TGF-β1 secreted *in vivo* might suggest that genetically determined low TGF-β production might be one of the factors involved in the susceptibility for colon rectal cancer. On the other hand, data here presented should be considered preliminary data as the exiguous number of patients studied does not allow haplotype reconstruction for both IL-10 and TGF-β1 SNPs. Haplotypes are actually considered more powerful to detect susceptibility alleles than individual polymorphisms.[20] However, our data suggest that in spite of the well-defined powerful immunoregulatory IL-10 role, TGF-β1 might play a costarring role in the prevention of carcinoma in the colonic–rectal microenvironment.

ACKNOWLEDGMENTS

This work was supported by grants from the Ministry of Education, University and Research, ex 60% to D.L., G.C., C.C., and S.P. A.C. and G.I.F. are Ph.D students at the Pathobiology Ph.D course (directed by C.C.) of Palermo University; this work is in partial fulfillment of the requirement for the Ph.D.

REFERENCES

1. EATON, K.A., M. MEFFORD & T. THEVENOT. 2001. The role of T cell subsets and cytokines in the pathogenesis of *Helicobacter pylori* gastritis in mice. J. Immunol. **166:** 7456–7461.
2. ROTH, K.A. *et al.* 1999. Cellular immune responses are essential for the development of *Helicobacter felis*-associated gastric pathology. J. Immunol. **163:** 1490–1497.
3. JACKSON, P.A. *et al.* 1996. Lymphocyte subset infiltration patterns and HLA antigen status in colorectal carcinomas and adenomas. Gut. **38:** 85–89.
4. LANDI, S. *et al.* 2003. Association of common polymorphisms in inflammatory genes interleukin (IL)6, IL8, tumor necrosis factor α, NFKB1, and peroxisome proliferator-activated receptor γ with colorectal cancer. Cancer Res. **63:** 3560–3566.
5. MACARTHUR, M. *et al.* 2004. Inflammation and cancer. II. Role of chronic inflammation and cytokine gene polymorphisms in the pathogenesis of gastrointestinal malignancy. Am. J. Physiol. Gastrointest. Liver Physiol. **286:** G515–G520.
6. SUTTON, P. *et al.* 2000. Dominant nonresponsiveness to *Helicobacter pylori* infection is associated with production of interleukin 10 but not gamma interferon. Infect. Immun. **68:** 4802–4804.
7. RET, K. *et al.* 1993. Interleukin-10-deficient mice develop chronic enterocolitis. Cell **75:** 263–274.
8. CAPELO, A. 2005. Dual role for TGF-beta1 in apoptosis. Cytokine Growth Factor Rev. **16:** 15–34.
9. GHOSH, J. *et al.* 2005. The role of transforming growth factor beta1 in the vascular system. Cardiovasc. Pathol. **14:** 28–36.
10. LIPTON, L. *et al.* 2003. Germline mutations in the TGF-β and Wnt signalling pathways are a rare cause of the "multiple" adenoma phenotype. J. Med. Genet. **40:** 35–38.
11. BECKER, C., M.C. FANTINI & M.F. NEURATH. 2006. TGF-beta as a T cell regulator in colitis and colon cancer. Cytokine Growth Factor Rev. **17:** 97–106.
12. MILLER, S.A., D.D. DYKES & H.F. POLESKY. 1988. A simple salting out procedure for extracing DNA from human nucleated cells. Nucl. Acid Res. **16:** 1215.
13. GEWALTIG, J. *et al.* 2002. Association of polymorphisms of the transforming growth factor-beta1 gene with the rate of progression of HCV-induced liver fibrosis. Clin. Chim. Acta **316:** 83–94.
14. CRIVELLO, A. *et al.* 2006. Frequency of polymorphisms of signal peptide of TGF-β1 and −1082G/A SNP at the promoter region of IL-10 gene in patients with carotid stenosis. Ann. N.Y. Acad. Sci. **1067:** 288–293.
15. MACARTHUR, M. *et al.* 2005. The role of cytokine gene polymorphisms in colorectal cancer and their interaction with aspirin use in the northeast of Scotland. Cancer Epidemiol. Biomarkers Prev. **14:** 1613–1618.
16. REYNARD, M.P., D. TURNER & C.V. NAVARRETE. 2000. Allele frequencies of polymorphisms of tumor necrosis factor-α, interleukin-2 genes in a North European Caucasoid group from UK. Eur. J. Immunogenet. **27:** 241–249.
17. HOLLEGAARD, M.V. & J.L. BIDWELL. 2006. Cytokine gene polymorphism in human disease: on-line databases, Supplement 3. Genes Immun. **7:** 269–276.
18. TAGORE, A. *et al.* 1999. Interleukin-10 (IL-10) genotypes in inflammatory bowel disease. Tissue Antigens **54:** 386–390.

19. GRAINGER, D.J. *et al.* 1999. Genetic control of the circulating concentration of transforming growth factor type beta1. Hum. Mol. Genet. **8:** 93–97.
20. NEALE, B.M. & P.C. SHAM. 2004. The future of association studies: gene-based analysis and replication. Am. J. Hum. Genet. **75:** 353–362.

Cytokine Gene Polymorphisms and Breast Cancer Susceptibility

LETIZIA SCOLA,[a,b] MARINA VAGLICA,[c] ANTONINO CRIVELLO,[a,b]
LAURA PALMERI,[c] GIUSI IRMA FORTE,[a,b]
MARIA CATENA MACALUSO,[c] ANTONIO GIACALONE,[a,b]
LAURA DI NOTO,[c] ALBERTO BONGIOVANNI,[c] CRISTINA RAIMONDI,[c]
ANGELA ACCARDO,[c] ROBERTO VERNA,[d] GIUSEPPINA CANDORE,[b]
CALOGERO CARUSO,[b] DOMENICO LIO,[a,b] AND SERGIO PALMERI[c]

[a]Patologia Clinica, Departimento di Biopatologia e Metodologie Biomediche, Università di Palermo, Palermo, Italy

[b]Gruppo di Studio sull'Immunosenescenza-Dipartimento di Biopatologia e Metodologie Biomediche, Università di Palermo, Palermo, Italy

[c]U.O Terapie Oncologiche Innovative, Dipartimento di Discipline Chirurgiche e Oncologiche, Università di Palermo, Palermo, Italy

[d]Centro di ricerca per la sperimentazione clinica, Università degli Studidi Roma "La Sapienza" Rome, Italy

ABSTRACT: Human breast cancer (BC) is characterized by a considerable clinical heterogeneity. Steroid hormone receptor expression and growth factor receptor expression have been considered suitable diagnostic and prognostic markers, whereas mutations of oncosuppressor and gatekeeper genes have been found associated with an increased risk for this malignancy. To evaluate the role that polymorphisms of genes involved in the regulation of inflammatory response might play in BC susceptibility, we investigated associations between cytokine functionally relevant polymorphisms in 84 BC patients compared to 110 age- and sex-matched controls. TNF-α (-308G/A), TGF-β1 (+869C/T), IL-10 (−1117G/A; −854C/T; −627C/A), and IFN-γ (874T/A) single nucleotide polymorphisms (SNPs) were identified by sequence-specific primers (SSP)-PCR or restriction fragment length polymorphism (RFLP)-PCR. Genotype or haplotype distributions for each polymorphisms were consistent with the HWE in these populations. We were unable to demonstrate differences in genotype or allele frequencies between patient and control groups. Data obtained in this study indicate that none of the cytokine SNPs studied is likely to have

Address for correspondence: Prof. Domenico Lio, Chair of Clinical Pathology, Immunosenescence Study Group, General Pathology Section, Department of Pathobiology and Biomedical Methodologies, University of Palermo, Corso Tukory 211, 90134 Palermo, Italy. Voice: +39-09-1655-5913; fax. +39-09-1655-5933.

e-mail: dolio@unipa.it

Ann. N.Y. Acad. Sci. 1089: 104–109 (2006). © 2006 New York Academy of Sciences.
doi: 10.1196/annals.1386.017

predisposing or protective effects on BC susceptibility. On the other hand, both positive and negative association with BC have been reported for some of the studied genotypes by different research groups. In conclusion, further studies involving larger numbers of subjects are required.

KEYWORDS: breast cancer; cytokine polymorphisms; susceptibility

INTRODUCTION

The clinical features of human breast cancer (BC) are characterized by a considerable heterogeneity. Biological markers as steroid hormone receptor expression, angiogenesis, cell proliferation, and cytokine production regulation have been found associated with differences in development and clinical course of this malignancy.[1] Some single nucleotide polymorphisms (SNPs) in nontranscribing region of cytokine genes, as $-308G/A$ of TNF-α, or the IL-10 promoter region haplotypes composed by $-1117G/A$, $-819C/T$, and $-627C/A$ SNPs, or the intronic $+874T/A$ SNP of IFN-γ gene, may influence a differential production of the respective cytokine, modifying affinity of regulatory elements to transcription factors.[2] Other SNPs as the $+869$ C/T (Leu10Pro) of the TGF-β1 gene modify the sequence of critical elements in protein sequence, as the so-called signal peptide of the TGF-β1,[3] influencing cytokine production. These polymorphisms have been investigated by different research groups considering that a genetic regulation of cytokine production might play a role in cancer susceptibility.[3–5] Here are reported the genotype frequencies of some cytokine functional polymorphisms evaluated in a group of patients affected by BC compared to sex- and age-matched control.

MATERIALS AND METHODS

Eighty-four women with BC were recruited from the Department of Oncologic and Surgical Disciplines at the University of Palermo. The control group consisted of 226 unrelated sex- and age-matched healthy subjects, recruited in the same geographic area. The DNA was extracted with the salting out technique. Cytokine polymorphisms were identified by sequence-specific primers or RFLP-PCR. The three Caucasian haplotypes composed by $-854C/T$, $-627C/A$, and $-1117G/A$ IL-10 SNP[6] were identified using the haplotype-specific typing method described by Koss *et al.*[7] The Leu10Pro polymorphism was analyzed by SSP-PCR methodology employing two primers sense-specific for $+869T$ and $+869C$, a primer antisense common to two alleles according to Gewaltig *et al.*[8] $+874T/A$ IFN-γ alleles were identified using the amplification refractory mutation system methodology described by Pravica *et al.*[9] In the TNF-α promoter region, -308G/A SNP

TABLE 1. Genotype frequencies (percentage) of haplotypes obtained by combination of polymorphisms −627C/A, −854C/T, and −1117G/A of IL-10 gene and +869C/T, TGF-β1, +874T/A IFN-γ, −308G/A, and TNF-α SNPs in a group of patients with BC and in a group of control women

		Patients N = 84	Controls N = 106
	GCC/GCC	16 (19.05)	21 (19.81)
	GCC/ACC	24 (28.57)	24 (22.64)
IL-10	GCC/ATA	16 (19.05)	21 (19.81)
−1117G/A	ACC/ACC	9 (10.71)	14 (13.21)
−854C/T haplotypes	ACC/ATA	14 (16.67)	14 (13.21)
−627C/A	ATA/ATA	5 (5.95)	12 (11.32)
	+869CC	41 (48.81)	35 (33.02)
TGF-β1	+869CT	27 (32.14)	52 (49.06)
+869C/T	+869TT	16 (19.05)	19 (17.92)
	+874TT	30 (35.71)	39 (36.79)
IFN-γ	+874TA	29 (34.52)	38 (35.84)
+874T/A	+874AA	25 (29.76)	29 (27.36)
	−308GG	71 (84.52)	79 (74.53)
TNF-α	−308GA	12 (14.29)	26 (24.53)
−308G/A	−308AA	1 (1.19)	1 (0.94)

was performed as described by Lio et al.[10] Comparisons were made among individual genotype frequencies and genotype distributions in the patient group and in the control population, using 2×2 and 2×3 contingency tables and χ^2 analysis.

RESULTS

Clinical and biological characteristics of the patient were analyzed, evaluating estrogen and progesterone receptor status, lymph node involvement, and tumor size. No associations were found among cytokine polymorphisms and clinical status or grading (data not shown). The genotype distributions for each polymorphism were consistent with the HWE in both the populations. TABLE 1 shows the genotype and haplotype frequencies of cytokine regulatory SNPs in BC patients and healthy controls.

As reported by Eskdale et al.,[6] −854C/T and −627C/A IL-10 SNPs are in tight linkage, the linkage of allele −854C with allele −627C and of allele −854T with allele −627A, and the presence of only three different allele combinations of −1117G/A, −854C/T, and −627C/A allows identification of the GCC, ACC, and ATA haplotypes in Caucasians. No significant differences were observed among haplotype combination frequencies in patient versus control groups. Similar results were obtained evaluating +874T/A SNP at the first intron of IFN-γ genes, +869C/T (Leu10Pro) TGF-β1, and −308G/A SNP at TNFA gene regulatory region.

DISCUSSION

Both tumor and free stromal cells are able to produce cytokines that seem to affect the complex phenomena occurring at the tumor–host interface, thus leading to tumor invasion.[11] Serum levels of many cytokines have been measured in patients with tumors. In particular, abnormal circulating levels or mRNA of IL-10 were observed in ovarian cancer, prostate carcinoma, and BC patients.[12–15] The concentration of circulating IL-10 correlated with the severity of BC as reported by Merendino *et al.*[15] IL-10 has been demonstrated to affect macrophage functions in different ways, weakening and turning off tumor-associated inflammation. The studies on genetic regulation of IL-10 production in patients affected by BC show disagreement between different distributions of IL-10 −1117G/A SNPs in both control and patient populations. We investigated the above-cited polymorphism and IL-10, −854C/T, −627C/A SNPs, in linkage with −1117G/A SNP.[6]

We observed a nonsignificant association between haplotype combination of IL-10 SNPs, as identified by Eskdale *et al.*,[6] and the risk of BC. Thus, our data are at variance with those described by Giordani *et al.*[16] on a population of BC patients of Southern Italy, and so are not clear on the role of IL-10 SNPs studied in susceptibility to BC. We also investigated the polymorphism Leu10Pro of TGF-β1 signaling peptide, extensively described in genetic BC studies. Two large contrasting findings associate the Pro/Pro phenotype with a 64% decreased[17] and 21% increased[18] BC risk. Our data appear to conflict with both large studies, showing nonassociation with TGF-β1 Leu10Pro SNP. On the other hand, our data are confirmed by a large study in Germany.[19]

IFN-γ is a member of a family of cytokines with immunomodulatory and antiproliferative activity. This activity is observed in murine model and *in vitro* on breast tumor–derived cell lines.[20,21] Nevertheless, nonassociation was demonstrated when we investigated the possible correlation of IFN-γ +874T/A SNP with susceptibility to BC.

As well known, TNF-α causes cytolysis and cytostasis of BC cell lines and hemorrhagic necrosis of transplanted tumors.[22] It also mediates IL-1-induced upregulation of HLA class II and is involved in apoptotic pathways. Tumors infiltrating lymphocytes and cells of tumor stroma are able to produce TNF-α.[23] On the other hand, both positive and negative association with BC have been reported for −308G/A genotypes by different research groups.[22,24] The limited sample size characterizing our and other studies could be an important factor explaining the variability among different results obtained for cytokine polymorphisms in the evaluation of susceptibility factors for BC.

In conclusion, further studies are required above all with larger cohorts of patients, before definitive conclusions can be drawn.

ACKNOWLEDGMENTS

This work was supported by grants from the Ministry of Education, University and Research, ex 60% to D.L., G.C., C.C. and S.P. A.C. and G.I.F. are Ph.D. students at Pathobiology Ph.D. course (directed by C.C.) of Palermo University and this work is in partial fulfillment of the requirement for the Ph.D.

REFERENCES

1. LOKTIONOV, A. 2004. Common gene polymorphisms, cancer progression and prognosis. Cancer Lett. **208:** 1–33.
2. BIDWELL, J. *et al.* 1999. Cytokine gene polymorphism in human disease: on-line databases. Genes Immun. **1:** 3–19.
3. DUNNING, A.M. *et al.* 2003. A transforming growth factor beta1 signal peptide variant increases secretion in vitro and is associated with increased incidence of invasive breast cancer. Cancer Res. **63:** 2610–2615.
4. KAMALI-SARVESTANI, E., A. MERAT & A.-R. TALEI. 2005. Polymorphism in the genes of alpha and beta tumor necrosis factors (TNF-α and TNF-β) and gamma interferon (IFN-γ) among Iranian women with breast cancer. Cancer Lett. **223:** 113–119.
5. FORTIS, C. *et al.* 1996. Increased interleukin-10 serum levels in patients with solid tumours. Cancer Lett. **104:** 1–5.
6. ESKDALE, J. *et al.* 1999. Microsatellite alleles and single nucleotide polymorphisms (SNP) combine to form four major haplotype families at the human interleukin-10 (IL-10) locus. Genes Immun. **1:** 151–155.
7. KOSS, K. *et al.* 2000. Interleukin-10 gene promoter polymorphism in English and Polish healthy controls. Polymerase chain reaction haplotyping using 3′ mismatches in forward and reverse primers. Genes Immun. **1:** 321–324.
8. GEWALTIG, J. *et al.* 2002. Association of polymorphisms of the transforming growth factor-beta1 gene with the rate of progression of HCV-induced liver fibrosis. Clin. Chim. Acta **316:** 83–94.
9. PRAVICA, V. *et al.* 2000. A single nucleotide polymorphism in the first intron of the human IFN-gamma gene: absolute correlation with a polymorphic CA microsatellite marker of high IFN-gamma production. Human Immunol. **61:** 863–866.
10. LIO, D. *et al.* 2006. Tumor necrosis factor-alpha -308A/G polymorphism is associated with age at onset of Alzheimer's disease. Mech. Age. Dev. **127:** 567–571.
11. COUSSENS, L.M. & Z. WERB. 2002. Inflammation and cancer. Nature **420:** 860–867.
12. PISA, P. *et al.* 1992. Selective expression of interleukin 10, interferon gamma, and granulocyte-macrophage colony-stimulating factor in ovarian cancer biopsies. Proc. Natl. Acad. Sci. USA **89:** 7708–7712.

13. MAFFEZZINI, M., A. LIMONATO & C. FORTIS. 1996. Salvage immunotherapy with subcutaneous recombinant interleukin 2 (rIL-2) and alpha-interferon (A-IFN) for stage D3 prostate carcinoma failing second-line hormonal treatment. Prostate **28:** 282–286.
14. YAMAMURA, M. *et al.* 1993. Local expression of antiinflammatory cytokines in cancer. J. Clin. Invest. **91:** 1005–1010.
15. MERENDINO, R.A. *et al.* 1996. Serum levels of interleukin-10 in patients affected by breast cancer. Immunol. Lett. **53:** 59–60.
16. GIORDANI, L. *et al.* 2003. Association of breast cancer and polymorphisms of interleukin-10 and tumor necrosis factor-alpha genes. Clin. Chem. Acta **49:** 1664–1667.
17. ZIV, E. *et al.* 2001. Association between the T29→C polymorphism in the transforming growth factor h1 gene and breast cancer among elderly white women: the study of osteoporotic fractures. JAMA **285:** 2859–2863.
18. KAKLAMANI, V.G. *et al.* 2005. Combined genetic assessment of transforming growth factor-B signaling pathway variants may predict breast cancer risk. Cancer Res. **65:** 3454–3461.
19. KRIPPL, P. *et al.* 2003. The L10P polymorphism of the transforming growth factor-β1 gene is not associated with breast cancer risk. Cancer Lett. **201:** 181–184.
20. KIRCHHOFF, S. & H. HAUSER. 1999. Cooperative activity between HER oncogenes and the tumor suppressor IRF-1 results in apoptosis. Oncogene **18:** 3725–3736.
21. RUIZ-RUIZ, C., C. MUNOZ-PINEDO & A. LOPEZ-RIVAS. 2000. Interferon-gamma treatment elevates caspase-8 expression and sensitises human breast tumor cells to a death receptor-induced mitochondria-operated apoptotic program. Cancer Res. **60:** 5673–5680.
22. SMITH, K.C. *et al.* 2004. Cytokine gene polymorphisms and breast cancer susceptibility and prognosis. Eur. J. Immunogenet. **31:** 167–173.
23. LIND, D.S. *et al.* 1993. Expansion of tumor specific cytokine secretion of bryostatin-activated T-cells from cryopreserved axillary lymph nodes of breast cancer patients. Surg. Oncol. **2:** 273–282.
24. AZMY, I.A. *et al.* 2004. Role of tumour necrosis factor gene polymorphisms (−308 and −238) in breast cancer susceptibility and severity. Breast Cancer Res. **6:** 395–400.

Adjuvant Diet to Improve Hormonal and Metabolic Factors Affecting Breast Cancer Prognosis

FRANCO BERRINO, ANNA VILLARINI, MICHELA DE PETRIS, MILENA RAIMONDI, AND PATRIZIA PASANISI

Department of Preventive and Predictive Medicine, Istituto Nazionale Tumori, Via Venezian 1, 20133, Milan, Italy

ABSTRACT: **Western lifestyle, characterized by reduced physical activity and a diet rich in fat, refined carbohydrates, and animal protein is associated with high prevalence of overweight, metabolic syndrome, insulin resistance, and high plasma levels of several growth factors and sex hormones. Most of these factors are associated with breast cancer risk and, in breast cancer patients, with increased risk of recurrences. Recent trials have proven that such a metabolic and endocrine imbalance can be favorably modified through comprehensive dietary modification, shifting from Western to Mediterranean and macrobiotic diet.**

KEYWORDS: **breast cancer; hormonal and metabolic factors; diet**

METABOLIC, ENDOCRINE, AND DIETARY CORRELATES OF INCREASED BREAST CANCER

The metabolic, endocrine, and dietary correlates of increased breast cancer risk and of increased risk of recurrence in breast cancer patients are summarized in FIGURE 1.

Overweight and obesity are associated with an increased risk of breast cancer after menopause.[1,2] The association decreases markedly when adjusted for serum levels of endogenous estrogens,[3] suggesting that most of the effect of overweight is due to the aromatization of androgens into estrogens in the adipose tissue. Epidemiological studies of breast cancer and obesity showed either no association or slightly reduced breast cancer risk before menopause.[2] The reason for this paradoxical effect is not clear. As menstrual cycles in obese premenopausal women are frequently anovulatory, it has been hypothesized that the lack of endogenous progesterone production could be responsible for

Address for correspondence: Franco Berrino, Department of Preventive and Predictive Medicine, Istituto Nazionale Tumori, Via Venezian, 1, 20133, Milan, Italy. Voice: +39-02-23903515; fax: +39-02-23903516.

e-mail: berrino@istitutotumori.mi.it

Ann. N.Y. Acad. Sci. 1089: 110–118 (2006). © 2006 New York Academy of Sciences.
doi: 10.1196/annals.1386.023

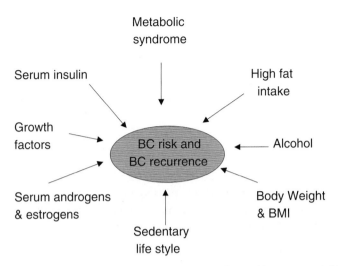

FIGURE 1. Hormonal, metabolic, and dietary correlates of breast cancer risk and recurrences.

the increased risk.[4] This hypothesis, however, has been shown to be false by the results of prospective studies showing that high endogenous progesterone levels are associated with significantly decreased breast cancer risk.[5,6] Anovulatory cycles are characterized by lower levels of both progesterone and estrogens, but studies measuring estrogens before menopause have not been able to find any clear association with the risk of breast cancer. Also, women who were overweight at the age of menarche experience a lower breast cancer risk in adulthood, independent of menstrual cycle characteristics.[7] Even if associated with early menarche, a moderate risk factor for breast cancer, early overweight might reflect well-functioning ovaries stimulating early breast epithelial cell differentiation. Preventing weight gain in adulthood, however, would decrease the overall burden of breast cancer,[8] as well as other "Western" diseases and premature mortality. Obese breast cancer patients appear to have a higher risk of lymph node metastasis and larger tumors, and many observational studies showed that, after adjustment for disease stage, overweight is associated with poorer prognosis.[9,10] Several studies, in particular, showed that weight gain in the course of adjuvant chemotherapy is a negative prognostic factor.[11–13]

Epidemiological studies consistently showed that a sedentary lifestyle is associated with increased risk of breast cancer, both before and after menopause.[1] Women who practice regularly at least some physical activity decrease their breast cancer risk by 30% or more.[1] There is evidence that physical activity may also protect against cancer recurrence. Daily physical activity corresponding to about half an hour of brisk walking may reduce breast cancer recurrences by 50%. More intense activity does not seem to add any benefit.[14]

Prospective studies with biological repositories have proven beyond reasonable doubt that the endogenous levels of serum sex hormones are associated with breast cancer risk. After menopause high serum levels of both estrogens and androgens predict the risk of breast cancer.[15,16] Women in the upper quintile of estradiol or testosterone showed the risk of breast cancer to be 2 to 3 times higher than women in the lower quintile, and the risk of androgens persisted after adjustment for estrogens and *vice versa*. Before menopause, the hormonal pattern at high risk of breast cancer is characterized by high serum levels of androgens and low levels of progesterone in the luteal phase of the menstrual cycle.[5,6] The risk of breast cancer in women with increased androgenic activity and luteal insufficiency may increase by 3 to 7 times.[6] Premenopausal estrogen levels do not seem associated with a subsequent risk of breast cancer, either because a single blood sample, as used in these prospective studies, may be insufficient to properly classify the hormonal pattern of premenopausal women, or because any level of estrogens, before menopause, is sufficiently high to promote breast cancer growth. Estrogen levels capable of promoting breast cancer after menopause, in fact, are still one order of magnitude lower than normal premenopausal levels. A recent prospective study, however, suggested that premenopausal breast cancer risk is associated with high serum levels of estrogens in the early follicular phase.[49] The role of estrogens in sustaining breast cancer cell proliferation, moreover, is clearly demonstrated by the efficacy of anti-estrogen therapies for treating and preventing recurrences.[17] Also, androgens proved to be strong predictors of recurrence. Patients with localized breast cancer with high testosterone levels show an increased risk of metastasis, local recurrence, and contralateral breast cancer.[18] Serum estradiol was also associated with recurrences, but the association became insignificant upon adjustment for testosterone.[18] Measuring testosterone levels, therefore, seems to be the most parsimonious endocrine examination to select women at high risk of breast cancer or patients at high risk of recurrence. Consistent with the elevation in risk by increasing endogenous testosterone level, women using estrogen plus testosterone therapies for menopausal symptoms have a significantly greater risk of invasive breast cancer than do women using estrogen only.[19]

Besides the synthesis of estrogens and androgens in the adipose tissue the association of obesity with breast cancer may be mediated by insulin resistance. Several epidemiological studies inconsistently showed an association between serum insulin or C-peptide and the risk of breast cancer.[20,21] This association is quite clear after menopause, while in young women it seems to be in the opposite direction.[22] Elevated serum insulin levels, however, are associated with an increased risk of recurrences in breast cancer patients.[23] IGF (insulin-like growth factor)-I is also likely to be involved in breast cancer incidence and prognosis. Several prospective cohort studies have suggested a strong association, especially for young premenopausal women.[24-28] (Some studies, however, failed to confirm such a strong association in young women).[29,30]

Insulin resistance and hyperinsulinemia are a feature of the so-called metabolic syndrome, defined by at least three of five metabolic factors, each of which has been found to be associated with breast cancer incidence: high plasma levels of glucose (>110 mg/100 mL), [26] high levels of triglycerides (>150 mg/100 mL),[31] low levels of HDL cholesterol (<50 mg/100 mL),[32] large waist circumference (>88 cm),[33] and hypertension (SBP > 130 mmHg or DBP >85 mmHg).[34] We examined the presence of metabolic syndrome in breast cancer patients and found that patients with metabolic syndrome have the worst prognosis, especially if it is associated with increased androgenic activity.[35]

The relationship between fat consumption and breast cancer risk is a highly controversial subject: several case–control studies suggested an association, but most prospective cohort studies did not. The WHI (Women's Health Initiative) randomized trial of dietary prevention, however, showed a borderline significant 9% decrease in breast cancer incidence in the low-fat arm.[36] Subgroup analyses showed a larger and significant effect in women characterized by high fat consumption at baseline, high white blood cell count, large waist circumference, hypertension, or diabetes, suggesting that women with markers of metabolic syndrome may be more likely to gain an advantage by dietary fat restriction. On the other hand, most observational studies analyzing the prognostic association of fat consumption at the time of diagnosis have found that fat intake negatively affects prognosis,[9] especially total and saturated fat,[37] whereas omega-3 might be protective.[38] Only a few observational studies considered the effect of diet after diagnosis with inconsistent results.[38] The WINS (Women's Initiative on Nutrition Study) randomized trial, however, showed that reducing fat consumption down to about 20% of calories significantly decreased the occurrence of recurrences by 22%.[39]

Most of the effect was due to the reduction of recurrences in estrogen receptor (ER)–negative patients, possibly because ER-positive patients were treated with tamoxifen, which may have conferred all the achievable preventive effect.

The consumption of alcoholic beverages has been consistently found to be associated with increased risk of breast cancer.[40] Only a few studies, however, examined its association with breast cancer prognosis, without significant associations with survival.[9]

MECHANISTIC CONSIDERATIONS

Various mechanisms by which diet and lifestyle may promote increased risk for and progression of breast cancer have been previously reviewed.[1,20,41] In short, sedentary lifestyle, overweight, and a fat-rich diet are major determinants of metabolic syndrome, which in turn is associated with insulin resistance and increased androgenic activity. Physical activity improves insulin sensitivity and decreases testosterone levels, and in the long term, IGF-I levels. Insulin

TABLE 1. DIANA-1: Hormonal changes after 5 months of diet in healthy postmenopausal women

	Change (%)	P		Change (%)	P
Testosterone	−18	**	Glucose	−6	*
Estradiol	−18	ns	Insulin	−10	ns
Free testosterone	−29	**	Insulin area	−8	*
Free estradiol	−23	*	C-peptide	−19	*
SHBG	+25	**	IGF-I	−6	ns
Triglycerides	−1	ns	IGFBP-1	+12	**
Total cholesterol	−14	**	IGFBP-2	+30	**
BMI	−6	**	Waist	−5	**

Note: See Berrino et al.[44] and Kaaks et al.[45]
*P < 0.05.
**P < 0.01

stimulates the synthesis of androgens in the ovary and the expression of GH receptors, and inhibits the liver production of SHBG and IGFBP1 and 2, thus increasing the bioavailability of both sex hormones and IGF-I. IGF-I is increased by a diet rich in protein, in particular, milk protein.[42] Alcohol intake increases the synthesis of androgens and estrogens.[43] Postmenopausal overweight is associated with increased peripheral conversion of androgens into estrogens, decreased SHBG, and increased insulin levels. A newer hypothesis suggests a critical role for the adipocyte production of adipokines, which may affect tumorigenesis through the upregulation of genes involved in proliferation, invasion, and metastasis.

THE DIANA STUDIES

The DIANA (DIet and ANdrogens) intervention trials demonstrated that a sustainable dietary modification aimed at lowering insulin levels, based on Mediterranean and macrobiotic dietary principles, can reduce body weight,

TABLE 2. DIANA-2: Hormonal changes after 12 months of diet in breast cancer patients

	Change (%)	P		Change (%)	P
Testosterone	−10	*	Glucose	−5	*
Estradiol	−6	*	Insulin	−17	*
SHBG	+5	*	IGF-I	−4	ns
Triglycerides	−14	*	PDGF	−38	**
Total cholesterol	−11	*	Systolic BP	−1	*
BMI	−5	**	Waist	−4	**

Note: Berrino et al.[18] and unpublished material.
*P < 0.05.
**P < 0.01.

metabolic syndrome, and the bioavailability of sex hormones and growth factors.[18,44,45] TABLES 1 and 2 summarize the results of these trials, showing the percentage of change in several metabolic and endocrine parameters after 5 months and 12 months, respectively, of dietary intervention. The prevalence of metabolic syndrome also decreased significantly. As a consequence of the highly satiating diet, women lost weight (about 4 kg) in both these studies. Part of the metabolic effects could have been just a consequence of this weight loss. Interestingly, however, the participating women lost weight just by changing the composition of the diet, without any recommendation to eat less. Together with other studies showing that a Mediterranean diet can reverse metabolic syndrome,[46,47] these results suggest that there is room for proposing adjuvant dietary changes both for breast cancer prevention and treatment. Patients with metabolic syndrome and high serum levels of testosterone, in particular, should be advised to modify their diet and to increase physical activity. Testosterone levels above 0.4 ng/mL (the upper tertile in our study populations) are associated with a significant increased risk. The prevalence of metabolic syndrome in adult Western populations ranges from 2 to 3% at 25 years of age to 25% above 70 years.[48] Metabolic screening for these two variables may identify subgroups of women and of breast cancer patients likely to benefit from dietary counselling.

DIETARY RECOMMENDATIONS FOR BREAST CANCER PATIENTS

At present our recommendations include:

1. Reduce calorie intake, through the preferred consumption of highly satiating foods, such as unrefined cereals, legumes, and vegetables.
2. Reduce high glycemic index and high insulinemic index food, such as refined flours, potatoes, white rice, corn flakes, sugar, and milk, using instead whole grain cereals (unrefined rice, barley, millet, oat, buckwheat, spelt, quinoa), legumes (any type, including soy products), and vegetables (any type, except potatoes).
3. Reduce sources of saturated fat (red and processed meat, milk, and dairy products) preferring instead unrefined vegetable fats, such as olive oil, nuts, and oleaginous seeds.
4. Reduce protein intake, mainly animal proteins (except fish).

REFERENCES

1. VAINIO, H. & F. BIANCHINI. 2002. Weight Control and Physical Activity, **Vol 6.**: IARC Handbooks of Cancer Prevention. Lyon, France.

2. LAHMANN, P.H., K. HOFFMANN, N. ALLEN et al. 2004. Body size and breast cancer risk: findings from the European Prospective Investigation into Cancer and Nutrition (EPIC). Intl. J. Cancer. **111:** 762–771.
3. KEY, T.J., P.N. APPLEBY, G.K. REEVES et al. 2003. Body mass index, serum sex hormones, and breast cancer risk in postmenopausal women. J. Natl. Cancer Inst. **95:** 1218–1226.
4. KEY, T.J. & M.C. PIKE. 1988. The role of oestrogens and progestagens in the epidemiology and prevention of breast cancer. Eur. J. Cancer Clin. Oncol. **24:** 29–43.
5. KAAKS, R., F. BERRINO, T. KEY, et al. 2005. Serum sex steroids in premenopausal women and breast cancer risk within the European Prospective Investigation into Cancer and Nutrition (EPIC). J. Natl. Cancer Inst. **97:** 755–765.
6. MICHELI, A., P. MUTI, G. SECRETO et al. 2004. Endogenous sex hormones and subsequent breast cancer in premenopausal women. Intl. J. Cancer **112:** 312–318.
7. BAER, H.J., G.A. COLDITZ, B. ROSNER, et al. 2005. Body fatness during childhood and adolescence and incidence of breast cancer in premenopausal women: a prospective cohort study. Breast Cancer Res. **7:** R314–R325.
8. LAHMANN, P.H., M. SCHULZ, K. HOFFMANN et al. 2005. Long-term weight change and breast cancer risk: the European prospective investigation into cancer and nutrition (EPIC). Br. J. Cancer **93:** 582–589.
9. ROCK, C.L. & W. DEMARK-WAHNEFRIED. 2002. Nutrition and survival after the diagnosis of breast cancer: a review of the evidence. J. Clin. Oncol. **20:** 3302–3316.
10. BERCLAZ, G., S. LI, K.N. PRICE et al. 2004. Body mass index as a prognostic feature in operable breast cancer: the International Breast Cancer Study Group experience. Ann. Oncol. **15:** 875–884.
11. CAMORIANO, J.K., C.L. LOPRINZI, J.N. INGLE, et al. 1990. Weight change in women treated with adjuvant therapy or observed following mastectomy for node-positive breast cancer. J. Clin. Oncol. **8:** 1327–1334.
12. KROENKE, C.H., W.Y. CHEN, B. ROSNER, M.D. HOLMES. 2005. Weight, weight gain, and survival after breast cancer diagnosis. J. Clin. Oncol. **23:** 1370–1378.
13. CHLEBOWSKI, R.T., J.M. WEINER, R. REYNOLDS, et al. 1986. Long-term survival following relapse after 5-FU but not CMF adjuvant breast cancer therapy. Breast Cancer Res. Treat. **7:** 23–30.
14. HOLMES, M.D., W.Y. CHEN, D. FESKANICH, et al. 2005. Physical activity and survival after breast cancer diagnosis. JAMA. **293:** 2479–2486.
15. KEY, T., P. APPLEBY, I. BARNES & G. REEVES. 2002. Endogenous sex hormones and breast cancer in postmenopausal women: reanalysis of nine prospective studies. J. Natl. Cancer Inst. **94:** 606–616.
16. KAAKS, R., S. RINALDI, T.J. KEY et al. 2005. Postmenopausal serum androgens, oestrogens and breast cancer risk: the European prospective investigation into cancer and nutrition. Endocr. Relat. Cancer **12:** 1071–1082.
17. ROY, V. & E.A. PEREZ. 2006. New therapies in the treatment of breast cancer. Semin. Oncol. **33:** S3–S8.
18. BERRINO, F., P. PASANISI, C. BELLATI, et al. 2005. Serum testosterone levels and breast cancer recurrence. Int. J. Cancer. **113:** 499–502.
19. TAMIMI, R.M., S.E. HANKINSON, W.Y. CHEN, et al. 2006. Combined estrogen and testosterone use and risk of breast cancer in postmenopausal women. Arch. Intern. Med. **166:** 1483–1489.

20. KAAKS, R. 1996. Nutrition, hormones, and breast cancer: is insulin the missing link? Cancer Causes Control. **7:** 605–625.

21. BRUNING, P.F., J.M. BONFRER, P.A. VAN NOORD, *et al.* 1992. Insulin resistance and breast-cancer risk. Int. J. Cancer **52:** 511–516.

22. VERHEUS, M., P.H. PEETERS, S. RINALDI *et al.* 2006. Serum C-peptide levels and breast cancer risk: results from the European prospective investigation into cancer and nutrition (EPIC). Int. J. Cancer. **119:** 659–667.

23. GOODWIN, P.J., M. ENNIS, K.I. PRITCHARD *et al.* 2002. Fasting insulin and outcome in early-stage breast cancer: results of a prospective cohort study. J. Clin. Oncol. **20:** 42–51.

24. HANKINSON, S.E., W.C. WILLETT, G.A. COLDITZ *et al.* 1998. Circulating concentrations of insulin-like growth factor-I and risk of breast cancer. Lancet **351:** 1393–1396.

25. TONIOLO, P., P.F. BRUNING, A. AKHMEDKHANOV *et al.* 2000. Serum insulin-like growth factor-I and breast cancer. Intl. J. Cancer. **88:** 828–832.

26. MUTI, P., T. QUATTRIN, B.J. GRANT *et al.* 2002. Fasting glucose is a risk factor for breast cancer: a prospective study. Cancer Epidemiol. Biomarkers Prev. **11:** 1361–1368.

27. ALLEN, N.E., A.W. RODDAM, D.S. ALLEN, *et al.* 2005. A prospective study of serum insulin-like growth factor-I (IGF-I), IGF-II, IGF-binding protein-3 and breast cancer risk. Br. J. Cancer. **92:** 1283–1287.

28. ROLLISON, D.E., C.J. NEWSCHAFFER, Y. TAO, *et al.* 2006. Premenopausal levels of circulating insulin-like growth factor I and the risk of postmenopausal breast cancer. Int. J. Cancer. **118:** 1279–1284.

29. RINALDI, S., P. TONIOLO, P. MUTI, *et al.* 2005. IGF-I, IGFBP-3 and breast cancer in young women: a pooled re-analysis of three prospective studies. Eur. J. Cancer Prev. **14:** 493–496.

30. SCHERNHAMMER, E.S., J.M. HOLLY, D.J. HUNTER, *et al.* 2006. Insulin-like growth factor-I, its binding proteins (IGFBP-1 and IGFBP-3), and growth hormone and breast cancer risk in The Nurses Health Study II. Endocr. Relat. Cancer. **13:** 583–592.

31. GOODWIN, P.J., N.F. BOYD, W. HANNA, *et al.* 1997. Elevated levels of plasma triglycerides are associated with histologically defined premenopausal breast cancer risk. Nutr. Cancer **27:** 284–292.

32. FURBERG, A.S., M.B. VEIEROD, T. WILSGAARD, *et al.* 2004. Serum high-density lipoprotein cholesterol, metabolic profile, and breast cancer risk. J. Natl. Cancer Inst. **96:** 1152–1160.

33. CONNOLLY, B.S., C. BARNETT, K.N. VOGT, *et al.* 2002. A meta-analysis of published literature on waist-to-hip ratio and risk of breast cancer. Nutr. Cancer. **44:** 127–138.

34. SOLER, M., L. CHATENOUD, E. NEGRI, *et al.* 1999. Hypertension and hormone-related neoplasms in women. Hypertension **34:** 320–325.

35. PASANISI, P., F. BERRINO, M. DE PETRIS, *et al.* 2006. Metabolic syndrome as a prognostic factor for breast cancer recurrences. Intl. J. Cancer **119:** 236–238.

36. PRENTICE, R.L., B. CAAN, R.T. CHLEBOWSKI *et al.* 2006. Low-fat dietary pattern and risk of invasive breast cancer: the Women's Health Initiative Randomized Controlled Dietary Modification Trial. JAMA **295:** 629–642.

37. HOLM, L.E., E. NORDEVANG, M.L. HJALMAR, *et al.* 1993. Treatment failure and dietary habits in women with breast cancer. J. Natl. Cancer Inst. **85:** 32–36.

38. HOLMES, M.D., M.J. STAMPFER, G.A. COLDITZ, *et al.* 1999. Dietary factors and the survival of women with breast carcinoma. Cancer **86:** 826–835.
39. CHLEBOWSKI, R.T., G.L. BLACKBURN, R.E. ELASHOFF, *et al.* 2005. Dietary fat reduction in postmenopausal women with primary breast cancer: Phase, III Women's Intervention Nutrition Study (WINS) [abstract]. J. Clin. Oncol. **23:**.
40. HAMAJIMA, N., K. HIROSE, K. TAJIMA *et al.* 2002. Alcohol, tobacco and breast cancer–collaborative reanalysis of individual data from 53 epidemiological studies, including 58,515 women with breast cancer and 95,067 women without the disease. Br. J. Cancer. **87:** 1234–1245.
41. LORINCZ, A.M. & S. SUKUMAR. 2006. Molecular links between obesity and breast cancer. Endocr. Relat. Cancer. **13:** 279–292.
42. NORAT, T., L. DOSSUS, S. RINALDI *et al.* 2006. Diet, serum insulin-like growth factor-I and IGF-binding protein-3 in European women. Eur. J. Clin. Nutr.
43. RINALDI, S., P.H. PEETERS, I.D. BEZEMER *et al.* 2006. Relationship of alcohol intake and sex steroid concentrations in blood in pre- and post-menopausal women: the European Prospective Investigation into Cancer and Nutrition. Cancer Causes Control **17:** 1033–1043.
44. BERRINO, F., C. BELLATI, G. SECRETO *et al.* 2001. Reducing bioavailable sex hormones through a comprehensive change in diet: the diet and androgens (DIANA) randomized trial. Cancer Epidemiol. Biomarkers Prev. **10:** 25–33.
45. KAAKS, R., C. BELLATI, E. VENTURELLI *et al.* 2003. Effects of dietary intervention on IGF-I and IGF-binding proteins, and related alterations in sex steroid metabolism: the Diet and Androgens (DIANA) Randomised Trial. Eur. J. Clin. Nutr. **57:** 1079–1088.
46. SERRA-MAJEM, L., B. ROMAN & R. ESTRUCH. 2006. Scientific evidence of interventions using the Mediterranean diet: a systematic review. Nutr. Rev. **64:** S27–S47.
47. ESPOSITO, K., R. MARFELLA, M. CIOTOLA *et al.* 2004. Effect of a Mediterranean-style diet on endothelial dysfunction and markers of vascular inflammation in the metabolic syndrome: a randomized trial. JAMA **292:** 1440–1446.
48. MICCOLI, R., C. BIANCHI, L. ODOGUARDI *et al.* 2005. Prevalence of the metabolic syndrome among Italian adults according to ATP III definition. Nutr. Metab. Cardiovasc. Dis. **15:** 250–254.
49. ELIASSEN, A.H., S.A. MISSMER, S.S., TWOROGER *et al.* 2006. Endogenous steroid hormone concentrations and risk of breast cancer among premenopausal women. J. Natl. Cancer Inst. **98:** 1406–1415.

TGF-Beta Signaling in Breast Cancer

MIRIAM B. BUCK AND CORNELIUS KNABBE

Department of Clinical Chemistry and Dr. Margarete Fischer-Bosch Institute of Clinical Pharmacology, Robert Bosch Hospital, Auerbachstrasse 110, 70376 Stuttgart, Germany

ABSTRACT: The antiestrogen tamoxifen is one of the most successful drugs in the endocrine treatment of breast cancer and significantly reduces the risk of recurrence and death. Antiestrogens act by inhibiting the production of growth-stimulatory factors as well as by activating peptides with growth-inhibitory effects like transforming growth factor-beta (TGF-β). In hormone-responsive breast cancer cells treatment with antiestrogens leads to the conversion of TGF-β1 into a biologically active form. Expression of TGF-β2 and TGF-β receptor (TβR) II is induced via a transcriptional mechanism involving p38 MAP kinase. Inhibition of p38 abolishes antiestrogen-dependent growth inhibition. However, the role of TGF-β in breast cancer progression is ambiguous, as it was shown to display both tumor-suppressing and -enhancing effects. A polymorphism in the promoter of TGF-β2 that enhances expression of the protein was associated with lymph node metastasis in breast cancer patients, pointing to a role of TGF-β2 in the process of invasion. An immunohistochemical study on TβRI and TβRII expression in breast cancer tissues indicates that the estrogen receptor (ER) status of a tumor is an important marker and a potential mediator of the transition of TGF-β from tumor suppressor to tumor promoter. In ER-negative tumors, expression of TβRII was associated with a subset of tumors that appeared to be highly aggressive, leading to strongly reduced overall survival times. Further characterization of the influence of ER expression on TGF-β signal transduction shows that ER-α plays a crucial role in TGF-β signaling.

KEYWORDS: antiestrogen; TGF-beta; breast cancer; growth inhibition; metastasis

INTRODUCTION

The most commonly used endocrine treatment for estrogen receptor (ER)–positive breast cancer is the antiestrogen tamoxifen. However, response to tamoxifen is variable and one-third of patients do not benefit from the treatment.[1]

Address for correspondence: Cornelius Knabbe, M.D., Department of Clinical Chemistry, Robert-Bosch-Hospital, Auerbachstrasse 110, 70376 Stuttgart, Germany. Voice: +49-711-81013501; fax: +49-711-81013618.

e-mail: cornelius.knabbe@rbk.de

Ann. N.Y. Acad. Sci. 1089: 119–126 (2006). © 2006 New York Academy of Sciences.
doi: 10.1196/annals.1386.024

The constitutive production of growth-promoting factors or a ligand-independent activation of survival pathways like the EGFR/erbB2 pathways are important factors promoting the escape from antihormonal growth-control.[2,3] Moreover, defects in autocrine growth-inhibitory loops involving transforming growth factor (TGF)-β proteins, their receptors, and signal transduction pathways have been recognized to play a central role in the development of antiestrogen resistance.[4,5]

TGF-β

TGF-β belongs to a large family of polypeptide growth factors that includes activins, inhibins, and bone morphogenetic proteins (BMPs).[6] Three human TGF-β isoforms have been described, which are structurally and functionally closely related. All three isoforms are secreted as latent precursor molecules. Latent TGF-β consists of the 25-kDa mature protein in a noncovalent association with the propeptide to which one of several latent TGF-β-binding proteins is linked. Latent TGF-β can be activated by proteolytic cleavage, interaction with integrins, or pH changes in the local environment.[7]

Active TGF-β has numerous regulatory activities that influence development, tissue repair, immune defense, inflammation, and tumorigenesis.[8] In order to initiate these biological effects TGF-β must bind to specific receptors, which are transmembrane serine/threonine kinases. TGF-β binds to TGF-β receptor type II (TβRII), which is a constitutively active kinase. TGF-β receptor type I (TβRI) is recruited into the complex and phosphorylated by TβRII. Phosphorylation of TβRI activates downstream signaling cascades.[9] Intracellular TGF-β signaling is complex and many different pathways can be activated. These include the Smad pathway, MAP kinase pathways, phosphoinositol-3-kinase, and PP2A. The Smad pathway appears to be the major TGF-β signal transduction pathway. Receptor-activated Smad2 or Smad3 proteins form complexes with Smad4. The resulting heteromeric Smad complexes are translocated to the nucleus, where they bind to specific promoter elements and regulate transcription of TGF-β-responsive genes.[10,11]

REGULATION OF TGF-β SIGNAL TRANSDUCTION BY ANTIESTROGENS

Treatment of hormone-sensitive MCF-7 cells with antiestrogens leads to an increased secretion of both biologically active TGF-β1 and TGF-β2. Detailed analysis of the underlying mechanisms showed that mRNA and protein expression levels of TGF-β1 remain constant, whereas the proportion of active versus latent TGF-β1 increases. Regulation of TGF-β2 secretion, on the other hand, primarily takes place at the transcriptional level. TGF-β2 expression is strongly induced by antiestrogens as demonstrated by quantification of mRNA and protein levels. No activation of TGF-β1 or induction of TGF-β2 is seen in antiestrogen-resistant MCF-7 variants or ER-negative human breast cancer cell lines under antiestrogen treatment.[4,12]

Analysis of MAP kinase signal transduction cascades showed that activation of p38-MAP kinase is a prerequisite for the antiestrogen induction of TGF-β2 mRNA. The promoter of TGF-β2 contains an ATF-2-binding site, and ATF-2 is a substrate of p38, suggesting that p38-activated ATF-2 participates in the hormonal regulation of TGF-β2-promoter activity.[4]

In general, the growth-inhibitory effect of any given antiestrogen correlates highly with the inducing effect on TGF-β2 and seems to be a direct function of the respective binding affinities for the ER. The very strong growth-inhibitory steroidal antiestrogen ICI 182.780 (fulvestrant), for example, has a stronger effect on TGF-β2 expression than the triphenylethylene-related antiestrogens like tamoxifen. Secretion of TGF-β2 appears to be tightly coupled to the hormonally controlled growth state and represents an indicator of the growth-inhibitory potential of a given antiestrogen.[13,14]

Only few in vivo studies have explored the regulation of TGF-β isoforms under treatment with antiestrogens. In one study, which included 37 breast cancer patients, tamoxifen was administered in a neo-adjuvant setting for a period of 3 to 10 months, at the end of which breast surgery was performed. Patients were classified as responders if there was a decrease in tumor volume of at least 20% between initial biopsy and final surgery. All three TGF-β isoforms were assessed by RNase protection assay before and following treatment. Almost all tumors expressed each TGF-β isoform and the majority of tumors did not show substantial changes in TGF-β isoform expression with treatment. However, significant changes in TGF-β2 were more frequently observed with therapy and a correlation between response to therapy and increasing TGF-β2 expression was observed.[15]

In a study from our group, which included 10 breast cancer patients, TGF-β1 and TGF-β2 mRNA expression was determined by quantitative RT-PCR. Tamoxifen was given initially over a short period of 1 to 12 days before breast surgery and continued afterward as adjuvant treatment. Relapse-free survival during the first 5 to 6 years of postoperative follow-up was considered as response to treatment. Expression of both TGF-β isoforms was detected in all samples examined. During neo-adjuvant treatment with tamoxifen a change of TGF-β2 mRNA expression was found in 8 of 10 cases, whereas TGF-β1 mRNA levels were stable. In this study prediction of response to tamoxifen was better when, in addition to the hormone receptor status of the tumor tissues, the tamoxifen-related induction of TGF-β2 mRNA was taken into consideration.[16]

We also observed an increase in TGF-β2 expression in plasma samples from patients with metastatic breast cancer who responded to tamoxifen therapy. In this study the TGF-β2 concentration in plasma from 20 patients was determined by enzyme-linked immunosorbent assay (ELISA) before and during treatment with tamoxifen and correlated to response. In patients who responded to treatment, TGF-β2 concentrations increased between the second and fourth week of treatment and decreased after the initial peak. Patients who did not respond did not show changes in TGF-β2 plasma levels in the first weeks of treatment, followed by an increase at the end of treatment, probably due to accumulating tumor burden. These data suggest, that in the first 4–8 weeks of treatment, the TGF-β2 plasma concentration is influenced mainly by tamoxifen, whereas later on it becomes a marker of progression.[17]

Taken together, these studies substantiate our observations made in breast cancer cell lines and suggest that upregulation of TGF-β2 expression on the transcriptional level may predict clinical response to tamoxifen.

In addition to the described effects on TGF-β1 and TGF-β2 antiestrogens strongly influence downstream TGF-β signal transduction. Similar to the ligands, expression of TGF-β receptors is differentially regulated. Expression of TβRII is induced by antiestrogens at the level of transcription and the degree of induction correlates directly with the growth-inhibitory potential of the respective antiestrogen used for stimulation. TβRI on the other hand is constitutively expressed at higher levels and not under hormonal influence.[18] Activation of p38 MAP kinase precedes the induction of TβRII and inhibition of p38 significantly blocks induction of both TGF-β2 and TβRII, pointing to a central role of this MAP kinase in the hormonal regulation of the TGF-β system.[4]

Downstream of the receptors a Smad pathway mediates antiestrogen effects. Smad2 is phosphorylated in response to antiestrogen treatment and Smad3 as well as Smad4 participate in antiestrogen action. However, promoter constructs containing only Smad-binding elements (SBEs) are less efficiently activated by antiestrogens than more complex promoters containing AP-1-binding sites as well as SBEs.[4] As Smad3 and Smad4 bind DNA only with low affinity, additional DNA contacts are necessary for specific and high-affinity binding of Smad complexes to target genes. This is achieved by cooperation of Smads with a large variety of different transcription factors.[10] The higher transcriptional activity of promoters that contain AP-1 in addition to Smad-binding sites suggests that AP-1 factors are additional mediators of antiestrogen-induced TGF-β responses.

TUMOR-PROMOTING ACTIVITY OF TGF-β IN BREAST CANCER

TGF-β is a very potent inhibitor of primary human mammary epithelial cells and most human breast cancer cell lines.[19,20] However, a large number of reports exist that indicate that TGF-β can turn into a promoter of progression in later tumor stages[21,22] and stimulation of angiogenesis, induction of extracellular matrix degradation, or inhibition of antitumor immune responses prevail over the inhibitory effects on proliferation.

Recently, our group has identified an insertion polymorphism in the *TGFB2* promoter located at -246 bp upstream of the transcriptional start site, which was significantly associated with the presence of lymph node metastases and advanced tumor stage in breast cancer patients. The risk of lymph node metastases was 4.7-fold higher for carriers of the *TGFB2*-246ins allele, suggesting that this polymorphism is associated with enhanced tumor growth and invasiveness. Transient transfection experiments in breast cancer cell lines showed that the -246ins polymorphism increases *TGFB2*-promoter activity. This effect was mediated by enhanced binding of the transcription factor Sp1 to the *TGFB2* -246ins allele.

In an immunohistochemical evaluation of TGF-β2 protein expression in tumor tissues we found that tumors that were heterozygous or homozygous for the -246ins allele showed a stronger staining intensity than did tumors with the wild-type sequence. Furthermore, the proportion of tumors showing expression for TGF-β2 was higher in patients with the -246ins allele. Staining for TGF-β2 was positive in 79% of the tumors with at least one -246ins allele, whereas only 32% of the tumors with wild-type genotype showed positive staining for TGF-β2 (15 of 19 vs. 19 of 59 respectively, $P = 0.0005$).[23]

Taken together, these data support the hypothesis that increased TGF-β2 expression levels in tumors with the -246ins allele may promote metastasis in breast cancer development.

An immunohistochemical study on TβRI and TβRII expression in breast cancer tissues indicates that the ER status of tumor cells can influence the outcome of TGF-β effects. In ER-negative tumors, expression of TβRII was associated with a subset of tumors that were highly aggressive, leading to strongly reduced overall survival times. Simultaneous loss of both ER and TβRII, on the other hand, was associated with longer overall survival times comparable with those of ER-positive patients. Thus, loss of ER expression might be a marker for the transition of TGF-β from tumor suppressor to tumor promoter.[24]

TGF-β AND ANTIHORMONE RESISTANCE

A breakdown of the inhibitory loops in which TGF-β participates might contribute to the development of antiestrogen resistance. The above-mentioned data point to a hormonal influence. Thus, in order to further characterize the impact of ER expression on TGF-β signal transduction, we transiently overexpressed ER-α in MDA435 ER-negative breast cancer cells. The TGF-β-sensitive reporter plasmid p3TP-lux, which contains Smad- and AP-1-binding sites, was used as an end point marker of TGF-β signal transduction. Expression of ER-α significantly attenuated TGF-β-dependent induction of p3TP-lux, indicating that ER-α is a crucial modulator of TGF-β signaling (M.B. Buck, unpublished data).

A cross-talk between growth factor and steroid hormone receptor signal transduction could be of general relevance for the regulation of growth and differentiation processes in hormone-responsive tissues and to changes in TGF-β signal transduction. It was shown previously, that the transcriptional activity of Smad3 can be suppressed by the ER, whereas ER-mediated transcriptional activity can be increased by activation of TGF-β signaling.[25]

Furthermore, several studies indicate that amplification of erbB2 confers antiestrogen resistance to ER-positive breast cancer cells.[26–29] TGF-β could be involved in this process, as it was shown that overexpression of erbB2 alters cellular responses to TGF-β and unmasks its promigratory and proinvasive effects.[30,31]

CONCLUSIONS

TGF-β is a hormonally regulated growth factor. Upregulation of TGF-β in hormone-responsive breast cancer cells by treatment with antiestrogens induces growth inhibitory effects of TGF-β. Loss of the hormonally controlled growth status, as seen in ER-negative cells, appears to modulate TGF-β effects, leading to enhanced tumor-promoting activities of TGF-β.

A number of questions still need to be addressed in order to completely understand the complex hormonal regulation of TGF-β, its interaction with survival pathways activated in the course of tumor progression, and the development of antihormone resistance.

REFERENCES

1. EARLY BREAST CANCER TRIALISTS' COLLABORATIVE GROUP. 2005. Effects of chemotherapy and hormonal therapy for early breast cancer on recurrence and 15-year survival: an overview of the randomised trials. Lancet **365:** 1687–1717.
2. DICKSON, R.B. & M.E. LIPPMAN. 1995. Growth factors in breast cancer. Endocr. Rev. **16:** 559–589.
3. HOUSTON, S.J., T.A. PLUNKETT, et al. 1999. Overexpression of c-erbB2 is an independent marker of resistance to endocrine therapy in advanced breast cancer. Br. J. Cancer **79:** 1220–1226.
4. BUCK, M.B., K. PFIZENMAIER, et al. 2004. Antiestrogens induce growth inhibition by sequential activation of p38 mitogen-activated protein kinase and transforming growth factor-beta pathways in human breast cancer cells. Mol. Endocrinol. **18:** 1643–1657.
5. KNABBE, C., M.E. LIPPMAN, et al. 1987. Evidence that transforming growth factor-beta is a hormonally regulated negative growth factor in human breast cancer cells. Cell **48:** 417–428.
6. KINGSLEY, D.M. 1994. The TGF-beta superfamily: new members, new receptors, and new genetic tests of function in different organisms. Genes Dev. **8:** 133–146.

7. ANNES, J.P., J.S. MUNGER, *et al.* 2003. Making sense of latent TGFbeta activation. J. Cell. Sci. **116:** 217–224.
8. ROBERTS, A.B. 1998. Molecular and cell biology of TGF-beta. Miner. Electrolyte Metab. **24:** 111–119.
9. DE CAESTECKER, M. 2004. The transforming growth factor-beta superfamily of receptors. Cytokine Growth Factor Rev. **15:** 1–11.
10. FENG, X.H. & R. DERYNCK.. 2005. Specificity and versatility in TGF-beta signaling through Smads. Annu. Rev. Cell. Dev. Biol. **21:** 659–693.
11. MOUSTAKAS, A. & C.H. HELDIN. 2005. Non-Smad TGF-beta signals. J. Cell. Sci. **118:** 3573–3584.
12. KNABBE, C., A. KOPP., *et al.* 1996. Regulation and role of TGF beta production in breast cancer. Ann. N.Y. Acad. Sci. **784:** 263–276.
13. KNABBE, C., G. ZUGMAIER, *et al.* 1991. Induction of transforming growth factor beta by the antiestrogens droloxifene, tamoxifen, and toremifene in MCF-7 cells. Am. J. Clin. Oncol. **14** (Suppl 2): S15–S20.
14. MULLER, V., E.V. JENSEN, *et al.* 1998. Partial antagonism between steroidal and nonsteroidal antiestrogens in human breast cancer cell lines. Cancer Res. **58:** 263–267.
15. MACCALLUM, J., J.C. KEEN, *et al.* 1996. Changes in expression of transforming growth factor beta mRNA isoforms in patients undergoing tamoxifen therapy. Br. J. Cancer **74:** 474–478.
16. BRANDT, S., A. KOPP, *et al.* 2003. Effects of tamoxifen on transcriptional level of transforming growth factor beta (TGF-beta) isoforms 1 and 2 in tumor tissue during primary treatment of patients with breast cancer. Anticancer Res. **23:** 223–229.
17. KOPP, A., W. JONAT, *et al.* 1995. Transforming growth factor beta 2 (TGF-beta 2) levels in plasma of patients with metastatic breast cancer treated with tamoxifen. Cancer Res. **55:** 4512–4515.
18. BUCK, M., J. VON DER FECHT, *et al.* 2002. Antiestrogenic regulation of transforming growth factor beta receptors I and II in human breast cancer cells. Ann. N.Y. Acad. Sci. **963:** 140–143.
19. BASOLO, F., L. FIORE, *et al.* 1994. Response of normal and oncogene-transformed human mammary epithelial cells to transforming growth factor beta 1 (TGF-beta 1): lack of growth-inhibitory effect on cells expressing the simian virus 40 large-T antigen. Int. J. Cancer **56:** 736–742.
20. ZUGMAIER, G., B.W. ENNIS, *et al.* 1989. Transforming growth factors type beta 1 and beta 2 are equipotent growth inhibitors of human breast cancer cell lines. J. Cell. Physiol. **141:** 353–361.
21. GORSCH, S.M., V.A. MEMOLI, *et al.* 1992. Immunohistochemical staining for transforming growth factor beta 1 associates with disease progression in human breast cancer. Cancer Res. **52:** 6949–6952.
22. MCEARCHERN, J.A., J.J. KOBIE, *et al.* 2001. Invasion and metastasis of a mammary tumor involves TGF-beta signaling. Int. J. Cancer **91:** 76–82.
23. BEISNER, J., M.B. BUCK, *et al.* 2006. A novel functional polymorphism in the transforming growth factor-beta2 gene promoter and tumor progression in breast cancer. Cancer Res. **66:** 7554–7561.
24. BUCK, M.B., P. FRITZ, *et al.* 2004. Prognostic significance of transforming growth factor beta receptor II in estrogen receptor-negative breast cancer patients. Clin. Cancer Res. **10:** 491–498.

25. MATSUDA, T., T. YAMAMOTO, *et al.* 2001. Cross-talk between transforming growth factor-beta and estrogen receptor signaling through Smad3. J. Biol. Chem. **276:** 42908–42914.
26. BORG, A., B. BALDETORP, *et al.* 1994. ERBB2 amplification is associated with tamoxifen resistance in steroid-receptor positive breast cancer. Cancer Lett. **81:** 137–144.
27. CARLOMAGNO, C., F. PERONE, *et al.* 1996. c-erb B2 overexpression decreases the benefit of adjuvant tamoxifen in early-stage breast cancer without axillary lymph node metastases. J. Clin. Oncol. **14:** 2702–2708.
28. HOUSTON, S.J., T.A. PLUNKETT, *et al.* 1999. Overexpression of c-erbB2 is an independent marker of resistance to endocrine therapy in advanced breast cancer. Br. J. Cancer **79:** 1220–1226.
29. WRIGHT, C., S. NICHOLSON, *et al.* 1992. Relationship between c-erbB-2 protein product expression and response to endocrine therapy in advanced breast cancer. Br. J. Cancer **65:** 118–121.
30. SETON-ROGERS, S.E., Y. LU, *et al.* 2004. Cooperation of the ErbB2 receptor and transforming growth factor beta in induction of migration and invasion in mammary epithelial cells. Proc. Natl. Acad. Sci. USA **101:** 1257–1262.
31. UEDA, Y., S. WANG, *et al.* 2004. Overexpression of HER2 (erbB2) in human breast epithelial cells unmasks transforming growth factor beta-induced cell motility. J. Biol. Chem. **279:** 24505–24513.

Recent Results from Clinical Trials Using SERMs to Reduce the Risk of Breast Cancer

VICTOR G. VOGEL

Departments of Medicine and Epidemiology, University of Pittsburgh Cancer Institute, Magee-Womens Hospital, Pittsburgh, Pennslyvania, USA

ABSTRACT: Selective estrogen receptor modulators (SERMs) are used for the treatment of invasive breast cancer. Chemoprevention is the use of specific natural or synthetic chemical agents to reverse, suppress, or prevent the progression of premalignant lesions to invasive carcinoma. The finding of a decrease in contralateral breast cancer incidence following tamoxifen administration for adjuvant therapy led to its use in breast cancer prevention. Four large trials have used tamoxifen, the prototypical SERM, as a breast cancer chemopreventive agent with differing results. In the National Surgical Adjuvant Breast and Bowel Project's (NSABP) Breast Cancer Prevention Trial (BCPT), tamoxifen reduced the risk of invasive breast cancer by 49%. Tamoxifen also reduced the incidence of benign breast disease as well as the number of breast biopsies in the treated women. Three other randomized prevention trials comparing tamoxifen with placebo have been reported and show a reduction in breast cancer incidence of 38%. Serum levels of estrone sulfate and testosterone are significantly associated with breast cancer risk, and estradiol appears to be more strongly associated with breast cancer in high-risk women. Raloxifene is comparable to tamoxifen in its ability to reduce the risk of breast cancer in postmenopausal, high-risk women and has fewer side effects, as shown in the study of tamoxifen and raloxifene. Several ongoing and planned studies will evaluate the ability of aromatase inhibitors to reduce the risk of breast cancer in women at increased risk.

KEYWORDS: breast neoplasms; risk assessment; prevention; tamoxifen; raloxifene; gonadal steroid hormones

INTRODUCTION

Selective estrogen receptor modulators (SERMs) are a class of drugs available since the 1970s for the treatment of invasive breast cancer. Their use has

Address for correspondence: Prof. Victor G. Vogel, M.D., M.H.S., F.A.C.P., University of Pittsburgh Cancer Institute Magee-Womens Hospital, 300 Halket Street, Room 3524, Pittsburgh, PA 15213. Voice: 412-641-6500; fax: 412-641-6461.
e-mail: vvogel@mail.magee.edu

Ann. N.Y. Acad. Sci. 1089: 127–142 (2006). © 2006 New York Academy of Sciences.
doi: 10.1196/annals.1386.010

recently expanded to include treatment of *in situ* breast cancer as well as of individuals who are at increased risk of the disease. The first task in considering SERMs for reduction of breast cancer risk is to identify individuals who are at increased risk of the disease and then to review recent results from prospective clinical trials that have evaluated SERMs for reduction of breast cancer risk. Finally, one needs to devise a plan to identify women who are at increased risk.

Factors that are known to affect the chances of developing breast cancer can be divided by the degree to which they elevate risk.[1] Many factors that are linked to hormone exposure (early menarche, late menopause, hormone replacement therapy, body mass index, alcohol intake) elevate risk only slightly. Family history carries a greater degree of risk, especially in women with a first-degree relative with premenopausal breast cancer, or with two or more relatives with breast cancer. The increased risk in nulliparous women or women experiencing a first live birth after the age of 30 years may result from the absence or delay in undergoing the final epithelial differentiation that occurs during the first full-term pregnancy and lactation. Radiation exposure (e.g., multiple chest fluoroscopies, atomic bomb survivors) has been known for many years to increase the risk of breast cancer. Quantitative methods for assessing risk have been published[2,3] and are commonly used in clinical settings to stratify the risk of developing invasive breast cancer.

Three types of histology—ductal carcinoma *in situ* (DCIS), lobular carcinoma *in situ* (LCIS), and atypical hyperplasia (AH)—are associated with a high risk of invasive breast cancer. A model of breast carcinogenesis suggests that AH of either the lobular or ductal type is an early developmental stage in the process that transforms normal cells into cancerous ones.[4] Whether all or even most cancers follow this developmental pathway, it has nonetheless been demonstrated that histological AH is a strong risk factor for future breast cancer development. Dupont *et al.*[5] have shown that women with biopsy-proven atypia have 5.3 times the risk of women with no proliferative disease, and 2.8 times the risk of women who show proliferative disease without atypia. At especially high risk (relative risk [RR] = 11) are women with AH who also have a first-degree family history of breast cancer.

Although the connection between atypia and increased breast cancer risk was first demonstrated by histologic examination of breast biopsy specimens, similar findings have been reported in studies examining cytologic abnormalities. Wrensch *et al.*[6] reported an increased risk of breast cancer associated with abnormal cells found in nipple aspiration fluid (NAF) in 2,701 cancer-free women 25 to 54 years of age. At an average follow-up time of 12.7 years, they found that women with cytologically atypical cells were 4.9 times more likely to develop breast cancer than those in whom no NAF could be obtained. In those with atypical cells and a positive family history of breast cancer, this risk increased to 18-fold when compared with women with no NAF and a negative family history, although confidence intervals (CI) were wide (4.6 to 70.2) because of the small number of subjects in this category.

TABLE 1. European tamoxifen prevention trials: Comparison with the NSABP BCPT

Trial	Sample size	Risk of breast cancer	Woman– years of follow-up	Number of invasive breast cancers	Breast cancers per 1,000 woman–years	
					Placebo	Tamoxifen
Italian[10,11]	5,408	Low to normal	20,731	41	2.3	2.1
Royal Marsden[12]	2,471	Based on family history	12,355	70	5.0	4.7
IBIS I [13]	7,152	High	~14,900	148	5.7	4.2
NSABP BCPT[14,15]	13,388	High	52,401	264	6.8	3.4

Similar findings have also been reported with random cellular samples from the breasts of high-risk women. Fabian et al.[7] performed random periareolar fine-needle aspiration (FNA) cytology on 480 high-risk women. At an average follow-up of 45 months, they found that women with atypical cells had a five-fold increased risk of developing breast cancer, though this risk may actually be understated in light of the fact that control women with no atypia had other risk factors for the development of breast cancer. In all three approaches just reviewed (one histologic and two cytologic), the estimated increase in risk was consistently similar (fourfold to fivefold). Nonetheless, there are conflicting reports about whether histologic atypia is the biologic equivalent of cytologic atypia. King et al.[8] detected AH in NAF in 67% of patients with an underlying malignancy, a finding that correlated significantly with the histologic presence of atypical proliferative disease. In contrast, Krishnamurthy et al.[9] were able to detect atypical or malignant cells in only 23% of NAF samples taken from patients with biopsy-proven malignancies from whom adequate samples were available. From the standpoint of risk stratification, however, cytologic atypia seems to be comparable with histologic AH.

Review of SERM Risk Reduction Trials

Chemoprevention is the use of specific natural or synthetic chemical agents to reverse, suppress, or prevent the progression of premalignant lesions to invasive carcinoma. The finding of a decrease in contralateral breast cancer incidence following tamoxifen administration for adjuvant therapy led to the concept that the drug might play a role in breast cancer prevention. Four large trials have used tamoxifen, the prototypical SERM, as a breast cancer chemopreventive agent with differing results. These trials are listed in TABLE 1, and the data from the largest of these trials will be reviewed first in some detail.

The Breast Cancer Prevention Trial (BCPT)

The National Surgical Adjuvant Breast and Bowel Project (NSABP) initiated the BCPT, P-1 in 1992 to evaluate the ability of tamoxifen to reduce the incidence of breast cancer.[14] Women ($n = 13{,}388$) were judged to be at increased risk for breast cancer if they (1) were 60 years of age or older, (2) were 35–59 years of age with a 5-year predicted risk for breast cancer of at least 1.66%, or (3) had a history of LCIS. They were randomly assigned to receive placebo ($n = 6{,}707$) or tamoxifen 20 mg per day orally ($n = 6{,}681$) for 5 years. Gail's risk model, based on a multivariate logistic regression model using combinations of risk factors, was used to estimate the risk of occurrence of breast cancer over time.[2] Factors in Gail's model include the number of first-degree female relatives (mother, sister[s], and daughter[s] with breast cancer; age at first live birth or the presence of nulliparity; the lifetime number of breast biopsies showing benign pathology (with or without AH); the age at menarche; and race.

With 54 months of average follow-up at the time of the initial report, tamoxifen reduced the risk of invasive breast cancer by 49% (two-sided $P < 0.00001$), with cumulative incidence through 69 months of follow-up of 43.4 versus 22.0 per 1,000 women in the placebo and tamoxifen groups, respectively. The decreased risk occurred in women aged 49 years or younger (44%), 50 to 59 years (51%), and 60 years or older (55%). Risk was also reduced in women with a history of LCIS (56%) or AH (86% for either lobular or ductal atypia) and in those with any category of predicted 5-year risk. Tamoxifen reduced the risk of noninvasive breast cancer by 50% (two-sided $P < 0.002$). Consistent with its known mechanism of action, tamoxifen reduced the occurrence of estrogen receptor (ER)-positive tumors by 69%, and there was no difference in the occurrence of ER-negative tumors. Tamoxifen administration did not alter the average annual rate of ischemic heart disease, but there was a reduction in hip, radius (Colles'), and spine fractures. The rate of endometrial cancer was increased in the tamoxifen group (risk ratio [RR] = 4.01; 95% CI = 1.70–10.90) among women aged 50 years or older. All cases of endometrial cancer in the tamoxifen group were stage I (localized disease), and no endometrial cancer deaths have occurred in this group. The rates of stroke, pulmonary embolism, and deep-vein thrombosis (DVT) were elevated in the tamoxifen group only among women aged 50 years or older. These data demonstrated that tamoxifen decreased the incidence of both invasive and noninvasive breast cancer among women at increased risk.

The BCPT was unblinded because of positive results, and follow-up continued for 7 years. At the time of this more extended follow-up, the cumulative rate of invasive breast cancer was reported to be reduced from 42.5 per 1,000 women in the placebo group to 24.8 per 1,000 women in the tamoxifen group (RR = 0.57, 95% CI = 0.46 to 0.70), a 43% reduction in risk compared to the original report of a 49% reduction. The cumulative rate of noninvasive breast cancer was reduced from 15.8 per 1,000 women in the placebo group to 10.2 per 1,000 women in the tamoxifen group (RR = 0.63, 95% CI = 0.45 to 0.89). Tamoxifen led to a 32% reduction in osteoporotic fractures (RR = 0.68, 95% CI = 0.51 to 0.92). RR of stroke, DVT, and cataracts (which increased with tamoxifen) and of ischemic heart disease and death (which were not changed with tamoxifen) were also similar to those initially reported. Risks of pulmonary embolism were approximately 11% lower than in the original report, and risks of endometrial cancer were about 29% higher, but these differences were not statistically significant. The net benefit achieved with tamoxifen varied according to age, race, and level of breast cancer risk. Despite the potential bias caused by the unblinding of the BCPT, the magnitudes of all beneficial and undesirable treatment effects of tamoxifen after 7 years of follow-up were similar to those initially reported, with notable reductions in breast cancer and increased risks of thromboembolic events and endometrial cancer. Readily identifiable subsets of individuals at increased risk for breast cancer comprising 2.5 million women in the United States could derive a net benefit from the drug.[16]

Benign Breast Disease in BCPT

Tamoxifen reduced the incidence of benign breast disease in the BCPT as well as the number of breast biopsies in the treated women.[17] Medical records were examined from 13,203 women with follow-up who participated in the NSABP BCPT. Women were included who had undergone a breast biopsy and had histologic diagnoses of adenosis, cyst, duct ectasia, fibrocystic disease, fibroadenoma, fibrosis, hyperplasia, or metaplasia. The RR for each histologic diagnosis was estimated for women who received tamoxifen and for women who received placebo. The number of biopsies was recorded for women in both the placebo and tamoxifen groups. Overall, tamoxifen treatment reduced the risk of benign breast disease by 28% (RR = 0.72, 95% CI = 0.65 to 0.79). Tamoxifen therapy resulted in statistically significant reductions in the risk of adenosis (RR = 0.59, 95% CI = 0.47 to 0.73), cyst (RR = 0.66, 95% CI = 0.58 to 0.75), duct ectasia (RR = 0.72, 95% CI = 0.53 to 0.97), fibrocystic disease (RR = 0.67, 95% CI = 0.58 to 0.77), hyperplasia (RR = 0.60, 95% CI = 0.50 to 0.71), and metaplasia (RR = 0.51, 95% CI = 0.41 to 0.62). Tamoxifen therapy also reduced the risk for fibroadenoma (RR = 0.77, 95% CI = 0.56 to 1.04) and fibrosis (RR = 0.86, 95% CI = 0.72 to 1.03). Compared with the placebo group, the tamoxifen group had 29% (95% CI = 23% to 34%) fewer biopsies (1,048 vs. 1,469) and 19% fewer women who underwent a biopsy (811 vs. 1,019). This resulted in a 29% reduction in the risk of biopsy in women treated with tamoxifen (RR = 0.71, 95% CI = 0.66 to 0.77). This risk reduction occurred predominantly, however, in women younger than 50 years.

Summary of Data with Tamoxifen for Risk Reduction

Three other randomized prevention trials comparing tamoxifen with placebo have been reported, and their results have been summarized.[18] The combined data from the prevention trials support a reduction in breast cancer incidence of 30% to 40% with tamoxifen. When analyzed by a fixed-effect model, the reduction is 38% (95% CI = 28–46; $P < 0.0001$) and all studies were compatible with this result. When analyzed by a random-effects model, the reduction was 34% (16–48; $P = 0.0007$). The adjuvant treatment studies show a slightly greater reduction (46%, $P < 0.0001$) when using the incidence of second, contralateral primary tumors as the end point. As reported by NSABP, there is no effect for breast cancers negative for ER; hazard ratio 1.22 (0.89–1.67); $P = 0.21$, but ER-positive cancers are decreased by 48% (36–58; $P < 0.0001$) in the tamoxifen prevention trials. Age has no apparent effect. Rates of endometrial cancer were increased in all tamoxifen prevention trials (consensus RR 2.4 [1.5–4.0]; $P = 0.0005$) and in the adjuvant trials (RR 3.4 [1.8–6.4]; $P = 0.0002$). Venous thromboembolic events are also increased in all tamoxifen studies (RR 1.9 [1.4–2.6] in the prevention trials; $P < 0.0001$).

Overall, there is no effect of tamoxifen on non–breast cancer mortality, and the only cause of death showing a mortality increase is pulmonary embolism. On the basis of this overview, the evidence now clearly shows that tamoxifen can reduce the risk of ER-positive breast cancer, and tamoxifen can be recommended as a preventive agent (except possibly in older women with a high risk of side effects).

Plasma Levels of Endogenous Sex Hormones and Breast Cancer Risk

An ancillary study was conducted within the NSABP BCPT trial to determine whether plasma levels of estradiol, testosterone, or SHBG were associated with breast cancer risk in a high-risk population. The investigators also tested the hypothesis that women with the highest levels of estradiol and testosterone would achieve the greatest risk reduction with tamoxifen. Using a case–cohort design, Beattie and her colleagues studied 135 women with postmenopausal breast cancer and 275 postmenopausal women without breast cancer who were enrolled in the NSABP BCPT and who had been treated with tamoxifen or placebo.[19] They measured estradiol, testosterone, and sex hormone–binding globulin by using radioimmunoassay in baseline plasma samples. RR and 95% CI for invasive breast cancer were estimated for each quartile of sex hormone level using Cox proportional hazards models. Median plasma levels of estradiol, testosterone, and sex hormone–binding globulin (SHBG) were similar between the case and cohort groups.

These data showed that the RR of breast cancer for women in the placebo group was not associated with measured sex hormone levels. The risks of

ER-positive breast cancer in women by quartile of estradiol were: Q1 [lowest], RR = 1.0; Q2, RR = 1.16, 95% CI = 0.49 to 2.7; Q3, RR = 1.08, 95% CI = 0.45 to 2.61; and Q4, RR = 1.29, 95% CI = 0.59 to 2.82). Furthermore (and, again, unlike the results in the MORE trial), the reduced risk of invasive breast cancer in tamoxifen-treated women compared with placebo-treated women was not associated with sex hormone levels. Unexpectedly, testosterone and SHBG showed a trend toward the opposite effect seen in prior studies, most of which showed increased risk with increased testosterone and decreased SHBG. There was no clear indication of increasing effectiveness of tamoxifen for ER-positive breast cancer prevention in women with the highest plasma estradiol levels. These data did not support, therefore, the use of endogenous sex hormone levels to identify women who are at particularly high risk of breast cancer and who are most likely to benefit from chemoprevention with tamoxifen.

Other Data Related to Sex Hormones and the Risk of Breast Cancer

The seeming paradox in the data just reviewed from the BCPT may be more completely explained by another recently published study. To examine whether the associations of endogenous estrogens and testosterone with breast cancer risk differ between high- and low-risk women, as determined by quantitative risk models, and by family history of breast cancer, Eliassen and her colleagues conducted a prospective, nested case–control study within the Nurses' Health Study.[20] From 1989 or 1990 until June 2000, blood samples were collected, 418 breast cancer patient cases were identified, and two controls (total $n =$ 817) were matched to each case. Women were classified as being at either high or low risk of breast cancer on the basis of their family history and other risk factors. Multivariate RR and 95% CIs were calculated by unconditional logistic regression, adjusting for matching and breast cancer risk factors.

The investigators found that estrone sulfate was statistically significantly associated with breast cancer risk among women with low ($<1.66\%$) and high ($\geq2.52\%$; 75th percentile) quantitative risk of breast cancer (fourth vs. first quartile RR = 3.6; 95% CI, 1.9 to 7.0; RR = 2.5; 95% CI, 1.2 to 5.1, respectively). Testosterone results were similar across the strata of predicted risk, with two times the risk in the fourth (vs. first) quartile. Estradiol appeared to be more strongly associated with breast cancer in women with higher predicted risk (RR = 4.5; 95% CI, 2.1 to 9.5) compared with women with lower risk (RR = 2.1; 95% CI, 1.2 to 3.6), but the differences were not statistically significant. These data suggest that higher levels of endogenous estrogens and testosterone are associated with increased breast cancer risk, regardless of predicted risk or family history of breast cancer. They also indicate that while endogenous estrogen and testosterone levels increase linearly across low and intermediate levels of quantitative risk, there is a plateau at the highest levels of risk. This may explain the apparently negative findings seen in the NSABP BCPT cohort.[21]

The worldwide data from prospective studies of the relationship between the levels of endogenous sex hormones and breast cancer risk in postmenopausal women also show multiple and complex relationships. Nine prospective studies of women not taking exogenous sex hormones when their blood was collected to determine hormone levels showed that the risk for breast cancer increased significantly with increasing concentrations of all sex hormones examined: total estradiol, free estradiol, non-SHBG-bound estradiol, estrone, estrone sulfate, androstenedione, dehydroepiandrosterone, dehydroepiandrosterone sulfate, and testosterone.[22] The RR for women with increasing quintiles of all hormone concentrations, relative to the lowest quintile, ranged from 1.04 to 2.58, and high SHBG was associated with a decrease in breast cancer risk. Interestingly, estradiol levels are generally higher in North American women than Asian women, and urinary estrogens are higher in North American teenagers, who face higher lifetime risks for breast cancer.

Eliassen et al.[20] tested the hypothesis that the risk of breast cancer, quantitatively assessed using either of the two multivariate risk models, is associated with measured levels of circulating endogenous estrogen and related compounds in postmenopausal women. Their findings strongly support the conclusion that the traditional risk factors for breast cancer mediate their effect through synthesis and/or metabolism pathways of endogenous human estrogen, and give credence to a possible association between hormone levels and tumor receptor status or invasive versus in situ tumor status. Their data are supported, in part, by another study showing a statistically significant association between breast cancer risk and the levels of both estrogens and androgens, but no statistically significant associations between this risk and the level of progesterone or SHBG.[23] When that analysis was limited to case subjects with ER-positive/progesterone receptor (PR)-positive breast tumors, and compared the highest with the lowest fourths of plasma hormone concentration, there were large increased risks of breast cancer associated with estradiol (RR = 3.3), testosterone (RR = 2.0), androstenedione (RR = 2.5), and dehydroepiandrosterone sulfate (RR = 2.3), and all hormones tended to be associated most strongly with in situ disease.

In agreement with these observations, earlier studies among women who had traditional risk factors for breast cancer showed that the risk for breast cancer was more than three times greater among women with the highest concentrations of bioavailable estradiol compared with women with the lowest concentration.[24]

Older postmenopausal women with the highest estradiol levels (≥ 12 pmol/L) in a prospective trial had a twofold increased risk for invasive breast cancer compared with women with lower levels of estradiol.[25] In the placebo group, women with estradiol levels greater than 10 pmol/L had a 6.8 times higher rate of breast cancer than breast cancer risk of women with undetectable estradiol levels.[26] Women with estradiol levels greater than 10 pmol/L in the raloxifene group had a rate of breast cancer that was 76% lower than that of women with estradiol levels greater than 10 pmol/L in the placebo group. Importantly, raloxifene reduced breast cancer risk in both the low- and high-estrogen subgroups for all risk factors examined, but the reduction was greatest in those with the highest estradiol levels. In contrast, women with undetectable estradiol levels had similar breast cancer risk whether or not they were treated with raloxifene. Older postmenopausal women whose testosterone levels were in the highest two quintiles had a fourfold increased risk of ER-positive breast cancer.[27]

A recent evaluation among women who were using postmenopausal HRT found that HRT users had statistically significantly higher estradiol, free estradiol, sex hormone–binding globulin, and testosterone, and lower free testosterone concentrations than non-HRT users.[28] Among the HRT users, there were modest associations with breast cancer risk when comparing the highest versus lowest quartiles of free estradiol, free testosterone, and SHBG, but not of estradiol or of testosterone. However, estradiol and free estradiol were significantly and positively associated with breast cancer risk among women older than 60 years (with a RR of nearly three) and among women with a body mass index of less than 25 kg/m.[2] The etiological issues are complex, however, given the findings of the clinical trials of the Women's Health Initiative, which showed an increased risk of breast cancer among women taking conjugated equine estrogens plus progesterone,[29] but not among those women with hysterectomy who were taking only conjugated equine estrogens.[30]

Although the data from BCPT did not suggest that hormone levels can further stratify risk, the data from Eliassen et al.[20] indicate a continuum of serum hormone levels that are directly correlated with the quantitative risk of developing invasive breast cancer. It is likely that there was a plateau in circulating hormone concentrations in BCPT, given that the mean quantitative risk scores among the participants was high (average 5-year Gail risk = 4); the Eliassen et al. study suggests a continuum of hormone levels that peaks among those women who are at highest risk.

Taken together, these observations suggest that endogenous sex hormones will serve better to select women at moderate risk for SERMs) or aromatase risk reduction interventions than quantitative risk assessment alone. Sex hormone levels require further evaluation, however, in order to assess breast cancer risk in high-risk women. Sex hormone levels may be able to determine which women may achieve the most benefit from SERMs when used to assess probable benefits from SERM therapy.

The NSABP Study of Tamoxifen and Raloxifene (STAR Trial)

The Multiple Outcomes Raloxifene Evaluation (MORE) Study, a multicenter, randomized, placebo-controlled, double-blind clinical trial completed in

1999, was designed to test whether raloxifene, at a daily dose of either 60 mg or 120 mg, reduced the risk of fracture in postmenopausal women with osteoporosis.[31] The primary end point was the development of fracture. Eligible women had a history of at least one vertebral body fracture. At 36 months of follow-up in 6,828 women, the risk of vertebral fracture was reduced 30% in the women who received raloxifene. These women had increased risk of venous thromboembolus when compared to those assigned to placebo (RR = 3.1, 95% CI, 1.5–6.2), but raloxifene did not cause an increase in either vaginal bleeding or endometrial cancer.

A secondary end point in the MORE trial was invasive breast cancer.[32] After 4 years of follow-up, there were 22 cases among 5,129 postmenopausal women randomized to raloxifene, compared with 39 cases among 2,576 postmenopausal women assigned to placebo. The MORE trial concluded that among older postmenopausal women with osteoporosis, the risk of ER-positive invasive breast cancer was decreased by 72% during 4 years of raloxifene treatment, with no apparent decrease in the incidence of ER-negative tumors.

The Continuing Outcomes Relevant to Evista (CORE) Trial examined the effect of four additional years of raloxifene therapy on the incidence of invasive breast cancer in women in the MORE trial who agreed to continue therapy.[33] After 4 years of participation in the CORE trial by 5,213 participants, the risk of invasive breast cancer was reduced by 69% (HR = 0.41, 95% CI 0.24–0.71) in the raloxifene group compared with the placebo group. During the 8 years of both the MORE and CORE trials, the incidence of invasive breast cancer (and of ER-positive invasive breast cancer in particular) were reduced by 66% (HR = 0.34, 95% CI 0.22–0.50) and 76% (HR = 0.24, 95% CI 0.15–0.40), respectively, in the raloxifene group compared with the placebo group. During the CORE trial, the RR of thromboembolism in the raloxifene group compared with that in the placebo group was 2.17 (95% CI 0.83–5.70). No increase in the risk of endometrial cancer was observed with raloxifene.

On the basis of the findings from the NSABP BCPT, tamoxifen was approved by the U.S. Food and Drug Administration for reducing breast cancer risk in high-risk women aged 35 years or older. STAR trial was launched to compare the relative effects and safety of raloxifene and tamoxifen on the risk of developing invasive breast cancer and other disease outcomes in high-risk, postmenopausal women.[34,35] To be eligible for participation in the STAR trial, a woman had to have at least a 5-year predicted breast cancer risk of 1.66% based on the Gail model; be at least 35 years of age and postmenopausal; not be taking tamoxifen, raloxifene, hormone therapy, oral contraceptives, or androgens for at least the previous 3 months; not currently be taking either warfarin or cholestyramine; have no history of stroke, pulmonary embolism, or DVT and no history of any malignancy diagnosed less than 5 years before randomization except basal or squamous cell carcinoma of the skin or carcinoma *in situ* of the cervix; have no uncontrolled atrial fibrillation, uncontrolled diabetes, or uncontrolled hypertension; and have no psychiatric condition that would interfere with adherence or a performance status that would restrict normal activity for a significant portion of each day.

The mean age of participants at the time of randomization was 58.5 years. Nine percent were younger than 50 years, 49.8% were between 50 and 59 years, and 41.2% were 60 years or older. More than 93% of participants were white, 2.5% were African American, 2.0% were Hispanic, and the remainder was of other racial/ethnic populations. Race information was collected as self-reported by the participants because it is a risk factor for breast cancer and is one of the factors used in the Gail model to determine the predicted risk of breast cancer. More than half of the participants reported having undergone a hysterectomy prior to randomization. Almost 19% reported a family history of breast cancer in two or more first-degree relatives, and more than 71% reported a history of invasive breast cancer in one or more. More than 9% reported a personal history of LCIS prior to enrollment in the trial, and 22.7% had breast biopsy results prior to trial enrollment that showed either atypical ductal or lobular hyperplasia. The mean predicted 5-year risk of developing breast cancer among the study population was 4.0%.

The STAR trial was designed to have a final analysis after 327 incident invasive breast cancers occurred. Nearly 200 clinical centers throughout North America participated, and 19,747 postmenopausal women with increased 5-year breast cancer risk were enrolled in slightly more than 5 years from 1999 through 2005. The mean age of the participants was 58.5 ± 7.4 years, and they were randomly assigned to receive either 5 years of daily oral tamoxifen 20 mg or raloxifene 60 mg daily. The primary outcomes of interest were invasive breast cancer, uterine cancer, noninvasive breast cancer, bone fractures, and thromboembolic events. At the time of the analysis of the trial in December 2005, there were 163 cases of invasive breast cancer in women assigned to tamoxifen and 168 in those assigned to raloxifene (incidence, 4.30 per 1,000 vs. 4.41 per 1,000; RR, 1.02; 95% CI = 0.82–1.28). In contrast to the findings for invasive breast cancer, there were fewer noninvasive breast cancers in the tamoxifen group than in the raloxifene group, although this difference did not reach statistical significance. There were 57 incident cases of noninvasive breast cancer among the women who took tamoxifen and 80 among the women who took raloxifene. (Rate for noninvasive breast cancer, 1.51 per 1,000 women assigned to tamoxifen and 2.11 per 1,000 women assigned to raloxifene [RR = 1.40; 95% CI = 0.98–2.00].) Cumulative incidence through 6 years was 8.1 per 1,000 in the tamoxifen group and 11.6 in the raloxifene group ($P = 0.052$). About 36% of the cases were LCIS and 54% were DCIS), with the balance being mixed types. The pattern of fewer cases among the tamoxifen group was evident for both LCIS and DCIS.

There were 36 cases of uterine cancer with tamoxifen and 23 with raloxifene (RR = 0.62, 95% CI = 0.35–1.08). No differences were found for other invasive cancer sites, for ischemic heart disease events, or for stroke. The number of osteoporotic fractures in the groups was similar. There were fewer cataracts

(RR = 0.79, 95% CI = 0.68–0.92) and cataract surgeries (RR = 0.82, 95% CI = 0.68–0.99) in the women taking raloxifene. There was no difference in the total number or causes of deaths ($n = 101$ vs. 96).

There were important differences when comparing the rates of thromboembolic vascular events reported with the two agents. Pulmonary emboli (RR = 0.64. 95% CI = 0.41–1.00) and DVT (RR = 0.74, 95% CI = 0.53–1.03) occurred less often in the raloxifene group. Although stroke or transient ischemic attack (TIA) did not differ statistically significantly between arms, there was a statistically significant 30% reduction in the risk of thromboembolic events in the raloxifene arm versus the tamoxifen arm (RR = 0.70, 0.54–0.91). For pulmonary embolism, the reduction in risk was 36% and for DVT, 26%. Compared with placebo in the MORE trial,[36] raloxifene demonstrated a threefold increase in the risk of pulmonary embolism (RR = 3.0, 95% CI = 1.2–9.3) and a 60% increased risk of DVT (RR = 1.6, 95% CI = 0.91–2.86). These data indicate that both tamoxifen and raloxifene increase the risk of thromboembolic events, but raloxifene less so.[37,38]

The Women's Health Initiative (WHI) trial indicated that estrogen plus progestin hormonal replacement therapy had hazard ratios of 1.41 (95% CI = 1.07–1.85) for stroke, 2.07 (95% CI = 1.49–2.87) for DVT, and 2.13 (95% CI = 1.39–3.25) for pulmonary embolism compared with placebo in postmenopausal women. Venous thromboembolic events occurred at similar rates among the postmenopausal women who took HRT in the WHI study and the postmenopausal women who took raloxifene in STAR.[39,40]

There was no statistically significant difference between raloxifene and tamoxifen in the risk of noninvasive disease (LCIS and DCIS) (incidence, 1.51 vs. 2.11 per 1,000 per year; RR, 1.40; 95% CI, 0.98–2.00). However, the STAR trial may have been underpowered to detect such a difference. Therefore, the clinical impact of this finding remains to be further evaluated. The mechanism that would allow for a decrease in invasive breast cancers but a lesser impact on noninvasive disease is unknown. Similar results were seen, however, in the MORE[32] and CORE[33] studies and the RUTH[41] trial, in which raloxifene did not reduce the risk of noninvasive breast cancer, although the number of events in those studies was very small. These results taken together suggest that different SERMs have unique and specific mixes of benefits and risks and that neither a benefit nor a risk seen with one SERM can be generalized across the entire class.

Most of the STAR cases of *in situ* carcinoma were diagnosed as a result of mammograms that demonstrated increasing calcifications. The individuals in STAR were undergoing careful follow-up, and, as a result, their lesions were small; most were treated surgically with lumpectomy. Approximately 36% of the cases were LCIS and 64% were DCIS or mixed LCIS and DCIS. The difference between the tamoxifen- and the raloxifene-treated individuals with DCIS was quite small (0.4 per 1,000 per year). The CORE results through 8 years of follow-up show that raloxifene continues to offer a significant reduction in invasive disease,[33] suggesting that raloxifene has a durable benefit despite this lesser impact on noninvasive disease.

Remaining Questions Related to SERM Therapy

Despite a number of large, prospective randomized trials having been conducted over the course of two decades to evaluate the ability of SERMs to decrease the risk of breast cancer in high-risk women, a number of questions remain. How long to use SERMs to achieve optimal benefit remains unanswered by the STAR trial and other relevant published data. Continued follow-up is both required and ongoing among STAR participants, who agreed to undergo follow-up indefinitely after unblinding; this follow-up will assist in answering questions about the duration of raloxifene treatment for breast cancer risk reduction.

The BCPT demonstrated that tamoxifen could reduce the risk of invasive breast cancer by 49% and established proof of principle that the chemoprevention of breast cancer is possible. Tamoxifen lowered the incidence of breast cancer in three randomized trials involving women at increased risk and is effective chemoprevention against the development of breast cancer in women at high risk. It remains unknown whether this demonstrated reduction in incidence of breast cancer will ultimately lead to an increased survival or overall health benefit for women at risk. Identifying women who are likely to develop ER-positive breast cancer is important when attempting to maximize the net benefits of tamoxifen use.

As we described, measurement of serum estradiol and testosterone levels may achieve this goal. Newer agents being evaluated for breast cancer risk reduction, such as aromatase inhibitors, may offer increased efficacy in the future.[42,43] The NSABP is planning a new prospective, randomized trial comparing raloxifene to letrozole, an aromatase inhibitor, in high-risk, postmenopausal women. The trial is to commence in late 2006 or early 2007 and will enroll 14,000 women in the United States and Canada. Support for the trial will come from the U.S. National Cancer Institute, Eli Lilly and Company, and Novartis Oncology.

REFERENCES

1. HOLLINGSWORTH, A.B., S.E. SINGLETARY, M. MORROW, et al. 2004. Current comprehensive assessment and management of women at increased risk for breast cancer. Am. J. Surg. **187:** 349–362.
2. GAIL, M.H., L.A. BRINTON, D.P. BYAR, et al. 1989. Projecting individualized probabilities of developing breast cancer for white females who are being examined annually. J. Natl. Cancer Inst. **81:** 1879–1886.
3. TYRER, J., S.W. DUFFY & J. CUZICK. 2004. A breast cancer prediction model incorporating familial and personal risk factors. Stat. Med. **23:** 1111–1130.

4. O'SHAUGHNESSY, J.A. 1996. Chemoprevention of breast cancer. JAMA **275:** 1349–1353.

5. DUPONT, W.D. & D.L. PAGE. 1985. Risk factors for breast cancer in women with proliferative breast disease. N. Engl. J. Med. **312:** 146–151.

6. WRENSCH, M.R., N.L. PETRAKIS, E.B. KING, *et al.* 1992. Breast cancer incidence in women with abnormal cytology in nipple aspirates of breast fluid. Am. J. Epidemiol. **135:** 130–141.

7. FABIAN, C.J., B.F. KIMLER, C.M. ZALLES, *et al.* 2000. Short-term breast cancer prediction by random periareolar fine-needle aspiration cytology and the Gail risk model. J. Natl. Cancer Inst. **92:** 1217–1227.

8. KING, E.B., K.L. CHEW, N.L. PETRAKIS & V.L. ERNSTER. 1983. Nipple aspirate cytology for the study of breast cancer precursors. J. Natl. Cancer Inst. **71:** 1115–1121.

9. KISHNAMURTHY, S., N. SNEIGE, P.A. THOMPSON, *et al.* 2003. Nipple aspirate fluid cytology in breast cancer. Cancer **99:** 97–104.

10. VERONESI, U., P. MAISONNEUVE, A. COSTA, *et al.* 1998. Prevention of breast cancer with tamoxifen: preliminary findings from the Italian randomised trial among hysterectomised women. Lancet **352:** 93–97.

11. VERONESI, U., P. MAISONNEUVE, V. SACCHINI, *et al.* 2002. Tamoxifen for breast cancer among hysterectomised women. Lancet **359:** 1122–1124.

12. POWLES, T.J., R. EELES, S. ASHLEY, *et al.* 1998. Interim analysis of the incidence of breast cancer in the Royal Marsden Hospital tamoxifen randomised chemo-prevention trial. Lancet **352:** 98–101.

13. IBIS INVESTIGATORS. 2002. First results from the International Breast Cancer Intervention Study (IBIS-I): a randomised prevention trial. Lancet **360:** 817–824.

14. FISHER, B., J.P. COSTANTINO, D.L. WICKERHAM, *et al.* 1998. Tamoxifen for prevention of breast cancer: report of the National Surgical Adjuvant Breast and Bowel Project P-1 Study. J. Natl. Cancer Inst. **90:** 1371–1388.

15. FISHER, B., J.P. COSTANTINO, D.L. WICKERHAM, *et al.* 2005. Tamoxifen for the prevention of breast cancer: current status of the National Surgical Adjuvant Breast and Bowel Project P-1 Study. J. Natl. Cancer Inst. **97:** 1652–1662.

16. FREEDMAN, A., B.I. GRAUBARD, S.R. RAO, *et al.* 2003. Estimates of the number of U.S. women who could benefit from tamoxifen for breast cancer chemopreven-tion. J. Natl. Cancer Inst. **95:** 526–532.

17. TAN-CHIU, E., J. WANG, J.P. COSTANTINO, *et al.* 2003. Effects of tamoxifen on benign breast disease in women at high risk for breast cancer. J. Natl. Cancer Inst. **95:** 302–307.

18. CUZICK, J., T. POWLES, U. VERONESI, *et al.* 2003. Overview of the main outcomes in breast-cancer prevention trials. Lancet **361:** 296–300.

19. BEATTIE, M.S., J.P. COSTANTINO, V. VOGEL, *et al.* 2006. Endogenous sex hormones and response to tamoxifen: an ancillary study in the Breast Cancer Prevention Trial (P-01). J. Natl. Cancer Inst. **98:** 110–115.

20. ELIASSEN, A.H., S.A. MISSMER, S.S. TWOROGER & S.E. HANKINSON. 2006. Endoge-nous steroid hormone concentrations and risk of breast cancer. J. Clin. Oncol. **24:** 1824–1830.

21. VOGEL, V.G. & E TAIOLI. 2006. Have we found the ultimate risk factor for breast cancer? J. Clin. Oncol. **24:** 1791–1793.

22. THE ENDOGENOUS HORMONES AND BREAST CANCER COLLABORATIVE. 2002. En-dogenous sex hormones and breast cancer in postmenopausal women: reanalysis of nine prospective studies. J. Natl. Cancer Inst. **94:** 606–616.

23. MISSMER, S.A., A.H. ELIASSEN, R.L. BARBIERI, *et al.* 2004. Endogenous estrogen, androgen, and progesterone concentrations and breast cancer risk among postmenopausal women. J. Natl. Cancer Inst. **96:** 1856–1865.

24. CAULEY, J.A., F.L. LUCAS, L.H. KULLER, *et al.* 1999. Elevated serum estradiol and testosterone concentrations are associated with a high risk for breast cancer. Ann. Intern. Med. **130:** 270–277.

25. LIPPMAN, M.E., K.A. KRUEGER, S. ECKERT, *et al.* 2001. Indicators of lifetime estrogen exposure: effect on breast cancer incidence and interaction with raloxifene therapy in the multiple outcomes of raloxifene evaluation study participants. J. Clin. Oncol. **19:** 3111–3116.

26. CUMMINGS, S.R., T. DUONG., E. KENYON, *et al.* 2002. Serum estradiol level and risk of breast cancer during treatment with raloxifene. JAMA **287:** 216–220.

27. CUMMINGS, S.R., J.S. LEE, L-Y LUI, *et al.* 2005. Sex hormones, risk factors, and risk of estrogen receptor-positive breast cancer in older women: a long-term prospective study. Cancer Epidemiol. Biomarkers Prev. **14:** 1047–1051.

28. TWOROGER, S.S., S.A. MISSMER, R.L. BARBIERI, *et al.* 2005. Plasma sex hormone concentrations and subsequent risk of breast cancer among women using postmenopausal hormones. J. Natl. Cancer Inst. **97:** 595–602.

29. THE WOMEN'S HEALTH INITIATIVE INVESTIGATORS. 2002. Risks and benefits of estrogen plus progestin in healthy postmenopausal women: principal results from the Women's Health Initiative randomized controlled trial. JAMA **288:** 321–333.

30. THE WOMEN'S HEALTH INITIATIVE STEERING COMMITTEE. 2004. Effects of conjugated equine estrogen in postmenopausal women with hysterectomy: The Women's Health Initiative Randomized Controlled Trial. JAMA **291:** 1701–1712.

31. ETTINGER, B., D.M. BLACK, B.H. MITLAK, *et al.* 1999. Multiple outcomes of raloxifene evaluation investigators. Reduction of vertebral fracture risk in postmenopausal women with osteoporosis treated with raloxifene: results from a 3-year randomized clinical trial. JAMA **282:** 637–645.

32. CUMMINGS, S.R., S. ECKERT, K.A. KRUEGER, *et al.* 1999. The effect of raloxifene on risk of breast cancer in postmenopausal women: results from the MORE randomized trial: Multiple Outcomes of Raloxifene Evaluation. JAMA **281:** 2189–2197.

33. MARTINO, S., J.A. CAULEY, E. BARRETT-CONNOR, *et al.* 2004. Continuing outcomes relevant to evista: breast cancer incidence in postmenopausal osteoporotic women in a randomized trial of raloxifene. J. Natl. Cancer Inst. **96:** 1751–1761.

34. VOGEL, V.G., J.P. COSTANTINO, D.L. WICKERHAM, *et al.* 2006. Effects of tamoxifen vs raloxifene on the risk of developing invasive breast cancer and other disease outcomes: the NSABP Study of Tamoxifen and Raloxifene (STAR) P-2 Trial. JAMA **295:**2727–2741.

35. LAND, S.R., D.L. WICKERHAM, J.P. COSTANTINO, *et al.* 2006. Patient-reported symptoms and quality of life during treatment with tamoxifen or raloxifene for breast cancer prevention: The NSABP Study of Tamoxifen and Raloxifene (STAR) P-2 Trial. JAMA **295:** 2742–2751.

36. BARRETT-CONNOR, E., D. GRADY, A. SASHEGYI, *et al.* 2002. Raloxifene and cardiovascular events in osteoporotic postmenopausal women: four-year results from the MORE (Multiple Outcomes of Raloxifene Evaluation) randomized trial. JAMA **287:** 847–857.

37. DECENSI, A., P. MAISONNEUVE, N. ROTMENSZ, *et al.* 2005. Effect of tamoxifen on venous thromboembolic events in a Breast Cancer Prevention Trial. Circulation **111:** 650–656.
38. BUSHNELL, C.D. & L.B. GOLDSTEIN. 2004. Risk of ischemic stroke with tamoxifen treatment for breast cancer: a meta-analysis. Neurology **63:** 1230–1233.
39. ANDERSON, G.L., M. LIMACHER, A.R. ASSAF, *et al.* 2004. Women's Health Initiative Steering Committee. Effects of conjugated equine estrogen in postmenopausal women with hysterectomy: the Women's Health Initiative Randomized Controlled Trial. JAMA **291:** 1701–1712.
40. WASSERTHEIL-SMOLLER, S., S. HENDRIX, M. LIMACHER, *et al.* 2003. WHI Investigators: effect of estrogen plus progestin on stroke in postmenopausal women: the Women's Health Initiative: a randomized trial. JAMA **289:** 2673–2684.
41. BARRETT-CONNOR, E., L. MOSCA, P. COLLINS, *et al.* 2006. Effects of raloxifene on cardiovascular events and breast cancer in postmenopausal women. N. Engl. J. Med. **355:** 125–137.
42. CUZICK, J. 2003. Aromatase inhibitors in prevention–data from the ATAC (Arimidex, tamoxifen alone or in combination) trial and the design of IBIS-II (the Second International Breast Cancer Intervention Study). Recent Results Cancer Res. **163:** 96–103.
43. GOSS, P.E. & K. STRASSER-WEIPPL. 2004. Prevention strategies with aromatase inhibitors. Clinical Cancer Res. **10**(1 Pt 2): 372S–379S.

Antihormones in Prevention and Treatment of Breast Cancer

RICCARDO PONZONE, NICOLETTA BIGLIA, MARIA ELENA JACOMUZZI, LUCA MARIANI, ANNELISE DOMINGUEZ, AND PIERO SISMONDI

Academic Unit of Gynaecological Oncology, University of Turin, Institute for Cancer Research and Treatment (IRCC) of Candiolo and A.S.O. Ordine Mauriziano, Turin, Italy

ABSTRACT: Breast cancer has the highest incidence of all types of cancer in women. Age and family history are the strongest risk factors, but sex hormones also play an important role, as demonstrated by epidemiological studies reporting a consistent association by reproductive personal history and breast cancer risk. The acceptability of preventive strategies by healthy women is closely related to their lifetime risk of developing breast cancer. Although surgical prevention may be considered in carriers of BRCA1/2 mutation, this option cannot be advocated for the majority of women whose risk is only moderately increased. In these women, chemoprevention with tamoxifen may reduce the incidence of estrogen receptor (ER)-positive breast carcinoma by 30–50%. Other drugs such as raloxifen and aromatase inhibitors (AIs) are currently being tested in this setting. Tamoxifen has been the most successful hormonal treatment over the last 30 years and, until recently, the most active drug in endocrine-sensitive breast cancer. In premenopausal breast cancer, tamoxifen still represents the therapy of choice, alone or in association with ovarian suppression. Conversely, in postmenopausal women it has been overtaken by third-generation AIs as first-choice drugs both in the adjuvant and metastatic settings. Many other issues, such as the optimal sequence between tamoxifen and AIs, the duration of AIs treatment, and the association of ovarian suppression and AIs in premenopausal patients still await the completion of randomized clinical trials. Furthermore, it is likely that treatment tailoring will be increased by the definition of patient subgroups that could derive larger benefits from AIs (progesterone receptor–negative, HER-2-overexpressing) or other new drugs.

KEYWORDS: breast; cancer; endocrine; treatment; prevention

Address for correspondence: Piero Sismondi, Institute for Cancer Research and Treatment (IRCC), Strada Provinciale 142, 10060 Candiolo, Turin, Italy. Voice: +39-011-9933444; fax: +39-011-9933447.
e-mail: sismondi@mauriziano.it

Ann. N.Y. Acad. Sci. 1089: 143–158 (2006). © 2006 New York Academy of Sciences.
doi: 10.1196/annals.1386.037

INTRODUCTION: RISK ASSESSMENT

Breast cancer has the highest incidence of all types of cancer in women and it is the second largest cause of cancer death in women.[1] Therefore, all women can be considered at risk for breast cancer. Furthermore, only 20% of cases of breast cancer diagnosed in the age group of 30–50 years and one-third of those in women older than 50 years of age develop in women with one or more risk factor(s).

On the other hand, both age and family history are strong risk factors and may certainly help in selecting those women most likely to develop breast cancer. Many other risk factors confer a lower increase of the risk and are mainly related to women's reproductive personal history such as age at menarche, menopause, and first pregnancy, breast feeding, and use of exogenous sex hormones.

The risk of developing breast cancer is perceived quite differently depending on whether it is presented in relative or absolute terms.[2] As an example, a 40% increase in the risk of developing breast cancer associated with two daily alcoholic drinks sounds frightening, yet in absolute terms this translates to only one additional case of breast cancer occurring among about 1,500 women.[3] Accordingly, the impressive 1 in 8 cumulative lifetime breast cancer risk of U.S. women only pertains to those who reach 75–80 years of age and escape other major causes of death (especially cardiovascular disease).

To overcome these problems, mathematical tools have been developed to project breast cancer risk over a definite period of time (usually 10 years). They take into account age, family history, reproductive factors and previous breast diseases,[4] have been extensively validated, and may assist physicians and patients in decision-making on preventive or screening strategies.

Conversely, such models are not applicable to families with an unusual concentration of breast and ovarian cancer cases, in which the presence of a hereditary component, typically the mutation of the BRCA1/2 genes, can be suspected. Specific tools have been developed to assess the likelihood of detecting germ-line mutations (BRCA Pro, Cyrillic, etc) and to select the individuals at risk who are candidates for genetic testing.[5]

It is increasingly clear that the genetic hereditabilty of breast cancer cannot be entirely ascribed to the mutation of single tumor-suppressor genes with high penetrance such as BRCA1/2, p53, or PTEN. Instead, many other genes with lower penetrance are likely implicated in determining the overall breast cancer risk, which could also be modified by reproductive or environmental factors. The most promising approach to assess this "background" genetic risk is represented by the simultaneous analysis of thousands of genes, with the definition of molecular signatures associated with different cancer risks (genomics, transcriptomics, proteomics).

PREVENTION

Lifestyle and/or environmental factors play an important role in influencing breast cancer risk. Their importance is suggested by the impressive difference in the incidence rates of populations living in undeveloped versus developed areas of the world, combined with the fact that the migration of individuals from low-risk populations to industrialized countries is associated with an increase of breast cancer risk in the next generation.

Many factors, such as physical exercise, low-fat diet, and reduction of alcohol use as well as early and/or multiple pregnancies, prolonged breast feeding, and avoidance of exogenous estrogens may account for at least part of these differences, while it is not clear whether environmental factors, apart from ionizing radiation, significantly increase the risk of the general population.

From the perspective of breast cancer prevention, it is likely that the adherence to strict dietary and reproductive habits to avoid these modifiable risk factors may actually reduce breast cancer incidence. Although the magnitude of the relative risk reduction is not expected to be great, if applied to the general population, this policy may well result in a significant number of cancers prevented. Nevertheless, this option may not be appealing to women who face an exceptionally increased breast cancer risk or who have already reached an age when the modification of such risk factors is no more possible or effective.[6]

For example, even accepting that appropriate lifestyle and reproductive choices may produce a 30% risk reduction, women with a BRCA1/2 mutation would still face a greater than 50% breast cancer lifetime risk. Therefore, prophylactic surgery (prophylactic mastectomy and/or oophorectomy) has been advocated in women at genetic risk and is currently pursued by an increasing percentage of healthy carriers.[7]

On the other hand, for most of the women generically defined "at risk" because they have one or two relatives with postmenopausal breast cancer or because of a previous biopsy for a proliferative benign breast disease, the lifetime risk of developing breast cancer is below 20%. For these large group of women, chemoprevention with "antihormones" is a feasible and attractive option.[8]

Tamoxifen

The selective estrogen receptor modulator (SERM) tamoxifen has been the most successful hormonal treatment and, until recently, the most active drug in estrogen receptor (ER)- and/or progesterone receptor (PR)-positive breast cancer.[9] Since the publication of the ATAC trial with anastrozole,[10] third-generation aromatase inhibitors (AIs) have overtaken tamoxifen as first-choice drug, both in the adjuvant and metastatic settings. Nevertheless, in the preventive setting tamoxifen is the only approved drug and the only one for which large and long-term data are available.

The observed 53% decrease of contralateral disease in the early trials of adjuvant therapy included in the overview of the Early Breast Cancer Trialists' Collaborative Group (EBCTCG) suggested the potential use of tamoxifen for breast cancer prevention.[10] This finding prompted the launch of prospective randomized trials that specifically tested tamoxifen for breast cancer chemoprevention in healthy women.[11–14]

Although the small Royal Marsden[11] and Italian trials [12] did not show a significant reduction of breast cancer incidence, both the large NSABP-P1[13] and IBIS-I[14] trials clearly showed that tamoxifen may indeed prevent breast cancer. A summary of all trials showed a 34% reduction of overall breast cancer incidence (invasive and noninvasive, ER-positive and -negative, pre- and postmenopausal) (TABLE 1).

As expected, no protection was conferred against ER-negative tumors (hazard ratio [HR] 1.22, 95% confidence interval [CI] 0.89–1.67; $P = 0.21$), while ER-positive cancers were decreased by 48% (95% CI 36–58; $P < 0.0001$). Conversely, age did not affect the degree of breast cancer reduction (HR 0.66; 95% CI 0.52–0.85 for age <50 years vs. HR 0.63; 95% CI 0.51–0.77 for age ≥ 50 years; $P = 0.96$). Tamoxifen increased both endometrial cancer (HR 2.4; 95% CI 1.5–4.0; $P = .0005$) and venous thromboembolic events (HR 1.9; 95% CI 1.4–2.6; $P < 0.0001$) with similar relative risks, but higher absolute risks among older women. Finally, no effect was observed in non-breast cancer mortality.[15]

The lower protection reported in the European IBIS-1 trial as compared to the American NSABP-P1 trial accounts for the fact that in Europe tamoxifen is not yet recommended as a preventive agent, except in women at very high breast cancer risk without significant comorbidities, while in the United States this indication has received the Food and Drug Administration's (FDA) approval.

TABLE 1. Breast cancer prevention trials with tamoxifen 20 mg/day for 5 years versus placebo

Trial	Population	No. Randomized	No. of Breast Cancers	Hazard Ratio	P
Royal Marsden (11)	High-risk, family history	2471	62 vs. 75	0.83	ns
Italian (12)	Normal-risk, hysterectomy	5408	34 vs. 45	0.76	ns
NSABP-P1 (13)	>1.6% 5-year risk	13 388	124 vs. 244	0.51	<.00001
IBIS-I (14)	>2-fold relative risk	7139	69 vs. 101	0.68	.013
Total		28 356	289 vs. 465	0.66	.0007

ns = not significant.

Raloxifene

Several clinical trials have demonstrated that raloxifene, a second-generation SERM, is effective in the prevention and treatment of osteoporosis. Furthermore, these trials, as well as preclinical models,[16] suggested that raloxifene may also reduce breast cancer risk in postmenopausal women.

The Multiple Outcomes Raloxifene Evaluation (MORE) study is a multicenter, randomized, placebo-controlled, double blind clinical trial that was designed to test whether 60–120 mg/day of raloxifene for 4 years could reduce the risk of fracture in 7,705 postmenopausal women with osteoporosis.[17] At 36 months of follow-up, the risk of vertebral fractures was reduced by 30%; among the secondary endpoints, the study showed an impressive 72% reduction in the risk of ER-positive invasive breast cancer, with no apparent decrease in the incidence of ER-negative tumors. Like tamoxifen, raloxifene increased the risk of pulmonary embolism (RR, 3.0; 95% CI, 1.2–9.3) and deep venous thrombosis (RR, 1.6; 95% CI, 0.91–2.86) as compared to placebo. Conversely, the risk of endometrial cancer was not affected by raloxifene use.

Participants in the MORE trial who agreed to continue therapy were entered in the Continuing Outcomes Relevant to Evista (CORE) trial; the primary endpoint of this study was to assess the incidence of invasive breast cancer after 4 additional years of raloxifene. The risk of invasive breast cancer among the 5,213 participants in the CORE trial was reduced by 69% (HR 0.31; 95% CI, 0.24–0.71), while the study confirmed the increase of thromboembolic events (HR 2.17; 95% CI, 0.83–5.70) and the null effect on endometrial risk associated with raloxifene use.[18]

The results of the National Surgical Adjuvant Breast and Bowel Project (NSABP) Study of Tamoxifen and Raloxifene (STAR) trial were published early this year. This was a prospective, double-blind, randomized clinical trial of 5 years of tamoxifen versus 5 years of raloxifene in 19,747 postmenopausal women of a mean age of 58.5 years, with increased 5-year breast cancer risk.[19] No differences were observed between the tamoxifen and raloxifene arms in the number of invasive breast cancers (163 vs. 168, risk ratio [RR], 1.02; 95% CI 0.82–1.28), but tamoxifen was associated with a lower incidence of noninvasive breast cancer (57 vs. 80; RR, 1.40; 95% CI, 0.98–2.00). In the raloxifene arm there were fewer endometrial cancers (36 vs. 23 cases; RR, 0.62; 95% CI, 0.35–1.08) and thromboembolic events (RR, 0.70; 95% CI, 0.54–0.91) and similar osteoporotic fractures. Finally, no difference was reported in the total number of deaths (101 vs. 96 for tamoxifen vs. raloxifene).

In the Raloxifene Use for The Heart (RUTH) Trial, 10,101 postmenopausal women with coronary heart disease (CHD) or multiple risk factors for CHD were randomized to 60 mg of raloxifene daily or placebo and followed for a median of 5.6 years. The two primary outcomes were coronary events and invasive breast cancer. Raloxifene reduced the risk of invasive breast cancer (HR 0.56; 95% CI, 0.38–0.83), but not the risk of primary coronary events

(HR 0.95; 95% CI, 0.84–1.07). Deaths from any cause or total stroke did not vary according to group assignment, but raloxifene was associated with an increased risk of fatal stroke (HR 1.49; 95% CI 1.00–2.24) and venous thromboembolism (HR 1.44; 95% CI 1.06–1.95).[20]

If raloxifene obtains FDA approval for chemoprevention after the publication of these studies, it is likely that many women will be willing to take it in the light of its perceived more favorable risk/benefit profile as compared to tamoxifen.

Aromatase Inhibitors

All three major trials comparing various AIs with tamoxifen as adjuvant treatment for invasive breast cancer have reported significant reductions in the risk of contralateral cancer favoring AIs[10,21,22] (TABLE 2) and similar results were reported by two other trials also.[23,24]

Furthermore, AIs were associated with fewer thromboembolic events and cases of endometrial cancer, whereas, as expected, musculoskeletal disorders and fractures occurred at a significantly higher rate with AI. Lower contralateral breast cancer rates (14 vs. 26, P-value not reported) were also found in the MA.17 adjuvant trial of extended endocrine therapy with 5 years of letrozole after 5 years of tamoxifen versus 5 years of tamoxifen in ER+ breast cancer.[25]

No clinical controlled trials have been yet published with AIs in a preventive setting. The IBIS-II trial is an ongoing large international randomized trial consisting of two substudies designed around different high-risk populations. One of them (treatment) will compare anastrozole versus tamoxifen for 5 years in 4,000 women who undergo breast-conserving surgery for ductal carcinoma *in situ* (DCIS), whereas the other (prevention) will compare anastrozole versus placebo for 5 years in 6,000 women classified at "high-risk" according to several risk factors, including a previous DCIS treated with mastectomy.[26]

Aromatase Inhibitors plus Other Drugs

The steroidal third-generation AI exemestane is currently being tested by the National Cancer Institute of Canada in the Mammary Prevention 3 trial, which will randomly assign 5,100 high-risk postmenopausal women to placebo versus exemestane versus exemestane plus celecoxib. Celecoxib is a COX-2 inhibitor that belongs to the family of nonsteroidal anti-inflammatory drugs (NSAIDs). Actually, aspirin and NSAIDs indirectly inhibit estrogen biosynthesis by reducing the synthesis of prostaglandins, which in turn stimulate aromatase gene expression.[27] Although prospective controlled trials are still lacking, both epidemiological and biological studies support the potential activity of this class of drugs for the prevention of ER+ breast tumors.[28,29] Conversely, clinical trials are under way for ER– tumors to test drugs whose mechanism of action is not directed to interfere with the estrogenic pathways, such as ornithine decarboxylase inhibitors, retinoids, and statins.[30]

TREATMENT

Estrogenic deprivation is a key element of breast cancer treatment. Clinical evidence on the role of estrogens in breast cancer progression was provided as early as in 1886 by Sir George Beatson, who demonstrated that surgical oophorectomy was able to provide tumor regression in patients with locally advanced breast cancer.[31] This pivotal observation and the discovery of estrogen receptors[32] were instrumental in the development of many endocrine treatments over the last 50 years, among which tamoxifen has been the most successful.[33]

Tamoxifen

Tamoxifen is a SERM approved by the FDA in 1977 for the treatment of women with advanced breast cancer. Although many of its properties are still not fully elucidated, tamoxifen binds the nuclear ER and exerts estrogen-antagonist activity in breast tissue thus inhibiting tumor growth. On the other hand, tamoxifen has an estrogen-agonistic effect on bone and serum lipid concentrations, which accounts for its protective effect against osteoporosis in postmenopausal women and, possibly, against cardiovascular diseases, whereas its ability to stimulate the endometrium is associated with an increase of endometrial cancer risk.

According to the latest overview of the EBCTCG,[34] about 5 years of adjuvant tamoxifen reduce the annual relapse and death rates in ER+ tumors by 40% and 31%, respectively. This effect is largely irrespective of the use of chemotherapy, age, progesterone receptor status, or other tumor characteristics and persists after discontinuation of therapy ("carry-over effect"), so that the cumulative reduction in mortality is more than twice as large at 15 years as at 5 years after diagnosis. The most serious side effects of tamoxifen are the increase of thromboembolic events (about two times) and endometrial cancer (almost three times), although mortality due to these events or any other non-breast cancer-related event is not significantly different among tamoxifen and non-tamoxifen users.

As far as the issue of duration is concerned, the results of the NSABP B-14 trial[35] suggest that there is no benefit in continuing tamoxifen beyond 5 years of therapy, although only the completion of the large ATLAS (Adjuvant Tamoxifen—Longer against Shorter) and aTTom (Adjuvant Tamoxifen Treatment Offer More?) trials will allow definite conclusions to be drawn.

TABLE 2. Incidence of contralateral breast cancer in randomized adjuvant trials comparing aromatase inhibitors with tamoxifen

Study	ATAC[10]	IES[21]	BIG 1–98[22]
Subjects	9,366 postmenopausal women with HR + or HR unknown breast cancer following primary surgery and chemotherapy	4,742 postmenopausal women with HR + or HR unknown breast cancer following completion of 2–3 years of tamoxifen	8,010 postmenopausal women with HR+ breast cancer following primary surgery and chemotherapy
Intervention	A vs. T for 5 years	T for 2–3 years followed by E vs. T continued for 5 years	L vs. T for 5 years
Median follow-up	68 months	30.6 months	25.8 months
Contralateral breast cancer	35 vs. 59, 42% reduction; $P = 0.01$ (only HR+ patients: 53% reduction; $P = 0.001$)	9 vs. 20 56% reduction $P = 0.00005$	16 vs. 27 41% reduction P = not reported

A = anastrozole; T = tamoxifen; L = letrozole; E = exemestane; HR = hormone receptors.

Ovarian Ablation/Suppression

As already recalled, ovarian ablation was the first systemic treatment for breast cancer to be introduced, and several randomized trials in the adjuvant setting have been conducted over the last 50 years. The EBCTCG meta-analysis of these trials clearly established that ovarian ablation/suppression among women less than 50 years of age at the time of treatment is associated with significant improvement in recurrence-free (17%; $P = 0.00001$) and overall survival (13%; $P = 0.004$) after 15 years of follow-up.[34] No difference was reported whether ovarian ablation/suppression was induced by surgery or radiotherapy or achieved with luteinizing hormone- or gonadotropin hormone-releasing hormone (LHRH or GnRH) agonists.

Although these gains may appear relatively small in absolute terms (4.3% and 3.2% respectively), it must be emphasized that 63% of the participants were ER-untested, and thus at least some ER-negative patients were included in these trials. Furthermore, a considerable proportion of women also received chemotherapy, which is known to reduce the benefit of other ovarian treatments through its toxic effect on ovarian activity. For instance, in the absence of chemotherapy, ovarian ablation/suppression was associated with a 25.7% ($P = 0.0005$) and 24.7% ($P = 0.0006$) reduction in the odds of recurrence and death, respectively, whereas the corresponding figures were 10% ($P > 0.1$) and 8% ($P > 0.1$) in the presence of chemotherapy. Accordingly, the benefit of adding ovarian ablation after chemotherapy was lower in the older (40–49 years) as compared to the younger (<40 years) premenopausal patients (ratio 0.95 vs 0.86, respectively) since the former experience higher rates of permanent ovarian suppression as a consequence of cytotoxic treatments.

Several head-to-head comparisons between chemotherapy and ovarian ablation showed that goserelin for 2 years is equivalent[36,37] or superior[38] to cyclophosphamide, methotrexate, and fluorouracil (CMF) for six courses in ER-positive patients, but inferior for the ER-negative population.

Ovarian Ablation/Suppression plus Tamoxifen

In premenopausal women with ER-positive advanced breast cancer, a meta-analysis of four clinical trials showed that the combined treatment of LHRH agonist plus tamoxifen confers a significant benefit in survival ($P = 0.02$), progression-free survival ($P = 0.0003$), and overall response rate ($P = 0.03$) over tamoxifen alone.[39]

In the adjuvant setting, several studies reported similar[40] or better[41] outcome with LH-RH agonist plus tamoxifen as compared to CMF or antracyclin-based combinations.[42] According to the Intergroup Trial 0101, in premenopausal, node-positive, ER-positive patients who received six courses of CMF, the addition of LH-RH inhibition alone after chemotherapy confers no benefit, whereas the combination of LH-RH inhibition plus tamoxifen does.[43] Conversely, in the Zoladex in Premenopausal Patients (ZIPP) trial, the association of LH-RH inibition and tamoxifen for 2 years was superior to tamoxifen alone for 2 years and no endocrine therapy.[44]

Taken together, these results suggest that ovarian inhibition in ER-positive breast cancer is at least as effective as chemotherapy. Furthermore, the contribution of ovarian inhibition is higher in the absence of previous chemotherapy or concomitant tamoxifen administration and also in the younger (< 40 years of age) patients, irrespective of the combination with other adjuvant treatments.[45]

Aromatase Inhibitors

Several phase III studies demonstrated that third-generation AIs are superior to tamoxifen as first-line therapy for metastatic breast cancer in postmenopausal women, with longer time to progression (anastrozole),[46] time to treatment failure (exemestane),[47] and survival (letrozole).[48]

The success of these early trials led to the comparison of AI against tamoxifen in the adjuvant setting either as single agents or given in combination or sequentially after tamoxifen (TABLE 3). Results from the three following strategies have been already published: (*a*) "upfront," comparing tamoxifen versus AIs as initial therapy for 5 years[10,22]; (*b*) "switch," comparing tamoxifen for 5 years versus tamoxifen for 2–3 years followed by AIs for 2–3 years[21,24]; and (*c*) "extended adjuvant," comparing tamoxifen for 5 years versus tamoxifen for 5 years followed by AIs for 5 years.[25]

With the notable exception of the combined therapy arm (anastrozole + tamoxifen) in the ATAC trial,[10] AIs showed superiority against tamoxifen in all of these trials, irrespective of study design, nodal status, and previous chemotherapy, with longer disease-free survival (TABLE 3) and time to distant metastasis rates. Although several thousands of patients have been involved in these trials, none of them has yet reached a sufficient number of events to demonstrate a significant overall survival benefit over tamoxifen.

A survival advantage for AI is expected to show up with longer follow-up also in the light of their favorable safety profile (fewer venous thromboembolic and ischemic cerebrovascular complications and endometrial cancer risk). The only worrying side effect associated with AI use is represented by a 50% increase in bone fractures, especially when compared with the positive effect of tamoxifen on bone mineral density.[50] More controversial is the potential detrimental effect of AI on serum lipids (especially hypercholesterolemia), which in turn could lead to an increase in deaths from cerebrovascular accident and cardiac incidents, as reported in the BIG 1-98 trial (7 vs. 1 and 13 vs. 6, respectively).[49] Finally, another minor characteristic and yet unexplained side effect of AIs is represented by musculoskeletal symptoms, whereas gynecological symptoms (endometrial polyps, vaginal discharge, and bleeding) are significantly lower as compared to occurring those with tamoxifen in all trials.

TABLE 3. Comparison of six adjuvant trials with aromatase inhibitors

	ATAC[9]	BIG 1-98[22]	ARNO 95/ABCSG 8[24]	ITA[23]	IES[21]	MA.17[25]
Design	A vs. T vs. AT × 5 yr, upfront	L vs. T × 5 yr, upfront	T→A vs. A, 5 yr, switch	T→A vs. A, 5 yr, switch	T→E vs T, 5 yr, switch	T × 5years vs. T→L × 10 yr, extended
No. of patients	6,186	8,010	3,224	448	4,742	5,187
Follow-up (months)	68	25.8	28	36	30.6	30
No. of events	1,226	647	177	45	449	247
Absolute benefit in DFS	3.7%	2.6%	3.1%	8.8%	4.7%	3.5%

DFS = disease-free survival; No. = number; yr = years; A = anastrozole; T = tamoxifen; L = letrozole; E = exemestane.

Many issues remain unresolved, such as the existence of a group of patients more likely to benefit from an upfront treatment with AIs. The latter hypothesis is supported by adjuvant and neoadjuvant studies, where the advantage of AIs over tamoxifen is particularly evident during the first 2–3 years of follow-up in PR-negative tumors[51] or in the presence of oncogene HER-2 overexpression.[52]

CONCLUSION

All variables that modify the exposure to endogenous or exogenous estrogens are known to influence a woman's lifetime risk of developing breast cancer. Given the availability of effective drugs like LH-RH analogues, SERMs, and AIs to prevent ER-positive cancers, more accurate methods must be developed to predict which high-risk women are most likely to develop this type of tumor.

Endocrine sensitivity has a major role in determining the chance of cure of breast cancer: according to recent microarray data, this single parameter discriminates truly different breast tumors. As a consequence, although the prognostic value of ER/PR expression is only weak, its predictive value is very strong and accounts for the overall more favorable prognosis of endocrine-sensitive tumors.

In premenopausal patients with ER/PR-positive disease, the benefit of the combination of ovarian ablation and tamoxifen is comparable to that of chemotherapy, while data are accumulating on the efficacy of the association of ovarian ablation plus AIs. In perimenopausal women, the sequential therapy with tamoxifen for 2–3 years followed by AIs is probably the most reasonable option, whereas in truly postmenopausal women the upfront treatment with AI is supported by their superior activity and more favorable side-effect profile.

With the advent of new alternatives to tamoxifen, the issue of the optimal duration of endocrine treatment is being investigated in several clinical trials, but in high-risk patients who completed 5 years of tamoxifen, the addition of further 5 years of letrozole may already be considered as the standard of care. Moreover, bisphosphonates are effective and safe drugs to counterbalance the loss of bone density and the consequent increase of osteoporotic fractures associated with AIs.

The future of breast cancer endocrine therapy, as well as that of many other oncological treatments, is directed to improve our way to "tailor" medical decisions by decrypting the specific "biological portrait" of each tumor. Toward this aim, it will be essential that the impressive improvements already achieved in the molecular characterization of the disease be backed by the development of new effective drugs.

REFERENCES

1. SMIGAL, C., A. JEMAL, E. WARD, *et al.* 2006. Trends in breast cancer by race and ethnicity: update 2006. CA Cancer. J. Clin. **56:** 168–183.

2. BUNKER, J.P., J. HOUGHTON & M. BAUM. 1998. Putting the risk of breast cancer in perspective. BMJ **317:** 1307–1309.
3. LONGNECKER, M.P., J.A. BERLIN, M.J. ORZA & T.C. CHALMERS. 1988. A meta-analysis of alcohol consumption in relation to risk of breast cancer. JAMA **260:** 652–656.
4. COSTANTINO, J.P., M.H. GAIL, D. PEE, *et al.* 1999. Validation studies for models projecting the risk of invasive and total breast cancer incidence. J. Natl. Cancer Inst. **91:** 1541–1548.
5. NELSON, H.D., L.H. HUFFMAN, R.M.S. FU, *et al.* 2005. Genetic risk assessment and BRCA mutation testing for breast and ovarian cancer susceptibility: systematic evidence review for the U.S. preventive services task force Ann. Intern. Med. **143:** 362–379.
6. DUNN, B.K., D.L. WICKERHAM & L.G. FORD. 2005. Prevention of hormone-related cancers: breast cancer. J. Clin. Oncol. **23:** 357–367.
7. NAROD, S.A., K. OFFIT. Prevention and management of hereditary breast cancer. J. Clin. Oncol. **23:** 1656–1663.
8. TSAO, A.S., E.S. KIM, W.K. HONG, *et al.* 2004. Chemoprevention of cancer. CA Cancer J. Clin. **54:** 150–180.
9. EARLY BREAST CANCER TRIALISTS' COLLABORATIVE GROUP. 1998. Tamoxifen for early breast cancer: an overview of the randomised trials. Lancet **351:** 1451–1467.
10. HOWELL, A., J. CUZICK, M. BAUM, *et al.* 2005. Results of the ATAC (Arimidex, Tamoxifen, Alone or in Combination) trial after completion of 5 years' adjuvant treatment for breast cancer. Lancet **365:** 60–62.
11. POWLES, T.J., R. EELES, S. ASHLEY, *et al.* 1998. Interim analysis of the incidence of breast cancer in the Royal Marsden Hospital tamoxifen randomised chemoprevention trial. Lancet **352:** 98–101.
12. VERONESI, U., P. MAISONNEUVE, A. COSTA, *et al.* 1998. Prevention of breast cancer with tamoxifen: preliminary findings from the Italian randomised trial among hysterectomised women. Lancet **352:** 93–97.
13. FISHER, B., J.P. COSTANTINO, D.L. WICKERHAM, *et al.* 1998. Tamoxifen for prevention of breast cancer: report of the national surgical adjuvant breast and bowel project P-1 Study. J. Natl. Cancer Inst. **90:** 1371–1387.
14. IBIS INVESTIGATORS. First results from the International Breast Cancer Intervention Study (IBIS-I): 2002. A randomised prevention trial. Lancet **360:** 817–824.
15. CUZICK, J., T. POWLES, U. VERONESI, *et al.* 2003. Overview of the main outcomes in breast-cancer prevention trials. Lancet **361:** 296–300.
16. SPORN, M.B., S.A. DOWSETT, J. MERSHON & H.U. BRYANT. 2004. Role of raloxifene in breast cancer prevention in postmenopausal women: clinical evidence and potential mechanisms of action. Clin. Ther. **26:** 830–840.
17. ETTINGER, B., D.M. BLACK & B.H. MITLAK, *et al.* 1999. Multiple Outcomes of Raloxifene Evaluation Investigators. Reduction of vertebral fracture risk in postmenopausal women with osteoporosis treated with raloxifene: results from a 3-year randomized clinical trial. JAMA **282:** 637–645.
18. MARTINO, S., J.A. CAULEY, E BARRETT-CONNOR, *et al.* 2004. Continuing outcomes relevant to Evista: breast cancer incidence in postmenopausal osteoporotic women in a randomized trial of raloxifene. J. Natl. Cancer Inst. **96:** 1751–1176.
19. VOGEL, V.G., J.P. COSTANTINO, D.L. WICKERHAM, *et al.* 2006. Effects of tamoxifen vs. raloxifene on the risk of developing invasive breast cancer and other disease

outcomes. The NSABP Study of Tamoxifen and Raloxifene (STAR) P-2 Trial. JAMA **295:** 2727–2741.

20. BARRETT-CONNOR, E., L. MOSCA, P. COLLINS, *et al.* 2006. Effects of raloxifene on cardiovascular events and breast cancer in postmenopausal women. N. Engl. J. Med. **355:** 125–137.

21. COOMBES, R.C., E. HALL, L.J. GIBSON, *et al.* 2004. A randomized trial of exemestane after two to three years of tamoxifen therapy in postmenopausal women with primary breast cancer. N. Engl. J. Med. **350:** 1081–1092.

22. THURLIMANN, B., A. KESHAVIAH & A.S. COATES, 2005. A comparison of letrozole and tamoxifen in postmenopausal women with early breast cancer. N. Engl. J. Med. **353:** 2747–2757.

23. BOCCARDO, F., A. RUBAGOTTI, M. PUNTONI, *et al.* 2005. Switching to anastrozole versus continued tamoxifen treatment of early breast cancer: preliminary results of the Italian Tamoxifen Anastrozole Trial. J. Clin. Oncol. **23:** 5138–5147.

24. JAKESZ, R., W. JONAT, M. GNANT *et al.* 2005. Switching of postmenopausal women with endocrine-responsive early breast cancer to anastrozole after 2 years' adjuvant tamoxifen: combined results of ABCSG trial 8 and ARNO 95 trial. Lancet **366:** 455–462.

25. GOSS, P.E., J.N. INGLE, S. MARTINO, *et al.* 2003. Randomized trial of letrozole in postmenopausal women after five years of tamoxifen therapy for early-stage breast cancer. N. Engl. J. Med. **349:** 1793–1802.

26. CUZICK, J.. 2003. Aromatase inhibitors in prevention–data from the ATAC (arimidex, tamoxifen alone or in combination) trial and the design of IBIS-II (the second International Breast Cancer Intervention Study). Recent Results Cancer Res. **163:** 96–103.

27. TERRY, M.B. M.D. GAMMON, F.F. Zhang, *et al.* 2004. Association of frequency and duration of aspirin use and hormone receptor status with breast cancer risk. JAMA **291:** 2433–2440.

28. DENKERT, C., K.J. WINZER & S. HAUPTMANN. 2004. Prognostic impact of cyclooxygenase-2 in breast cancer. Clin. Breast Cancer **4:** 428–433.

29. KUNDU, N. & A.M. FULTON. 2002. Selective cyclooxygenase (COX)-1 or COX-2 inhibitors control metastatic disease in a murine model of breast cancer. Cancer Res. **62:** 2343–2346.

30. CHEMOPREVENTION OF BREAST CANCER. 2006. Tamoxifen, raloxifene, and beyond. Am. J. Therap. **13:** 337–348.

31. BEATSON, G.T.. 1896. On the treatment of inoperable cases of carcinoma of the mamma: suggestions for a new method of treatment, with illustrative cases. Lancet **2:** 104–107.

32. JENSEN, E.V. & V.C. JORDAN. 2003. The estrogen receptor: a model for molecular medicine. Clin. Cancer Res. **9:** 1980–1989.

32. OSBORNE, C.K.. 1988. Tamoxifen in the treatment of breast cancer. N. Engl. J. Med. **339:** 1609–1618.

34. EARLY BREAST CANCER TRIALISTS' COLLABORATIVE GROUP (EBCTCG). 2005. Effects of chemotherapy and hormonal therapy for early breast cancer on recurrence and 15-year survival: an overview of the randomised trials. Lancet **365:** 1687–1717.

35. FISHER, B., J. DIGNAM, J. BRYANT, *et al.* 2001. Five versus more than five years of tamoxifen for lymph node-negative breast cancer: updated findings from the National Surgical Adjuvant Breast and Bowel Project B-14 randomized trial. J. Natl. Cancer Inst. **93:** 684–690.

36. JONAT, W., M. KAUFMANN, W. SAUERBREI, *et al.* 2002. Goserelin versus cyclophosphamide, methotrexate, and fluorouracil as adjuvant therapy in premenopausal patients with node-positive breast cancer: The Zoladex early breast cancer research association study. J. Clin. Oncol. **20:** 4628–4635.

37. INTERNATIONAL BREAST CANCER STUDY GROUP. 2003. Adjuvant chemotherapy followed by goserelin versus either modality alone for premenopausal lymph node-negative breast cancer: a randomised trial. J. Natl. Cancer Inst. **95:** 1833–1846.

38. THOMSON, C.S., C.J. TWELVES, E.A. MALLON, *et al.* 2002. Adjuvant ovarian ablation vs CMF chemotherapy in premenopausal breast cancer patients: trial update and impact of immunohistochemical assessment of ER status. Breast **11:** 419–429.

39. KLIJN, J.G., R.W. BLAMEY, F. BOCCARDO, *et al.* 2001. Combined tamoxifen and luteinizing hormone releasing hormone (LHRH) agonist versus LHRH agonist alone in premenopausal advanced breast cancer: a meta-analysis of four randomised trials. J. Clin. Oncol. **19:** 343–353.

40. BOCCARDO, F., A. RUBAGOTTI, D. AMOROSO, *et al.* 2000. Cyclophosphamide, methotrexate and fluorouracil versus tamoxifen plus ovarian suppression as adjuvant treatment of estrogen receptor positive pre-/perimenopausal breast cancer patients: results of the Italian breast cancer adjuvant study group 02 randomized trial. J. Clin. Oncol. **18:** 2718–2727.

41. JAKESZ, R., H. HAUSMANINGER, E. KUBISTA, *et al.* 2002. Randomized adjuvant trial of tamoxifen and goserelin versus cyclophosphamide, methotrexate, and fluorouracil: evidence for the superiority of treatment with endocrine blockade in premenopausal patients with hormone-responsive breast cancer—Austrian Breast and Colorectal Cancer Study Group Trial 5. J. Clin. Oncol. **20:** 4621–4627.

42. ROCHÉ, H.H., P. KERBRAT, J. BONNETERRE, *et al.* 2000. Complete hormonal blockade versus chemotherapy in premenopausal early-stage breast cancer patients (pts) with positive hormone-receptor (HR+) and 1-3 node-positive (N+) tumor: results of the FASG 06 trial [abstr 279]. Proc. Am. Soc. Clin. Oncol. **19:**72a.

43. DAVIDSON, N.E., A. O'NEILL, A. VUKOV, *et al.* 2003. Chemohormonal therapy in premenopausal node-positive, receptor-positive breast cancer: an Eastern Cooperative Oncology Group phase III intergroup trial (E5188,INT-0101) [abstr 15]. Proc. Am. Soc. Clin. Oncol. **22:**5.

44. RUTQVIST, L.E.. 1999. Zoladex and tamoxifen as adjuvant therapy in premenopausal breast cancer: a randomized trial by the Cancer Research Campaign (C.R.C.) Breast Cancer Trials Group, the Stockholm Breast Cancer Study Group, the South-East Sweden Breast Cancer Group & the Gruppo Interdisciplinare Valutazione Interventi in Oncologia (G.I.V.I.O) [abstr 251]. Proc. Am. Soc. Clin. Oncol. **18: 67a**.

45. DELLAPASQUA, S., M. COLLEONI, R.D. GELBER & A. GOLDHIRSCH. 2005. Adjuvant endocrine therapy for premenopausal women with early breast cancer. J. Clin. Oncol. **23:** 1736–1750.

46. BONNETERRE, J., A. BUZDAR, J.M.A. NABHOLTZ *et al.* 2001. Anastrozole is superior to tamoxifen as first-line therapy in hormone receptor positive advanced breast carcinoma: results of two randomized trials designed for combined analysis. Cancer **92:** 2247–2258.

47. PARIDAENS, R., P. THERASSE, L. DIRIX. 2004. et al. First line hormonal treatment (HT) for metastatic breast cancer (MBC) with exemestane (E) or tamoxifen (T)

in postmenopausal patients (pts)—a randomized phase III trial of the EORTC Breast Group. Proc. Am. Soc. Clin. Oncol. **23:** 6

48. MOURIDSEN, H., M. GERSHANOVICH, Y. SUN, *et al.* 2003. Phase III study of letrozole versus tamoxifen as first-line therapy of advanced breast cancer in postmenopausal women: analysis of survival and update of efficacy from the International Letrozole Breast Cancer Group. J. Clin. Oncol. **21:** 2101–2109.

49. THURLIMANN, B., A. KESHAVIAH & A.S. COATES, 2005. A comparison of letrozole and tamoxifen in postmenopausal women with early breast cancer. N. Engl. J. Med. **353:** 2747–2757.

50. HOWELL, A. on behalf of the ATAC Trialists Group. 2003. Effect of anastrozole on bone mineral density: 2-year results of the Arimidex (anastrozole), tamoxifen, alone or in combination (ATAC) trial. Breast Cancer Res. Treat. **82**(suppl 1): 27.

51. DOWSETT, M., J. CUZICK, C. WALE, *et al.* 2005. Retrospective analysis of time to recurrence in the atac trial according to hormone receptor status: an hypothesis-generating study J. Clin. Oncol. **23:** 7512–7517.

52. ELLIS, M.J., A. COOP, B. SINGH, *et al.* 2001. Letrozole is more effective neoadjuvant endocrine therapy than tamoxifen for ErbB-1- and/or ErbB2-positive, estrogen receptor-positive primary breast cancer: evidence from a phase III randomized trial. J. Clin. Oncol. **19:** 3808–3816.

HER2/neu Expression in Relation to Clinicopathologic Features of Breast Cancer Patients

ADELE TRAINA,[a] BIAGIO AGOSTARA,[b] LORENZO MARASÀ,[c]
MAURIZIO CALABRÒ,[a] MAURIZIO ZARCONE,[a]
AND GIUSEPPE CARRUBA[a]

[a]Experimental Oncology, Department of Oncology, P.O. "M. Ascoli,"
ARNAS-Civico, Palermo 90127, Italy

[b]Medical Oncology, Department of Oncology, P.O. "M. Ascoli," ARNAS-Civico,
Palermo 90127, Italy

[c]Pathology Units, Department of Oncology, P.O. "M. Ascoli," ARNAS-Civico,
Palermo 90127, Italy

ABSTRACT: We have evaluated HER2/neu expression in 1,355 breast cancer patients recruited at the Breast Cancer Registry in Palermo between
January 1999 and December 2004. In this retrospective study, HER2/neu
expression was related to clinicopathologic features of the disease, including tumor size, nodal and menopausal status, estrogen and progesterone receptors. Statistical analysis on all 1,355 patients showed a significant correlation between HER2/neu and nodal status ($P < 0.001$),
and a significant association between HER2/neu overexpression and estrogen and progesterone receptors status ($P < 0.001$). In 194 patients
without metastasis, with an average follow-up ≥ 5 years, only HER2/neu
3+ and histopathologic grading G3 were significantly associated with
overall survival.

KEYWORDS: HER2/neu; breast cancer; overall survival analysis

INTRODUCTION

Human epidermal growth factor receptor-2 is a proto-oncogene that encodes
a cell-surface receptor referred to as HER2/neu or c-erbB-2.[1] The HER2/neu
oncogene is located on chromosome 17q21[1] and encodes a 185-kDa transmembrane glycoprotein that is homologous to the other three members of the
family: HER1, HER3, and HER4.[2–7] These membrane proteins consist of a

Address for correspondence: Dr. Adele Traina, Experimental Oncology Unit, Department of Oncology, P.O. "M. Ascoli," via Parlavecchio n. 139, 90127 Palermo, Italy. Voice: +39-091-666-4346; fax:
+39-091-666-4352.

e-mail: registrotumori@ospedalecivicopa.org

Ann. N.Y. Acad. Sci. 1089: 159–167 (2006). © 2006 New York Academy of Sciences.
doi: 10.1196/annals.1386.029

tyrosine-protein kinase domain, a single membrane-spanning region, and two cysteine-rich extracellular domains.[8–9] Contrary to the latter three proteins, no ligand has been so far identified to bind HER2/neu. This receptor may act through heterodimerization with one of the other three family members after their activation upon ligand binding.[10–14] The heterodimerization ultimately leads to autophosphorylation as a result of intrinsic tyrosine kinase activity, and triggers a signaling cascade to the nucleus for subsequent gene transcription. HER2/neu gene amplification and/or protein overexpression occur in 14–30% of all cases of breast cancer.[15–16]

There is consistent evidence that amplification and/or overexpression of HER2/neu are associated with a worse clinical outcome in both node-positive and node-negative breast cancer patients.[17]

In the present study, we have inspected the expression of HER2/neu in relation to the clinical-pathological features of the disease, aiming to determine the potential impact of this oncogene product on the overall survival of patients.

MATERIALS AND METHODS

Patients

A total of 1,355 breast cancer patients were all recruited at our Breast Cancer Registry of Palermo between January 1999 and December 2004. All patients had a histologically documented adenocarcinoma of the breast. The mean age of patients involved in the study was 57 years (range 22–93 years). A total of 65 patients (4.8%) had a metastatic neoplasia *ab initio* (M1). The sites mostly affected by metastatic dissemination were bone, liver, and lung.

All patients affected by nonmetastatic breast cancer had undergone surgical treatment (mastectomy or quadrantectomy) and depletion of the homolateral axillary cavity and adjuvant therapy according to the guidelines of the Consensus Conference on Breast Cancer.[18] The most frequent histotype was the infiltrating ductal carcinoma, whereas 144 patients (~ 11%) were affected by infiltrating lobular carcinoma.

We also assessed overall survival in a subgroup of 208 patients having a follow-up time >5 years. These patients had undergone surgery between January 1999 and December 2001. The mean age of these patients was 54 years (range 29–85 years). A total of 14 of these patients (6.7%) had metastatic disease at the time of diagnosis and were censored for the survival analyses.

Immunohistochemistry (IHC) of HER2/neu Expression

Methodological procedures of HER2/neu have been previously described.[21] The 2–4-μM-thick tissue sections were cleared in xylene rehydrated in ethanol, and finally rinsed in distilled water. The slides were then incubated with primary antibody (rat polyclonal antibody anti-human HER2/neu protein) for 30 min at room temperature.

The reaction was subsequently revealed through incubation with the visualization reactant (EN Vision/ HRP Plus, rabbit) and samples were processed with a chromogen agent (DAB) for 10 min and counterstained with hematoxylin for 30 sec. The slides were then dehydrated and mounted using a natural resin. At the end of the procedure, membranes of the positive cells were stained in red-brown, while negative ones were stained in blue-violet. HER2/neu stain intensity was graded according to the following scale: cases showing no staining were scored 0; cases with less than 10% membrane scored staining 1+; cases with more than 10% weak-to-moderate complete membrane staining scored 2+; and cases with more than 10% strong complete membrane staining scored 3+.

FISH Analysis of HER2/neu Amplification

As reported elsewhere, 2–4-μM paraffin-embedded tissue sections were cleared and hydrated. Sample were then enzymatically digested, denatured and finally incubated for 12 h with the DNA HER2/neu gene probe (INFORM HER2/neu probe for automation, Ventana) labeled with biotin.

After hybridization, samples were washed in buffer and subsequently incubated with a detection system consisting of a first antibiotin rat monoclonal antibody labeled with fluorescein isothiocyanate (FITC) and a second FITC-labeled anti-IgG rat antibody, which further amplifies the signal.

The slides were finally counterstained with the VECTASHIELD system (Vector Laboratories, Burlingame, CA, USA), analyzed with fluorescence microscope, and the number of fluorescein signals counted in 20 nuclei of invasive tumor cells for each field. Cases were considered amplified if the mean number of fluorescence signals was greater than 4.

Statistical Methods

The correlation degree between the HER2/NEU expression and the histopathological characteristics of the patients was analyzed by Pearson's chi-square test. The overall survival curves were graphed using the Kaplan-Meyer method.

RESULTS

As reported in TABLE 1, of the 1,290 patients who did not show metastases at presentation, 62%, had a T1 primary tumor. The nodal status showed a slight

TABLE 1. Clinical features of 1,290 M0 breast cancer patients

Features		%
T, tumor size	T1	62.00
	T2	31.53
	T3	1.15
	T4	5.32
N, nodal status	N0	57.66
	N+	42.34
G, tumor grading	G1	10.36
	G2	53.83
	G3	35.80
ER/PR status[a]	+/+	62.42
	+/−	13.86
	−/+	4.88
	−/−	18.83
ER status (S/N)[b]	+/+	57.97
	+/0	2.90
	0/+	29.71
	0/0	9.42
Menopausal status (M)	PreM	31.99
	PostM	68.01

[a] Immunohistochemical assay.
[b] LBS of soluble (S) and nuclear (N) cell fractions.

prevalence of N0 (57.6%) with respect to N1 patients (42.4%). The distribution of the patients according to the number of involved nodes shows that 49.1% of the patients has a number of metastatic nodes that varied between 1 and 3; 34.7% between 3 and 10; and 16.2% had more than 10 metastatic nodes. A total of 53.8% of the patients had a G2 tumor, 35.8% were G3, and only 10.4% were G1.

The ER expression was determined by immunohistochemical (IHC) studies in 1,147 patients and by ligand binding assay (LBA) in 138 patients. As regards LBA, 58% of patients showed a homogenously positive ER status (+/+); 9.4% were receptor-negative (−/−); and the remaining 32.6% were ER-negative in the soluble (0/+, 29.7%) or nuclear cell fraction (+/0, 2.9%).

The IHC shows that 62.4% of the patients were both ER- and PR-positive; 13.9% had an ER-positive and PR-negative status; while 18.8% were negative for either receptor. Only 4.9% of cases showed an ER-negative and PR-positive status.

As shown in FIGURE 1 most of the M0 patients (72.5%) had a negative or +1 HER2/neu status, whereas the +2 and +3 cases were approximately 27.5% of the total.

On the contrary patients with metastases showed a considerably greater proportion of +2 and +3 cases (approximately 40%), and a total number of negative or +1 cases around 60%.

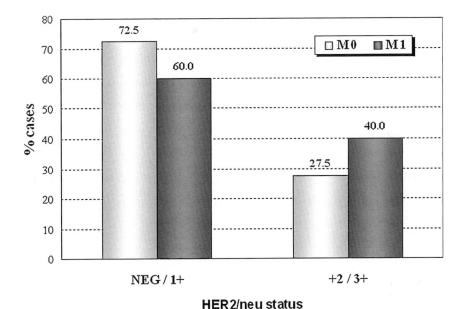

FIGURE 1. Distribution of HER2/neu expression in relation to metastatic disease ($P =$ 0.075).

In the 1,290 M0 patients, we have assessed the correlation between HER2/neu and other histopathological features of breast cancer. In particular, a statistically significant correlation ($P < 0.001$) was observed between HER2/neu +3 expression and a negative receptor status, as assessed by IHC studies (TABLE 2).

A statistically significant correlation was also found between a positive nodal status and HER2/neu overexpression ($P < 0.001$) (TABLE 3).

Furthermore, patients having HER2/neu +3 tumors were significantly associated with G3 tumor grade ($P < 0.001$) (TABLE 4).

The overall survival in relation to the HER2/neu status was assessed in a subgroup of 194 M0 patients operated between January 1999 and December 2001, having an average follow-up time of 58 months.

The expression of HER2/neu in these patients was comparable to that of the original group (1,290) of patients (TABLE 5).

TABLE 2. Percent distribution of HER2/neu expression in relation to receptor status

HER-2/neu	ER+/PgR+	ER+/PgR−	ER−/PgR+	ER−/PgR−
3+	12.85	16.35	14.29	25.00
0–2+	87.15	83.65	85.71	75.00

TABLE 3. Percent distribution of HER2/neu expression in relation to nodal status

HER-2 / neu	N0	N+
3+	11.96	20.83
0–2+	88.04	79.17

TABLE 4. Percent distribution of HER2/neu expression in relation to tumor grading

HER-2 / neu	G1	G2	G3
3+	7.32	14.20	21.70
2+	8.94	12.79	12.50
NEG/1+	83.74	73.01	65.80

TABLE 5. Comparison of HER2/neu distribution in the two groups of 1,290 and 194 breast cancer patients

HER-2/neu	1999–2004(1,290 cases)	%	1999–2001(194 cases)	%
0 / 1+	935	72.48	145	74.74
2+	154	11.94	22	11.34
3+	201	15.58	27	13.92

In univariate analysis, neither age at diagnosis nor menopausal status or tumor size had a significant influence on the overall survival. Overall, only histological grade ($P = 0.0428$) (FIG. 2) and HER2/neu status ($P = 0.0267$) (FIG. 3) were significant discriminants in univariate analysis of patients' survival.

DISCUSSION

The prognostic value of HER2/neu has always been controversial. Studies showing a shorter overall survival for HER2/neu-positive patients have been contradicted by others which failed to find such an association.[19] In any case, the actual role of HER2/neu as a predictive marker in breast cancer patients is still a matter of debate.[15] Several possible reasons could account for this inconsistency. One frequently quoted reason could be the rather small sample size of many studies.

However, probably the most important reason lies in the lack of standardized evaluation protocols in most earlier studies.

In this retrospective study, we have assessed the HER2/neu expression through IHC on 1,355 patients affected by breast cancer.

The overexpression of this oncogene in patients affected by localized and metastatic disease was 16% and 25%, respectively. These data are in substantial agreement with most of the data reported in the literature.[15]

The total percentage HER2/neu-positive (+2 and +3) cases through by IHC was considerably greater among metastatic patients (40%) than in patients without metastases (27.5%).

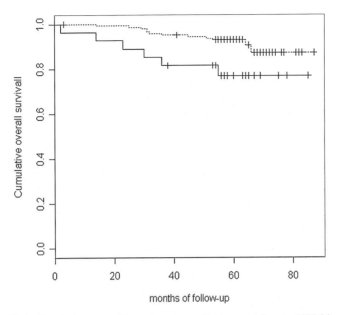

FIGURE 2. Survival curve of breast cancer patients according to HER2/neu status. Kaplan-Meyer analysis ($P = 0.0267$). *Dashed line* = 0/1+ patients; *solid line* = +3 patients.

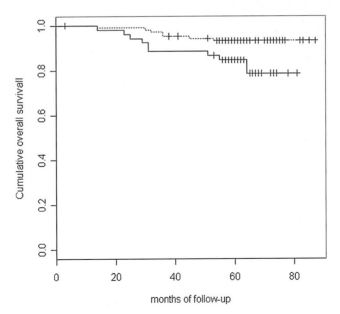

FIGURE 3. Survival curve in breast cancer patients according to tumor grading. Kaplan-Meyer analysis ($P = 0.0428$). *Dashed line* = G1 and G2 patients; *solid line* = G3 patients.

It is interesting to note that the HER2/neu cases, as classified by IHC are significantly associated with ER and PR status as determined by IHC ($P < 0.001$).

A very strong association ($P < 0.001$) was also observed between HER2/neu status and both nodal involvement and tumor grading ($P < 0.001$). On the contrary, no association was evidenced with other clinical-pathological parameters, such as tumor dimension, menopausal status, and age.

In a survival analysis of 194 breast cancer patients without metastases, whose average follow-up time was 58 months, the mortality risk observed was significantly higher in HER2/neu +3 cases than in negative and +1 cases ($P = 0.0267$). In addition, the mortality risk was markedly higher in G3 than in G1 and G2 tumors ($P = 0.0428$).

Long-term prospective studies are necessary to validate these findings and to ascertain whether monoclonal antibodies against HER2/neu (Herceptin) could be beneficial as an additional and/or alternative adjuvant therapy option in breast cancer patients overexpressing HER2/neu.[20]

REFERENCES

1. STERN, D.F., P.A. HEFFERNAN & R.A. WEINBERG. 1986. p185, a product of the neu proto-oncogene, is a receptorlike protein associated with tyrosine kinase activity. Mol. Cell Biol. **6:** 1729–1740.
2. HYNES, N.E. & D.F. STERN. 1994. The biology of erbB-2/neu/HER2/NEU and its role in cancer. Bioch. Biophys. Acta **1198:** 165–184.
3. AKIYAMA, T., C. SUDO, H. OGAWARA, et al. 1986. The product of human c-erbB-2 gene: a 185 Kilodalton glycoprotein with tyrosineKinase activity. Science **232:** 1644–1646.
4. BARGMANN, C.I., M.C. HUNG & R.A. WEINBERG. 1986. The neu oncogene encodes an epidermal growth factor receptor-related protein. Nature **319:** 226–230.
5. COUSSENS, L., T.L. YANG-FENG, Y.-C. LIAO, et al.1985. Tyrosine kinase receptor with extensive homology to EGF receptor shares chromosomal location with neu oncogene. Science **230:** 1132–1139.
6. SCHECHTER, A.L., D.F. STERN, L. VAIDYANATHAN, et al. 1984. The neu oncogene: an erbB-related gene encoding a 185,000-Mr tumour antigen. Nature **213:** 513–516.
7. RIESE, D.J. & D.F. STERN.1998. Specificity within the EGF family/ErbB receptor family signaling network. Bioessays **20:** 41–48.
8. MAGUIRE, H.C. & M.I. GREENE. 1989. The neu (c-erbB-2) oncogene. Semin. Oncol. **16:** 148–155
9. VAN DER GEER, P., T. HUNTER & R.A. LINDBERG. 1994. Receptor protein tyrosine kinases and their signal transduction pathways. Annu. Rev. Cell. Biol. **10:** 251–337.
10. PINKAS-KRAMARSKI, R., R. EILAM, I. ALROY, et al. 1997. Differential expression of NDF/neuregulin receptors ErbB-3 and ErbB-4 and involvement in inhibition of neuronal differentiation. Oncogene **15:** 2803–2815.
11. KLAPPER, L.N., S. GLATHE, N. VAISMAN, et al. 1999. The ErbB-2/HER2/NEU oncoprotein of human carcinomas may function solely as a shared coreceptor for

multiple stroma-derived growth factors. Proc. Natl. Acad. Sci. USA **96:** 4995–5000.

12. PINKAS-KRAMARSKI, R., M. SHELLY, B.C. GUARINO, *et al.* 1998. erbB Tyrosine kinases and two neuregulin families constitute a ligand receptor network. Mol. Cell. Biol. **18:** 6090–6101.

13. ALROY, I. & Y. YARDEN. 1997. The erbB signaling network in embryogenesis and oncogenesis: signal diversification through combinatorial ligand-receptor interaction. FEBS Lett. **410:** 83–86.

14. TZAHAR, E., G. LEVKOWITZ, D. KARUNAGARAN, *et al.* 1996. A hierarchical network of interreceptor interactions determines sal transduction by neu differentiation factor/neuregulin and epidermal growth factor. Mol. Cell. Biol. **16:** 5276–5287.

15. SLAMON, D.J., W. GODOLPHIN, L.A. JONES, *et al.* 1989. Studies of the HER2/neu proto-oncogene in human breast and ovarian cancer. Science **244:** 707–712.

16. SLAMON, D.J., G.M. CLARK, S.G. WONG, *et al.* 1987. Human breast cancer: correlation of relapse and survival with amplification of the HER2/neu oncogene. Science **235:** 177–182.

17. LÜFTNER, D., A. JUNG, P. SCHIMID, *et al.* 2003. Upregulation of HER2/neu by ovarian ablation: results of a randomized trial comparing leuproein to CMF as adjuvant therapy in node-positive breast cancer patient. Breast Cancer Res. Treat. **80:** 245–255.

18. GOLDHIRSCH, A., J.H. GLICK, W. R.D. GELBER,, *et al.* 2005. Meeting Highlights: International Expert Consensus on the Primary Therapy of Early Breast Cancer 2005. Ann. Oncol. **16:** 1569–1583.

19. REED, W. E. HANNISDAL, P.J. BOEHLER, *et al.* 1989. The prognostic value of p53 and c-erb B-2 immunostaining is overrated for patients with lymph node negative breast carcinoma: a multivariate analysis of prognostic factors in 613 patients with a follow-up of 14–30 years. Cancer **88:**804–813.

20. BASELGA, J., L. GIANNI, C. GEYER, *et al.* 2004. Future options with trastuzumab for primary systemic and adjuvant therapy. Semin. Oncol. **31**(5 Suppl. 10): 51–57. Review.

21. CASTAGNETTA, L.M. *et al.* 2002. Ligand binding and cytochemical analysis of estrogen and progesterone receptors in relation to follow-up in patients with breast cancer. Ann. N. Y. Acad. Sci. **963:** 98–103.

Sex Steroids and Prostate Carcinogenesis

Integrated, Multifactorial Working Hypothesis

MAARTEN C. BOSLAND[a,b]

[a]University of Illinois at Chicago, Chicago, Illinois 606129, USA

[b]New York University School of Medicine, New York, New York, USA

ABSTRACT: Androgens are thought to cause prostate cancer, but there is little epidemiological support for this notion. Animal studies, however, demonstrate that androgens are very strong tumor promotors for prostate carcinogenesis after tumor-initiating events. Even treatment with low doses of testosterone alone can induce prostate cancer in rodents. Because testosterone can be converted to estradiol-17β by the enzyme aromatase, expressed in human and rodent prostate, estrogen may be involved in prostate cancer induction by testosterone. When estradiol is added to testosterone treatment of rats, prostate cancer incidence is markedly increased and even a short course of estrogen treatment results in a high incidence of prostate cancer. The active testosterone metabolite 5α-dihydrotestosterone cannot be aromatized to estrogen and hardly induces prostate cancer, supporting a critical role of estrogen in prostate carcinogenesis. Estrogen receptors are expressed in the prostate and may mediate some or all of the effects of estrogen. However, there is also evidence that in the rodent and human prostate conversion occurs of estrogens to catecholestrogens. These can be converted to reactive intermediates that can adduct to DNA and cause generation of reactive oxygen species, and thus estradiol can be a weak DNA damaging (genotoxic) carcinogen. In the rat prostate DNA damage can result from estrogen treatment; this occurs prior to cancer development and at exactly the same location. Inflammation may be associated with prostate cancer risk, but no environmental carcinogenic risk factors have been definitively identified. We postulate that endogenous factors present in every man, sex steroids, are responsible for the high prevalence of prostate cancer in aging men, androgens acting as strong tumor promoters in the presence of a weak, but continuously present genotoxic carcinogen, estradiol-17β.

KEYWORDS: prostate; prostate cancer; estrogen, androgen; carcinogenesis; hormonal carcinogenesis

Address for correspondence: Maarten C. Bosland, Department of Pathology, University of Illinois at Chicago College of Medicine, 840 South Wood Street, Room 130 CSN, MC 847, Chicago, IL 60612, USA. Voice: +1-312-355-3724; fax: +1-312-996-7586.

e-mail: boslandm@uic.edu

Ann. N.Y. Acad. Sci. 1089: 168–176 (2006). © 2006 New York Academy of Sciences.

doi: 10.1196/annals.1386.040

INTRODUCTION

Prostate cancer is a very common cancer in males in most European and North American countries. In the United States it is the most frequently diagnosed nonskin malignancy in men and it is the most common cause of death from cancer. Small, microscopic-size (histologic) carcinomas in the prostate are exceedingly common in men over the age of 30 years and may occur in as many as 50% of men over 50 years of age and in 80% of men over 80 years; lifetime risk of such prostate cancer is on the order of 85%. However, clinically apparent cancer of the prostate is far less common, lifetime risk being in the range of 15–20% in most European and North American countries, and this malignancy is only clinically important in men over the age of 50 years. Why this cancer is so common and why the majority of histologic carcinomas do not progress to a clinically relevant stage within the lifetime of most men is not clear. In fact, the causes of prostate cancer are not understood even though the disease is highly prevalent (see Refs. 1, 2, 3, and 4 for reviews). Besides age, which is a strong risk factor, there are few other established risk factors, including a family history of prostate cancer, a Western lifestyle, and an African American heritage—worldwide, the incidence of clinically significant prostate cancer is highest among black Americans and is far more common in Western countries than in most Asian countries and most less-affluent societies. However, for neither risk factor are the underlying mechanisms known. Prostatitis (prostatic inflammation), which a very frequent condition as well, is suspected to be a risk factor.[5] Although hard evidence for an inflammatory hypothesis remains elusive, the oxidative stress associated with inflammation offers an attractive mechanism whereby prostatitis may contribute to cancer formation.[5] Another highly prevalent prostatic disease, benign prostatic hypertrophy (BPH), is not associated with prostate cancer.

Prostate cancer is a hormone-dependent malignancy that develops from an androgen-dependent tissue that contains androgen receptors. The vast majority of prostate carcinomas initially respond to androgen ablation therapy, but later relapse to an androgen-independent (hormone-refractory) state. Because of these features, androgens are thought to be involved in the causation of prostate cancer. However, there is very little support for this notion from a variety of epidemiological studies or tissue-based investigations.[6] For example, in a meta-analysis by Eaton et al.,[7] there was a total absence of a relation between prediagnostic androgen levels in serum or plasma. However, there are also data in support of such a relationship[8] and recent reports of an inverse relationship between risk and androgen levels.[9] Another example is that even hormone-refractory prostate cancers express androgen receptors that are activated.[10] While a ligand-independent mechanism is thought to be responsible for this phenomenon, it does not provide support for the hypothesis of androgens as a cause of prostate cancer in humans. The only support for a hormonal-causation hypothesis comes from the recently completed prevention study with the drug finasteride, which inhibits 5α-reductase, the enzyme that converts testosterone to the active androgen 5α-dehydrotestosterone.[11] A 7-year intervention with this drug reduced prostate cancer risk in healthy men by about 25%. However, more high-grade cancers were found in those men who did develop prostate cancer while on the drug than in men who received a placebo, undercutting the notion that androgens cause possible aggressive prostate carcinomas that are likely to become clinically evident. Two interpretations of the outcome of the finasteride study might be (1) that androgens cause clinically insignificant cancers, but not prostate carcinomas that progress to become aggressive, or (2) that androgen is necessary for prostate cancer causation, but not sufficient and that other factors are major determinants of progression to the aggressive stage.

Animal studies, on the other hand, clearly demonstrate that androgens are very strong tumor promotors for prostate carcinogenesis at very low, near physiological, concentrations. This may explain why it has been difficult to find significant associations between elevated levels of circulating androgens and risk of prostate cancer. Even treatment with low doses of testosterone alone can induce prostate cancer in rats, albeit at low incidence in most strains. A single prostate-targeted tumor-initiating dose of one of several chemical carcinogens causes a low incidence of prostate carcinomas in rats. Subsequent long-term, low-dose testosterone treatment markedly increases prostate cancer yields, demonstrating the strong tumor-promoting activity of androgens.[12]

Testosterone can be converted to estradiol-17β by the enzyme aromatase, which is expressed in the human prostate,[13] and there is indirect evidence for aromatase expression in rodent prostate (Vega and Bosland, unpublished data).[14–16] Therefore, estrogen may be involved in the induction of prostate cancer by this androgen. The Noble (NBL) rat strain is very sensitive to testosterone treatment. When estradiol is added to testosterone treatment of these NBL rats, prostate cancer incidence is increased from 35–40% with androgen alone to 90–100% within approximately 1 year.[17] Unpublished reports from our laboratory indicate that even a short course of estrogen treatment (for 2–4 months) is sufficient to result in a high incidence (approximately 70%) of prostate cancer in rats in the presence of chronic low-dose androgen treatment. The active testosterone metabolite 5α-dihydrotestosterone cannot be aromatized to estrogen and does not induce prostate cancer in more than 5% of treated rats, supporting the notion that estrogen plays a critical role in prostate carcinogenesis.[18] However, when estradiol is added to the androgen treatment, cancer formation does not nearly increase as much as when estradiol is given with testosterone. Unfortunately, experiments with just estrogen treatment result in the shutdown of endogenous androgen production due to reduction of LH production via the pituitary feedback, and this leads to prostate atrophy, which renders prostate carcinogenesis studies impossible. Studies with aromatase knockout mice[16] and aromatase-overexpressing mice[14,15] are potentially interesting, but these mice suffer from androgen abnormalities that make their interpretation limited. Aromatase knockout mice lack estrogen production, but have elevated testosterone levels and prostate enlargement but no cancer.[16] Aromatase-overexpressing mice have elevated estrogen production, but markedly reduced testosterone levels, and develop no prostate lesions related to cancer.[14,15] Both observations are consistent with the notion that both hormones are necessary for prostate cancer development.

The estrogen receptors-α and -β are expressed in the prostate and may mediate some or all of the effects of estrogen.[19-21] Indeed, simultaneous treatment of NBL rats with estradiol plus testosterone and an antiestrogen (ICI 182,780) inhibits the development of dysplasia in the prostate (or murine prostatic intraepithelial neoplasia), a putative preneoplastic lesion.[22] On the other hand, there is no effect of administration of another antiestrogen, tamoxifen, to rats treated with low-dose testosterone after exposure to a prostate-directed carcinogen; prostate cancer yield remained high in these rats.[23] One effect of estradiol treatment of rats is the estrogen receptor–mediated induction of enlargement and tumors of the pituitary gland, which leads to marked elevation of circulating prolactin. These effects are counteracted by treatment with antiestrogens. High circulating levels of prolactin are known to produce prostatic inflammation in rats,[24] and treatment with antiestrogens lowers prolactin in estrogen-treated rats and reduces inflammation.[22] Because inflammation may be associated with reactive hyperplasia similar to the aforementioned dysplasia, the inhibition of dysplasia development by antiestrogens in rats treated with estradiol plus testosterone may simply be due to the lowering of prolactin in these animals. Indeed, treatment of these steroid hormone–exposed rats with an antiprolactin drug, bromocryptin, not only lowers prolactin levels, but also inhibits the development of dysplasia and inflammation in the prostate.[25] Of note, the dysplasia and inflammation in NBL rats treated with estradiol plus estosterone occur in the same region of the prostate (dorsolateral prostate), whereas carcinomas in these animals originate in another region (the periurethral area);[17] the dysplasia in the dorsolateral prostate only rarely progresses to cancer (Bosland, unpublished results). The studies with the ICI antiestrogen and bromocryptin did not last sufficiently long to determine their effects on the induction of periurethral prostate carcinomas. Taken together, these data (1) do not support a major role of estrogen receptors in the induction of prostate cancer or dysplasia, but conclusive studies are lacking at present, and (2) indicate that prolactin appears to play a role in the generation of dorsolateral prostate dysplasia in NBL rats treated with estradiol plus testosterone, but it is not clear whether this hormone is involved in cancer formation. There is a notion that the estrogen receptor-β may mediate inhibition of the progression of prostate cancer,[21] but this is not a generally accepted and validated concept at present.

There is also evidence from partially published results of the author in collaboration with E. Cavalieri and E. Rogan (unpublished results)[26] that, in the rodent and human prostate, conversion occurs of estradiol and estrone to catecholestrogen, 2- and 4-hydroxyestrogens. These catecholestrogens can be converted to estrogen semiquinones and estrogen quinones by the process of redox cycling; these are reactive intermediates that can adduct to DNA and cause generation of reactive oxygen species.[27,28] The DNA adducts formed by the 4-hydroxyestrogen quinones depurinate, leading to apurinic sites in the DNA, which can lead to the generation of mutations by error-prone DNA repair processes.[29] Indeed, there is evidence from experiments in other tissues indicating that estradiol can be a weak DNA damaging (genotoxic) carcinogen.[30] Partially published results from studies by the author in collaboration with E. Cavalieri and E. Rogan indicate that these reactions can take place in the rat prostate[26] and possibly the human prostate. In addition, there is some evidence that in the NBL rat prostate DNA damage results from estrogen treatment and that this occurs prior to cancer development and at the exact same location within the rat prostate where carcinomas develop after treatment with estradiol plus testosterone.[31,27,26] There are enzymes, such as catechol-O-methyltransferase and glutathione reductase, that protect against these reactive estrogen metabolites. These protective enzymes appear to be more active in the dorsolateral prostate region, which does not develop cancer in NBL rats treated with estradiol plus testosterone, and less active in the periurethral prostate area, where carcinomas do develop.[26]

As indicated above, no environmental carcinogenic factors associated with prostate cancer risk have been definitively identified and the causes of this very prevalent malignancy remain elusive. Therefore, it is attractive to postulate that endogenous factors present in every man, namely sex steroids, are responsible for the high frequency of prostate cancer in aging men. If one hypothesizes that androgens act as strong tumor promotors, the presence within the prostate of a weak, but ubiquitously and continuously present genotoxic carcinogen, estradiol-17β, may be sufficient to cause prostate cancer at high prevalence in humans just as it appears to do in the NBL rat model. The increase in estrogen-to-androgen ratio that occurs in aging men [32] can be viewed as support for the notion that estrogens, in addition to androgens, are critical factors in prostate carcinogenesis. This hypothesis may explain why prostate cancer is so common. However, it does not explain why some tumors progress to be clinically evident and aggressive, while others remain apparently indolent. It also does not explain why this process of progression is far more common in Western countries, particularly among African American men, than in most Asian countries, while migrants from low-risk to high-risk countries acquire the risk of their new environment.[1-3] Clearly, there are other factors than hormones *per se* that play a decisive role. There may be genetic, hereditary factors as well as environmental factors determining (1) the sensitivity of the androgen receptor for 5α-dehydrotestosterone and (2) critical steps in the metabolism of androgens (5α-reductase) and estrogens (aromatase and the enzymes involved in generation of and protection against reactive estrogen metabolites). Indeed, prostate cancer risk appears associated with the length of

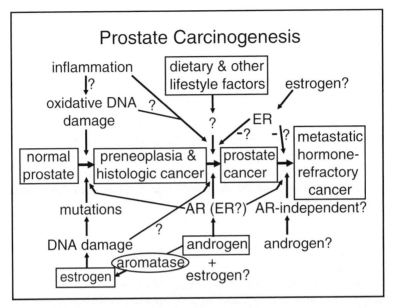

FIGURE 1. Summary of the proposed hypothesis of prostate carcinogenesis involving three steps: (1) the formation of preneoplasia (high-grade prostatic intraepithelial neoplasia) and histologic carcinoma; (2) progression to clinically significant (aggressive) carcinoma; and (3) further progression to metastatic and hormone-refractory carcinoma. Four proposed major determinants of these steps—estrogen, androgen, aromatase, and dietary and lifestyle factors—are indicated within text boxes. Less certain factors and mechanisms involved in prostate carcinogenesis, such as inflammation, androgen receptor (AR), and estrogen receptors (ER), are not placed within a text box and are identified with question marks.

a CAG repeat sequence in the coding region of the androgen receptor, which is known to affect androgen receptor activity. Short CAG repeat lengths in this region are associated with higher androgen receptor activity and higher prostate cancer risk, and they are more common in African Americans than in other racial groups.[1,4] There is also some evidence to suggest that 5α-reductase activity is lower in Asian men than in other ethnic groups.[33] However, both associations are not consistently found and there are contradictory reports and there are no consistent relationships between genetic polymorphisms in the 5α-reductase gene and prostate cancer risk.[1,4] There is no doubt that there are environmental factors, which are critical determinants of risk of clinically evident prostate cancer, explaining the changes in prostate cancer risk in migrants from low- to high-risk countries, but these factors have not been identified.

In conclusion, prostate carcinogenesis appears to be a highly multifactorial process in which hormones, both androgens and estrogen, play a central role. A causative role of inflammation has been proposed, but evidence for this notion is not very strong at present. Environmental and genetic factors may determine in large part the risk of clinically significant prostate cancer by affecting the rate of progression of early-stage carcinomas; steroid hormone effects may be responsible for the very high prevalence of prostate cancer. If one hypothesizes that androgens act as strong tumor promotors, the presence of a weak, but ubiquitously and continuously present genotoxic carcinogen, estradiol-17β, may be sufficient to cause prostate cancer at high prevalence. Although this hypothesis (FIG. 1) does not take into account some of the important intricacies of prostate biology such as stromal–epithelial interrelationships and factors such as the IGF axis, it provides a new framework on which to base novel approaches to understanding prostate carcinogenesis. Moreover, this proposed mechanism may offer opportunities for preventive interventions by agents that inhibit formation of reactive estrogen metabolites that damage DNA or enhance enzymatic factors that provide protection against these metabolites.

ACKNOWLEDGMENTS

The results from our laboratory have been supported in part by NIH Grants No. CA104334 and CA75293, and the collaborations between the author and E. Cavalieri and E. Rogan have been supported in part by NIH Grant No. CA49210 and DOD Grant No. DAMD 17-02-1-0660.

REFERENCES

1. BOSLAND, M.C. 2000. The role of steroid hormones in prostate carcinogenesis. J. Natl. Cancer Inst. Monogr. 27: 39–66.
2. CHAN, J.M., P.H. GANN & E.L. GIOVANNUCCI. 2005. Role of diet in prostate cancer development and progression. J. Clin. Oncol. 23: 8152–8160.
3. GANN, P.H. 2002. Risk factors for prostate cancer. Rev. Urol. 4(Suppl 5): S3–S10.
4. PLATZ, E.A. & E. GIOVANNUCCI. 2004. The epidemiology of sex steroid hormones and their signaling and metabolic pathways in the etiology of prostate cancer. J. Steroid Biochem. Mol. Biol. 92: 237–253.
5. PALAPATTU, G.S., S. SUTCLIFFE, P.J. BASTIAN, et al. 2005. Prostate carcinogenesis and inflammation: emerging insights. Carcinogenesis 26: 1170–1181.
6. MORGENTALER, A. 2006. Testosterone and prostate cancer: an historical perspective on a modern myth. Eur. Urol. 50: 935–939. Jul 27 [Epub ahead of print].
7. EATON, N.E., G.K. REEVES, P.N. APPLEBY & T.J. KEY. 1999. Endogenous sex hormones and prostate cancer: a quantitative review of prospective studies. Br. J. Cancer 80: 930–934.
8. GANN, P.H., C.H. HENNEKENS, J. MA, et al. 1996. Prospective study of sex hormone levels and risk of prostate cancer. J. Natl. Cancer Inst. 88: 1118–1126.
9. SEVERI, G., H.A. MORRIS, R.J. MACINNIS, et al. 2006. Circulating steroid hormones and the risk of prostate cancer. Cancer Epidemiol. Biomarkers Prev. 15: 86–91.
10. TAPLIN, M.E. & S.P. BALK. 2004. Androgen receptor: a key molecule in the progression of prostate cancer to hormone independence. J. Cell. Biochem. 91: 483–490.

11. THOMPSON, I.M., P.J. GOODMAN, C.M. TANGEN, *et al.* 2003. The influence of finasteride on the development of prostate cancer. N. Engl. J. Med. **349:** 215–224.

12. BOSLAND, M.C., H.C. DREEF-VAN DER MEULEN, S. SUKUMAR, *et al.* 1992. Multistage prostate carcinogenesis: the role of hormones. *In* Multistage Carcinogenesis. Proceedings of the 22nd International symposium of the Princess Takamatsu Cancer Research Fund. C.C. Harris, S. Hirohashi, N. Ito, H.C. Pitot, T. Sugimura, M. Terada, J. Yokota, Eds.: 109–123. Japan Sci. Soc. Press/Boca Raton, FL. CRC Press. Tokyo, Japan.

13. ELLEM, S.J., J.F. SCHMITT, J.S. PEDERSEN, *et al.* 2004. Local aromatase expression in human prostate is altered in malignancy. J. Clin. Endocrinol. Metab. **89:** 2434–2441.

14. FOWLER, K.A., K. GILL, N. KIRMA, *et al.* 2000. Overexpression of aromatase leads to development of testicular leydig cell tumors: an in vivo model for hormone-mediated testicular cancer. Am. J. Pathol. **156:** 347–353.

15. LI, X., E. NOKKALA, W. YAN, *et al.* 2001. Altered structure and function of reproductive organs in transgenic male mice overexpressing human aromatase. Endocrinology **142:** 2435–2442.

16. MCPHERSON, S.J., H. WANG, M.E. JONES, *et al.* 2001. Elevated androgens and prolactin in aromatase-deficient mice cause enlargement, but not malignancy, of the prostate gland. Endocrinology **142:** 2458–2467.

17. BOSLAND, M.C., H. FORD & L. HORTON. 1995. Induction of a high incidence of ductal prostate adenocarcinomas in NBL and Sprague Dawley rats treated with estradiol-17β or diethylstilbestrol in combination with testosterone. Carcinogenesis **16:** 1311–1317.

18. BOSLAND, M.C., H. FORD, L. HORTON, *et al.* 1995. Progression of putative precursor lesions of rat prostatic adenocarcinomas induced by estradiol-17β and androgens. Proc. Am. Assoc. Cancer Res. **36:** 271.

19. LATIL, A., I. BIECHE, D. VIDAUD, *et al.* 2001. Evaluation of androgen, estrogen (ER alpha and ER beta), and progesterone receptor expression in human prostate cancer by real-time quantitative reverse transcription-polymerase chain reaction assays. Cancer Res. **61:** 1919–1926.

20. LAU, K.M., I. LEAV & S.M. HO. 1998. Rat estrogen receptor-alpha and -beta, and progesterone receptor mRNA expression in various prostatic lobes and microdissected normal and dysplastic epithelial tissues of the Noble rat. Endocrinology **139:** 424–427.

21. LEAV, I., K.M. LAU, J.Y. ADAMS, *et al.* 2001. Comparative studies of the estrogen receptors beta and alpha and the androgen receptor in normal human prostate glands, dysplasia, and in primary and metastatic carcinoma. Am. J. Pathol. **59:** 79–92.

22. THOMPSON, C.J., N.N. TAM, J.M. JOYCE, *et al.* 2002. Gene expression profiling of testosterone and estradiol-17 beta-induced prostatic dysplasia in Noble rats and response to the antiestrogen ICI 182,780. Endocrinology **143:** 2093–2105.

23. MCCORMICK, D.L., W.D. JOHNSON, R.A. LUBET, *et al.* 2002. Differential chemopreventive activity of the antiandrogen, flutamide, and the antiestrogen, tamoxifen, in the rat prostate [abstract 3178]. Proc. Am. Assoc. Cancer Res.

24. TANGBANLUEKAL, L. & C.L. ROBINETTE. 1993. Prolactin mediates estradiol-induced inflammation in the lateral prostate of Wistar rats. Endocrinology **132:** 2407–2416.

25. LANE, K.E., I. LEAV, J. ZIAR, *et al.* 1997. Suppression of testosterone and estradiol-17beta-induced dysplasia in the dorsolateral prostate of Noble rats by bromocriptine. Carcinogenesis **18:** 1505–1510.

26. CAVALIERI, E.L., P.D. DEVANESAN, M.C. BOSLAND, *et al.* 2002. Catechol estrogen metabolites and conjugates in different regions of the prostate of Noble rats treated with 4-hydroxyestradiol: implications for estrogen-induced initiation of prostate cancer. Carcinogenesis **23:** 329–333.

27. CAVALIERI, E., K. FRENKEL, J.G. LIEHR, *et al.* 2000. Estrogens as endogenous genotoxic agents–DNA adducts and mutations. J. Natl. Cancer Inst. Monogr. **27:** 75–93.

28. CAVALIERI, E., D. CHAKRAVARTI, J. GUTTENPLAN, *et al.* 2006. Catechol estrogen quinones as initiators of breast and other human cancers: implications for biomarkers of susceptibility and cancer prevention. Biochim. Biophys. Acta **1766:** 63–78.

29. MAILANDER, P.C., J.L. MEZA, S. HIGGINBOTHAM & D. CHAKRAVARTI. 2006. Induction of A.T to G.C mutations by erroneous repair of depurinated DNA following estrogen treatment of the mammary gland of ACI rats. J. Steroid Biochem. Mol. Biol. **101:** 204–215. Sep 16 [Epub ahead of print].

30. LIEHR, J.G. 2000. Role of DNA adducts in hormonal carcinogenesis. Regul. Toxicol. Pharmacol. **32:** 276–282.

31. HAN, X., J.G. LIEHR & M.C. BOSLAND. 1995. Induction of a DNA adduct detectable by ^{32}P-postlabeling in the dorsolateral prostate of NBL/Cr rats treated with estradiol-17β and testosterone. Carcinogenesis **16:** 951–954.

32. VERMEULEN, A., J.M. KAUFMAN, S. GOEMAERE & I. VAN POTTELBERG. 2002. Estradiol in elderly men. Aging Male **5:** 98–102.

33. ROSS, R.K., L. BERNSTEIN, R.A. LOBO, *et al.* 1992. 5-alpha-reductase activity and risk of prostate cancer among Japanese and US white and black males. Lancet **339:** 887–889.

Estrogens and Antiestrogens as Etiological Factors and Therapeutics for Prostate Cancer

SHUK-MEI HO,[a,b] YUET-KIN LEUNG,[a,b] AND IRVING CHUNG[a,b]

[a]Department of Environmental Health, College of Medicine, University of Cincinnati, Cincinnati, Ohio 45267, USA

[b]Department of Surgery, University of Massachusetts Medical School, Worcester, Massachusetts 01605, USA

ABSTRACT: Mounting evidence supports a key role played by estrogen or estrogen in synergy with an androgen, in the pathogenesis of prostate cancer (PCa). New experimental data suggest that this process could begin as early as prenatal life. During adulthood, estrogen carcinogenicity is believed to be mediated by the combined effects of hormone-induced, unscheduled cell proliferation and bioactivation of estrogens to genotoxic carcinogens. Increased bioavailability of estrogen through age-dependent increases in conversion from androgen could also be a contributing factor. Individual variations and race-/ethnic-based differences in circulating or locally formed estrogens or in tissue estrogen responsiveness may explain differential PCa risk among individuals or different populations. Estrogen receptor (ER)-α and ER-β are the main mediators of estrogen action in the prostate. However, ER-β is the first ER subtype expressed in the fetal prostate. During cancer development, ER-β expression is first lost as tumors progress into high grade in the primary site. Yet, its reexpression occurs in all metastatic cases of PCa. A change in cytosine methylation in a regulatory CpG island located in the proximal promoter of ER-β may constitute an "on/off" switch for reversible regulation of ER-β expression. A variety of estrogenic/antiestrogenic/selective estrogen receptor modulator (SERM)-like compounds have been shown to use non-ERE pathways, such as tethering of ER-β to NF-κB binding proteins, Sp2, or Ap1 for gene transactivation. These findings open new avenues for drug design that now focuses on developing a new generation of estrogen-based PCa therapies with maximal proapoptotic action but few or no side effects.

Address for correspondence: Shuk-Mei Ho, Ph.D., Division of Environmental Genetics and Molecular Toxicology, Department of Environmental Health, College of Medicine, University of Cincinnati, Cincinnati, OH 45267. Voice: 513-558-5701; fax: 513-558-0071.
e-mail: shuk-mei.ho@uc.edu

Ann. N.Y. Acad. Sci. 1089: 177–193 (2006). © 2006 New York Academy of Sciences.
doi: 10.1196/annals.1386.005

KEYWORDS: estrogen receptor; antiestrogens; selective estrogen receptor modulator (SERM); nuclear receptor coregulators; DNA methylation; developmental reprogramming; licorice; apigenin; phytoestrogen; apoptosis; oxidative stress; genomic damages; prostate cancer risk; hormonal therapy

INTRODUCTION

Traditionally, androgens are considered to be the major sex hormones regulating normal and malignant growth of the prostate. However, recent literature suggests equally important roles for estrogenic compounds in these processes.[1-6] The primary objectives of this article are to summarize research findings from our laboratory and those from our collaborators that (*a*) address mechanisms by which estrogens, endogenous or environmental, contribute to prostate carcinogenesis, and (*b*) evaluate the potentials of estrogens, phytoestrogens, and antiestrogens as therapeutics for the prevention and treatment of prostate cancer (PCa).

DO ESTROGENS CONTRIBUTE TO THE PATHOGENESIS OF PCa?

Epidemiological findings have suggested a role of estrogen in the pathogenesis of PCa in men. An earlier study found that African Americans, who have the highest incidence of PCa in the United States, also have significantly higher levels of serum estrogens than their Caucasian American peers, even at a young age.[7] In contrast, lower circulating estrogen levels have been noted in Japanese men, who are known to have a low risk of PCa in comparison with a higher-risk group, Caucasian Dutch men.[8] Furthermore, the incidence of PCa rises exponentially in elderly men, in whom the ratio of estrogen to androgen may increase by up to 40%.[9-14] This age-related hormonal shift is primarily due to a decline in testicular function and an increase in aromatization of adrenal androgens by peripheral adipose tissue during aging. At the cellular level, significant declines in 5-α-dihydrotestosterone levels and increases in estrogen [estradiol (E2) and estrone (E1)] levels have been observed in prostatic epithelial cells.[14,15] Collectively, these endocrine changes at midlife, termed *andropause*, may significantly augment estrogenic stimulation of the prostatic epithelium, leading to reactivation of growth and subsequent neoplastic transformation.

Experimental models have helped establish estrogens, alone or synergistically with androgens, as potent inducers of aberrant growth and neoplastic transformation in the prostate.[1-3,6] Prenatal exposure to maternal estrogens or adult exposure to pharmacological doses of estrogens induces a benign lesion termed *squamous metaplasia*, which is derived from basal cell proliferation of the prostates in various species, including humans.[16] Using a susceptible rat strain (the Noble rat), we demonstrated that chronic exposure to testosterone (T) plus E2 in adulthood leads to the evolution of a precancerous lesion similar to human prostatic intraepithelial neoplasia (PIN) and full-blown PCa at high incidences.[2,17–19] Cellular and molecular changes implicated as mechanisms leading to carcinogenesis include: (1) a dramatic increase in epithelial cell proliferation[19]; (2) upregulation of growth factor signaling pathways (e.g., TGF/EGF receptor signaling,[20] prolactin/prolactin receptor signaling,[21] MAP kinase activation[22]); (3) increased cell survival potentials through overexpression of antiapoptotic mediators (e.g., metallothionein,[23] TRPM-2/clusterin[24]); (4) elevations in oxidative stress (OS)-induced DNA damages[25–27]; (5) genome-wide and specific changes in gene expression[28]; (6) breakdown of epithelial basement membrane and stromal extracellular matrix due to increases in gelatinolytic proteinase activities[29]; and (7) altered expression of glycoconjugates in smooth muscles and their associated extracellular matrix.[30,31]

DOES ESTROGEN BIOACTIVATION OR DETOXIFICATION AFFECT PCa RISK?

In addition to promoting aberrant cell growth, estrogens may initiate carcinogenesis by acting as chemical carcinogens via metabolic bioactivation. Natural estrogens (E1 and E2) are converted to potential genotoxic metabolites, 2-hydroxyl and 4-hydroxyl catechol estrogens and their quinone/semiquinone intermediates, by cytochrome P450 enzymes (CYP) 1A1 and CYP1B1, respectively, whereas the enzyme catechol-*O*-methyl-transferase (COMT) is responsible for their removal via methoxylation.[32–34] Estrogen-derived genotoxic intermediates can directly cause genomic damage by DNA adduct formation or indirectly inflict damage via induction of OS, which results in accumulation of reactive oxygen species (ROS). Thus, several isoforms of glutathione *S*-transferases (GSTs) that detoxify ROS could also afford protection against estrogen genotoxicity. Genetic polymorphisms that alter enzyme activity, or DNA hypermethylation or mutations that silence cognate genes, are therefore expected to influence life-long exposures of target cells/tissues to genotoxic estrogen metabolites, consequently having an impact on PCa risk.[35]

Molecular epidemiology studies have implicated the *CYP1A1-M1* allele, the *CYP1B1 Leu432Val*, polymorphisms of *COMT* (codon 62 and 158), and the *GSTM1-null* genotype as important modifiers of PCa risk in specific populations.[36–43] Recently, we identified a novel *CYP1A1* variant (*CYP1A1v*) that resides preferentially in the nucleus and mitochondria and we have discovered overexpression of CYP1A1 associated with the development of human epithelial ovarian cancer.[44] Ectopic expression of *CYP1A1v* in nontumorigenic ovarian surface epithelial cells led to neoplastic transformation *in vitro*. We recently obtained new evidence that a similar phenomenon exists for prostate carcinogenesis (Leung *et al.*, unpublished material). These findings support the hypothesis that intranuclear production of genotoxic estrogen metabolites could cause tumor initiation. These data are in agreement with our earlier findings that estrogen carcinogenicity results in genomic damage, as illustrated by our observation of increased DNA strand breakage[26] and increased nuclear 8-oxy-deguanosine staining[45] in the prostates of T plus E2–treated Noble rats. In contrast, increased COMT expression or activities may offer protection against carcinogenesis as the enzyme is responsible for the metabolic inactivation of catechol estrogens through conversion to methoxyestrogens. Furthermore, 2-methoxyestradiol has recently been shown to exhibit potent apoptotic activity against rapidly growing PCa cells.[46] Future research efforts focusing on correlating expression levels of estrogen-metabolizing enzymes and functional roles of their various polymorphic isoforms may shed new light on differential PCa risks observed among different individuals or populations.

Similarly, *in situ* production of estrogen from androgen via the activity of aromatase, encoded by *CYP19*, may be an important risk modifier for PCa.[47] Both the aromatase protein and its enzyme activity have been demonstrated in specimens of PCa and benign prostatic hyperplasia (BPH).[48–50] Earlier clinical trials that sought to test aromatase inhibitors as therapeutics have been focused on their efficacy in treating BPH,[51,52] and attention to its use to treat PCa has only emerged recently.[53] Population studies now showed that polymorphisms in *CYP19,* such as intron 4[TTTA]n repeat[54,55] and *C/T* versus *T/T* genotype,[55] are associated with familial PCa. These new clinical and epidemiological findings, in combination with those obtained from preclinical mouse models,[29,56] have provided a strong basis for testing aromatase inhibitors as monotherapies or adjuvant treatments for PCa.

COULD PCa RISKS BE DETERMINED DURING EARLY LIFE STAGES?

Experimental evidence has long suggested that the risk of developing PCa in adulthood could be determined by early life exposure to natural or environmental estrogens—a phenomenon referred to as "estrogen imprinting."[57] Perinatal and neonatal exposure of rats[58–61] or mice[62–64] to estrogens or estrogen mimics induces development of various proliferative lesions in the adult gland. These changes may be partially explained by permanent changes in androgen receptor levels, estrogen receptor (ER) statuses, interacinar stromal tissue volume, and the proliferative potential of the prostatic epithelium.[60,65–67] The "estrogenized" adult glands also demonstrate a lack of differentiation, disorganization of the acini, and excessive luminal sloughing. Recently, we have provided convincing data to link early estrogen exposure to increased PCa risk in an animal model.[68] Neonatal exposure of Sprague–Dawley rats to low doses of E2 or an environment estrogen, bisphenol A (BPA), sensitizes the adult prostate to later life T plus E2–induced dysplasia and neoplasia development. Using a genome-wide screening protocol, we identified phosphodiesterase 4D4, an enzyme responsible for regulating cellular cAMP, as a target for "epigenetic reprogramming." Failure of its cognate gene to be silenced by DNA methylation during aging could be a contributing factor for increased PIN and tumor incidences in the exposed gland.

Whether analogous phenomena exist in humans remains unclear. However, it has been shown that circulating E2 levels of pregnant African American women are higher than those of Caucasian American women.[69,70] Furthermore, Ekbom and associates[71,72] have reported that indicators of high levels of endogenous pregnancy hormones, such as high birth weight and jaundice in the offspring, are associated with increased risk of PCa, while indicators of low levels, like pre-eclampsia, are associated with decreased risk.[71] If intrauterine or perinatal environments are important for PCa risk in adulthood, cancer prevention strategies should be directed to these early developmental stages. Of relevance to this line of argument is a concern about exposure to estrogenic mimics in early development. Several human studies now show significant exposures of human fetuses to BPA, likely caused by maternal use of consumer products that leach this estrogen mimic, and BPA transfer from maternal to fetal circulation via the placenta.[73–77]

ERs AS FUNCTIONALLY DIVERGENT MEDIATORS OF ESTROGEN ACTION IN THE PROSTATE

It is now known that the effects of estrogens on all tissues, including the prostate, are mediated by ER-α and ER-β.[78,79] These two ER subtypes are structurally similar, consisting of the six common domains (A–F) found in all steroid hormone receptors. The DNA-binding domain of ER-α is very similar to that of ER-β, differing only by three amino acids. In contrast, the N-terminal A/B domain of both receptors share only a 15.5% homology, the ligand binding domains are 58% homologous, and the C-terminal F domains are distinctly different. These structural dissimilarities confer significant functional differences between the two-receptor subtypes. Depending on the binding ligand, the two receptors interact with different coregulators and enhancer elements to achieve the broadest degree of functional diversity and specificity.[80–82] Adding to the complexity of estrogen action is the recent discovery of five isoforms of ER-β with distinct functional differences and unique patterns of tissue- and cell-type-specific distribution.[80]

The precise biological functions of the two ER subtypes in the normal prostate and their involvement in prostate carcinogenesis remain incompletely understood. We[83] and others[76,84–89] have reported differential expression patterns of the two receptors between the epithelial and stromal compartments of the normal and malignant adult human prostate. ER-β is localized predominantly to the basal epithelial cell compartment of the normal human prostate, where ER-α is rarely found. ER-α is mainly expressed in the stroma of the normal gland. Results from experimental models[90–92] suggest that ER-β may exert an antiproliferative effect on basal epithelial cells, thus affording a protective effect against PCa.[93] Findings in ER-β knockout mice indicate that these animals develop prostatic hyperplasia in old age, a phenomenon that does not occur in ER-α knockout mice.[94] Jiang et al.[90] observed an age-dependent decline in ER-β expression in the canine prostate. Prins and associates[95] reported that neonatal exposure of rats to estrogen causes downregulation of ER-β, upregulation of ER-α, and development of hyperplastic, dysplastic, and neoplastic lesions in the adult ventral prostates. Others suggested that functions of ER-β in the normal prostate are related to its role in protecting tissues against oxidative injury. ER-β was found to be more effective than ER-α in transactivation of the electrophile/antioxidant response element, and to act as a better inducer of antioxidant enzymes, including quinone reductase and GSTs.[96–98] The antioxidant function of ER-β, though not yet demonstrated in the prostate, has been widely speculated to offer protection against cardiovascular diseases,[99] neural degeneration,[100–102] and breast cancer development.[103] An analogous function of ER-β in the prostate would be a fruitful area of future investigation.

During fetal development of the human prostate, ER-β is the first to appear in the fetal prostate (by the seventh week of gestation) and is the only ER subtype expressed in the epithelial and stromal cells during early ductal morphogenesis.[16,104] By week 15 of gestation, ER-α expression appears and is strongly associated with squamous metaplasia in the distal periurethral ducts and utricle. These findings suggest ER-β, perhaps in concert with androgen receptors, mediates the very early stage of fetal prostate development, followed by the action of ER-α. These findings should be given serious consideration in any design of prevention strategies for lowering PCa risk due to prenatal estrogen imprinting in the future.

ER-β APPEARS TO PLAY A DUAL ROLE IN PROSTATE CARCINOGENESIS

In an earlier study,[83] we have compared the expression of androgen receptor (AR), ER-α, and ER-β in PINs, primary carcinomas and metastatic PCa in bone and lymph nodes. Compared to its levels in normal basal epithelial cells, ER-β was downregulated in high-grade PIN lesions, while the expression of ER-α or AR in these lesions remained unchanged. Interestingly, ER-β was strongly expressed in Gleason grade 3 carcinoma, but its expression was markedly diminished in higher-grade carcinomas (grade 4/5). Our observation that ER-β expression is lost during tumor progression in the primary site was confirmed by results from other groups.[76,85,86,105,106] A speculative interpretation of these findings is that ER-β serves as a "brake" for carcinogenesis[93] by acting as an antiproliferative mediator in the basal epithelial compartment along with its antioxidant action to prevent oxidative genomic damages. Disruption of this equilibrium may trigger or be required for neoplastic transformation in the human prostate.

Ironically, we observed high levels of ER-β but little or no ER-α expression in the majority of cases of PCa metastasized to the bone and regional lymph nodes.[83] Its levels in these metastases were lowered by antiestrogen-based therapies involving diethylstilbestrol (DES) or PC-SPES.[107] Potential action of ER-β in metastatic PCa remains unknown, but it is reasonable to speculate that its expression offers survival advantages to the PCa cells in these distant sites. Reexpression of ER-β in PCa metastases could be due to induction by *in situ* factors produced in the metastatic sites. Alternatively, PCa cells that fail to lose ER-β expression might have a higher potential to escape from the prostate and establish themselves in distant sites through clonal expansion. The mechanism responsible for inactivating and reactivating the *ER-β* gene *in vivo* has been deciphered. The cytosine methylation status of a novel CpG island in the proximal promoter of *ER-β* has been shown to inversely correlate with ER-β expression across the entire spectrum of normal, precancerous, cancerous, and metastatic lesions of PCa.[108] Thus, reversible regulation of *ER-β* expression via an epigenetic mechanism serves to "flip" the gene on and off during PCa development and progression.[109]

Finally, ER-α, expressed mainly in the stromal compartment of the prostate, may also contribute to the pathogenesis of PCa. Higher levels of ER-α was observed in the prostatic stroma of Hispanic and Asian men than in Caucasian and African American men, who are at higher risk for PCa.[110] In a genotyping and allelic frequency analysis of six different polymorphic loci of ER-α in a Japanese population, polymorphism in codon 10 was found associated with higher PCa risk.[111]

In summary, it has become apparent that ER-β is a key determinant of the genesis, progression, and metastasis of PCa. Therapeutic approaches targeting its activation/inactivation may have important ramifications in PCa treatment.

SERMS, PHYTOESTROGENS, AND NEW ESTROGENIC/ANTIESTROGENIC AGENTS AS THERAPIES FOR PCa

DES, a xenoestrogen, was used as the first standard therapy for PCa treatment.[112] It fell out of favor on account of cardiac toxicity and other major side effects.[6,113,114] Similarly, clinical trials have found that the first generation of antiestrogens or SERMs, such as tamoxifen, toremifene, and raloxifene, have limited efficacy as alternative therapies to DES.[6,115–119] Despite these setbacks, the likelihood of developing effective and less toxic SERMs/estrogen-based therapies for PCa has improved substantially, coincident with our growing knowledge on the differential actions and expression of the two ER subtypes in PCas.

Traditionally, estrogen-induced PCa regression is believed to be mediated by its action on the hypothalamic-pituitary axis, thereby inhibiting testosterone synthesis.[120] However, it is now known that many estrogens/antiestrogens/phytoestrogens/SERMs, including DES, 2-methoxy-E_2, genistein, resveratrol, licochalcone, raloxifene, ICI 182,780 (ICI), and estramustine, have antitumor effects independent of this pathway. Their ability to suppress PCa cell growth has been attributed to a broad range of actions including direct cytotoxicity,[121] interruption of cell cycle progression,[122,123] induction of apoptosis,[123–125] depolymerization of microtubules,[126] inhibition of DNA synthesis,[127] inhibition of topoisomerase II,[128] blockade of tyrosine kinase,[128,129] disruption of apoptotic regulators,[130] and activation of death domain receptors.[131,132] Some of these estrogenic/antiestrogenic compounds are also potent inhibitors of angiogenesis and metastasis,[133] through their actions in upregulating expression of genes with antiangiogenesis or antimetastasis properties,[133] activating the cell adhesion signaling molecule focal adhesion kinase,[134] and reduction in metastatic spreading via the lymphatic system.[135]

We have recently found that the pure antiestrogen ICI,[136] the flavonoid apigenin,[137] and a water-soluble extract of licorice (Chung *et al.*, unpublished material) exert their antiproliferative effects on PCa cells via a ER-β-mediated mechanism, as validated by selective ER-β knockdown experiments using siRNA and antisense oligonucleotides against the receptor. Furthermore, we have learnt that they can use noncanonical mechanisms in gene activation. For example, ICI activates genes, such as *IL-8, IL-12, embryonic growth/differentiation factor,* and *tyrosine kinase-related* (*RYK*) that lack classical estrogen-responsive elements (*EREs*) in their promoters. Instead, the mode of action involves tethering of ER-β on NF-κB binding proteins or Sp1, and activation of these pathways rather than signaling via the classical *ERE*.[80] These findings have prompted us to apply a rational drug design strategy to identify novel estrogen-derived chemicals that have enhanced proapoptotic activity (likely mediated by noncanonical signaling) but reduced estrogenic action (probably mediated via *ERE*) in order to customize a potent anti-PCa drug with few side effects. To this end, we recently reported the successful use of nanomolar concentrations of an ER-β-selective ligand, APVE2, to achieve cell kill of PCa cells *in vitro*.[138] When tested in human prostate and pancreatic cancer xenografts in nude mice this compound was found to exhibit extremely favorable antitumor efficacies and minimal side effects in dose escalation experiments (Bakshi *et al.*, unpublished material).

OVERALL CONCLUSION

A key role played by estrogens and estrogen mimics in prostate carcinogenesis is well supported by epidemiological findings and experimental data.

Our recent data strongly argue that the process may begin as early as prenatal and perinatal life stages. Complex interplay between hormonal and chemical actions and between genomic and epigenetic mechanisms likely drive the full spectrum of events involved in PCa initiation, promotion, and progression. Individuals or ethnic/racial groups expressing particular polymorphisms in genes encoding specific estrogen-metabolizing enzymes that affect bioactivation, bioavailability, and degradation of estrogens probably possess different PCa risks due to differential life-long exposure to the active carcinogens. The predominance of ER-β in fetal and adult prostate functions offers new opportunities for designing high-efficacy therapies or intervention strategies based on our understanding of the biology of this ER subtype. The fact that the actions of SERMs, antiestrogens, and phytoestrogens can exert their antitumor actions through noncanonical pathways opens avenues for the development of a new generation of PCa treatment regimens, with high antitumor potency and minimal systemic side effects caused by their innate estrogenicity.

ACKNOWLEDGMENTS

This work is supported in part by the NIH Grants DK DK61084, CA112532, CA15776, ES013071, ES12281, and a DOD Grant DAMD-W81XWH-04-1-0165.

REFERENCES

1. BOSTWICK, D.G., H.B. BURKE, D. DJAKIEW, *et al.* 2004. Human prostate cancer risk factors. Cancer **101:** 2371–2490.
2. HO, S.M., K. LANE & K. LEE. 1997. Neoplastic transformation of the prostate. *In* Prostate: Basic and Clinical Aspects. Rajesh K Naz, Ed.: 74–114. CRC Press. New York.
3. HO, S.M. 2004. Estrogens and anti-estrogens: key mediators of prostate carcinogenesis and new therapeutic candidates. J. Cell Biochem. **91:** 491–503.
4. PRINS, G.S. 2000. Molecular biology of the androgen receptor. Mayo Clin. Proc. **75**(Suppl): S32–S35.
5. RISBRIDGER, G.P., J.J. BIANCO, S.J. ELLEM & S.J. MCPHERSON. 2003. Oestrogens and prostate cancer. Endocr. Relat. Cancer **10:** 187–191.
6. TAPLIN, M.E. & S.M. HO. 2001. Clinical review 134: The endocrinology of prostate cancer. J. Clin. Endocrinol. Metab. **86:** 3467–3477.
7. ROSS, R., L. BERNSTEIN, H. JUDD, *et al.* 1986. Serum testosterone levels in healthy young black and white men. J. Natl. Cancer Inst. **76:** 45–48.
8. DE JONG, F.H., K. OISHI, R.B. HAYES, *et al.* 1991. Peripheral hormone levels in controls and patients with prostatic cancer or benign prostatic hyperplasia: results from the Dutch-Japanese case-control study. Cancer Res. **51:** 3445–3450.
9. DESLYPERE, J.P. & A. VERMEULEN. 1985. Influence of age on steroid concentrations in skin and striated muscle in women and in cardiac muscle and lung tissue in men. J. Clin. Endocrinol. Metab. **61:** 648–653.

10. FELDMAN, H.A., C. LONGCOPE, C.A. DERBY, *et al.* 2002. Age trends in the level of serum testosterone and other hormones in middle-aged men: longitudinal results from the Massachusetts Male Aging Study. J. Clin. Endocrinol. Metab. **87:** 589–598.

11. GRAY, A., J.A. BERLIN, J.B. MCKINLAY & C. LONGCOPE. 1991. An examination of research design effects on the association of testosterone and male aging: results of a meta-analysis. J. Clin. Epidemiol. **44:** 671–684.

12. GRAY, A., H.A. FELDMAN, J.B. MCKINLAY & C. LONGCOPE. 1991. Age, disease, and changing sex hormone levels in middle-aged men: results of the Massachusetts Male Aging Study. J. Clin. Endocrinol. Metab. **73:** 1016–1025.

13. GRIFFITHS, K. 2000. Estrogens and prostatic disease. International Prostate Health Council Study Group. Prostate **45:** 87–100.

14. VERMEULEN, A., R. RUBENS & L. VERDONCK. 1972. Testosterone secretion and metabolism in male senescence. J. Clin. Endocrinol. Metab. **34:** 730–735.

15. KRIEG, M., R. NASS & S. TUNN. 1993. Effect of aging on endogenous level of 5 alpha-dihydrotestosterone, testosterone, estradiol, and estrone in epithelium and stroma of normal and hyperplastic human prostate. J. Clin. Endocrinol. Metab. **77:** 375–381.

16. ADAMS, J.Y., I. LEAV, K.M. LAU, *et al.* 2002. Expression of estrogen receptor beta in the fetal, neonatal, and prepubertal human prostate. Prostate **52:** 69–81.

17. HO, S.M., I. LEAV, F.B. MERK, *et al.* 1995. Induction of atypical hyperplasia, apoptosis, and type II estrogen-binding sites in the ventral prostates of Noble rats treated with testosterone and pharmacologic doses of estradiol-17 beta. Lab. Invest. **73:** 356–365.

18. LEAV, I., S.M. HO, P. OFNER, *et al.* 1988. Biochemical alterations in sex hormone-induced hyperplasia and dysplasia of the dorsolateral prostates of Noble rats. J. Natl. Cancer Inst. **80:** 1045–1053.

19. LEAV, I., F.B. MERK, P.W. KWAN & S.M. HO. 1989. Androgen-supported estrogen-enhanced epithelial proliferation in the prostates of intact Noble rats. Prostate **15:** 23–40.

20. KAPLAN, P.J., I. LEAV, J. GREENWOOD, *et al.* 1996. Involvement of transforming growth factor alpha (TGFalpha) and epidermal growth factor receptor (EGFR) in sex hormone-induced prostatic dysplasia and the growth of an androgen-independent transplantable carcinoma of the prostate. Carcinogenesis **17:** 2571–2579.

21. LEAV, I., F.B. MERK, K.F. LEE, *et al.* 1999. Prolactin receptor expression in the developing human prostate and in hyperplastic, dysplastic, and neoplastic lesions. Am. J. Pathol. **154:** 863–870.

22. LEAV, I., C.M. GALLUZZI, J. ZIAR, *et al.* 1996. Mitogen-activated protein kinase and mitogen-activated kinase phosphatase-1 expression in the Noble rat model of sex hormone-induced prostatic dysplasia and carcinoma. Lab. Invest. **75:** 361–370.

23. GHATAK, S., P. OLIVERIA, P. KAPLAN & S.M. HO. 1996. Expression and regulation of metallothionein mRNA levels in the prostates of noble rats: lack of expression in the ventral prostate and regulation by sex hormones in the dorsolateral prostate. Prostate **29:** 91–100.

24. HO, S.M., I. LEAV, S. GHATAK, *et al.* 1998. Lack of association between enhanced TRPM-2/clustering expression and increased apoptotic activity in sex-hormone-induced prostatic dysplasia of the Noble rat. Am. J. Pathol. **153:** 131–139.

25. GHATAK, S. & S.M. HO. 1996. Age-related changes in the activities of antioxidant enzymes and lipid peroxidation status in ventral and dorsolateral prostate lobes of Noble rats. Biochem. Biophys. Res. Commun. **222:** 362–367.

26. HO, S.M. & D. ROY. 1994. Sex hormone-induced nuclear DNA damage and lipid peroxidation in the dorsolateral prostates of Noble rats. Cancer Lett. **84:** 155–162.

27. TAM, N.N., S. GHATAK & S.M. HO. 2003. Sex hormone-induced alterations in the activities of antioxidant enzymes and lipid peroxidation status in the prostate of Noble rats. Prostate **55:** 1–8.

28. THOMPSON, C.J., N.N. TAM, J.M. JOYCE, *et al.* 2002. Gene expression profiling of testosterone and estradiol-17 beta-induced prostatic dysplasia in Noble rats and response to the antiestrogen ICI 182,780. Endocrinology **143:** 2093–2105.

29. LI, X., E. NOKKALA, W. YAN, *et al.* 2001. Altered structure and function of reproductive organs in transgenic male mice overexpressing human aromatase. Endocrinology **142:** 2435–2442.

30. CHAN, F.L. & S.M. HO. 1999. Comparative study of glycoconjugates of the rat prostatic lobes by lectin histochemistry. Prostate **38:** 1–16.

31. CHAN, F.L., H.L. CHOI & S.M. HO. 2001. Analysis of glycoconjugate patterns of normal and hormone-induced dysplastic Noble rat prostates, and an androgen-independent Noble rat prostate tumor, by lectin histochemistry and protein blotting. Prostate **46:** 21–32.

32. CAVALIERI, E., K. FRENKEL, J.G. LIEHR, *et al.* 2000. Estrogens as endogenous genotoxic agents—DNA adducts and mutations. J. Natl. Cancer Inst. Monogr. 75–93.

33. YAGER, J.D. & J.G. LIEHR. 1996. Molecular mechanisms of estrogen carcinogenesis. Annu. Rev. Pharmacol. Toxicol. **36:** 203–232.

34. YAGER, J.D. 2000. Endogenous estrogens as carcinogens through metabolic activation. J. Natl. Cancer Inst. Monogr. 67–73.

35. NOCK, N.L., M.S. CICEK, L. LI, *et al.* 2006. Polymorphisms in estrogen bioactivation, detoxification and oxidative DNA base excision repair genes and prostate cancer risk. Carcinogenesis **27:** 1842–1848.

36. ACEVEDO, C., J.L. OPAZO, C. HUIDOBRO, *et al.* 2003. Positive correlation between single or combined genotypes of CYP1A1 and GSTM1 in relation to prostate cancer in Chilean people. Prostate **57:** 111–117.

37. CACERES, D.D., J. ITURRIETA, C. ACEVEDO, *et al.* 2005. Relationship among metabolizing genes, smoking and alcohol used as modifier factors on prostate cancer risk: exploring some gene-gene and gene-environment interactions. Eur. J. Epidemiol. **20:** 79–88.

38. QUINONES, L.A., C.E. IRARRAZABAL, C.R. ROJAS, *et al.* 2006. Joint effect among p53, CYP1A1, GSTM1 polymorphism combinations and smoking on prostate cancer risk: an exploratory genotype-environment interaction study. Asian J. Androl. **8:** 349–355.

39. SILIG, Y., H. PINARBASI, S. GUNES, *et al.* 2006. Polymorphisms of CYP1A1, GSTM1, GSTT1, and prostate cancer risk in Turkish population. Cancer Invest. **24:** 41–45.

40. SOBTI, R.C., K. ONSORY, A.I. AL BADRAN, *et al.* 2006. CYP17, SRD5A2, CYP1B1, and CYP2D6 gene polymorphisms with prostate cancer risk in North Indian population DNA. Cell Biol. **25:** 287–294.

41. SUZUKI, M., M.R. MAMUN, K. HARA, *et al.* 2005. The Val158Met polymorphism of the catechol-O-methyltransferase gene is associated with the

PSA-progression-free survival in prostate cancer patients treated with estramustine phosphate. Eur. Urol. **48:** 752–759.

42. TANAKA, Y., M. SASAKI, H. SHIINA, *et al.* 2006. Catechol-O-methyltransferase gene polymorphisms in benign prostatic hyperplasia and sporadic prostate cancer. Cancer Epidemiol. Biomarkers Prev. **15:** 238–244.

43. TANG, Y.M., B.L. GREEN, G.F. CHEN, *et al.* 2000. Human CYP1B1 Leu432Val gene polymorphism: ethnic distribution in African-Americans, Caucasians and Chinese; oestradiol hydroxylase activity; and distribution in prostate cancer cases and controls. Pharmacogenetics **10:** 761–766.

44. LEUNG, Y.K., K.M. LAU, J. MOBLEY, *et al.* 2005. Overexpression of cytochrome P450 1A1 and its novel spliced variant in ovarian cancer cells: alternative subcellular enzyme compartmentation may contribute to carcinogenesis. Cancer Res. **65:** 3726–3734.

45. TAM, N.N., Y. GAO, Y.K. LEUNG & S.M. HO. 2006. Induction of NAD(P)H oxidases and nitric oxide synthetases leading to oxidative and nitrosative stresses in hormonal carcinogenesis of the prostate gland in Noble rats [abstract]. Proceedings of the 95th annual meeting of the American Association of Cancer Research, Orlando, Florida, 2004.

46. LAKHANI, N.J., M.A. SARKAR, J. VENITZ & W.D. FIGG. 2003. 2-Methoxyestradiol, a promising anticancer agent. Pharmacotherapy **23:** 165–172.

47. ELLEM, S.J. & G.P. RISBRIDGER. 2006. Aromatase and prostate cancer. Minerva Endocrinol. **31:** 1–12.

48. DI, S.E., G. BRIATICO, D. GIUDICI, *et al.* 1994. Endocrine properties of the testosterone 5 alpha-reductase inhibitor turosteride (FCE 26073). J. Steroid Biochem. Mol. Biol. **48:** 241–248.

49. HIRAMATSU, M., I. MAEHARA, M. OZAKI, *et al.* 1997. Aromatase in hyperplasia and carcinoma of the human prostate. Prostate **31:** 118–124.

50. MATZKIN, H. & M.S. SOLOWAY. 1992. Response to second-line hormonal manipulation monitored by serum PSA in stage D2 prostate carcinoma. Urology **40:** 78–80.

51. RADLMAIER, A., H.U. EICKENBERG, M.S. FLETCHER, *et al.* 1996. Estrogen reduction by aromatase inhibition for benign prostatic hyperplasia: results of a double-blind, placebo-controlled, randomized clinical trial using two doses of the aromatase-inhibitor atamestane. Atamestane Study Group. Prostate **29:** 199–208.

52. SUZUKI, K., H. OKAZAKI, Y. ONO, *et al.* 1998. Effect of dual inhibition of 5-alpha-reductase and aromatase on spontaneously developed canine prostatic hypertrophy. Prostate **37:** 70–76.

53. KRUIT, W.H., G. STOTER & J.G. KLIJN. 2004. Effect of combination therapy with aminoglutethimide and hydrocortisone on prostate-specific antigen response in metastatic prostate cancer refractory to standard endocrine therapy. Anticancer Drugs **15:** 843–847.

54. SUZUKI, K., H. NAKAZATO, H. MATSUI, *et al.* 2003. Genetic polymorphisms of estrogen receptor alpha, CYP19, catechol-O-methyltransferase are associated with familial prostate carcinoma risk in a Japanese population. Cancer **98:** 1411–1416.

55. SUZUKI, K., H. NAKAZATO, H. MATSUI, *et al.* 2003. Association of the genetic polymorphism of the CYP19 intron 4[TTTA]n repeat with familial prostate cancer risk in a Japanese population. Anticancer Res. **23:** 4941–4946.

56. McPherson, S.J., H. Wang, M.E. Jones, *et al*. 2001. Elevated androgens and prolactin in aromatase-deficient mice cause enlargement, but not malignancy, of the prostate gland. Endocrinology **142:** 2458–2467.

57. Rajfer, J. & D.S. Coffey. 1978. Sex steroid imprinting of the immature prostate. Long-term effects. Invest. Urol. **16:** 186–190.

58. Arai, Y., Y. Suzuki & Y. Nishizuka. 1977. Hyperplastic and metaplastic lesions in the reproductive tract of male rats induced by neonatal treatment with diethylstilbestrol. Virchows. Arch. A. Pathol. Anat. Histol. **376:** 21–28.

59. Arai, Y., T. Mori, Y. Suzuki & H.A. Bern. 1983. Long-term effects of perinatal exposure to sex steroids and diethylstilbestrol on the reproductive system of male mammals. Int. Rev. Cytol. **84:** 235–268.

60. Prins, G.S. 1992. Neonatal estrogen exposure induces lobe-specific alterations in adult rat prostate androgen receptor expression. Endocrinology **130:** 3703–3714.

61. Vorherr, H., R.H. Messer, U.F. Vorherr, *et al*. 1979. Teratogenesis and carcinogenesis in rat offspring after transplacental and transmammary exposure to diethylstilbestrol. Biochem. Pharmacol. **28:** 1865–1877.

62. McLachlan, J.A., R.R. Newbold & B. Bullock. 1975. Reproductive tract lesions in male mice exposed prenatally to diethylstilbestrol. Science **190:** 991–992.

63. McLachlan, J.A. 1977. Prenatal exposure to diethylstilbestrol in mice: toxicological studies. J. Toxicol. Environ. Health **2:** 527–537.

64. Pylkkanen, L., R. Santti, R. Newbold & J.A. McLachlan. 1991. Regional differences in the prostate of the neonatally estrogenized mouse. Prostate **18:** 117–129.

65. Prins, G.S., R.J. Sklarew & L.P. Pertschuk. 1998. Image analysis of androgen receptor immunostaining in prostate cancer accurately predicts response to hormonal therapy. J. Urol. **159:** 641–649.

66. Prins, G.S., L. Birch, J.F. Couse, *et al*. 2001. Estrogen imprinting of the developing prostate gland is mediated through stromal estrogen receptor alpha: studies with alphaERKO and betaERKO mice. Cancer Res. **61:** 6089–6097.

67. vom Saal, F.S., B.G. Timms, M.M. Montano, *et al*. 1997. Prostate enlargement in mice due to fetal exposure to low doses of estradiol or diethylstilbestrol and opposite effects at high doses. Proc. Natl. Acad. Sci. USA **94:** 2056–2061.

68. Ho, S.M., W.Y. Tang, D.F. Belmonte & G.S. Prins. 2006. Developmental exposure to estradiol and bisphenol a increases susceptibility to prostate carcinogenesis and epigenetically regulates phosphodiesterase type 4 variant 4. Cancer Res. **66:** 5624–5632.

69. Henderson, B.E. & H.S. Feigelson. 2000. Hormonal carcinogenesis. Carcinogenesis **21:** 427–433.

70. Potischman, N., R. Troisi, R. Thadhani, *et al*. 2005. Pregnancy hormone concentrations across ethnic groups: implications for later cancer risk. Cancer Epidemiol. Biomarkers Prev. **14:** 1514–1520.

71. Ekbom, A., C.C. Hsieh, L. Lipworth, *et al*. 1996. Perinatal characteristics in relation to incidence of and mortality from prostate cancer. BMJ **313:** 337–341.

72. Ekbom, A., J. Wuu, H.O. Adami, *et al*. 2000. Duration of gestation and prostate cancer risk in offspring. Cancer Epidemiol. Biomarkers Prev. **9:** 221–223.

73. IKEZUKI, Y., O. TSUTSUMI, Y. TAKAI, *et al.* 2002. Determination of bisphenol A concentrations in human biological fluids reveals significant early prenatal exposure. Hum. Reprod. **17:** 2839–2841.

74. KURODA, N., Y. KINOSHITA, Y. SUN, *et al.* 2003. Measurement of bisphenol A levels in human blood serum and ascitic fluid by HPLC using a fluorescent labeling reagent. J. Pharm. Biomed. Anal. **30:** 1743–1749.

75. SCHONFELDER, G., W. WITTFOHT, H. HOPP, *et al.* 2002. Parent bisphenol A accumulation in the human maternal-fetal-placental unit. Environ. Health Perspect. **110:** A703–A707.

76. TSURUSAKI, T., D. AOKI, H. KANETAKE, *et al.* 2003. Zone-dependent expression of estrogen receptors alpha and beta in human benign prostatic hyperplasia. J. Clin. Endocrinol. Metab. **88:** 1333–1340.

77. YAMADA, H., I. FURUTA, E.H. KATO, *et al.* 2002. Maternal serum and amniotic fluid bisphenol A concentrations in the early second trimester. Reprod . Toxicol. **16:** 735–739.

78. NILSSON, S. & J.A. GUSTAFSSON. 2000. Estrogen receptor transcription and transactivation: basic aspects of estrogen action. Breast Cancer Res. **2:** 360–366.

79. PETTERSSON, K. & J.A. GUSTAFSSON. 2001. Role of estrogen receptor beta in estrogen action. Annu. Rev. Physiol. **63:** 165–192.

80. LEUNG, Y.K., P. MAK, S. HASSAN & S.M. HO. 2006. Estrogen receptor (ER) β isoforms: a key to understanding ER-β signaling. Proc. Natl. Acad. Sci. USA **103:** 13162–13167.

81. OSBORNE, C.K., R. SCHIFF, S.A. FUQUA & J. SHOU. 2001. Estrogen receptor: current understanding of its activation and modulation. Clin. Cancer Res. **7:** 4338s–4342s.

82. TREMBLAY, G.B. & V. GIGUERE. 2002. Coregulators of estrogen receptor action. Crit. Rev. Eukaryot. Gene Expr. **12:** 1–22.

83. LEAV, I., K.M. LAU, J.Y. ADAMS, *et al.* 2001. Comparative studies of the estrogen receptors beta and alpha and the androgen receptor in normal human prostate glands, dysplasia, and in primary and metastatic carcinoma. Am. J. Pathol. **159:** 79–92.

84. FIXEMER, T., K. REMBERGER & H. BONKHOFF. 2003. Differential expression of the estrogen receptor beta (ERbeta) in human prostate tissue, premalignant changes, and in primary, metastatic, and recurrent prostatic adenocarcinoma. Prostate **54:** 79–87.

85. HORVATH, L.G., S.M. HENSHALL, C.S. LEE, *et al.* 2001. Frequent loss of estrogen receptor-beta expression in prostate cancer. Cancer Res. **61:** 5331–5335.

86. LATIL, A., I. BIECHE, D. VIDAUD, *et al.* 2001. Evaluation of androgen, estrogen (ER alpha and ER beta), and progesterone receptor expression in human prostate cancer by real-time quantitative reverse transcription-polymerase chain reaction assays. Cancer Res. **61:** 1919–1926.

87. ROYUELA, M., M.P. DE MIGUEL, F.R. BETHENCOURT, *et al.* 2001. Estrogen receptors alpha and beta in the normal, hyperplastic and carcinomatous human prostate. J. Endocrinol. **168:** 447–454.

88. TORLAKOVIC, E., W. LILLEBY, G. TORLAKOVIC, *et al.* 2002. Prostate carcinoma expression of estrogen receptor-beta as detected by PPG5/10 antibody has positive association with primary Gleason grade and Gleason score. Hum. Pathol. **33:** 646–651.

89. WEIHUA, Z., M. WARNER & J.A. GUSTAFSSON. 2002. Estrogen receptor beta in the prostate. Mol. Cell Endocrinol. **193:** 1–5.

90. JIANG, J., H.L. CHANG, Y. SUGIMOTO & Y.C. LIN. 2005. Effects of age on growth and ERbeta mRNA expression of canine prostatic cells. Anticancer Res. **25:** 4081–4090.

91. POELZL, G., Y. KASAI, N. MOCHIZUKI, *et al.* 2000. Specific association of estrogen receptor beta with the cell cycle spindle assembly checkpoint protein, MAD2. Proc. Natl. Acad. Sci. USA **97:** 2836–2839.

92. WEIHUA, Z., S. MAKELA, L.C. ANDERSSON, *et al.* 2001. A role for estrogen receptor beta in the regulation of growth of the ventral prostate. Proc. Natl. Acad. Sci. USA **98:** 6330–6335.

93. SIGNORETTI, S. & M. LODA. 2001. Estrogen receptor beta in prostate cancer: brake pedal or accelerator? Am. J. Pathol. **159:** 13–16.

94. KREGE, J.H., J.B. HODGIN, J.F. COUSE, *et al.* 1998. Generation and reproductive phenotypes of mice lacking estrogen receptor beta. Proc. Natl. Acad. Sci. USA **95:** 15677–15682.

95. CHANG, W.Y. & G.S. PRINS. 1999. Estrogen receptor-beta: implications for the prostate gland. Prostate **40:** 115–124.

96. MONTANO, M.M. & B.S. KATZENELLENBOGEN. 1997. The quinone reductase gene: a unique estrogen receptor-regulated gene that is activated by antiestrogens. Proc. Natl. Acad. Sci. USA **94:** 2581–2586.

97. MONTANO, M.M., B.M. WITTMANN & N.R. BIANCO. 2000. Identification and characterization of a novel factor that regulates quinone reductase gene transcriptional activity. J. Biol. Chem. **275:** 34306–34313.

98. MONTANO, M.M., H. DENG, M. LIU, *et al.* 2004. Transcriptional regulation by the estrogen receptor of antioxidative stress enzymes and its functional implications. Oncogene **23:** 2442–2453.

99. DIMITROVA, K.R., K.W. DEGROOT, J.P. SUYDERHOUD, *et al.* 2002. 17-beta estradiol preserves endothelial cell viability in an in vitro model of homocysteine-induced oxidative stress. J. Cardiovasc. Pharmacol. **39:** 347–353.

100. GELINAS, S., G. BUREAU, B. VALASTRO, *et al.* 2004. Alpha and beta estradiol protect neuronal but not native PC12 cells from paraquat-induced oxidative stress. Neurotox. Res. **6:** 141–148.

101. MIZE, A.L., R.A. SHAPIRO & D.M. DORSA. 2003. Estrogen receptor-mediated neuroprotection from oxidative stress requires activation of the mitogen-activated protein kinase pathway. Endocrinology **144:** 306–312.

102. TREUTER, E., M. WARNER & J.A. GUSTAFSSON. 2000. Mechanism of oestrogen signalling with particular reference to the role of ER beta in the central nervous system. Novartis Found. Symp. **230:** 7–14.

103. BIANCO, N.R., L.J. CHAPLIN & M.M. MONTANO. 2005. Differential induction of quinone reductase by phytoestrogens and protection against oestrogen-induced DNA damage. Biochem. J. **385:** 279–287.

104. SHAPIRO, E., H. HUANG, R.J. MASCH, *et al.* 2005. Immunolocalization of estrogen receptor alpha and beta in human fetal prostate. J. Urol. **174:** 2051–2053.

105. PASQUALI, D., S. STAIBANO, D. PREZIOSO, *et al.* 2001. Estrogen receptor beta expression in human prostate tissue. Mol. Cell. Endocrinol. **178:** 47–50.

106. PASQUALI, D., V. ROSSI, D. ESPOSITO, *et al.* 2001. Loss of estrogen receptor beta expression in malignant human prostate cells in primary cultures and in prostate cancer tissues. J. Clin. Endocrinol. Metab. **86:** 2051–2055.

107. LAI, J.S., L.G. BROWN, L.D. TRUE, *et al.* 2004. Metastases of prostate cancer express estrogen receptor-beta. Urology **64:** 814–820.

108. ZHU, X., I. LEAV, Y.K. LEUNG, et al. 2004. Dynamic regulation of estrogen receptor-beta expression by DNA methylation during prostate cancer development and metastasis. Am. J. Pathol. **164:** 2003–2012.
109. DOMANN, F.E. & B.W. FUTSCHER. 2004. Flipping the epigenetic switch. Am. J. Pathol. **164:** 1883–1886.
110. HAQQ, C., R. LI, D. KHODABAKHSH, et al. 2005. Ethnic and racial differences in prostate stromal estrogen receptor alpha. Prostate **65:** 101–109.
111. TANAKA, Y., M. SASAKI, M. KANEUCHI, et al. 2003. Polymorphisms of estrogen receptor alpha in prostate cancer. Mol. Carcinogen. **37:** 202–208.
112. HUGGINS, C. & C.V. HODGES. 1972. Studies on prostatic cancer. I. The effect of castration, of estrogen and androgen injection on serum phosphatases in metastatic carcinoma of the prostate CA. Cancer J. Clin. **22:** 232–240.
113. COX, R.L. & E.D. CRAWFORD. 1995. Estrogens in the treatment of prostate cancer. J. Urol. **154:** 1991–1998.
114. DENIS, L.J. & K. GRIFFITHS. 2000. Endocrine treatment in prostate cancer. Semin. Surg. Oncol. **18:** 52–74.
115. BERGAN, R.C., E. REED, C.E. MYERS, et al. 1999. A phase II study of high-dose tamoxifen in patients with hormone-refractory prostate cancer. Clin. Cancer Res. **5:** 2366–2373.
116. HAMILTON, M., W. DAHUT, O. BRAWLEY, et al. 2003. A phase I/II study of high-dose tamoxifen in combination with vinblastine in patients with androgen-independent prostate cancer. Acta Oncol. **42:** 195–201.
117. LISSONI, P., P. VIGANO, M. VAGHI, et al. 2005. A phase II study of tamoxifen in hormone-resistant metastatic prostate cancer: possible relation with prolactin secretion. Anticancer Res. **25:** 3597–3599.
118. SHAZER, R.L., A. JAIN, A.V. GALKIN, et al. 2006. Raloxifene, an oestrogen-receptor-beta-targeted therapy, inhibits androgen-independent prostate cancer growth: results from preclinical studies and a pilot phase II clinical trial. BJU Int. **97:** 691–697.
119. STEIN, S., B. ZOLTICK, T. PEACOCK, et al. 2001. Phase II trial of toremifene in androgen-independent prostate cancer: a Penn cancer clinical trials group trial. Am. J. Clin. Oncol. **24:** 283–285.
120. EL-RAYES, B.F. & M.H. HUSSAIN. 2002. Hormonal therapy for prostate cancer: past, present and future. Expert. Rev. Anticancer Ther. **2:** 37–47.
121. SCHULZ, P., H.W. BAUER, W.P. BRADE, et al. 1988. Evaluation of the cytotoxic activity of diethylstilbestrol and its mono- and diphosphate towards prostatic carcinoma cells. Cancer Res. **48:** 2867–2870.
122. KUMAR, A.P., G.E. GARCIA & T.J. SLAGA. 2001. 2-methoxyestradiol blocks cell-cycle progression at G(2)/M phase and inhibits growth of human prostate cancer cells. Mol. Carcinogen. **31:** 111–124.
123. QADAN, L.R., C.M. PEREZ-STABLE, C. ANDERSON, et al. 2001. 2-Methoxyestradiol induces G2/M arrest and apoptosis in prostate cancer. Biochem. Biophys. Res. Commun. **285:** 1259–1266.
124. KIM, I.Y., B.C. KIM, D.H.SEONG, et al. 2002. Raloxifene, a mixed estrogen agonist/antagonist, induces apoptosis in androgen-independent human prostate cancer cell lines. Cancer Res. **62:** 5365–5369.
125. SHIMADA, K., M. NAKAMURA, E. ISHIDA, et al. 2003. Requirement of c-jun for testosterone-induced sensitization to N-(4-hydroxyphenyl)retinamide-induced apoptosis. Mol. Carcinogen. **36:** 115–122.

126. DAHLLOF, B., A. BILLSTROM, F. CABRAL & B. HARTLEY-ASP. 1993. Estramustine depolymerizes microtubules by binding to tubulin. Cancer Res. **53:** 4573–4581.

127. KUWAJERWALA, N., E. CIFUENTES, S. GAUTAM, *et al.* 2002. Resveratrol induces prostate cancer cell entry into s phase and inhibits DNA synthesis. Cancer Res. **62:** 2488–2492.

128. MATSUKAWA, Y., N. MARUI, T. SAKAI, *et al.* 1993. Genistein arrests cell cycle progression at G2-M. Cancer Res. **53:** 1328–1331.

129. MISRA, R.R., S.D. HURSTING, S.N. PERKINS, *et al.* 2002. Genotoxicity and carcinogenicity studies of soy isoflavones. Int. J. Toxicol. **21:** 277–285.

130. RAFI, M.M., R.T. ROSEN, A. VASSIL, *et al.* 2000. Modulation of bcl-2 and cytotoxicity by licochalcone-A, a novel estrogenic flavonoid. Anticancer Res. **20:** 2653–2658.

131. LAVALLEE, T.M., X.H. ZHAN, M.S. JOHNSON, *et al.* 2003. 2-methoxyestradiol up-regulates death receptor 5 and induces apoptosis through activation of the extrinsic pathway. Cancer Res. **63:** 468–475.

132. MOR, G., F. KOHEN, J. GARCIA-VELASCO, *et al.* 2000. Regulation of fas ligand expression in breast cancer cells by estrogen: functional differences between estradiol and tamoxifen. J. Steroid Biochem. Mol. Biol. **73:** 185–194.

133. LI, Y. & F.H. SARKAR. 2002. Gene expression profiles of genistein-treated PC3 prostate cancer cells. J. Nutr. **132:** 3623–3631.

134. LIU, Y., E. KYLE, R. LIEBERMAN, *et al.* 2000. Focal adhesion kinase (FAK) phosphorylation is not required for genistein-induced FAK-beta-1-integrin complex formation. Clin. Exp. Metastasis **18:** 203–212.

135. NEUBAUER, B.L., K.L. BEST, D.F. COUNTS, *et al.* 1995. Raloxifene (LY156758) produces antimetastatic responses and extends survival in the PAIII rat prostatic adenocarcinoma model. Prostate **27:** 220–229.

136. LAU, K.M., M. LASPINA, J. LONG & S.M. HO. 2000. Expression of estrogen receptor (ER)-alpha and ER-beta in normal and malignant prostatic epithelial cells: regulation by methylation and involvement in growth regulation. Cancer Res. **60:** 3175–3182.

137. MAK, P., Y.K. LEUNG, W.Y. TANG, *et al.* 2006. Apigenin suppresses cancer cell growth via ERβ. Neoplasia. In press.

138. MOBLEY, J.A., J.O. L'ESPERANCE, M. WU, *et al.* 2004. The novel estrogen 17alpha-20Z-21-[(4-amino)phenyl]-19-norpregna-1,3,5(10),20-tetraene-3,17beta-diol induces apoptosis in prostate cancer cell lines at nanomolar concentrations in vitro. Mol. Cancer Ther. **3:** 587–595.

Crosstalk between EGFR and Extranuclear Steroid Receptors

ANTIMO MIGLIACCIO, GABRIELLA CASTORIA,
MARINA DI DOMENICO, ALESSANDRA CIOCIOLA,
MARIA LOMBARDI, ANTONIETTA DE FALCO,
MERLIN NANAYAKKARA, DANIELA BOTTERO, ROSINA DE STASIO,
LILIAN VARRICCHIO, AND FERDINANDO AURICCHIO

*Dipartimento di Patologia Generale, Facoltà di Medicina e Chirurgia,
II Università di Napoli, Via L. De Crecchio, 7-80138 Naples, Italy*

ABSTRACT: Epidermal growth factor (EGF) stimulates DNA synthesis
and cytoskeletal rearrangement in human breast cancer (MCF-7) and
human prostate cancer (LNCaP) cells. Both effects are inhibited by estrogen (ICI 182,780) and androgen (Casodex) antagonists. This supports the
view that crosstalk exists between EGF and estradiol (ER) and androgen
(AR) receptors and suggests that these receptors are directly involved in
the EGF action. Our recent work shows that EGF stimulates ER phosphorylation on tyrosine and promotes the association of a complex between EGFR, AR/ER, and the kinase Src. The complex assembly triggers
Src activity, epidermal growth factor receptor (EGFR) phosphorylation
on tyrosine, and the EGF-dependent signaling pathway activation. In
these cells, the AR/ER/Src complex is required for the EGF action, as the
growth factor effects are abolished upon receptor silencing by specific
SiRNAs and steroid antagonists or Src inhibition by the kinase inhibitor
PP2.

KEYWORDS: androgen receptor; estrogen receptor; signal transduction;
epidermal growth factor

INTRODUCTION

Crosstalk between growth factors and steroid receptors in the nuclear
compartment leads to ligand-independent activation of the steroid receptor–
dependent transcription. Serine phosphorylation of steroid receptors by growth
factor–activated signaling kinases triggers this activation. Recent data and findings described herein reveal that a crosstalk between growth factors and steroid

Address for correspondence: Ferdinando Auricchio, Dipartimento di Patologia Generale, Facoltà
di Medicina e Chirurgia, II Università di Napoli, Via L. De Crecchio, 7-80138 Naples, Italy. Voice:
+39-081-566-5676; fax: +39-081-291-327.
e-mail:ferdinando.auricchio@unina2.it

Ann. N.Y. Acad. Sci. 1089: 194–200 (2006). © 2006 New York Academy of Sciences.
doi: 10.1196/annals.1386.006

receptors occurs in a bidirectional way also at a nontranscriptional level. Interestingly, epidermal growth factor (EGF) signaling is strongly enhanced by the functional interplay between the EGF receptor/erb-B2 heterodimer and the estradiol receptor (ER)–androgen receptor (AR) complex in MCF-7 cells. ER tyrosine phosphorylation, triggered by growth factors, causes the assembly of the EGFR/ER/AR/Src signaling complex, which, in turn, induces EGFR phosphorylation on tyrosine. Since growth factors and steroid receptors are known to dramatically contribute to breast cancer progression, these findings contribute to the understanding of their action.

EGF activity converges on the ER in human mammary cancer–derived cells as well as in uterus, thereby triggering DNA synthesis and cell proliferation. EGF can also activate genes regulated by estrogen-responsive elements.[1–3] An increase in uterine weight and proliferation of the uterine epithelial cells follows EGF or insulin-like growth factor-I (IGF-I) treatment of ovariectomized mice. Interestingly, these effects are not observed in ER-α knockout mice, indicating that ER-α is required in this growth factor activity.[3] Elevated Src activity has been found in breast tumor specimens and cell lines.[4] Moreover, both EGFR and Src are overexpressed in a subset of human breast tumors and a wealth of evidence indicates physical and functional associations between EGFR and Src (reviewed in Ref. 5). Expression of dominant negative Src in murine fibroblasts interferes with EGF-induced mitogenesis and cytoskeletal changes.[6] Therefore, steroid receptors and Src seem to be components of the signaling pathway elicited by EGF.

In MCF-7 and LNCaP cells, ER and AR, once activated by steroid hormones, stimulate a mitogenic signaling network known to be engaged by growth factors.[7,8] We recently observed in these cells an unexpected crosstalk between EGFR and the extranuclear steroid receptors, which will be analyzed in the course of this report.

Epidermal Growth Factor Signaling in Mammary Cancer Cells is Upregulated by Steroid Receptors and Src

Recent evidence from our laboratory[9] indicates that steroid receptors and Src play a key role in EGF-triggered DNA synthesis and stress fiber breakdown. EGF stimulates the S-phase entry of MCF-7 cells maintained in phenol red–free medium supplemented with charcoal-treated serum. In accordance with a previous report,[1] the effect of EGF is abolished by ICI 182,780, a pure antiestrogen. Interestingly, the pure antiandrogen Casodex also abolishes the growth hormone effect. Effects similar to those of the two steroid antagonists are observed in the presence of the Src kinase family inhibitor, PP2, as well as in cells transiently transfected with siRNA silencing ER-α or AR. EGF rapidly induces fan-like membrane protrusions and ruffles in MCF-7 cells. Also in this case, both steroid antagonists prevent EGF-induced cytoskeletal changes. Src activity is also involved in these responses as indicated by the PP2 inhibitory effect on EGF-induced cytoskeletal changes. In conclusion, the two steroid receptors and Src have a key role in the EGF-elicited responses in MCF-7 cells.

EGF-Triggered Src Activation in MCF-7 Cells is Inhibited by Steroid Antagonists

Src family tyrosine kinases are involved in signaling of different growth factor receptors including EGFR. They can promote initiation of signaling pathways required for DNA synthesis and actin cytoskeleton rearrangements.[10] In MCF-7 cells EGF activates Src, whereas ICI 182,780 prevents this activation as well as the EGF-induced Ras and Erk-2 activities. Therefore, ER-α plays a major role in the regulation of EGF-elicited signal transducing pathway in MCF-7 cells. Casodex also prevents the EGF-induced activation of Src in MCF-7 cells, which express AR. Lack of effect of ICI 182,780 on EGF signaling in ER-negative MDA-MB231 cells indicates that inhibition of EGF-induced Src activation by ICI 182,780 in human mammary cancer cells requires ER-α expression.

EGF Triggers Association of ER-α and AR with Src and EGFR

Simultaneous to Src activation, EGF induces association of ER-α and AR with Src and EGFR in MCF-7 cells. A selective inhibitor of the EGFR tyrosine kinase, Iressa (ZD 1839), and the anti-erb-B2 antibody herceptin (Trastuzumab), block the EGF-elicited Src activation and ER-α tyrosine phosphorylation and prevent the association of Src with ER and AR. Transient transfection of Cos cells with hAR and either hER-α (HEG0) cDNAs or the HEG537 cDNA mutant, lacking the only phosphorylatable tyrosine, that in position 537,[11] shows that this phosphotyrosine is required for the coexpressed receptors/Src complex assembly.

AR and ER-α are Associated with Unstimulated MCF-7 and LNCaP Cells

Co-immunoprecipitations of either AR or ER indicate that 8% of the two receptors are associated in MCF-7 cells under basal conditions. Interestingly, a similar association occurs in LNCaP cells between ERβ and AR. Pull-down experiments with glutathione S-transferase (GST) fusion protein constructs show that the association between the two receptors is direct. Association was previously observed between ERα and progesterone receptor-B in human mammary cancererived cells under basal conditions and in vitro. It is required in different cell lines for progestin stimulation of signal transducing pathway, which triggers G1-S transition.[12,13,14]

Ligand-Stimulated Epidermal Growth Factor Receptor Tyrosine Phosphorylation in MCF-7 Cells is Uupregulated by Steroid Receptors and Src

The above described experiments show that EGF induces ligand-independent extranuclear steroid receptor activation. Remarkably, steroid receptors, in turn, regulate the EGFR. In fact, EGFR phosphorylation in EGF-stimulated MCF-7 cells is strongly reduced when the cells are stimulated by the growth factor in the presence of either ER or AR antagonists. This finding suggests a novel, steroid-independent regulatory role of steroid receptors on EGFR. This conclusion is supported by the strong inhibitory effect on EGFR phosphorylation observed after the knockdown of ERa or AR gene in MCF-7 cells. In addition to the steroid receptors, Src is required for EGFR phosphorylation in MCF-7 cells. EGFR tyrosine phosphorylation triggered by EGF is much weaker in cells expressing kinase-inactive Src. On this basis we propose that Src kinase activity plays a key role in the EGF-dependent EGFR phosphorylation in MCF-7 cells and that this activity is under the control of the Src-associated steroid receptors. This possibility is strongly corroborated by the experiments in Cos cells transiently co-transfected with hAR and the wild-type hERα, or its mutant HEG537. In fact, EGF strongly stimulates EGFR tyrosine phosphorylation in Cos cells expressing HEG0, whereas a much weaker stimulation was detected in cells expressing HEG537, which is not able to interact with Src and induce association of AR/ER/Src. Remarkably, comparison of EGFR tyrosine phosphorylation in cells transfected with the empty vector or ERα- and AR-expressing plasmids shows that in the presence of the two steroid receptors a much stronger EGFR phosphorylation is triggered by EGF. This provides additional evidence that the expression of the two steroid receptors upregulates EGFR phosphorylation.

EGF-Elicited Effects Are Inhibited by Steroid Antagonists in LNCaP Cells

In LNCaP cells, as in MCF-7 cells, EGF induces DNA synthesis. Antiandrogen and antiestrogen abolish this stimulation. The antagonists also prevent EGF-induced cytoskeletal changes and the growth factortimulated Src activation. These findings indicate that also in prostate cancer cells EGF signaling is regulated by the two steroid receptors.

CONCLUSIONS

On the basis of the results presented, one may envisage a new model of crosstalk between extranuclear steroid receptors and EGFR. a central role being played by the physical and functional interactions between EGFR, steroidal

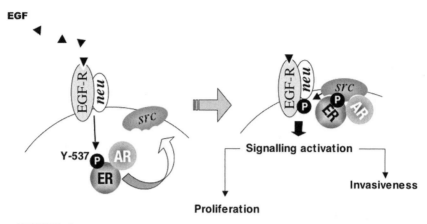

FIGURE 1.

receptors, and Src (FIG. 1). The EGF-activated Src, which is associated with the ER/AR complex, strongly acts on the EGFR phosphorylation. Conversely, when ER and/or AR are locked in an inactive conformation by hormone antagonists or when the steroid receptor levels are downregulated by siRNA, their action on Src and EGFR is missing or heavily impaired and EGF-induced EGFR tyrosine phosphorylation is minimal. Interestingly, in MCF-7 cells, silencing of steroid receptor genes abolishes the EGF-elicited DNA synthesis, further indicating that such an effect requires steroid receptors. Similarly, ER-α is required for EGF-triggered DNA synthesis in uterine epithelial cells *in vivo*.[3] The complexity of the described crosstalk between EGF and the steroid receptor/Src complex is underlined by the observation that steroid receptors also control, through Src, the EGF-elicited cytoskeletal changes, a classic nongenomic effect in breast and prostate cancer cells. Association of AR with ER in MCF-7 and LNCaP cells under basal conditions represents a novel and important crosstalk between the two receptors, which are linked in their responses to growth factors or steroid hormones. This study also reveals other aspects of the molecular assembly that regulates nongenomic steroid receptor action. In the ER/Src complex triggered by estradiol or androgen in MCF7, LNCaP or T47D cells,[8] phosphotyrosine in position 537 of ER-α is crucial for the hormone-induced association of ER-α with Src-SH2 and consequent Src activation and mitogenesis.[8] The same phosphotyrosine residue is required for the association of ER-α with Src triggered by EGF. On the basis of previous and present findings, the ER/AR/Src association is crucial for proliferation triggered by steroid hormone[8] or EGF in hormone-responsive cells. This is a point with important implications since a large number of mammary and prostate cancers respond to steroid hormones and growth factors. This association represents a target for a novel, rational, and specific therapy of cancers expressing steroid receptors.

ACKNOWLEDGMENTS

This research has been supported by: "Associazione Italiana per la Ricerca sul Cancro," Ministero dell'Università e della Ricerca Scientifica (Cofinanziamenti Ministero dell'Università e Ricerca Scientifica a Tecnologica 2003 and 2004; Fondo per gli Investimenti della Ricerca di Base 2001), Ministero della Sanità (Programmi Speciali; Lgs. 229/99), and a Fondazione Italiana per la Ricerca sul Cancro fellowship (M. Lombardi).

REFERENCES

1. VIGNON, F., M.M. BOUTON & H. ROCHEFORT. 1987. Antiestrogens inhibit the mitogenic effect of growth factors on breast cancer cells in the total absence of estrogens. Biochem. Biophys. Res. Commun. **146:** 1502–1508.
2. IGNAR-TROWBRIDGE, D.M., K.G. NELSON, M.C. BIDWELL, *et al.* 1992. Coupling of dual signaling pathways: epidermal growth factor action involves the estrogen receptor. Proc. Natl. Acad. Sci. USA **89:** 4658–4662.
3. HEWITT, S., J.C. HARRELL & K.S. KORACH. 2005. Lessons in estrogen biology from knockout and transgenic animals. Annu. Rev. Physiol. **67:** 285–308.
4. OTTENHOFF-KALFF, A.E., G. RIJKSEN, E.A. VAN BEURDEN, *et al.* 1992. Characterization of protein kinases from human breast cancer: involvement of the c-Src oncogene product. Cancer Res. **52:** 4773–4778.
5. ISHIZWAR, R. & S.J. PARSONS. 2004. c-Src and cooperating partners in human cancer. Cancer Cell **6:** 209–214.
6. ROCHE, S., M. KOEGL, M.V. BARONE, *et al.* 1995. DNA synthesis induced by some but not all growth factors requires Src family protein tyrosine kinases. Mol. Cell. Biol. **15:** 1102–1109.
7. MIGLIACCIO, A., M. DI DOMENICO, G. CASTORIA, *et al.* 1996. Tyrosine kinase/p21ras/MAP-kinase pathway activation by estradiol-receptor complex in MCF-7 cells. EMBO J. **15:** 1292–1300.
8. MIGLIACCIO, A., G. CASTORIA, M. DI DOMENICO, *et al.* 2000. Steroid-induced androgen receptor-oestradiol receptor-Src complex triggers prostate cancer cell proliferation. EMBO J. **19:** 5406–5417.
9. MIGLIACCIO, A., M. DI DOMENICO, G. CASTORIA, *et al.* 2005. Steroid receptor regulation of epidermal growth factor through Src in breast and prostate cancer cells: steroid anatgonist action. Cancer Res. **65:** 10585–10593.
10. BROMANN, A.P., H. KORKAYA & S.A. COURTNEIGE. 2004. The interplay between Src family kinases and receptor tyrosine kinases. Oncogene **23:** 7957–7968.
11. CASTORIA, G., A. MIGLIACCIO, S. GREEN, *et al.* 1993. Properties of a purified estradiol-dependent calf uterus tyrosine kinase. Biochemistry **32:** 1740–1750.
12. MIGLIACCIO, A., D. PICCOLO, G. CASTORIA, *et al.* 1998. Activation of the Src/p21ras/Erk pathway by progesterone receptor via cross-talk with estrogen receptor. EMBO J. **17:** 2008–2018.
13. BALLARE, C., M. UHRIG, T. BECHTOLD, *et al.* 2003. Two domains of the progesterone receptor interact with the estrogen receptor and are required for progesterone

activation of the c-Src/Erk pathway in mammalian cells. Mol. Cell. Biol. **23:** 1994–2008

14. VALLEJO, G., C. BALLARE, J.L. BARANAO, *et al.* 2005. Progestin activation of nongenomic pathways via cross talk of progesterone receptor with estrogen receptor beta induces proliferation of endometrial stromal cells. Mol. Endocrinol. **19:** 3023–3037.

Estrogens and Mechanisms of Prostate Cancer Progression

GIUSEPPE CARRUBA

Experimental Oncology, Department of Oncology, ARNAS-Civico, Palermo, Italy

ABSTRACT: Prostate cancer is a major health issue in westernized countries, being considered a prototypical age-related, androgen-dependent tumor. However, data on the association between circulating androgens and prostate cancer have been inconsistent and mostly not compatible with the androgen hypothesis. In addition, plasma androgen-to-estrogen ratio appears to decrease with age, suggesting that estrogens may also have a role. Results from our own and others' studies suggest that circulating steroids cannot be considered representative of their actual intraprostatic levels. This is a consequence of the expression and/or activity of steroid enzymes, including 17β-hydroxysteroid dehydrogenase (17β-HSD), 5α-reductase, $3\alpha/3\beta$-HSD, and aromatase, which may eventually lead to a differential tissue accumulation of steroid derivatives having distinct biological activities. Interestingly, many of the genes encoding for steroid enzymes are highly polymorphic in nature, although only a few studies have investigated their relation with prostate cancer and the data presently available are inconclusive. Locally produced or metabolically transformed estrogens may differently affect proliferative activity of prostate cancer cells. In our studies, estrogen may either stimulate or decrease prostate cancer cell growth, also depending on the receptor status. In particular, an imbalance of ERα and ERβ expression may be critical to determine the ultimate estrogen effects on prostate cancer cell growth. Furthermore, evidence is accumulating that estrogens regulate gene transcription through an array of estrogen-response elements (EREs) and non-EREs, either ligand-dependent or -independent. This is further complicated by the presence of receptor isoforms, distinct cofactor interaction, and potential heterodimerization. Based on this combined evidence, a hypothetical model of prostate cancer progression is presented.

KEYWORDS: estrogen; receptor; metabolism; prostate cancer; progression

Address for correspondence: Giuseppe Carruba, M.D., Ph.D., Department of Oncology, P.O. M. Ascoli, ARNAS-Civico, Piazzale N. Leotta 2, 90127 Palermo, Italy. Voice: +39-091-666-4348; fax: +39-091-666-4352.

e-mail: lucashbl@unipa.it

Ann. N.Y. Acad. Sci. 1089: 201–217 (2006). © 2006 New York Academy of Sciences.
doi: 10.1196/annals.1386.027

INTRODUCTION

Prostate cancer is a major health issue in westernized countries. Although it represents a common cause of morbidity and mortality in men in the developed world, it ought to be preventable and curable. However, the molecular pathology of prostate cancer is intricate: endogenous sex steroids along with environmental factors (e.g., diet) and host immune and inflammatory responses are likely to cooperate in the pathogenesis of prostate cancer.

In the last decades, both epidemiologists and cancer researchers have been struggling to identify the etiological factors that could explain the nearly 40-fold difference in incidence and the 12-fold difference in mortality of prostate cancer across different geographic areas and ethnicities.[1] In this framework, migrant population studies have emphasized the role that environmental and lifestyle factors, notably diet, may have in both development and progression of this neoplasm.[2] Although a variable, though minor, proportion (up to 9%) of prostate cancer can be based on genetic, heritable factors, the effects of environment and lifestyle appear to be essential for the manifestation of disease, even in men carrying strong cancer-susceptibility genes. It is noteworthy that environmental and dietary factors are highly likely to induce significant changes in endogenous hormone levels and metabolism and this may eventually lead prostate cancer to develop and/or to progress. In this respect, sex steroids may be implicated as intermediaries between exogenous effectors, either environmental or nutritional, and molecular targets in the process of initiation, promotion, and progression of prostate cancer.

EPIDEMIOLOGY

Prostate cancer is currently the most common neoplasm and the second leading cause of cancer death in men in the United States, with an estimate of 234,460 new cases and 27,350 deaths from this disease to be expected in the year 2006.[3] In Europe, in a figure similar to that of the United States, human prostate cancer has exhibited a steady increase of incidence over the years. However, incidence rates have now leveled off in men aged over 65 years and mortality rates have been consistently declining since 1990. Interestingly enough, incidence rates for prostate cancer vary considerably across northern and southern Europe, respectively being 80.1/100,000 and 44.7/100,000 in 2000 (IARC databases). In particular, Sweden has the highest incidence rates (139.3/100,000), while Greece has the lowest (43.4/100,000), with a cumulative risk that ranges from 0.5 up to 2.2 across European countries.

There is a nearly 40-fold and a 12-fold difference, respectively, in incidence and mortality rates from prostate cancer between African American men and men in Hong Kong and Japan. Although both genetic and environmental factors may contribute to explaining this large geographic variation, the causes remain largely unknown. Previous studies on migrants who moved from countries with low incidence/mortality rates of prostate cancer (i.e., China or Japan) to countries with higher prostate cancer rates (United States) showed, within a generation, a significant increase in prostate cancer incidence/mortality as compared with their counterparts in the countries of origin.[4–7]

On the other hand, prostate cancer incidence is rising rapidly in Asian countries, including Japan, as Asians gradually adopt westernized diet and lifestyle.[8,9] This evidence suggests that environmental and, especially, lifestyle factors play a dominant role in prostate cancer development. For example, sedentary lifestyle and high-fat diet have been associated with an increase in prostate cancer risk.[10] An explanation of the linkage between environmental and/or lifestyle factors and prostate cancer risk might be the influence of these factors on sex steroid metabolism, in particular estrogen metabolism.

Age, ethnicity, and family history, however, remain the few, well-established risk factors for prostate cancer.

SEX STEROIDS AND PROSTATE CANCER

Early studies, conducted in clinical settings, support the postulated link between gonadal steroids and prostate cancer by showing that eunuchs, whose testes were removed or never developed, do not suffer from prostate cancer or even benign prostatic hyperplasia.[11,12] On the other hand, a higher incidence of prostate cancer has been found in men who used androgens as anabolic agents or therapeutics.[13–15] Furthermore, either pharmacological or surgical castration is effective as palliative treatment of prostate cancer.[16] High levels of endogenous gonadal steroids have been considered as risk factors for prostate cancer.

There is clear-cut experimental evidence that sex hormones, both androgens and estrogens, may be important in prostate cancer. *In vitro* studies have shown that androgens and estrogens sustain and regulate prostate epithelial cell growth.[17–20] One of the most relevant pieces of evidence in favor of the causal association between sex steroids and prostate cancer has been provided by animal studies. Long-term administration of testosterone and estradiol to Noble rats results in a high incidence of adenocarcinomas in the dorsolateral prostate.[22] Leav and associates[23] indicated that the combined treatment of intact Noble rats with testosterone and estradiol, but not the separate administration of these gonadal steroids alone, induced florid dysplasia and markedly elevated mitotic index in the rat dorsolateral prostates. The authors suggested that protracted androgen-supported estrogen-enhanced stimulation of cell proliferation may be required for dysplastic lesions to develop in the rat prostate. This evidence is of particular interest since prostate adenocarcinoma was found to be very difficult to experimentally induce. More recently, using an elegant model system, Cunha and colleagues revealed that a 5–8-week treatment with testosterone and estradiol induced atypical hyperplasia and carcinoma in the male nude mouse grafted with Rb-null mouse embryonic prostates, suggesting that deletion of the Rb gene predisposes prostatic epithelium to hyperplasia and enhances its susceptibility to hormonal carcinogenesis.[23,24]

Nevertheless, while the association of sex steroids with prostate cancer is supported by biological evidence, epidemiological studies have reported inconclusive data. Analytical studies using direct measurement of serum steroid levels in relation to prostate cancer risk have, in fact, shown inconsistent results. Measurement of endogenous hormones in blood poses many methodological and/or logistic problems, including variations in biological specimen collection and assay methods. These problems may explain, at least in part, the inconsistency of previous study results.

Circulating Steroids

Human prostate cancer is widely recognized as a paradigm of age-related, androgen-dependent tumor. However, there is consistent evidence that both total and bioavailable serum testosterone significantly decline with age, eventually leading to an inverse association between circulating testosterone and the risk of developing prostate cancer (FIG. 1). Although this appears as contradictory evidence, it is important to point out that the time scale of prostate carcinogenesis and cancer progression can be up to 35–40 years or longer (FIG. 2). Therefore, the timing for the impact of androgen and/or estrogen on prostate cancer development and progression should be allocated in an

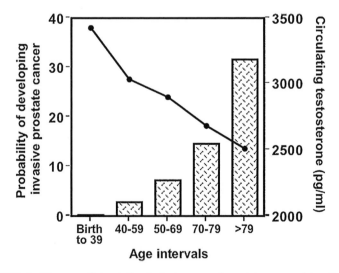

FIGURE 1. Changes of circulating testosterone and prostate cancer risk with age.

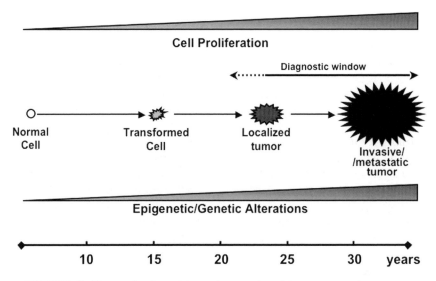

FIGURE 2. Time scale of prostate carcinogenesis and tumor progression.

approximate range of 15–25 years prior to clinical manifestation of the tumor, when serum androgens are still potentially relevant. Furthermore, there is convincing evidence that exposure of prostate cells to elevated estrogens early in uterine or perinatal life (a process referred to as developmental estrogenization or estrogen imprinting[25]) may be responsible for permanent perturbations of prostate development that may eventually result in predisposition to development of precancerous or malignant lesions in the prostate (see also the article by Prins and associates in this volume).

Several epidemiologic studies have investigated the association between circulating androgens and prostate cancer incidence, but the resulting data have been largely inconclusive and mostly not compatible with the androgen hypothesis. Only results from the Physicians' Health Study[26] show a significant trend of increasing prostate cancer risk with increasing levels of plasma testosterone when hormone and steroid hormone–binding globulin (SHBG) levels were simultaneously adjusted. In contrast, a subsequent meta-analysis by Eaton and colleagues,[27] presenting a quantitative review of the data from eight prospective epidemiological studies, clearly indicates that there are no large differences in circulating hormones between men who subsequently develop prostate cancer and those who remain free of disease. This inconsistency may be a consequence of several issues related to measurement of plasma androgens. In the first place, it remains to be established whether a single assay of plasma androgens can be considered representative of average androgen levels over an etiologically relevant time of life. Other methodological issues would include standardization of time of the day for blood collection, optimization of sample storage, and mutual statistical adjustment of circulating hormones and SHBG to estimate their free (bioavailable) fraction. In men, the balance between systemic levels of androgens and estrogens is altered significantly upon aging.[28] Plasma androgen levels decline, whereas estrogen levels remain relatively constant, eventually leading to a decrease in the androgen-to-estrogen ratio with age, suggesting that estrogens may also have a role in prostate cancer.

Despite the fact that this complexity may, at least in part, justify the inconsistency of data on the association of serum androgens and prostate cancer risk, a major question remains: to what extent do levels of circulating androgens associate with respective intraprostatic concentrations? In this respect, intra-tissue levels of sex steroids have been reported to be several times (10 to 100) greater than the respective plasma values. Furthermore, metabolic profiles of intra-tissue steroids may substantially diverge from their plasmatic counterpart as they are governed by key enzymes of steroid metabolism. Therefore, circulating levels of individual steroids can hardly be considered representative of the actual amounts of bioavailable hormones to target cells.

Tissue Steroids

In specific tissues of the body, the balance between androgens and estrogens may differ significantly from that in the plasma, being strictly dependent upon the expression and the activity of steroid-metabolizing enzymes, including 5α-reductase and aromatase.[29–31] The role of local synthesis of steroids has assumed an increasing importance in some disease states, particularly in target glandular tissue such as that of breast or prostate, wherein abnormal levels of estradiol and/or estrone and some of their hydroxylated derivatives may promote tumor development and progression.[32–34] In this framework, a divergent expression and/or activity of key steroid enzymes (including dehydrogenases, hydroxylases, sulfotransferases, sulfatases, and aromatase) may eventually lead to a differential accumulation of biologically active hormone derivatives in individual target tissues. This is of crucial importance to predict the overall biological impact that sex steroids may have on peripheral target tissues and, hence, their potential role in cancer development and/or progression.

In our previous studies, we have compared intra-tissue estrogen content in *nontumoral* and malignant human breast tissues. We have observed that hydroxy estrogen derivatives represent the majority of tissue estrogens, with the so-called *classical estrogens* (estradiol, estrone, estriol) representing a mere 5% of the total. Markedly greater amounts of 2-hydroxy-estradiol, 4-hydroxy-estradiol, and 16α-hydroxy-estrone (16α-OHE1) were found in cancer tissues with respect to nontumoral breast, while elevated 16α-OHE1 and a low 2-OHE1:16α-OHE1 ratio were associated with a prolonged survival of breast cancer patients. Although this evidence apparently conflicts with the implication of 16αOHE1 as either initiator or promoter of human mammary cancer,[35,36] the potential role of this metabolite, as well as that of other hydroxyestrogens, on the onset and the clinical progression of breast cancer may well be different, if not opposite. A few early studies have also assessed intra-tissue concentrations of sex steroids in the human prostate and produced comparable results.[37,38]

Local Biosynthesis and Metabolism

Human prostate epithelial cells are endowed with key enzymes of steroid metabolism and, hence, have the ability to locally produce and transform gonadal steroids. In our previous work[39] we have assessed rates and direction of androgen metabolism in cultured human prostate cancer cells using an original HPLC approach that allows the simultaneous measurement of several enzyme activities in *intact* cells in culture. In brief: androgen-resistant PC3 cells show a marked oxidative activity leading to the accumulation of androstenedione and other 17-keto androgens when incubated with testosterone as a precursor, with the biologically relevant dihydrotestosterone (DHT) remaining undetectable. Conversely, androgen-responsive LNCaP cells exhibited a much lower extent of 17β oxidation, with relatively high formation rates of DHT and its derivatives, 3α/3β-androstanediol. Interestingly enough, metabolic profiles of estrogens were strictly comparable, with a massive 17β oxidation of estradiol (E2) to estrone (E1) being seen in PC3 cells but not in LNCaP cells (FIG. 3). This highly divergent extent of 17β oxidation of both androgen and estrogen (as illustrated in FIGURE 4) is simply a reflection of a differential expression and activity of 17β-hydroxysteroid dehydrogenase (17β-HSD) enzyme isoforms having distinct catalytic preferences. In a further study[40] we have in fact clearly

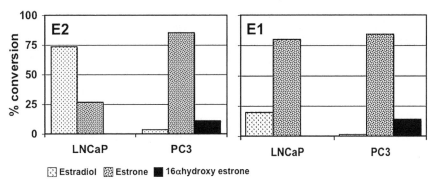

FIGURE 3. Estrogen metabolism in human prostate cancer cells. Cultured cells were incubated with tritiated estradiol (E2, left) or estrone (E1, right) as precursor. Rates and direction of metabolic pathways were assessed using our intact cell analysis approach, as extensively described elsewhere.[39] Data represent average percentages of two experiments performed in triplicate.

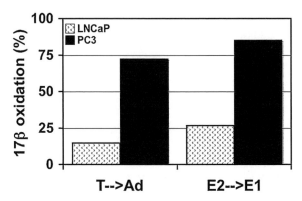

FIGURE 4. Extent of 17β-oxidation in human prostate cancer cells. LNCaP cells and PC3 cells were incubated with either testosterone (T) or estradiol (E2) as a precursor and the formation of the respective 17β-oxidized derivative androstenedione (Ad) or estrone (E1) was measured as previously reported.[40]

indicated that 17β-HSD type 2 isoform (HSD2), which has a major oxidative activity, is exclusively expressed in PC3 cells, thus being responsible for the remarkable 17β-oxidation seen in this cell line. This finding is of outmost importance, since preferential pathways of estrogen metabolism (mainly reductive in LNCaP cells, but almost solely oxidative in PC3 cells) ultimately favor cell growth by respectively maintaining or removing estradiol that has an opposite impact on the proliferative activity of these cell lines (see the next section of this paper).

Estrogen synthesis may occur via aromatization of androgens through the aromatase enzyme; therefore the aromatase is a critical regulator of the balance between androgens and estrogens that contributes to both circulating and tissue levels of these hormones. Aberrant expression of aromatase is believed to contribute to the development and/or progression of human breast cancer.[32,33] As there is increasing evidence that the prostate gland is a primary target for direct estrogenic activity[41–43] it might be important to determine whether or not aromatase is expressed locally and to identify any changes that may occur with prostate disease. Our *in vitro* studies have revealed that LNCaP cells contain aromatase activity, even though to a significantly lower extent than that observed in MCF7 human mammary carcinoma cells.[44] Although evidence on the expression and activity of aromatase in prostate tissues and cells is conflicting, there is a clear indication that local synthesis of estrogen in the prostate gland may be significant in prostate tumor development and/or progression.

It is noteworthy that many of the genes encoding for key steroid enzymes are highly polymorphic in nature.[45] The functional significance of these polymorphisms remains unknown. They may theoretically help to determine the impact of production, stability, or activity of steroid enzymes on individual risk of prostate cancer. Clearly, further work is needed to better distinguish the influence of variants in the normal sequence of these genes on prostate cancer risk.

ESTROGENS AND PROSTATE CANCER CELL GROWTH

Although androgens have been historically implicated as primary regulators of the growth of normal and malignant human prostate, there is consistent evidence that estrogens play a significant role in the normal development, differentiation, and growth of the prostate gland. Furthermore, both *in vitro* and *in vivo* studies have provided data to support the potential role of estrogen in the development and progression of prostate cancer.[46–48]

Early studies originally reported that the administration of pharmacological doses of estrogen, alone or in combination with androgens, results in the development of a well-defined proliferative prostatic lesion, referred to as squamous metaplasia.[22,49] In addition, the treatment of Noble rats with both estrogens and androgens determines the induction of a pre-cancerous lesion similar to human intraepithelial neoplasia (PIN) and an elevated incidence of prostatic adenocarcinomas.[21,50]

We have previously investigated the proliferative effects of estrogens on cultured human prostate cancer cells.[19,20] In particular, we have observed that the growth of androgen-responsive LNCaP cells is significantly stimulated by physiological concentrations of estradiol (E2) and that this effect appears to be receptor-mediated, being completely abolished by the simultaneous addition of the pure antiestrogen ICI-182,780 (FIG. 5A). Conversely, E2 shows a significant, dose-dependent inhibition of the proliferative activity of androgen-resistant PC3 cells; once again, this effect appears to be receptorial, being abrogated by the combination of E2 with its antagonist ICI-182 (FIG. 5B). Intriguingly, the growth of PC3 cells is markedly increased by an antibody neutralizing transforming growth factor-β (TGF-β) activity. This effect is opposed by the simultaneous addition of E2 (0.01–100 nM), being almost completely reversed at the dose of 100 nM (FIG. 6). Although we failed to demonstrate any increase of TGF-β mRNA after estradiol administration, we observed a significant rise of TGF-β (notably TGF-β2) protein levels in PC3 cells after E2 addition (FIG. 7), suggesting that the estrogen-induced growth inhibition of PC3 cells may occur at post-transcriptional or translational level. Given that the proliferative effects of estrogens on human prostate cancer cells appear to be predominantly receptor-mediated, it would be important to assess sex steroid receptor content and the balanced expression of different steroid receptors and their variants.

ESTROGEN RECEPTORS AND PROSTATE CANCER

It is largely recognized that many classical effects of sex steroids are mediated through specific intracellular receptors that belong to the superfamily

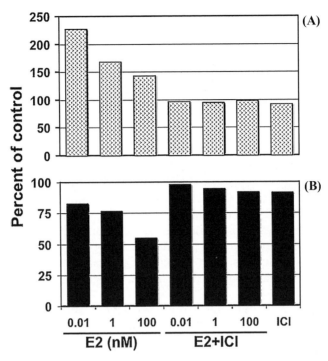

FIGURE 5. Growth effects of estrogen and antiestrogen in human prostate cancer cells. LNCaP (**A**) and PC3 (**B**) cells were treated with estradiol (E2) alone or in combination with its antagonist, ICI-182,780, as reported elsewhere.[19,20]

of nuclear receptors.[51] On the other hand, there is accumulating evidence that steroids, especially estrogens, and their receptors may combine or act unconnectedly to exploit a large array of both genomic and nongenomic, either ligand-dependent or -independent, actions.[52,53] As far as estrogens are concerned, two main receptor forms exist: the classical estrogen receptor (ER) α and the recently discovered ERβ. These two receptors have diverse physiological effects on a variety of human tissues, including the reproductive system, the bone, the cardiovascular system, and the central and peripheral nervous systems.[54] Both receptors act as nuclear transcription factors, but their respective patterns of gene regulation and function are strictly dependent upon their tissue-specific expression. Furthermore, selective ligands for either receptor have been recently developed and designated as selective estrogen receptor modulators (SERMs), since their agonist or antagonist activity depends specifically on the cellular context and promoter sequences of regulated genes.[55,56] This picture is further complicated by the presence of receptor splicing variants and mutants whose function is still uncertain.[57] However,

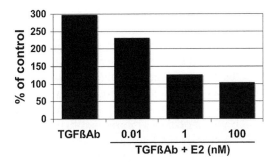

FIGURE 6. Estrogen reverts the growth increase induced by neutralizing transforming growth factor-β (TGFβ) activity in PC3 prostate cancer cells. Cells were treated with a neutralizing anti-TGF-β antibody alone or in combination with increasing estradiol concentrations.[19]

differential characteristics in terms of ligand binding, estrogen-response element (ERE) activity, and heterodimerization may ultimately direct estrogen action in target tissues and cells. In this respect, the most striking feature is that the balance of ERα and ERβ may be critical to generating tissue-specific estrogenic responses: an alteration of this physiological equilibrium may well be implicated in the development and/or progression of major hormone-related tumors, including those of the prostate.

Both ERα and ERβ are expressed in the adult human prostate, although ERα appears to be predominantly located in the stromal compartment and ERβ is mostly localized to the basal epithelial compartment and, to a much lesser

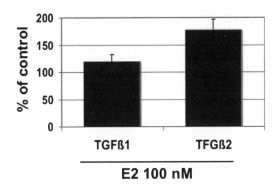

FIGURE 7. Estrogen induces TGFβ synthesis in PC3 human prostate cancer cells. Cultured PC3 cells were treated with 100 nM estradiol (E2) and the expression of both TGF-β1 and TGF-β2 assessed using Western blot and densitometric analysis (unpublished data).

extent, to stromal cells. The use of knockout mice for both ER types (ERKO) has provided relevant information to better understand the function of either receptor. In particular, βERKO mice develop prostate hyperplasia in adulthood, while αERKO mice do not.[58] Overall, there seems to be evidence to support the view that ERβ may be protective against abnormal proliferation of prostate epithelial cells. It has been reported that both toremifene[59] and genistein[60] prevent the development of prostate cancer in the transgenic adenocarcinoma mouse prostate (TRAMP) model: it is intriguing that these two agents exert their protective effect acting as ERβ agonists.

The expression of both ERα and ERβ (at either transcript or protein level) has been the subject of different studies comparing nontumoral, benign, and malignant human prostate. Overall, most studies indicate that ERβ expression is reduced in cancer as compared to benign or normal tissues, whereas ERα expression persists (reviewed by Bardin and colleagues[61]). In this respect, the protective role of ERβ may be based on direct (ERβ-specific) and/or indirect (through ERα regulation) effects limiting cell proliferation. Therefore, the loss of ERβ expression may represent a crucial step in estrogen-dependent prostate cancer progression.

We have assessed steroid receptor content of cultured LNCaP and PC3 human prostate cancer cells.[18,19] Results of these studies are summarized in TABLE 1. The two cell lines displayed a strikingly different ER status, with LNCaP cells having a predominant expression of ERα and PC3 cells of ERβ. Also, LNCaP cells exhibited greater amounts of both androgen and progesterone receptors with respect to PC3 cells. This finding provides a convincing explanation for the divergent effects of estradiol on growth of these two cell lines. The predominant expression of ERα in LNCaP cells and of ERβ in PC3 cells may in fact be responsible for the E2-induced increase and reduction of proliferative activity observed in LNCaP and PC3 cells, respectively. Once again, the balance of the two ER types appears to be essential for the growth control of prostate cancer cells, suggesting that an accurate assessment of ER status in the prognostic and therapeutic definition of prostate cancer patients should include ERα and ERβ, if not their isoforms.

TABLE 1. Steroid receptor status of human prostate cancer cells

	ERα	ERβ	AR	PR
LNCaP	+++	+	++	+
PC3	±	+++	+	ND

Receptor content was measured by immunocytochemical assay and quantitative image analysis estimating both the percentage of stained cells and the intensity of staining.

AR, androgen receptor; PR, progesterone receptor; ND, not detectable.

CONCLUSIONS

Since the pioneering work of Charles Huggins, androgens have been universally considered pivotal in the regulation of normal prostatic function and malignant prostate growth. However, a bulk of experimental evidence has accumulated to support an equally important role for estrogens in the development and/or progression of human prostate cancer.

Progression of prostatic adenocarcinoma, similar to its cognate mammary cancer, is usually described as featured by an initial hormone-responsive phase, wherein androgens are thought to play a major role in sustaining tumor growth, almost invariably followed by a hormone-refractory phase, where cancer cell growth becomes independent of androgens and is mostly maintained by other mitogens, including growth factors and cytokines. However, this categorization is merely based on the progressive loss of response of prostate cancer patients to endocrine treatment. This "clinical" definition would better correspond to a different type of growth control and a distinct hormone-sensitive status of prostate cancer cells during tumor progression (FIG. 8). Based on the combined evidence reported, a hypothetical model of prostate cancer progression is here presented (see FIG. 9). In this model, the hormone-responsive phase is characterized by a steroid-induced cell proliferation where classical, receptor-mediated effects of both androgens and estrogens are prevalent. In the following phase, tumor cells become androgen-resistant as a consequence of AR mutation or alteration of other androgen-signaling mechanisms. The concurrent loss of ERβ, possibly induced by hypermethylation in the gene promoter region,[62] creates an estrogen-sensitive condition where the growth of cancer cells is stimulated by estrogen via ERα. Finally, a hindrance in

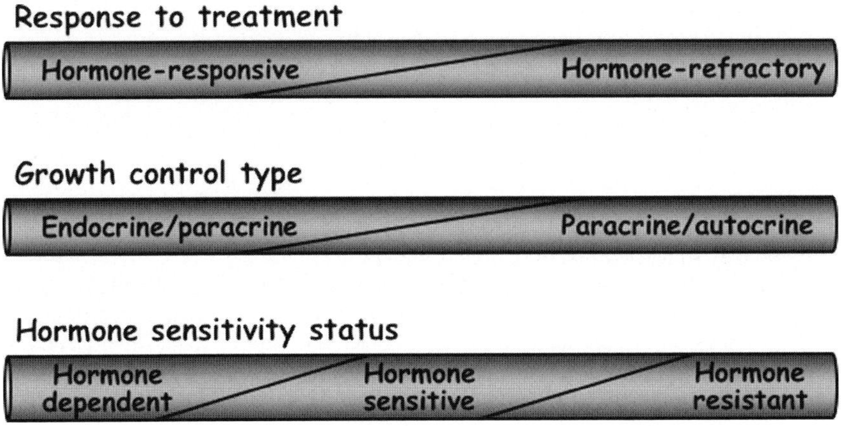

Response to treatment

Hormone-responsive	Hormone-refractory

Growth control type

Endocrine/paracrine	Paracrine/autocrine

Hormone sensitivity status

Hormone dependent	Hormone sensitive	Hormone resistant

FIGURE 8. Categories of prostate cancer progression. For explanation see text.

Steroid-induced   Estrogen-induced   Growth factor-induced
cell proliferation   cell proliferation   cell proliferation

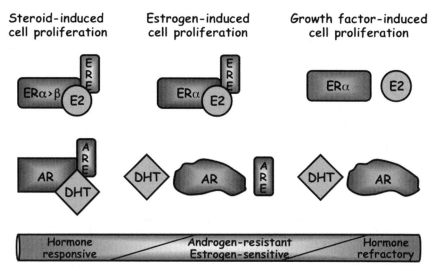

FIGURE 9. Prostate cancer progression: a hypothetical model. For explanation see text.

estrogen action (either at the receptor level or ERE, or both) may result in a hormone-refractory phase where prostate cancer cells proliferate in response to locally produced growth factors and/or cytokines.

Should this speculative depiction be confirmed by future *in vivo* studies and/or by using suitable animal model systems, an accurate assessment of estrogen function in benign and cancerous human prostate might be important to design effective strategies for both prevention and treatment of this malignancy. In this respect, the use of aromatase inhibitors, ERα antagonists, and ERβ-specific ligands, alone or in combination, may be in turn exploited, depending on individual prostate sensitivity to estrogen.

REFERENCES

1. HSING, A.W. & S.S. DEVESA. 2001. Trends and patterns of prostate cancer: what do they suggest? Epidemiol. Rev. **23:** 3–13.
2. KOLONEL, L.N., D. ALTSHULER & B.E. HENDERSON. 2004. The multiethnic cohort study: exploring genes, lifestyle and cancer risk. Nat. Rev. Cancer **4:** 519–527.
3. AMERICAN CANCER SOCIETY. 2006. Cancer facts and figures 2006. American Cancer Society. Atlanta, GA.
4. KOLONEL, L.N. 1985. Cancer incidence among Filipinos in Hawaii and the Philippines. Natl. Cancer Inst. Monogr. **69:** 93–98.
5. TOMINAGA, S. 1985. Cancer incidence in Japanese in Japan, Hawaii, and western United States. Natl. Cancer Inst. Monogr. **69:** 83–92.

6. STELLMAN, S.D. & Q.S. WANG. 1994. Cancer mortality in Chinese immigrants to New York city. Comparison with Chinese in Tianjin and with United States-born whites. Cancer **73:** 1270–1275.

7. COOK, L.S., M. GOLDOFT, S.M. SCHWARTZ & N.S. WEISS. 1999. Incidence of adenocarcinoma of the prostate in Asian immigrants to the United States and their descendants. J. Urol. **161:** 152–155.

8. WYNDER, E.L., Y. FUJITA, R.E. HARRIS, *et al.* 1991. Comparative epidemiology of cancer between the United States and Japan. A second look. Cancer **67:** 746–763.

9. LIU, M.C., A. HAI & A.T. HUANG. 1993. Cancer epidemiology in the Far East-contrast with the United States. Oncology (Huntingt) **7:** 99–110.

10. TYMCHUK, C.N., R.J. BARNARD, T.H. NGO & W.J. ARONSON. 2002. Role of testosterone, estradiol, and insulin in diet- and exercise-induced reductions in serum-stimulated prostate cancer cell growth *in vitro*. Nutr. Cancer **42:** 112–116.

11. HUGGINS, C. & C.V. HODGES. 2002. Studies on prostatic cancer: I. The effect of castration, of estrogen and of androgen injection on serum phosphatases in metastatic carcinoma of the prostate. 1941. J. Urol. **168:** 9–12.

12. HENDERSON, B.E., R.K. ROSS, M.C. PIKE & J.T. CASAGRANDE. 1982. Endogenous hormones as a major factor in human cancer. Cancer Res. **42:** 3232–3239.

13. GUINAN, P.D., W. SADOUGHI, H. ALSHEIK, *et al.* 1976. Impotence therapy and cancer of the prostate. Am. J. Surg. **131:** 599–600.

14. ROBERTS, J.T. & D.M. ESSENHIGH. 1986. Adenocarcinoma of prostate in 40-year-old body-builder (letter). Lancet **2:** 742.

15. JACKSON, J.A., J. WAXMAN & A.M. SPIEKERMAN. 1989. Prostatic complications of testosterone replacement therapy. Arch. Intern. Med. **149:** 2365–2366.

16. GARNICK, M.B. 1993. Prostate cancer: screening, diagnosis, and management. Ann. Intern. Med. **118:** 804–818.

17. IGUCHI, T., Y. FUKAZAWA, N. TANI, *et al.* 1990. Effect of some hormonally active steroids upon the growth of LNCaP human prostate tumour cells *in vitro*. Cancer J. **3:** 184–191.

18. SONNENSCHEIN, C., N. OLEA, M.E. PASANEN & A.M. SOTO. 1989. Negative controls of cell proliferation: human prostate cancer cells and androgens. Cancer Res. **49:** 3474–3481.

19. CARRUBA, G., U. PFEFFER, E. FECAROTTA, *et al.* 1994. Estradiol inhibits growth of hormone non responsive PC3 human prostate cancer cells. Cancer Res. **54:** 1190–1193.

20. CASTAGNETTA, L., M.D. MICELI, C. SORCI, *et al.* 1995. Growth of LNCaP human prostate cancer cells is stimulated by estradiol via its own receptor. Endocrinology **136:** 2309–2319.

21. NOBLE, R.L. 1977. The development of prostatic adenocarcinoma in Nb rats following prolonged sex hormone administration. Cancer Res. **37:** 1929–1933.

22. LEAV, I., F.B. MERK, P.W. KWAN & S.M. HO. 1989. Androgen supported estrogen-enhanced epithelial proliferation in the prostates of intact Noble rats. Prostate **15:** 23–40.

23. WANG, Y., S.W. HAYWARD, A.A. DONJACOUR, *et al.* 2000. Sex hormone-induced carcinogenesis in Rb-deficient prostate tissue. Cancer Res. **60:** 6008–6017.

24. CUNHA, G.R., Y.Z. WANG, S.W. HAYWARD & G.P. RISBRIDGER. 2001. Estrogenic effects on prostatic differentiation and carcinogenesis. Reprod. Fertil. Dev. **13:** 285–296.

25. SANTTI, R., R.R. NEWBOLD, S. MAKELA, *et al.* 1994. Developmental estrogenization and prostatic neoplasia. Prostate **24:** 67–78.

26. GANN, P.H., C.H. HENNEKENS, J. MA, *et al.* 1996. Prospective study of sex hormone levels and risk of prostate cancer. J. Natl. Cancer Inst. **88:** 1118–1126.
27. EATON, N.E., G.K. REEVES, P.N. APPLEBY & T.J. KEY. 1999. Endogenous sex hormones and prostate cancer: a quantitative review of prospective studies. Br. J. Cancer **80:** 930–934.
28. VERMEULEN, A., J.M. KAUFMAN, S. GOEMAERE & I. VAN POTTELBERG. 2002. Estradiol in elderly men. Aging Male **5:** 98–102.
29. NEGRI-CESI, P., A. POLETTI, A. COLCIAGO, *et al.* 1998. Presence of 5-alpha-reductase isozymes and aromatase in human prostate cancer cells and in benign prostate hyperplastic tissue. Prostate **34:** 283–291.
30. WEBER, K.S., N.A. JACOBSON, K.D. SETCHELL & E.D. LEPHART. 1999. Brain aromatase and 5alpha-reductase, regulatory behaviors and testosterone levels in adult rats on phytooestrogen diets. Proc. Soc. Exp. Biol. Med. **221:** 131–135.
31. STEERS, W.D. 2001. 5-Alpha-reductase activity in the prostate. Urology **58:** 17–24.
32. SIMPSON, E.R., M.S. MAHENDROO, J.E. NICHOLS & S.E. BULUN. 1994. Aromatase gene expression in adipose tissue: relationship to breast cancer. Int. J. Fertil. Menopausal Stud. **39:** 75–83.
33. SANTEN, R.J., S.J. SANTNER, R.J. PAULEY, *et al.* 1997. Oestrogen production via the aromatase enzyme in breast carcinoma: which cell type is responsible? J. Steroid Biochem. Mol. Biol. **61:** 267–271.
34. CASTAGNETTA, L., O.M. GRANATA, A. TRAINA, *et al.* 2002. Tissue content of hydroxyestrogens in relation to survival of breast cancer patients. Clin. Cancer Res. **8:** 3146–3155.
35. BRADLOW, H.L., R.J. HERSHCOPF, C.P. MARTUCCI & J. FISHMAN. 1985. Estradiol 16α-hydroxylation in the mouse correlates with mammary tumor incidence and presence of murine mammary tumor virus: a possible model for the hormonal etiology of breast cancer in humans. Proc. Natl. Acad. Sci. USA **82:** 6295–6299.
36. BRADLOW, H., N. TELANG, D. SEPKOVIC & M. OSBORNE. 1996. 2-hydroxyestrone: the "good" estrogen. J. Endocrinol. **150**(Suppl.): S259–S265.
37. FARNSWORTH, W.E. & J.R. BROWN. 1976. Androgen of the human prostate. Endocr. Res. Commun. **3:** 105–117.
38. GELLER, J., J. ALBERT, D. DE LA VEGA, *et al.* 1978. Dihydrotestosterone concentration in prostate cancer tissue as a predictor of tumor differentiation and hormonal dependency. Cancer Res. **38:** 4349–4352.
39. CASTAGNETTA, L., O.M. GRANATA, L. POLITO, *et al.* 1994. Different conversion metabolic rates of testosterone are associated to hormone-sensitive status and -response of human prostate cancer cells. J. Steroid Biochem. **49:** 351–357.
40. CARRUBA, G., J. ADAMSKI, M. CALABRÒ, *et al.* 1997. Molecular expression of 17βhydroxysteroid dehydrogenase types in relation to their activity in human prostate cancer cells. Mol. Cell. Endocrinol. **135:** 51–57.
41. JARRED, R.A., B. CANCILLA, G.S. PRINS, *et al.* 2000. Evidence that estrogens directly alter androgen-regulated prostate development. Endocrinology **141:** 3471–3477.
42. PRINS, G.S., L. BIRCH, H. HABERMANN, *et al.* 2001. Influence of neonatal estrogens on rat prostate development. Reprod. Fertil. Dev. **13:** 241–252.
43. PUTZ, O., C.B. SCHWARTZ, S. KIM, *et al.* 2001. Neonatal low- and high-dose exposure to estradiol benzoate in the male rat. I. Effects on the prostate gland. Biol. Reprod. **65:** 1496–1505.
44. CASTAGNETTA, L., O.M. GRANATA, V. BELLAVIA, *et al.* 1997. Product of aromatase activity in intact LNCaP and MCF7 human cancer cells. J. Steroid Biochem. Mol. Biol. **61:** 287–292.

45. PLATZ, E.A. & E. GIOVANNUCCI. 2004. The epidemiology of sex steroid hormones and their signaling and metabolic pathways in the etiology of prostate cancer. J. Steroid Biochem. Mol. Biol. **92:** 237–253.

46. BOSLAND, M.C. 2000. The role of steroid hormones in prostate carcinogenesis. J. Natl. Cancer Inst. Monogr. **27:** 39–66.

47. TAPLIN, M.E. & S.M. HO. 2001. Clinical review 134: the endocrinology of prostate cancer. J. Clin. Endocrinol. Metab. **86:** 3467–3477.

48. RISBRIDGER, G.P., J.J. BIANCO, S.J. ELLEM & S.J. MCPHERSON. 2003. Oestrogens and prostate cancer. Endocr. Relat. Cancer **10:** 187–191.

49. MERK, F.B., M.J. WARHOL, P.W. KWAN, *et al.* 1986. Multiple phenotypes of prostatic glandular cells in castrated dogs after individual or combined treatment with androgen and estrogen. Morphometric, ultrastructural, and cytochemical distinctions. Lab. Invest. **54:** 442–456.

50. LEAV, I., S.M. HO, P. OFNER, *et al.* 1988. Biochemical alterations in sex hormone-induced hyperplasia and dysplasia of the dorsolateral prostates of Noble rats. J. Natl. Cancer Inst. **80:** 1045–1053.

51. ESCRIVA, H., S. BERTRAND & V. LAUDET. 2004. The evolution of the nuclear receptor superfamily. Essays Biochem. **40:** 11–26.

52. LEVIN, E.R. 2001. Cell localization, physiology and nongenomic actions of estrogen receptors. J. Applied Physiol. **91:** 1860–1867.

53. BJÖRNSTRÖM, L. & M. SJÖBERG. 2005. Mechanisms of estrogen receptor signaling: convergence of genomic and nongenomic actions on target genes. Mol. Endocrinol. **19:** 833–842.

54. GUSTAFSSON, J.A. 2003. What pharmacologists can learn from recent advances in estrogen signalling. Trends Pharmacol. Sci. **24:** 479–485.

55. FRASOR, J., D.H. BARNETT, J.M. DANES, *et al.* 2003. Response-specific and ligand dose-dependent modulation of estrogen receptor (ER) alpha activity by ERbeta in the uterus. Endocrinology **144:** 3159–3166.

56. MUTHYALA, R.S., S. SHENG, K.E. CARLSON, *et al.* 2003. Bridged bicyclic cores containing a 1,1-diarylethylenemotif are high-affinity subtype-selective ligands for the estrogen receptor. J. Med. Chem. **46:** 1589–1602.

57. MATTHEWS, J. & J.A. GUSTAFSSON. 2003. Estrogen signaling: a subtle balance between ER alpha and ER beta. Mol. Interv. **3:** 281–292.

58. KREGE, J.H., J.B. HODGIN, J.F. COUSE, *et al.* 1998. Generation and reproductive phenotypes of mice lacking estrogen receptor beta. Proc. Natl. Acad. Sci. USA **95:** 15677–15682.

59. RAGHOW, S., M.Z. HOOSHDARAN, S. KATIYAR & M.S. STEINER. 2002. Toremifene prevents prostate cancer in the transgenic adenocarcinoma of mouse prostate model. Cancer Res. **62:** 1370–1376.

60. MENTOR-MARCEL, R., C.A. LAMARTINIERE, I.E. ELTOUM, *et al.* 2001. Genistein in the diet reduces the incidence of poorly differentiated prostatic adenocarcinoma in transgenic mice (TRAMP). Cancer Res. **61:** 6777–6782.

61. BARDIN, A., N. BOULLE, G. LAZENNEC, *et al.* 2004. Loss of ERβ expression as a common step in estrogen-dependent tumor progression. Endocr. Related Cancer **11:** 537–551.

62. LI, L.C., S.T. OKINO, R. DAHIYA. 2004. DNA methylation in prostate cancer. Biochim. Biophys. Acta **1704:** 87–102.

Monocyte–Macrophage System as a Target for Estrogen and Selective Estrogen Receptor Modulators

PIRKKO L. HÄRKÖNEN[a] AND H. KALERVO VÄÄNÄNEN[b]

[a]Lund University, Department of Laboratory Medicine, Tumor Biology, Malmö University Hospital, CRC Entrance 72, 205 02 Malmö, Sweden

[b]University of Turku, Institute of Biomedicine, Department of Anatomy, FI-20520 Turku 52, Finland

ABSTRACT: Postmenopausal decline of estrogen production is associated with development of several degenerative disorders such as osteoporosis, neuroinflammatory diseases and vascular wall degeneration. These are associated with the activation of the cells of the monocyte–macrophage system in a context-dependent manner. Estrogen regulates differentiation, maturation and function of many cell types in this system directly or indirectly via other cells by autocrine/paracrine mechanisms. Estrogen effects on the monocyte–macrophage system are primarily repressive. Most of these effects are mediated by repression of expression of genes for cytokines or modulation of other inflammatory mediators by the estrogen receptor (ER)-dependent or nongenomic pathways. The ER-dependent mechanisms mostly involve modulation of the nuclear factor kappa B (NF-kappaB) pathway for transcriptional regulation of cytokine or other mediator genes. In the context of hormone-regulated cancer, estrogen can influence production of cytokines or other inflammatory mediators by both tumor cells and tumor-invading macrophages. The interactions of breast and prostate cancer cells with tumor-associated macrophages (TAMs) may play an important role in tumor progression and even in the development of resistance to hormonal treatment. Regulation of the monocyte–macrophage system by estrogen and cross-talk between the ER and cytokine-mediated pathways provides multiple novel targets for development of selective ER modulator (SERM) molecules for prevention and treatment of postmenopausal degenerative and neoplastic diseases.

KEYWORDS: estrogen; estrogen receptor; selective estrogen receptor modulator (SERM); monocyte–macrophage system; osteoclast; dendritic cell; microglia; tumor-associated macrophage (TAM); breast cancer; prostate cancer

Address for correspondence: Pirkko L. Härkönen, Lund University, Department of Laboratory Medicine, Tumor Biology, Malmö University Hospital, CRC Entrance 72, 205 02 Malmö, Sweden. Voice: +46-40-391-106; fax: +46-40-33-7043.
e-mail: pirkko.harkonen@med.lu.se

Ann. N.Y. Acad. Sci. 1089: 218–227 (2006). © 2006 New York Academy of Sciences.
doi: 10.1196/annals.1386.045

INTRODUCTION

The monocyte–macrophage system (previously called the reticuloendothelial system) includes circulating monocytes, their precursors in the bone marrow and various tissue macrophages, either free macrophages or so-called histiocytes or tissue-fixed macrophages. Well-known examples of the latter are Küpffer cells in the liver, microglia in the central nervous system, dendritic or antigen-presenting cells in lymphoid tissues, Langerhans cells in the skin, and osteoclasts in bone. This cellular system was previously called the reticuloendothelial system, and the old classification also included vascular endothelial cells and some fibroblasts of lymphoid organs. There are, however, new data suggesting that, indeed, some cells of the vascular endothelium may be derived from the same lineage as the members of the monocyte–macrophage system.[1]

The monocyte–macrophage system consists of many different cell types. The final phenotype and functions of these cells are obviously very much dependent on the local environment in specific tissues. However, even if macrophages in different tissues show very different phenotypes, they clearly share several common functional features that are common to all of them. For example, they all have retained a marked capacity for phagocytosis and secretion of various proinflammatory and anti-inflammatory cytokines which have both autocrine and paracrine functions.

Many cell types in the monocyte–macrophage system express estrogen receptors (ERs) and they have also been shown to be regulated by estrogen.[2,3] Thus they provide multiple targets for estrogen and selective ER modulators (SERMs) for regulation of their activity, either directly or indirectly via surrounding cells, and for modulation of the physiological and pathological tissue processes that they are involved in.

ASSOCIATION OF SEVERAL DISEASE STATES WITH POSTMENOPAUSAL DECLINE OF ESTROGEN

Declining levels of estrogen in menopause are associated with several degenerative processes in various tissues. Although cellular and molecular mechanisms in most cases are still far from clear, clinical experience and a huge body of data from experimental and clinical studies clearly suggest that many of these degenerative processes can be slowed down or at least modulated by estrogen replacement therapy, thus suggesting that a promoting and/or causal factor could be estrogen deficiency (FIG. 1).

One of the best examples of menopause-related tissue degeneration is postmenopausal osteoporosis. In all mammalian species studied, including human, lack of estrogen induces increase of bone resorption due to an increased number and activity of osteoclasts.[4] This leads to deterioration of

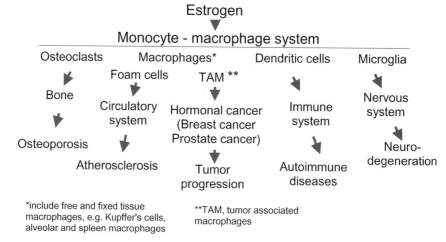

FIGURE 1. Scheme for the cell types of the monocyte-macrophage system that are regulated by estrogen and that are involved in development of several degenerative and neoplastic diseases.

bone tissue, increases risk for fractures, and can be prevented by estrogen. In addition to bone, other skeletal tissues such as striated muscle and articular cartilage show degenerative changes that are caused by estrogen deficiency.[5–7]

In addition to the skeleton, several other organ systems show increased rate of deterioration that is associated with decrease of sex steroids.[8] This is exemplified by a rapid increase in the incidence of degeneration of vascular wall and atherosclerosis and degenerative neural diseases in postmenopausal women. In many tissues cells of the monocyte–macrophage system are closely linked to these catabolic events, leading to various signs and consequences of tissue degeneration.

ESTROGEN REGULATION OF THE MONOCYTE–MACROPHAGE SYSTEM

Estrogen regulates several cell types of the monocyte–macrophage system by controlling production of proinflammatory and/or immunosuppressive cytokines and growth factors (FIG. 1). Estrogen is particularly known to inhibit expression of TNFα, IL-1, and IL-6, which are key mediators of the activated macrophages and several other cell types including microglial and dendritic cells (DCs) of the monocyte–macrophage system. Production of macrophage colony-stimulating factor (M-CSF) and granulocyte–macrophage colony-stimulating factor, which control differentiation and function of the cells of the monocyte–macrophage lineage by bone marrow cells, is also rapidly increased after estrogen withdrawal in both *in vivo* and *in vitro* experiments.[9,10] Another major pathway of estrogen regulation of the monocyte–macrophage system is stimulation of production of members of the immunosuppressive transforming growth factor (TGF) beta family.[2,11] In addition, estrogen modulates cytokine production and function of target inflammatory/immune cells via nongenomic mechanisms that cause rapid changes, for example, in NO metabolism.

The mediators of estrogen effect are possibly best understood in differentiation of osteoclasts. It is now well documented that the receptor activator of nuclear factor kappa B (RANK), its ligand, RANKL (also known as TRANCE, osteoclast differentiation factor and osteoprotegerin ligand) and the natural RANKL inhibitor, osteoprotegerin, are the key factors regulating osteoclast formation in normal bone. This pathway is also involved in mediating effect of estrogen on osteoclasts.[12]

MECHANISMS OF ESTROGEN REGULATION OF CELLS OF THE MONOCYTE–MACROPHAGE LINEAGE

Estrogen effects that lead to modulation of the monocyte–macrophage system cells are primarily repressive. A major mechanism of estrogen action in this context is a transcriptional repression of expression of cytokine genes. The best characterized pathway is regulation of activity of the transcription factor NF-kappaB. The estrogen–ER complex has been reported to inhibit binding of the NF-kappaB complex to regulatory areas of target genes,[13,14] or to prevent nuclear translocation and a transcriptional activation of the TNF alpha gene by a component of NF-kappaB (p65).[15] The known mechanisms primarily involve ER alpha. An interesting recent paper reported that in the absence of a ligand ER binds as a component of the activating transcription complex to the TNF alpha promoter, whereas the ligand-bound ER recruits another cofactor (GRIP1) to the complex, which leads to repression of TNF alpha gene expression.[16]

Other transcription factors (such as C/EBP and AP-1) and mechanisms are also important in ER-dependent transrepression of important inflammatory target genes. In addition, rapid nongenomic pathways such as NO-mediated mechanisms may have a very important although so far poorly characterized role in estrogen modulation of expression, function or degradation of inflammatory and immune mediators.[2]

ACTIVATION OF THE MONOCYTE–MACROPHAGE SYSTEM AS A COMMON DENOMINATOR FOR DISEASES THAT ARE RELATED TO ESTROGEN DEFICIENCY

The activation of the monocyte–macrophage system seems to take place in several organs and organ systems not only during inflammation, but also during tissue degeneration that is related to aging. Probably the best characterized example is osteoporosis, which is associated with menopause and/or aging. It is now well established that estrogen deficiency induces osteoclast formation from bone marrow precursors. Recent evidence suggests that estrogen inhibition of osteoclastogenesis is mainly indirect and probably mediated via mesenchymal cells.[17,18] Stromal mesenchymal cells of bone marrow as well as more differentiated osteoblastic cells stimulate osteoclastogenesis by secreting RANKL. Estrogen increases their capacity to produce osteoprotegerin, a decoy receptor for RANKL. It may also regulate the capacity of osteoblastic cells to produce RANKL. Thus, estrogen effect on osteoclastogenesis is inhibitory and mainly indirect.

Besides the development of postmenopausal osteoporosis the OPG/RANKL/RANK system has been implicated in immune-mediated and malignant bone diseases such as rheumatoid arthritis and osteolytic bone metastases.[19] In these conditions the estrogen-increased OPG may protect against bone damage. Interestingly, the OPG/RANKL/RANK has also been associated with vascular diseases and arterial calcification although presently the capacity of estrogen and/or OPG to protect in this context is not clear.

Estrogen has been shown to slow down the development of atherosclerosis both in animal models and in humans.[20] It has been suggested that this is mainly due to its inhibitory effect on the accumulation of lipid-loaded foamy macrophages in the vessel wall. Estrogen inhibits expression of vascular monocyte chemotactic protein-1, which results in decreased recruitment of macrophages to the vessel wall, which is an early event in atherosclerosis.[21] The data further suggest that estrogen acts in several ways to reduce the accumulation of cholesteryl esters in macrophages.[22] In addition, estrogen may have a direct antioxidative effect, thus reducing activation of macrophages by oxidized low-density lipoprotein (LDL).[23] Although the cellular and molecular effects of estrogen on the development of atherosclerosis are still far from clear, several lines of data support the conclusion that estrogen has a protective effect against atherosclerosis.

DCs are professional antigen-presenting cells. DCs, macrophages, and B lymphocytes all express both types of ERα and β, indicating that estrogen might directly modulate immune responses. Serum levels of estrogen also correlate with the severity of certain autoimmune diseases, which supports the idea that estrogen could specifically modulate DC function. There are both *in vitro* and *in vivo* results suggesting that estrogen regulates both DC differentiation and their capacity for antigen presentation.[24–26] There is also increasing evidence that estrogen modulates secretion of various cytokines and chemokines from DCs and thus also indirectly regulates T cell and B cell responses.[27]

The neuroprotective effect of estrogen has been demonstrated in several experimental models. Accordingly, estrogen replacement therapy has been associated with decreased severity of age-related neurodegenerative diseases such as Alzheimer's disease[28] although there are also conflicting results. The neuroprotective mechanism of estrogen is not clear, but a bulk of evidence suggests that estrogen inhibits microglial activation.[29–32] Most of the neuroprotective effects seem to be mediated through ER alpha.[29] This conclusion is supported by a number of studies showing that estrogen can decrease the neurotoxicity of the factors released by microglia. It has also been shown that estrogen treatment of aged female mice significantly lowered the number of astrocytes and microglial cells.[33]

TUMOR-ASSOCIATED MACROPHAGES (TAMs) AND HORMONAL CANCER

TAMs and other immune cells are involved in a complex way in the development and growth of tumors, hormonal cancer included.[34,35] They are also considered to have an important role in stromal activation, invasion and metastasis of the tumor. Cancer cells recruit macrophages by producing cytokines, whose process can be accelerated when estrogen suppression of cytokine expression disappears upon estrogen decline, for example, postmenopausally. In addition, TAMs themselves are targets for estrogen action. The hormone regulates production of proinflammatory and/or anti-inflammatory cytokines by TAMs in a context-dependent manner.[36] Furthermore, macrophages may even modulate responsiveness of tumor cells to hormonal treatment. In an interesting study[37] Zhu et al. reported that macrophage-produced inflammatory signals (IL-1β) can reverse ER (and androgen receptor) repression of growth stimulatory target genes by relevant antihormone and cause resistance to hormonal treatment. It is thus clear that macrophage-related inflammatory mechanisms play an important, even if a very complex role in regulation of growth and progression of hormonal cancer.

REGULATION OF CELLS OF THE MONOCYTE–MACROPHAGE SYSTEM WITH SERMs

Estrogen regulation of the monocyte–macrophage system and expression of genes for immune and inflammatory mediators offer obvious possibilities for ER modulation by selective ligands of ER α and β. Possibilities of preventing activation of osteoclasts and development of osteoporosis with SERMs have been studied most and several SERM molecules have been shown to be osteo-protective.[38,39] As could be expected the ER-mediated SERM effects seem to be targeted to differentiation of osteoclastic precursors. They are also mostly mediated by surrounding osteoblastic or stromal cells. The well-demonstrated bone-protective effect of raloxifene as well as some other compounds[39,40] is associated with decreased osteoclastogenesis. It is associated with a modulated production of cytokines such as IL-6 and TNF-alpha, as shown in experimental and clinical studies.[41] Some SERMs such as tamoxifen and toremifene have also direct effects on osteoclasts.[42,43]

The possibility of modulating DC function with certain SERMs has also been evaluated. The antiestrogens tamoxifen and toremifene[44,45] as well as ralox-ifene[27] are able to inhibit the differentiation and maturation of DCs. While this capacity could possibly be exploited in the treatment of autoimmune diseases it might, on the other hand, interfere with useful immune responses in association with breast cancer treatment or prevention of osteoporosis with tamoxifen or toremifene[44,45] and raloxifene, respectively.[27] Tamoxifen and raloxifene were also shown to exert anti-inflammatory effects in neuroglial cells, but so far the mechanisms are not understood.[32,33,46]

Raloxifene, tamoxifen, and toremifene were developed to inhibit estrogen-stimulated cell proliferation and prevent growth and development of estrogen-regulated cancer. In case of the monocyte–macrophage system and production of immune or inflammatory mediators, the effects of estrogen are often in-hibitory and mediated by transcriptional or nongenomic repression of cytokine gene expression. Recently, considerable efforts have been taken to develop lig-ands of the ER that would selectively mimic the anti-inflammatory and anti-immune effects of estrogen without stimulating proliferation or causing other unwanted effects of the hormone. A ligand that selectively inhibits NF-kappaB transcriptional activation but fails to promote conventional estrogen effects has recently been reported.[47,48] Considering the complicated pattern of the cell- and tissue-specific NF-kappaB-mediated anti-inflammatory effects that estrogen elicits, it is clear that a detailed knowledge of the mechanisms of specific cel-lular responses would be needed to develop and exploit "repression-selective" SERM molecules[16] for prevention and treatment of degenerative diseases that are associated with estrogen deficiency.

REFERENCES

1. ZHAO, Y. & T. MAZZONE. 2005. Human umbilical cord blood-derived f-macrophages retain pluripotentiality after thrombopoietin expansion. Exp. Cell. Res. **310:** 311–318.
2. PFEILSCHIFTER, J., R. KODITZ, M. PFOHL, *et al.* 2002. Changes in proinflammatory cytokine activity after menopause. Endocr. Rev. **23:** 90–119. Review.
3. LANG, T.J. 2004. Estrogen as an immunomodulator. Clin. Immunol. **113:** 224–230.

4. VÄÄNÄNEN, H.K. & P.L. HÄRKÖNEN. 1996. Estrogen and bone metabolism [review]. Maturitas (Suppl.): S65–S69.
5. RICHETTE, P., M. CORVOL & T. BARDIN. 2003. Estrogens, cartilage, and osteoarthritis. Joint Bone Spine **70:** 257–262.
6. SIROLA, J. & T. RIKKONEN. 2005. Muscle performance after the menopause. J. Br. Menopause Soc. **11:** 45–50.
7. SIROLA, J., M. TUPPURAINEN, R. HONKANEN, *et al.* 2005. Associations between grip strength change and axial postmenopausal bone loss–a 10-year population-based follow-up study. Osteoporos. Int. **16:** 1841–1848.
8. SKOUBY, S.O., F.F. AL-AZZAWI, D. BARLOW, *et al.* 2005. Climacteric medicine: European Menopause and Andropause Society (EMAS) 2004/2005 position statements on peri- and postmenopausal hormone replacement therapy. Maturitas **51:** 8–14.
9. LEA, C.K., U. SARMA & A.M. FLANAGAN. 1999. Macrophage colony stimulating-factor transcripts are differentially regulated in rat bone-marrow by gender hormones. Endocrinology **140:** 273–279.
10. KIMBLE, R.B., S. SRIVASTAVA, F.P. ROSS, *et al.* 1996. Estrogen deficiency increases the ability of stromal cells to support murine osteoclastogenesis via an interleukin-1 and tumor necrosis factor-mediated stimulation of macrophage colony-stimulating factor production. J. Biol. Chem. **271:** 28890–28897.
11. HEINO, T.J., T.A. HENTUNEN & H.K. VAANANEN. 2002. Osteocytes inhibit osteoclastic bone resorption through transforming growth factor-beta: enhancement by estrogen. J. Cell. Biochem. **85:** 185–197.
12. SHEVDE, N.K., A.C. BENDIXEN, K.M. DIENGER, *et al.* 2000. Estrogens suppress RANK ligand-induced osteoclast differentiation via a stromal cell independent mechanism involving c-Jun repression. Proc. Natl. Acad. Sci. USA **97:** 7829–7834.
13. STEIN, B. & M.X. YANG. 1995. Repression of the interleukin-6 promoter by estrogen receptor is mediated by NF-kappa B and C/EBP beta. Mol. Cell. Biol. **15:** 4971–4979.
14. KASSEM, M., S.A. HARRIS, T.C. SPELSBERG, *et al.* 1996. Estrogen inhibits interleukin-6 production and gene expression in a human osteoblastic cell line with high levels of estrogen receptors. J. Bone Miner. Res. **11:** 193–199.
15. GHISLETTI, S., C. MEDA, A. MAGGI, *et al.* 2005. 17beta-estradiol inhibits inflammatory gene expression by controlling NF-kappaB intracellular localization. Mol. Cell. Biol. **25:** 2957–2968.
16. CVORO, A., C. TZAGARAKIS-FOSTER, D. TATOMER, *et al.* 2006. Distinct roles of unliganded and liganded estrogen receptors in transcriptional repression. Mol. Cell. **21:** 555–564
17. CLOWES, J.A., B.L. RIGGS & S. KHOSLA. 2005. The role of the immune system in the pathophysiology of osteoporosis. Immunol. Rev. **208:** 207–227.
18. MICHAEL, H., P.L. HÄRKÖNEN, H.K. VÄÄNÄNEN, *et al.* 2005. Estrogen and testosterone use different cellular pathways to inhibit osteoclastogenesis and bone resorption. J. Bone Miner. Res. **20:** 2224–2232.
19. HOFBAUER, L.C. & M. SCHOPPET. 2004. Clinical implications of the osteoprotegerin/RANKL/ RANK system for bone and vascular diseases [review]. JAMA **292:** 490–495.
20. HANKE, H., C. LENZ & G. FINKING. 2001. The discovery of the pathophysiological aspects of atherosclerosis: a review. Acta Chir. Belg. **101:** 162–169.

21. SELI, E., U.A. KAYISLI, B. SELAM, *et al.* 2002. Estradiol suppresses vascular monocyte chemotactic protein-1 expression during early atherogenesis. Am. J. Obstet. Gynecol. **187:** 1544–1549.
22. NAPOLITANO, M., I. BLOTTA, A. MONTALI, *et al.* 2001. 17beta-estradiol enhances the flux of cholesterol through the cholesteryl ester cycle in human macrophages. Biosci. Rep. **21:** 637–652.
23. TSUDA, M., M. IWAI, J.M. LI, *et al.* 2005. Inhibitory effects of AT1 receptor blocker, olmesartan, and estrogen on atherosclerosis via anti-oxidative stress. Hypertension **45:** 545–551.
24. PAHARKOVA-VATCHKOVA, V., R. MALDONADO & S. KOVATS. 2004. Estrogen preferentially promotes the differentiation of CD11c+ CD11b (intermediate) dendritic cells from bone marrow precursors. J. Immunol. **172:** 1426–1436.
25. BENGTSSON, A.K., E.J. RYAN, D. GIORDANO, *et al.* 2004. 17beta-estradiol (E2) modulates cytokine and chemokine expression in human monocyte-derived dendritic cells. Blood **104:** 1404–1410.
26. PETTERSSON, A., C. CIUMAS, V. CHIRSKY, *et al.* 2004. Dendritic cells exposed to estrogen in vitro exhibit therapeutic effects in ongoing experimental allergic encephalomyelitis. J. Neuroimmunol. **156:** 58–65.
27. NALBANDIAN, G., V. PAHARKOVA-VATCHKOVA, A. MAO, *et al.* 2005. The selective estrogen receptor modulators, tamoxifen and raloxifene, impair dendritic cell differentiation and activation. J. Immunol. **175:** 2666–2675.
28. BRINTON, R.D. 2004. Impact of estrogen therapy on Alzheimer's disease: a fork in the road? CNS Drugs **18:** 405–422.
29. VEGETO, E., S. BELCREDITO, S. ETTERI, *et al.* 2003. Estrogen receptor-alpha mediates the brain anti-inflammatory activity of estradiol. Proc. Natl. Acad. Sci. USA **100:** 9614–9619.
30. VEGETO, E., S. BELCREDITO, S. GHISLETTI, *et al.* 2006. The endogenous estrogen status regulates microglia reactivity in animal models of neuroinflammation. Endocrinology **147:** 2263–2272.
31. MORALE, M.C., P.A. SERRA, F. L'EPISCOPI, *et al.* 2006. Estrogen, neuroinflammation and neuroprotection in Parkinson's disease: glia dictates resistance versus vulnerability to neurodegeneration. Neuroscience **138:** 869–878.
32. BAKER, A.E., V.M. BRAUTIGAM & J.J. WATTERS. 2004. Estrogen modulates microglial inflammatory mediator production via interactions with estrogen receptor beta. Endocrinology **145:** 5021–5032.
33. LEI, D.L., J.M. LONG, J. HENGEMIHLE, *et al.* 2003. Effects of estrogen and raloxifene on neuroglia number and morphology in the hippocampus of aged female mice. Neuroscience **121:** 659–666.
34. COUSSENS, L.M. & Z. WERB. 2002. Inflammation and cancer. Nature **420:** 860–867.
35. LEWIS C.F. & J.W. POLLARD. 2006. Distinct role of macrophages in different tumor microenvironments. Cancer Res. **66:** 605–612.
36. ROBINSON, S.C. COUSSENS, L.M. 2005. Soluble mediators of inflammation during tumor development. Adv. Cancer Res. **93:**159–187.
37. ZHU, P., S.H. BAEK, E.M. BOURK, *et al.* 2006. Macrophage/cancer cell interactions mediate hormone resistance by a nuclear receptor derepression pathway. Cell **124:** 615–629.
38. QU, Q., H. ZHENG, J. DAHLLUND, *et al.* 2000. Selective estrogenic effects of a novel triphenylethylene compound, FC1271a, on bone, cholesterol level, and reproductive tissues in intact and ovariectomized rats. Endocrinology **141:** 802–820.

39. KUNG SUTHERLAND, M.S., S.G. LIPPS, N. PATNAIK, *et al.* 2003. SP500263, a novel SERM, blocks osteoclastogenesis in a human bone cell model: role of IL-6 and GM-CSF. Cytokine **23:** 1–14.

40. RIGGS, B.L. & L.C. HARTMANN. 2003. Selective estrogen-receptor modulators—mechanisms of action and application to clinical practice. N. Engl. J. Med. **348:** 618–629.

41. GIANNI, W., A. RICCI, P. GAZZANIGA, *et al.* 2004. Raloxifene modulates interleukin-6 and tumor necrosis factor-alpha synthesis in vivo: results from a pilot clinical study. J. Clin. Endocrinol. Metab. **89:** 6097–6099

42. PARIKKA, V., Z. PENG, T. HENTUNEN, *et al.* 2005. Estrogen responsiveness of bone formation in vitro and altered bone phenotype in aged estrogen receptor-alpha-deficient male and female mice. Eur. J. Endocrinol. **152:** 301–314.

43. LEHENKARI, P., V. PARIKKA, T.J. RAUTIALA, *et al.* 2003. The effects of tamoxifen and toremifene on bone cells involve changes in plasma membrane ion conductance. J. Bone Miner. Res. **18:** 473–481.

44. KOMI, J. & O. LASSILA. 2000. Nonsteroidal anti-estrogens inhibit the functional differentiation of human monocyte-derived dendritic cells. Blood **95:** 2875–2882.

45. KOMI, J., M. MÖTTÖNEN, R. LUUKKAINEN, *et al.* 2001. Non-steroidal anti-oestrogens inhibit the differentiation of synovial macrophages into dendritic cells. Rheumatology **40:** 185–191.

46. SUURONEN, T., T. NUUTINEN, J. HUUSKONEN, *et al.* 2005. Anti-inflammatory effect of selective estrogen receptor modulators (SERMSs) in microglial cells. Inflamm. Res. **54:** 194–203.

47. CHADWICK, C.C., S. CHIPPARI, E. MATELAN, *et al.* 2005. Identification of pathway-selective estrogen receptor ligands that inhibit NF-kappaB transcriptional activity. Proc. Natl. Acad. Sci. USA **102:** 2543–2548.

48. KEITH, J.C., JR., ALBERT, L.M., Y. LEATHURBY, *et al.* 2005. The utility of pathway selective estrogen receptor ligands that inhibit nuclear factor-kappa B transcriptional activity in models of rheumatoid arthritis. Arthritis Res. Ther. **7:** R427–R438.

Sex Hormones and Risk of Liver Tumor

L. GIANNITRAPANI,[a] M. SORESI,[a] E. LA SPADA,[a] M. CERVELLO,[b]
N. D'ALESSANDRO,[c] AND G. MONTALTO[a]

[a]Dipartimento di Medicina Clinica e Patologie Emergenti, Università di
Palermo, Palermo, Italy

[b]Istituto di Biomedicina e Immunologia Molecolare "A. Monroy," C.N.R.,
Palermo, Italy

[c]Dipartimento di Scienze Farmacologiche, Universita di Palermo, Palermo, Italy

ABSTRACT: The liver is morphologically and functionally modulated by
sex hormones. Long-term use of oral contraceptives (OCs) and anabolic
androgenic steroids (AASs) can induce both benign (hemangioma, adenoma, and focal nodular hyperplasia [FNH]) and malignant (hepatocellular carcinoma [HCC]) hepatocellular tumors. Hepatic adenomas
(HAs) are rare, benign neoplasms usually occurring in young women,
the development and the complications of which have been related to the
strength of OCs and the duration of their use. HA incidence has fallen
since the introduction of pills containing smaller amounts of estrogens.
FNH is a benign lesion, most commonly seen in young women, which is
thought to represent a local hyperplastic response of hepatocytes to a vascular abnormality. Because of the female predominance and the young
age at onset, a role of female hormones has been suggested. Furthermore,
a large proportion of women with FNH (50–75%) are OC users. Liver
hemangiomas (LHs) are the most common benign liver tumors and are
seen more commonly in young adult females. The female predilection
and clinical observations of LH growth under conditions of estrogenic
exposure suggest a possible role for estrogen in the pathogenesis of LHs.
HCC has become one of the most widespread tumors in the world in
recent years, representing the sixth leading cancer and the third most
common cause of death from cancer. Apart from liver cirrhosis, numerous other factors responsible for its onset have been proposed: hepatitis
infections from virus B (HBV) and C (HCV), alcohol, smoking, and aflatoxin. However, regardless of etiology, chronic liver diseases progress at
unequal rates in the two sexes, with the major sequelae, such as cirrhosis
and HCC, being more frequent in men than in women. These epidemiological data have prompted researchers to investigate the relationship
between sex hormones and liver tumors. The human liver expresses estrogen and androgen receptors and experimentally both androgens and

Address for correspondence: Prof. Giuseppe Montalto, Ordinario di Medicina Interna, Policlinico
Universitario di Palermo, via del Vespro, 141, Palermo, Italy. Voice: +39-0916552991; fax: +39-
0916552847.

e-mail: gmontal@unipa.it

Ann. N.Y. Acad. Sci. 1089: 228–236 (2006). © 2006 New York Academy of Sciences.
doi: 10.1196/annals.1386.044

estrogens have been implicated in stimulating hepatocyte proliferation and may act as liver tumor inducers or promoters.

KEYWORDS: benign liver tumors; HCC; estrogens; androgens; aromatase

INTRODUCTION

The liver is a hormone-sensitive organ, and in fact both normal liver and hepatocellular carcinoma (HCC) tissues from male and female mammals have been shown to express specific estrogen receptors (ERs). Experimentally, estrogens may act as liver tumor inducers or promoters *in vivo*,[1,2] and are involved in stimulating hepatocyte proliferation *in vitro*.[3] Moreover, anti-estrogens like tamoxifen have been shown to reduce levels of ERs and to inhibit hepatocyte proliferation following partial hepatectomy.[4]

As regards the role of androgens, it has also been observed that androgen receptors (ARs), specifically activated by testosterone, are present in normal liver tissue from both males and females and that their expression is increased in tumor tissue and in the surrounding liver of individuals with HCC.[5]

In addition, observations from clinical and epidemiological studies have highlighted that the long-term use of OCs and anabolic androgenic steroids (AASs) can induce benign and malignant hepatocellular tumors. Benign tumors of the liver are often discovered incidentally in asymptomatic individuals during diagnostic imaging or exploratory laparotomy performed for other reasons. Hemangiomas are the most common benign liver tumors, followed in prevalence by focal nodular hyperplasia (FNH) and the rarer condition of adenoma; their growth and development have been linked to hormonal stimulation.

However, although evidence from the literature concurs to a great extent on the role of sex hormones in the development of benign liver tumors and in particular liver adenoma, in the field of HCC this role is much more controversial. In fact, HCC usually occurs in individuals with chronic liver disease with a clear disadvantage for the male sex, thus suggesting a possible causal importance of androgens. Male cirrhotics who develop HCC, however, present a characteristic imbalance with a relative hyperestrogenic state, so that a role of estrogen in liver cancer has been hypothesized as well.

SEX HORMONES AND BENIGN LIVER TUMORS

Liver hemangiomas (LHs) are the most common benign liver neoplasms. They are diagnosed more commonly in young adult females, with a female:male ratio of 5:1. In around 70% of patients they are multiple. Variants include giant hemangiomas, which can occupy up to the entire hepatic lobe and may expand the liver contour.

From an anatomic point of view LHs consist of large, well-defined blood-filled spaces, lined by a single layer of endothelium and separated by fibrous septae. Pathologically, they comprise vascular lakes and channels, some of which can develop thrombosis and fibrosis.

Several case studies in the past have proposed that tumor growth may be related to estrogens. This hypothesis comes from observations that estrogen replacement therapy may play a role in the pathogenesis of recurrent LHs,[6] that a prolonged administration of oral contraceptive (OCs) may facilitate the growth of LHs,[7] and that LHs can grow and become symptomatic during pregnancy.[8]

However, despite these premises, in the last 2 years two studies have been published yielding contradictory results.[9,10] In a recent case–control study by Gemer et al. the possible association of OCs with LHs was explored. Several parameters, such as age, age at menarche, age at first pregnancy, number of pregnancies, age at menopause and OC use, were compared in women with and without LH and there was no significant difference between the two groups. From these results the authors concluded that there was no association between oral contraception, menstrual or reproductive history, and development of LH and, as a consequence, that there were no indications for the withdrawal of oral contraception in women with LH.[9]

On the contrary, in a study by Glinkova et al., the impact of female sex hormones on the natural history of LH was prospectively evaluated, with the conclusions that age at first period was inversely associated with the size of LHs, age at menopause was positively correlated with the number of LHs, and that hormone therapy increased the risk of LH enlargement.[10]

Other molecular studies have tended to explain the mechanisms by which estrogens may regulate endothelial cell turnover, again with somewhat controversial results. In fact, it has been shown that estrogens can enhance endothelial cell proliferation, migration, and organization into capillary-like structures in vitro and augment experimental angiogenesis in vivo.[11] In contrast, in vitro studies have suggested that certain steroids may inhibit angiogenesis.[12]

FNH is a rare benign lesion which is seen more frequently in young adult females, with a women:men ratio of 8:1. Although the risk factors for FNH are largely unknown, a role for female hormones has been suggested in view of the female predominance and the young age at onset. FNH forms as an unencapsulated mass, which consists of multiple pseudolobules around a central area of fibrous tissue. The etiology of these lesions is unclear, but the histopathological findings may be related to an underlying developmental abnormality with a hyperplastic response of the liver parenchyma and a disorganized growth pattern of hepatocytes and ducts. They can be multiple; hemorrhage is exceedingly rare; and they apparently have no malignant potential.

To obtain more information about the association of FNH and OC use a case–control study was recently conducted by Scalori et al. in an area of northern

Italy.[13] In this study the distribution of cases and controls and the corresponding OR according to OC use, duration of use, age at starting use, and time since stopping use, were evaluated. This study provided definite and quantitative evidence that OC use was significantly, although modestly associated with FNH. The time–risk relation gave convincing support to the existence of a real association, given that there was a direct trend in risk with duration and an inverse trend with age at first use.[13]

However, in a previous study a few years ago, Mathieu *et al.* studied the relationship between the number and size of FNH lesions in women divided into five groups: no OC use; high-dose OC use; low-dose OC use; low-dose and high-dose OC use; and pure progestagen use.[14] They found no differences between these groups as regards the number and size of the lesions. These data showed that neither the size nor the number of FNH lesions were influenced by OC use and that size changes during follow-up were rare and did not seem to depend on OC use, so they concluded that low-dose OC can be maintained in young women with FNH.[14]

Finally, hepatic adenomas (HAs) are uncommon benign neoplasms usually occurring in young women. They are considered noncancerous lesions with little clinical significance; however, even though rarely, they can become cancerous. Moreover, they can become large-sized during pregnancy, presumably as a result of estrogen stimulation, and under these circumstances they can rupture, resulting in acute bleeding and peritonitis. Liver cell adenomas are usually well demarcated, but the capsule may not be clearly obvious. They are large when detected (25–30 cm in diameter). The histological appearance is of benign-looking hepatocytes often arranged in cords.

HA has been strongly associated with the use of OCs; in fact, it has been calculated that about 320 new cases are diagnosed each year, mostly attributable to OC use. This association was first suggested by Baum *et al.*,[15] who in 1973 reported seven cases of HA, all related to OC, and has been supported by many other subsequent publications.[16,17] In women who have never used OCs or who have used them for less than 24 months, HA develops at an annual rate ranging from 1 to 1.3 per million in the age ranges of 16–30 and 31–44 years, respectively.[17] Its incidence, however, has fallen since the introduction of pills containing smaller amounts of estrogens.

Consequently, in contrast with what happens for LH and FNH, at least for HA there is an agreement among authors about the fact that the association between OCs and HA is strong and depends on the duration of use. Furthermore, unresected lesions may decrease in size in young women once they stop OC use. All these data taken together suggest that the association between HA and OC use is one of cause and effect.

In recent times AASs have also been proven to be involved in the development of HA.[18] Apparently, androgen-induced HAs are relatively rare. However, the possibility that an oral AAS can induce liver cell proliferation must be taken into account and sportsmen taking AASs over a long period should be considered a group at risk for developing hepatic sex hormone–related tumors.

SEX HORMONES AND HCC

HCC has become one of the leading causes of death for cancer worldwide, being the fifth most frequent neoplasia in the world, with 564,300 new cases in 2000 (5.6%) and more than 12,000 new cases per year in Italy.[19,20] Its incidence is now increasing all over the world with a variable geographical distribution according to the spread of the main risk factors, namely hepatitis B and C viruses (HBV, HCV) and liver cirrhosis (LC) whatever the cause. In fact, in areas like India, Southeast Asia, and the developing countries in general, where the prevalence of HBV infection is still high, the incidence of HCC is more than 20 per 100,000 inhabitants.[20] On the contrary, HCV predominates as a cause of HCC in the developed countries, with an intermediate (Italy, Spain) to low (USA) incidence of tumor.[21,22] Other risk factors (Aflatoxin B1, alcohol, hereditary diseases) may play a significant role in specific contexts. Finally, among the other factors associated with an increased risk of development of HCC regardless of the geographical setting, there is male gender. In most published series a striking predominance of the tumor in males has been described, with a male-to-female ratio ranging from 2 to 11:1. Moreover, the prognosis seems to be more benign in females than in males because women have a better survival rate and a reduced recurrence of the disease after treatment.[23]

However, it has to be considered that in Western countries 80–90% of HCCs develop in a liver with an underlying cirrhosis and this complicates the understanding of the role of sex hormones in liver carcinogenesis, especially because male cirrhotics present a so-called "feminization" of their phenotype due to a relatively hyperestrogenic condition. These premises make it necessary to distinguish between HCC with and HCC without underlying LC to try to eliminate this confounding factor. In women without underlying LC there is a great deal of evidence for the responsibility of OC use in the development of HCC. In a recent meta-analysis of eight studies, which confirms previous data,[24,25] it was stated that OC use increases the risk of HCC with an overall OR of 2.5 in ever- versus never-users of OCs and an overall OR of 5.8 for the longest duration of use.[26]

Evidence for the role of sex hormones in the development of LC-correlated HCC is much more controversial. LC determines an alteration in sex hormone balance, which is more evident in males as the activity of ERs is increased in the liver with an enhancement of its response to estrogens.[27] Our group has published a study in which it was observed that the serum estradiol-to-testosterone ratio was higher in individuals with HCC and LC than in normal individuals or individuals with LC alone.[28] In contrast, two recent studies from Korea and Japan suggested that elevated serum testosterone levels or an imbalanced testosterone–estradiol rate is associated with an increased risk of HCC,[29,30] but trials using different antiandrogenic compounds to treat or reduce the progression of liver cancer have shown quite disappointing results, with an almost complete lack of effect for this therapeutic approach.[31,32] However, studies also using antiestrogen drugs have yielded controversial results. In fact, most of the studies published in the early 1990s reported reduced tumor growth rates and prolonged survival in subjects treated with tamoxifen compared to untreated controls, but they were based on small numbers of patients. Two recent papers, a multicentric trial including 496 patients with HCC at any stage and a trial with 119 patients with unresectable HCC, in which the patients were randomized to receive tamoxifen or placebo, concluded that tamoxifen was not effective in HCC treatment.[33,34] A possible explanation for the failure of the therapeutic approach with antiestrogen drugs can be found in some experimental and clinical observations of the presence of a variant form of ER (vER), deriving from an exon 5-deleted transcript, which lacks the hormone-binding domain, also in the liver.[35] It has been observed that in HCC vER largely predominates and sometimes becomes the only form expressed and that it is also expressed by the peritumoral cirrhotic tissues of patients with HCC, especially males.[36] Moreover, the growth rate of HCC in subjects with vER is significantly higher than in patients with tumors expressing the wild-type form (wtER), and the spontaneous survival in patients with wtER is exceedingly better than in patients with HCC characterized by vER.[36] Another explanation could be that estrogen has been described as exerting a possible role in the growth regulation of both normal and cancer human liver cells by alternative, nonreceptorial mechanisms.[37] Finally, our group recently published a study in which the activity and expression of aromatase enzyme (the one that converts androgens into estrogens) was investigated in nontumoral, cirrhotic, and malignant human liver tissues and cells. Our observations were that human HCC tissues showed elevated aromatase activity, with consequently higher estrogen formation rates than in nontumoral liver tissues. If it can be assumed that estrogen plays a role in hepatoma cell growth via nonreceptor pathways, a strategy reducing estrogen concentration in the tumor with the use of aromatase inhibitors could be attempted.[38]

CONCLUSIONS

Benign liver neoplasms, such as LH and FNH, whose growth and development have been variably linked to sex hormones, have a benign course and can be managed conservatively; only HA must be followed up more carefully on account of its potential malignancy.

As regards the role of estrogens in HCC, it seems that in the physiological status of premenopausal women, in the absence of other risk factors for liver disease, they have a somewhat protective role against the development of HCC.

On the contrary, the hyperestrogenic status of the cirrhotic male or the high concentrations of estrogens in the old formulations of OCs, together with the presence of vER in the liver and/or other risk factors, may increase the risk of developing HCC.

Finally, if the evidence of a local estrogen formation from androgens is confirmed to have a role in the development and progression of human HCC, this may provide a basis to improve endocrine treatment of HCC patients using antiaromatase drugs.

REFERENCES

1. REZNIK-SCHULLER, H. 1979. Carcinogenic effects of diethylstilbestrol in male Syrian golden hamsters and European hamsters. J. Natl. Cancer Inst. **62:** 1083–1088.
2. LI, J.J. & S.A. LI. 1984. High incidence of hepatocellular carcinomas after synthetic estrogen administration in Syrian golden hamsters fed alpha-naphthoflavone: a new tumor model. J. Natl. Cancer Inst. **73:** 543–547.
3. FRANCAVILLA, A., L. POLIMENO, M. BARONE, et al. 1993. Hepatic regeneration and growth factors. J. Surg. Oncol. Suppl. **3:** 1–7.
4. FRANCAVILLA, A., L. POLIMENO, A. DI LEO, et al. 1989. The effect of estrogen and tamoxifen on hepatocyte proliferation *in vivo* and in vitro. Hepatology **9:** 614–620.
5. OHNISHI, S., T. MURAKAMI, T. MORIYAMA, et al. 1986. Androgen and estrogen receptors in hepatocellular carcinoma and in the surrounding noncancerous liver tissue. Hepatology **6:** 440–443.
6. CONTER, R.L. & W.P. LONGMIRE, JR. 1988. Recurrent hepatic hemangiomas. Possible association with estrogen therapy. Ann. Surg. **207:** 115–119.
7. MATHIEU, D., E.S. ZAFRANI, M.C. ANGLADE, et al. 1989. Association of focal nodular hyperplasia and hepatic hemangioma. Gastroenterology **97:** 154–157.
8. SAEGUSA, T., K. ITO, N. OBA, et al. 1995. Enlargement of multiple cavernous hemangioma of the liver in association with pregnancy. Intern. Med. **34:** 207–211.
9. GEMER, O., O. MOSCOVICI, C.L. BEN-HORIN, et al. 2004. Oral contraceptives and liver hemangioma: a case-control study. Acta Obstet. Gynecol. Scand. **83:** 1199–1201.
10. GLINKOVA, V., O. SHEVAH, M. BOAZ, et al. 2004. Hepatic haemangiomas: possible association with female sex hormones. Gut **53:** 1352–1355.
11. SCHNAPER, H.W., K.A. MCGOWAN, S. KIM-SCHULZE, et al. 1996. Oestrogen and endothelial cell angiogenic activity. Clin. Exp. Pharmacol. Physiol. **23:** 247–250.
12. JAGGERS, D.C., W.P. COLLINS & S.R. MILLIGAN. 1996. Potent inhibitory effects of steroids in an in vitro model of angiogenesis. J. Endocrinol. **150:** 457–464.
13. SCALORI, A., A. TAVANI, S. GALLUS, et al. 2002. Oral contraceptives and the risk of focal nodular hyperplasia of the liver: a case-control study. Am. J. Obstet. Gynecol. **186:** 195–197.
14. MATHIEU, D., H. KOBEITER, D. CHERQUI, et al. 1998. Oral contraceptive intake in women with focal nodular hyperplasia of the liver. Lancet **352:** 1679–1680.
15. BAUM, J.K., F. HOLTZ, J.J. BOOKSTEIN, et al. 1976. Possible association between benign hepatomas and oral contraceptives. Lancet **2:** 926–929.
16. EDMONSON, H.A., B. HENDERSON & B. BENTON. 1976. Liver-cell adenomas association with use of oral contraceptives. N. Engl. J. Med. **294:** 470–472.

17. ROOKS, J.B., H.W. ORY, K.G. ISHAK, *et al.* 1979. Epidemiology of hepatocellular adenoma. The role of oral contraceptive use. JAMA **242:** 644–648.
18. NAKAO, A., K. SAKAGAMI, Y. NAKATA, *et al.* 2000. Multiple hepatic adenomas caused by long-term administration of androgenic steroids for aplastic anemia in association with familial adenomatous polyposis. J. Gastroenterol. **35:** 557–562.
19. LANDIS, S.H., T. MURRAY, S. BOLDEN, *et al.* 1998. Cancer statistics, 1998. CA Cancer J. Clin. **48:** 6–29.
20. MONTALTO, G., M. CERVELLO, L. GIANNITRAPANI, *et al.* 2002. Epidemiology, risk factors, and natural history of hepatocellular carcinoma. Ann. N.Y. Acad. Sci. **963:** 13–20.
21. STROFFOLINI, T., P. ANDREONE, A. ANDRIULLI, *et al.* 1998. Characteristics of hepatocellular carcinoma in Italy. J. Hepatol. **29:** 944–952.
22. EL-SERAG, H.B. & A.C. MASON. 1999. Rising incidence of hepatocellular carcinoma in the United States. N. Engl. J. Med. **340:** 745–750.
23. EL-SERAG, H.B. 2001. Epidemiology of hepatocellular carcinoma. Clin. Liver Dis. **5:** 87–107.
24. NEUBERGER, J., D. FORMAN, R. DOLL, *et al.* 1986. Oral contraceptives and hepatocellular carcinoma. Br. Med. J. (Clin. Res. Ed.). **292:** 1355–1357.
25. FORMAN, D., T.J. VINCENT & R. DOLL. 1986. Cancer of the liver and the use of oral contraceptives. Br. Med. J. (Clin. Res. Ed.). **292:** 1357–1361.
26. YU, M.C. & J.M. YUAN. 2004. Environmental factors and risk for hepatocellular carcinoma. Gastroenterology **127:** S72–S78.
27. ROSSINI, G.P., G.M. BALDINI, E. VILLA, *et al.* 1989. Characterization of estrogen receptors from human liver. Gastroenterology **96:** 1102–1109.
28. MONTALTO, G., M.D. MICELI, M. SORESI, *et al.* 1997. Sex hormones in patients with liver cirrhosis and hepatocellular carcinoma. Oncol Rep. **4:** 1–4.
29. YU, M.W., S.W. CHENG, M.W. LIN, *et al.* 2000. Androgen-receptor gene CAG repeats, plasma testosterone levels, and risk of hepatitis B-related hepatocellular carcinoma. J. Natl. Cancer Inst. **92:** 2023–2028.
30. TANAKA, K., H. SAKAI, M. HASHIZUME, *et al.* 2000. Serum testosterone:estradiol ratio and the development of hepatocellular carcinoma among male cirrhotic patients. Cancer Res. **60:** 5106–5110.
31. CHAO, Y., W.K. CHAN, Y.S. HUANG, *et al.* 1996. Phase II study of flutamide in the treatment of hepatocellular carcinoma. Cancer **77:** 635–639.
32. GRIMALDI, C., H. BLEIBERG, F. GAY, *et al.* 1998. Evaluation of antiandrogen therapy in unresectable hepatocellular carcinoma: results of a European Organization for Research and Treatment of Cancer multicentric double-blind trial. J. Clin. Oncol. **16:** 411–417.
33. CLIP GROUP (CANCER OF THE LIVER ITALIAN PROGRAMME). 1998. Tamoxifen in treatment of hepatocellular carcinoma: a randomised controlled trial. Lancet **352:** 17–20.
34. LIU, C.L., S.T. FAN, I.O. NG, *et al.* 2000. Treatment of advanced hepatocellular carcinoma with tamoxifen and the correlation with expression of hormone receptors: a prospective randomized study. Am. J. Gastroenterol. **95:** 218–222.
35. VILLA, E., L. CAMELLINI, A. DUGANI, *et al.* 1995. Variant estrogen receptor messenger RNA species detected in human primary hepatocellular carcinoma. Cancer Res. **55:** 498–500.
36. VILLA, E., A. GROTTOLA, A. COLANTONI, *et al.* 2002. Hepatocellular carcinoma: role of estrogen receptors in the liver. Ann. N. Y. Acad. Sci. **963:** 37–45.

37. JIANG, S.Y., R.Y. SHYU, M.Y. YEH, *et al.* 1995. Tamoxifen inhibits hepatoma cell growth through an estrogen receptor independent mechanism. J. Hepatol. **23:** 712–719.
38. CASTAGNETTA, L.A., B. AGOSTARA, G. MONTALTO, *et al.* 2003. Local estrogen formation by nontumoral, cirrhotic, and malignant human liver tissues and cells. Cancer Res. **63:** 5041–5045.

Aromatase Inhibitors

Structural Features and Biochemical Characterization

YANYAN HONG AND SHIUAN CHEN

Department of Surgical Research, Beckman Research Institute of the City of Hope, Duarte, California 91010, USA

ABSTRACT: Aromatase is the enzyme synthesizing estrogens from androgens. In estrogen-dependent breast tumors, estrogens induce the expression of growth factors responsible for cancer cell proliferation. *In situ* estrogen synthesis by aromatase ¨is thought to play a key role in the promotion of breast cancer growth. Aromatase inhibitors (AIs) provide new approaches for the prevention and treatment of breast cancer by inhibiting estrogen biosynthesis. Through reverse transcription polymerase chain reaction (RT-PCR) and immunohistochemical techniques, aromatase has been found to be expressed in many endocrine tissues and tumors originating from these tissues. Unexpectedly, this enzyme is now known to also be expressed in liver, lung, and colon cancers. Such findings suggest a potential role for endocrine manipulation of these types of cancer using AIs. Three Food and Drug Administration (FDA)-approved AIs, anastrozole (Arimidex), letrozole (Femara), and exemestane (Aromasin), effectively challenging tamoxifen, have been used as first-line drugs in the treatment of hormone-dependent breast cancer, and possibly other aromatase-expressing cancers. In addition, natural anti-aromatase chemicals, such as flavones and coumarins, have been identified. Efforts to develop new lines of AIs derived from these phytochemicals have been initiated in several laboratories. Finally, significant progress has been made in the understanding of the structure–function relationship of aromatase. Such information has helped the examination of binding characteristics of AIs, the evaluation of reaction mechanism of aromatase, and the explanation of the molecular basis for a low catalytic activity of the natural variant, M364T.

KEYWORDS: breast cancer; aromatase inhibitors; flavonoid phytoestrogen; mechanism-based inhibitor; structural model

Address for correspondence: Dr. Shiuan Chen, Department of Surgical Research, Beckman Research Institute of the City of Hope, 1500 E. Duarte Rd., Duarte, CA 91010. Voice: 626-359-8111; ext. 63454; fax: 626-301-8972.

e-mail: schen@coh.org

Ann. N.Y. Acad. Sci. 1089: 237–251 (2006). © 2006 New York Academy of Sciences.

doi: 10.1196/annals.1386.022

INTRODUCTION

Aromatase, a cytochrome P450, catalyzes three consecutive hydroxylation reactions converting C19 androgens to aromatic C18 estrogens. Upon receiving electrons from NADPH-cytochrome P450 reductase, aromatase converts androstenedione and testosterone to estrone and estradiol, respectively. The aromatization of androgen is the terminal and rate-limiting step in estrogen synthesis. Pathologically, an abnormal overexpression of aromatase in breast tissue plays an important role in breast cancer development.[1–9] Inhibition of aromatase is a new strategy for reducing growth-stimulatory effects of estrogen in breast cancer by decreasing circulating levels of estrogen. During the last several years, a significant number of articles have been published to demonstrate the presence of aromatase in several endocrine tissues (such as ovary, uterus, prostate, and bone) and cancer associated with these tissues. It is, however, unexpected to find aromatase in cancer not associated with endocrine function, such as that of the liver,[10–13] lung,[14,15] colon,[16,17] and oral keratinocytes.[18] These findings suggest potential endocrine manipulation in the treatment of these types of cancer, and support adjuvant and sequential systemic treatment including AIs. Although AIs are now accepted to be important drugs for hormonal therapy of cancers, their action at the molecular level is not yet described.

FIRST-, SECOND-, AND THIRD-GENERATION INHIBITORS

Effective AIs developed as therapeutic agents are described as first-, second-, and third-generation inhibitors according to the order of their clinical development. The first-generation inhibitor refers to the nonsteroidal inhibitor aminoglutethimide (AG) (FIG. 1), which was the first AI to be studied in patients,[19] but the reports of adrenal insufficiency led to withdrawal from clinical use. AG is less specific and inhibits other CYP450 enzymes involved in cortisol and aldosterone biosynthesis, which results in toxicity. Its efficacy in inhibiting aromatase activity stimulated the development of various new inhibitors during the 1980s and 1990s.

The second-generation inhibitors include the imidazole derivative fadrozole[20] and steroid analogue formestane (4-hydroxyandrostenedione)[21,22] (FIG. 1). Fadrozole is more selective and potent than AG, but it still has inhibitory effects on aldosterone, progesterone, and corticosterone biosynthesis. Formestane was the first selective AI to be used clinically and was effective and well tolerated.[23] However, the fact of its requirement of intramuscular administration limited its clinical use.

The third-generation inhibitors, developed in the early 1990s, including two triazole derivatives anastrozole (Arimidex)[24] and letrozole (Femara)[25] and one steroid analogue exemestane (Aromasin)[26] (FIG. 1), are widely used as the first-line drugs in the endocrine treatment of hormone-dependent breast cancer

First-generation   **Second-generation**

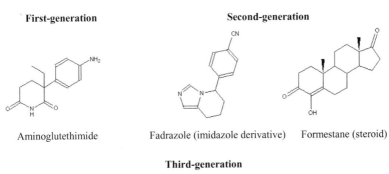

Aminoglutethimide   Fadrazole (imidazole derivative)   Formestane (steroid)

Third-generation

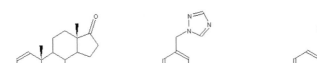

Exemestane (steroid)   Anastrozole (triazole derivative)   Letrozole (triazole derivative)

FIGURE 1. First-, second-, and third-generation aromatase inhibitors.

in postmenopausal patients. Anastrozole, letrozole, and exemestane are administered orally with 1 mg, 2.5 mg, and 25 mg once daily, respectively. Compared to the first- and second-generation inhibitors, the third-generation inhibitors produce greater clinical benefit with near-complete specificity at clinical use. These drugs were also found to be better tolerated than tamoxifen and were associated with lower incidences of endometrial cancer, vaginal bleeding and discharge, cerebrovascular events, venous thromboembolic events, and hot flashes.[27,28] In addition, the incidence of contralateral breast cancer occurrence was found to be significantly lower in the AI group than the tamoxifen group.[27,29,30] However, the long-term effects of these drugs on skeletal problems, cardiovascular disease, and Alzheimer's disease need to be carefully followed up.

Anastrozole and letrozole are nonsteroidal derivatives that have the triazole functional which interacts with the heme prosthetic group of aromatase, and they act as competitive inhibitors with respect to the androgen substrates. Exemestane is a steroidal and mechanism-based inhibitor that is catalytically converted into a chemically reactive species, leading to irreversible inactivation of aromatase.

MECHANISM-BASED INHIBITORS

A mechanism-based inhibitor is a steroidal inhibitor that is recognized by the enzyme as a pseudo-substrate, and is then converted to reactive intermediates,

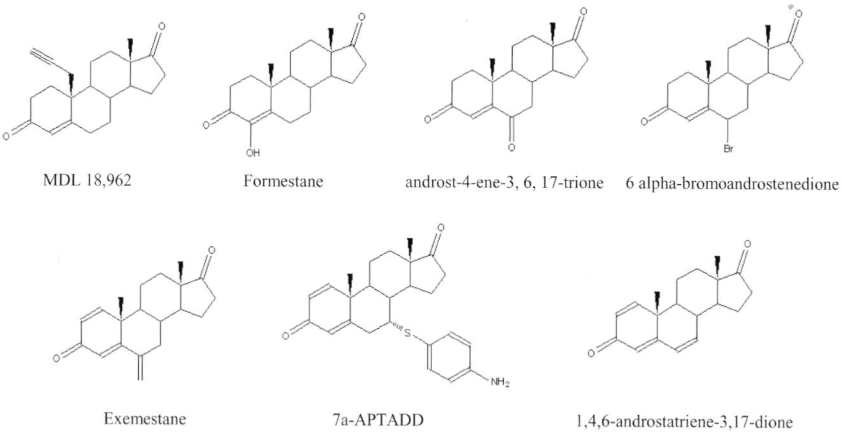

MDL 18,962   Formestane   androst-4-ene-3, 6, 17-trione   6 alpha-bromoandrostenedione

Exemestane   7a-APTADD   1,4,6-androstatriene-3,17-dione

FIGURE 2. Mechanism-based inhibitors.

which irreversibly bind to the enzyme to produce suicide inhibition. Mechanism-based inhibitors cause time-dependent inhibition of aromatase only in the presence of its redox partner NADPH-P450 reductase and co-factor NADPH. These inhibitors are generally classified into several groups (FIG. 2): C-10 substituted androstendione (i.e., MDL 18,962,); 4-substituted androstenedione (i.e., formestane); 6-substituted androstenedione (i.e., androst-4-ene-3, 6, 17-trione, 6 alpha-bromoandrostenedione); substituted androsta-1, 4-diene-3, 17-diones (i.e., 7α-APTADD, exemestane); substituted androsta-1, 4, 6-diene-3, 17-diones (i.e., 1,4,6-androstatriene-3,17-dione). These inhibitors have recently been discussed in a review by Brueggemeier et al.[31] Several evidences have supported the fact that the reactive intermediates result from enzymatic oxidation at the C-19 group of mechanism-based inhibitors: compounds lacking a C-19 methyl group did not cause a time-dependent inhibition;[32] tritium release from [19-^{3}H]-19,19-difluoroandrost-4-ene-3,17-dione during inactivation of aromatase[33]; and incubation of androst-4-ene-3,6,17-trione (AT) with human placental microsome yielded the 19-hydroxy-AT and 19-oxo-AT.[34] Moreover, experimental results from radioactive inhibitor probe studies demonstrate that a mechanism-based inhibitor can be covalently bound to aromatase.[35] Mechanism-based inhibitors provide promising perspectives for drug design because these steroid analogue inhibitors are highly selective and less toxic.

Among these mechanism-based inhibitors, as discussed above, exemestane has been approved by the FDA for the treatment of hormone-dependent breast cancer. It causes a time-dependent inactivation of human placental aromatase with a $t1/2$ of 13.9 min and K_i of 26 nM.[36] Our laboratory has recently found that exemestane (as well as formestane) can further induce a degradation of aromatase by proteasome, which occurs after the irreversible inactivation step,[37] indicating that these mechanism-based inhibitors not only can inactivate aromatase, but also can eliminate the enzyme protein. The exact nature of the interaction of these mechanism-based inhibitors with aromatase protein and amino acids involved has yet to be elucidated. The ability of exemestane and formestane to induce enzyme degradation could explain why it has been difficult to identify the amino acids/peptides that participated in the mechanism-based inhibition of aromatase by these inhibitors. However, recent advances in structure–function studies of aromatase have generated valuable structure information for the evaluation of the interaction of steroid ligands (including the substrate and inhibitors such as exemestane) with the aromatase enzyme (discussed in the next section).

BINDING NATURE OF THE ANDROGEN SUBSTRATE/STEROIDAL INHIBITOR

Extensive computer modeling, site-directed mutagenesis, and proteomic analysis from this and other laboratories have helped to define the active site region of aromatase and to evaluate the reaction mechanism of this enzyme.[38–51] On the basis of the crystal structure of human CYP2C9, and taking our laboratory findings into consideration, Favia et al.[52] recently generated a three-dimensional model of aromatase. After careful evaluation, we feel that the model by Favia et al.[52] is more reliable than those previously generated in this and other laboratories because it can adequately explain most of our experimental data. By carefully examining this new model and the results from our recent structure–function studies of aromatase, a new clamping mechanism of substrate/steroidal inhibitor, binding to the active site, has been proposed.[53] The heme iron is ligated by a conserved cysteine (C437) and the propionates of the heme interact with the side chains of R115, W141, R145, R375, and R435. The steroid substrate/inhibitor sits above the heme, with its C19 methyl group pointing to the heme iron, and is positioned next to the I helix (FIG. 3). Our site-directed mutagenesis data allow us to identify three additional important regions in the active site of aromatase. Together with D309, S478, and H480 in the β-4 sheet at the carboxy-terminus are thought to participate in a charge relay system that lead to the aromatization of the A ring of the substrate.[53] I133 and F134 in the B′-C loop are hypothesized to interact with the D ring of the substrate/inhibitor through van der Waals forces.[53] The 3′-flanking loop (P368-M374) of the K helix is thought to participate in forming the hydrophobic ligand-binding pocket and hence possibly residue V373 interacts specifically with the B ring of the substrate/inhibitor. This loop (P368-M374), together with the B′-C loop and β4-including loop, holds the steroid substrate/inhibitor at the correct orientation. Exemestane, the FDA-approved mechanism-based AI, is hypothesized to be converted to reactive intermediates by heme through the hydroxylation of the C-19 group, helped by D309. Finally, the intermediates,

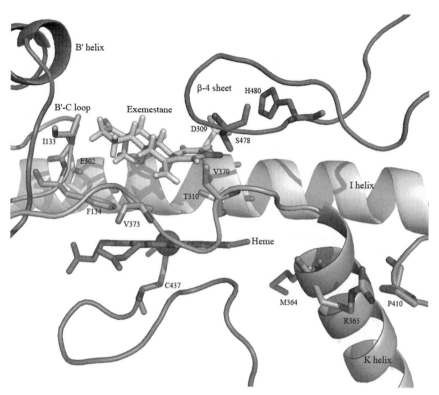

FIGURE 3. Clamping mechanism of exemestane binding provided by the heme, I helix, B'-C loop, β-4 sheet, and the 3'-flanking loop of the K helix.

irreversibly bound to the enzyme, cause suicide inhibition in which D309 may be involved.

In a recent study, Ma *et al.* identified and characterized genetic polymorphisms in the human aromatase gene.[54] There are four coding single nucleotide polymorphisms (cSNPs) in the coding region. These cSNPs alter the following amino acids: W39R, T201M, R264C, and M364T. Interestingly, the M364T variant was found to be less stable and to have significantly lower affinities for the androgen substrate and for the inhibitor exemestane. Our laboratory previously generated two mutants, R365A and R365K.[41] These mutants were not active. The immunoprecipitation analysis revealed that these mutants were expressed, but at levels lower than that of the wild-type enzyme. These results indicate that R365 plays a very critical role during the enzyme catalysis because it cannot be replaced with a lysine residue. Computer modeling analysis has revealed that M364 and R365 are situated in the K helix (FIG. 3). It is thought that the side chain of R365 forms a hydrogen bond with the backbone carbonyl oxygen of P410, which is located in the loop between the β-1/β-2 two sheets (R375-I395) and L helix (G439-R456). C437, the heme-binding cysteine residue, is located at the end of this loop. Possibly, R365 stabilizes this loop structure. M364 faces toward the inside of the active site, although it is not close to the heme and steroidal ligand. It is likely that M364 helps to form the hydrophobic pocket together with the loop P368-M374.

The availability of a reliable three-dimensional model of aromatase has helped us better understand the molecular features of the active site and catalytic mechanism of the enzyme. The model will enable the application of the structure-based design (SBD) of the next generation of selective and potent AIs.

PHYTOCHEMICAL INHIBITORS

Studies have suggested that diet sources, including cruciferous vegetables, soy, rye flour, grapes, and mushrooms, are associated with a decreased risk of breast cancer.[55–59] Bioactive food components present in these diet sources demonstrate various biological activities and are being investigated for the prevention of both ER+ and ER– breast tumors. Some phytochemicals, isolated from the plant kingdom, such as flavonoids and lignans, are known to be competitive inhibitors of aromatase, resulting in a decrease in the level of estrogen. For example, isolicoflavonol/prenylated flavonoid (Fig. 4), isolated from

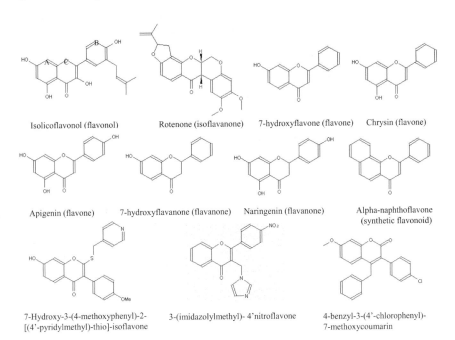

Isolicoflavonol (flavonol)   Rotenone (isoflavanone)   7-hydroxyflavone (flavone)   Chrysin (flavone)

Apigenin (flavone)   7-hydroxyflavanone (flavanone)   Naringenin (flavanone)   Alpha-naphthoflavone (synthetic flavonoid)

7-Hydroxy-3-(4-methoxyphenyl)-2-[(4'-pyridylmethyl)-thio]-isoflavone   3-(imidazolylmethyl)- 4'nitroflavone   4-benzyl-3-(4'-chlorophenyl)-7-methoxycoumarin

FIGURE 4. Flavonoid aromatase inhibitors.

the paper mulberry, was found to suppress aromatase with IC_{50} values near 0.1 μM[60]; nectandrin-B/lignan, with anti-aromatase activity, was isolated from *Myristicaceae*;[61] Procyanidin B dimers, isolated from red wine and grape seeds, were shown to be aromatase inhibitors; and the *in vivo* studies in an aromatase-transfected MCF-7 breast cancer xenograft model also demonstrated that these chemicals reduced androgen-dependent tumor growth.[58] These studies indicate that procyanidin B dimers could be used as chemopreventive agents against breast cancer.

The most comprehensive studies of phytochemical aromatase inhibitors are focused on flavonoid phytoestrogens. Phytoestrogens are plant-derived nonsteroidal compounds that possess estrogen-like biological activity, and may function as antiestrogens or weak estrogens by competing with estrogens for binding to ER. Flavonoids include flavanones/isoflavanones, flavones/isoflavones, and flavonols/isoflavonols, characterized as containing the benzopyranone ring system. Some flavanoids are capable of inhibiting aromatase (Fig. 4). For example, IC_{50} values for the inhibition of aromatase by the isoflavanone derivative rotenone (from *Derris*) was 0.3 μM; the flavones 7-hydroxyflavone, chrysin (from *Passiflora coerulea*), and apigenin (from *Matricaria chamomilla*) were 4, 7, 20 μM; and the flavanones 7-hydroxyflavanone and naringenin (from *Petunia*) were 65 and 85 μM, respectively.[62] Some flavanoids are poorer inhibitors or possess no effect on aromatase activity. Genistein (Fig. 5), an isoflavone phytoestrogen abundant in soy products with numerous biochemical activities, elevates the conversion of the most physiologically active form of estrogen (estradiol) to an estrogenically weaker metabolite (estrone) by increasing 17-betahydroxysteroid dehydrogenase activity,[63] but slightly inhibits aromatase activity.[63–65] Flavonoids exerting no effect on aromatase activity are baicalein, 6-hydroxylavone, daidzein, quercetin, catechin, and equol (Fig. 5).[64,66] Generally, natural flavones are more potent than isoflavones in inhibiting aromatase. The binding characteristics by flavone and isoflavone have been studied using computer modeling and site-directed mutagenesis. It was found that these compounds bind to the active site of aromatase in an orientation in which their ring–A and –C mimic ring–D and –C of the steroidal substrate, respectively.[64,67] These studies also provide a molecular basis describing why isoflavones are significantly poorer inhibitors of aromatase than flavones.

Although flavonoid natural products have weak aromatase inhibitory activity, the benzopyranone-ring system of flavonoid provides a molecular scaffold for designing potential aromatase inhibitors for future drug development. The synthetic flavonoid, alpha-naphthoflavone (Fig. 4), is a potent aromatase inhibitor with an IC_{50} value of 0.5 μM.[66] Brueggemeier *et al.*[63] reported that several compounds in the initial benzopyranone libraries, which were constructed by diversifying the benzopyranone scaffold and utilizing combinatorial chemistry approaches, inhibit aromatase activity in screening assays. Kim *et al.*[68] reported the synthesis of several pyridine-containing isoflavones.

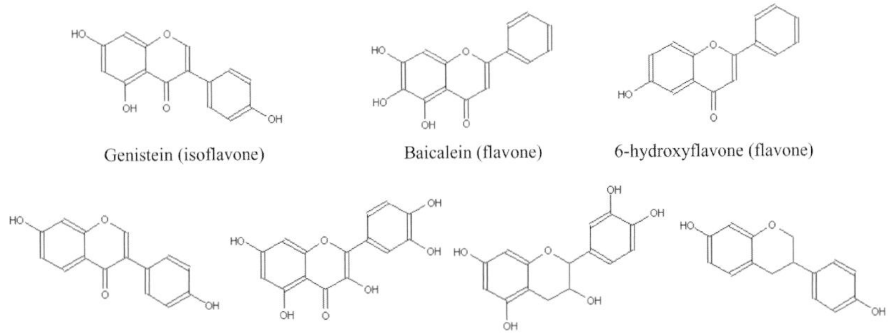

Genistein (isoflavone) Baicalein (flavone) 6-hydroxyflavone (flavone)

Daidzein (isoflavone) Quercetin (flavanol) Catechin Equol (isoflavandiol)

FIGURE 5. Flavonoid noninhibitors of aromatase.

The best inhibitors in this series, such as 7-hydroxy-3-(4-methoxyphenyl)-2-[(4'-pyridylmethyl)-thio]-isoflavone (FIG. 4), inhibited the human placental aromatase with K_i values around 0.3 μM. Gobbi et al.[69] also reported the synthesis of a series of flavone derivatives as AIs, with the removal of the 7-methoxy group leading to compounds showing inhibitory activity in the nanomolar range. Among them, 3-(imidazolylmethyl)- 4'nitroflavone (FIG. 4) had an IC_{50} value of 45 nM when the assay was performed with the substrate (androstenedione) concentration of 500 nM. Recanatini et al.[70] have synthesized chromone and xanthone derivatives. Several xanthone derivatives were found to inhibit aromatase with IC_{50} values around 50 nM in the presence of 2.5 μM of the androgen substrate. Interestingly, our laboratory has found a series of coumarins that can act as competitive inhibitors of aromatase with respect to the androgen substrate.[71] The best inhibitor in this series, 4-benzyl-3-(4'-chlorophenyl)-7-methoxycoumarin (FIG. 4), inhibits aromatase with a K_i value of 84 nM. These results suggest that it is possible to generate new potent AIs that are derived from natural anti-aromatase chemicals.

There are two considerations for the development of a new generation of AIs from natural anti-aromatase chemicals. The specificity of chemicals has to be carefully examined. Many phytochemicals have been shown to have more than one activity in the body. In addition, it is important to confirm the results generated from the assay using placental microsomes (a noncellular assay) with the in-cell assay. The in-cell assay is performed using cells that express aromatase and will determine whether the inhibitor can enter the cells. Some AIs, identified by noncellular assays, have been found to be inactive when tested with in-cell assay.[72] It is also important to demonstrate that potential AIs can actually suppress androgen (converted to estrogen by aromatase)-mediated cell proliferations. 4-Benzyl-3-(4'-chlorophenyl)-7-methoxycoumarin, an anti-aromatase chemical identified in our laboratory, was found not only to be active by the in-cell assay, but also to suppress the proliferation of aromatase and estrogen receptor–positive MCF-7aro breast cancer cells through a Matrigel thread three-dimensional cell culture.[71]

CHEMOPREVENTION STUDIES USING GRAPE SEED EXTRACT AND MUSHROOMS

Our laboratory has found that grapes, mushrooms, and red wine contain chemicals that can suppress aromatase activity.[57–59,73,74] Therefore, a diet that includes grapes, mushrooms, and red wine would be considered preventative against breast cancer. We are purifying and characterizing these natural anti-aromatase chemicals and evaluating their *in vivo* effects using animal experiments. The active chemicals in grapes and red wine have been found to be procyanidin dimers that are present at high concentrations in grape seeds.[58] Recently, grape seed extract (GSE) was found to inhibit aromatase activity in a dose-dependent manner and reduce androgen-dependent tumor growth in an aromatase-transfected MCF-7 (MCF-7aro) breast cancer xenograft model,[59] agreeing with our previous findings. More interestingly, through the suppression of the expression of CREB-1 and GR, GSE has been found to decrease the expression of aromatase in breast cancer tissue by reducing the activity of promoters I.3, II, and I.4.[59] Therefore, GSE can suppress estrogen production in breast cancer through at least two mechanisms: inhibition of the expression of aromatase and functioning as an AI. On the basis of results of preclinical studies from this and other laboratories, a phase I chemoprevention clinical trial involving GSE in postmenopausal women has been initiated at our institution, the City of Hope (<http://clinicaltrials.coh.org/study_display.aspx?pid=3713861>). GSE is a common dietary supplement that is widely used. Additional experiments to determine the mechanisms of inhibition of aromatase activity and downregulation of its expression through breast cancer–specific promoters by GSE would help in designing prevention strategies that selectively suppress its expression and activity in breast tumor tissue while also maintaining estrogen levels in normal tissues.

PERSPECTIVES

The potent and highly selective third-generation AIs are the approved therapeutic agents for the treatment of estrogen-dependent breast cancer in postmenopausal women. Furthermore, a combination of aromatase inhibitors with signal transduction inhibitors (i.e., HER1/2 kinase inhibitors and COX2 inhibitors) is being developed in an attempt to increase the efficacy of AIs. This type of therapy will also be useful for other aromatase-expressing cancers.

The design and synthesis of derivatives using natural bioactive chemicals as scaffolds with aromatase inhibitory activity would provide a new series of potent and selective agents for cancer prevention and treatment. The availability of the active-site structural information has assisted the examination of binding characteristics of AIs and the evaluation of the reaction mechanism of aromatase. Such information will also be critical for the design of new selective and potent AIs. At the present time, the weak inhibitory effects on aromatase of natural products may require a high level of exposure to get a significant impact in cancer patients, and the diverse biological activities with various enzymes and receptor systems of these phytochemicals limit their therapeutic use. However, a diet containing bioactive chemicals that decrease aromatase activity and expression offers an intriguing prevention strategy to reduce the incidence of breast cancer and other hormone-dependent cancers. Therefore, identification of diet sources that contain anti-aromatase chemicals is very interesting and important. Furthermore, it is critical to translate the findings from the laboratory research into clinical use. As the first step, our institution has initiated a clinical trial to examine whether GSE intake will result in the reduction of circulating estrogen levels in postmenopausal women, leading to a decrease of the incidence of breast cancer.

ACKNOWLEDGMENTS

The research projects described in this article have been supported by NIH grants ES08258, CA44735 and CA33572 (the COH Cancer Center grant), UC Breast Cancer Research Grants 4PB-0115 and 10PB-0140, AICR Grant 99B054, and a predoctoral fellowship from the UC Breast Cancer Research Program (to Y.H.).

REFERENCES

1. ESTEBAN, J.M. *et al*. 1992. Detection of intratumoral aromatase in breast carcinomas. An immunohistochemical study with clinicopathologic correlation. Am. J. Pathol. **140:** 337–343.
2. BULUN, S.E. *et al*. 1993. A link between breast cancer and local estrogen biosynthesis suggested by quantification of breast adipose tissue aromatase cytochrome P450 transcripts using competitive polymerase chain reaction after reverse transcription. J. Clin. Endocrinol. Metab. **77:** 1622–1628.
3. HARADA, N. 1997. Aberrant expression of aromatase in breast cancer tissues. J. Steroid. Biochem. Mol. Biol. **61:** 175–184.
4. JAMES, V.H. *et al*. 1987. Aromatase activity in normal breast and breast tumor tissues: *in vivo* and *in vitro* studies. Steroids **50:** 269–279.
5. LU, Q. *et al*. 1996. Expression of aromatase protein and messenger ribonucleic acid in tumor epithelial cells and evidence of functional significance of locally produced estrogen in human breast cancers. Endocrinology **137:** 3061–3068.
6. MILLER, W.R. & J. O'NEILL. 1987. The importance of local synthesis of estrogen within the breast. Steroids **50:** 537–548.
7. SANTEN, R.J. *et al*. 1994. Stromal spindle cells contain aromatase in human breast tumors. J. Clin. Endocrinol. Metab. **79:** 627–632.

8. SUN, X.Z., D. ZHOU & S. CHEN. 1997. Autocrine and paracrine actions of breast tumor aromatase. A three-dimensional cell culture study involving aromatase transfected MCF-7 and T-47D cells. J. Steroid Biochem. Mol. Biol. **63:** 29–36.

9. VERMEULEN, A. et al. 1986. Aromatase, 17 beta-hydroxysteroid dehydrogenase and intratissular sex hormone concentrations in cancerous and normal glandular breast tissue in postmenopausal women. Eur. J. Cancer Clin. Oncol. **22:** 515–525.

10. CASTAGNETTA, L.A. et al. 2003. Local estrogen formation by nontumoral, cirrhotic, and malignant human liver tissues and cells. Cancer Res. **63:** 5041–5045.

11. KAO, Y.C. et al. 1999. Induction of aromatase expression by aminoglutethimide, an aromatase inhibitor that is used to treat breast cancer in postmenopausal women. Anticancer Res. **19:** 2049–2056.

12. AGARWAL, V.R. et al. 1998. Molecular basis of severe gynecomastia associated with aromatase expression in a fibrolamellar hepatocellular carcinoma. J. Clin. Endocrinol. Metab. **83:** 1797–1800.

13. HARADA, N. et al. 1998. Localized aberrant expression of cytochrome P450 aromatase in primary and metastatic malignant tumors of human liver. J. Clin. Endocrinol. Metab. **83:** 697–702.

14. WEINBERG, O.K. et al. 2005. Aromatase inhibitors in human lung cancer therapy. Cancer Res. **65:** 11287–11291.

15. ZHOU, X.D., W.Q. CAI & H.W. CAO. 2002. Relationship between level of sexual hormone in external blood and aromatase expression in cancer tissues of male patients with lung cancer. Ai Zheng. **21:** 259–262.

16. ENGLISH, M.A. et al. 1999. Loss of estrogen inactivation in colonic cancer. J. Clin. Endocrinol. Metab. **84:** 2080–2085.

17. FIORELLI, G. et al. 1999. Estrogen synthesis in human colon cancer epithelial cells. J. Steroid Biochem. Mol. Biol. **71:** 223–230.

18. CHENG, Y.S. et al. 2006. Aromatase expression in normal human oral keratinocytes and oral squamous cell carcinoma. Arch. Oral. Biol. **51:** 612–620.

19. SANTEN, R.J. 1981. Suppression of estrogens with aminoglutethimide and hydrocortisone (medical adrenalectomy) as treatment of advanced breast carcinoma: a review. Breast Cancer Res. Treat. **1:** 183–202.

20. BERETTA, K.R. et al. 1990. CGS 16949A, a new aromatase inhibitor in the treatment of breast cancer—a phase I study. Ann Oncol. **1:** 421–426.

21. DOWSETT, M. et al. 1989. Dose-related endocrine effects and pharmacokinetics of oral and intramuscular 4-hydroxyandrostenedione in postmenopausal breast cancer patients. Cancer Res. **49:** 1306–1312.

22. BRODIE, A.M. 1994. Aromatase inhibitors in the treatment of breast cancer. J. Steroid. Biochem. Mol. Biol. **49:** 281–287.

23. COOMBES, R.C. et al. 1984. 4-Hydroxyandrostenedione in treatment of postmenopausal patients with advanced breast cancer. Lancet. **2:** 1237–1239.

24. PLOURDE, P.V. et al. 1995. ARIMIDEX: a new oral, once-a-day aromatase inhibitor. J. Steroid Biochem. Mol. Biol. **53:** 175–179.

25. LIPTON, A. et al. 1995. Letrozole (CGS 20267). A phase I study of a new potent oral aromatase inhibitor of breast cancer. Cancer **75:** 2132–2138.

26. EVANS, T.R. et al. 1992. Phase I and endocrine study of exemestane (FCE 24304), a new aromatase inhibitor, in postmenopausal women. Cancer Res. **52:** 5933–5939.

27. BAUM, M. et al. 2002. Anastrozole alone or in combination with tamoxifen versus tamoxifen alone for adjuvant treatment of postmenopausal women with early

breast cancer: first results of the ATAC randomised trial. Lancet **359**: 2131–2139.

28. SMITH, I.E. & M. DOWSETT. 2003. Aromatase inhibitors in breast cancer. N. Engl. J. Med. **348**: 2431–2442.

29. COOMBES, R.C. *et al*. 2004. A randomized trial of exemestane after two to three years of tamoxifen therapy in postmenopausal women with primary breast cancer. N. Engl. J. Med. **350**: 1081–1092.

30. GOSS, P.E. *et al*. 2003. A randomized trial of letrozole in postmenopausal women after five years of tamoxifen therapy for early-stage breast cancer. N. Engl. J. Med. **349**: 1793–1802.

31. BRUEGGEMEIER, R.W., J.C. HACKETT & E.S. DIAZ-CRUZ. 2005. Aromatase inhibitors in the treatment of breast cancer. Endocr. Rev. **26**: 331–345.

32. COVEY, D.F. & W.F. HOOD. 1981. Enzyme-generated intermediates derived from 4-androstene-3,6,17-trione and 1,4,6-androstatriene-3,17-dione cause a time-dependent decrease in human placental aromatase activity. Endocrinology **108**: 1597–1599.

33. FURTH, P.S. & C.H. ROBINSON. 1989. Tritium release from [19-3H]-19,19-difluoroandrost-4-ene-3,17-dione during inactivation of aromatase. Biochemistry **28**: 1254–1259.

34. NUMAZAWA, M., K. MIDZUHASHI & M. NAGAOKA. 1994. Metabolic aspects of the 1 beta-proton and the 19-methyl group of androst-4-ene-3,6,17-trione during aromatization by placental microsomes and inactivation of aromatase. Biochem Pharmacol. **47**: 717–726.

35. BRUEGGEMEIER, R.W. 1993. Steroidal inhibitors as chemical probes of the active sites of aromatase. J. Steroid Biochem. Mol. Biol. **44**: 357–365.

36. GIUDICI, D. *et al*. 1988. 6-Methylenandrosta-1,4-diene-3,17-dione (FCE 24304): a new irreversible aromatase inhibitor. J Steroid Biochem. **30**: 391–394.

37. WANG, X. & S. CHEN. 2006. Aromatase destablizer: novel action of exemestane, an FDA approved aromatase inhibitor. Cancer Res. In press.

38. ZHOU, D.J., D. POMPON & S.A. CHEN. 1990. Stable expression of human aromatase complementary DNA in mammalian cells: a useful system for aromatase inhibitor screening. Cancer Res. **50**: 6949–6954.

39. ZHOU, D.J., D. POMPON & S.A. CHEN. 1991. Structure-function studies of human aromatase by site-directed mutagenesis: kinetic properties of mutants Pro-308—Phe, Tyr-361—Phe, Tyr-361—Leu, and Phe-406—Arg. Proc. Natl. Acad. Sci. USA **88**: 410–414.

40. ZHOU, D.J. *et al*. 1992. A site-directed mutagenesis study of human placental aromatase. J. Biol. Chem. **267**: 762–768.

41. CHEN, S. & D. ZHOU. 1992. Functional domains of aromatase cytochrome P450 inferred from comparative analyses of amino acid sequences and substantiated by site-directed mutagenesis experiments. J. Biol. Chem. **267**: 22587–22594.

42. KADOHAMA, N. *et al*. 1993. Catalytic efficiency of expressed aromatase following site-directed mutagenesis. Biochim. Biophys. Acta **1163**: 195–200.

43. AMARNEH, B. *et al*. 1993. Functional domains of human aromatase cytochrome P450 characterized by linear alignment and site-directed mutagenesis. Mol. Endocrinol. **7**: 1617–24.

44. CHEN, S. *et al*. 1993. Structure–function studies of human aromatase. J. Steroid. Biochem. Mol. Biol. **44**: 347–356.

45. ZHOU, D. *et al*. 1994. Mutagenesis study at a postulated hydrophobic region near the active site of aromatase cytochrome P450. J. Biol. Chem. **269**: 19501–19508.

46. GRAHAM-LORENCE, S. *et al.* 1995. A three-dimensional model of aromatase cytochrome P450. Protein Sci. **4:** 1065–1080.
47. CHEN, S. *et al.* 2003. Structure-function studies of aromatase and its inhibitors: a progress report. J. Steroid. Biochem. Mol. Biol. **86:** 231–237.
48. KAO, Y.C. *et al.* 1996. Binding characteristics of seven inhibitors of human aromatase: a site-directed mutagenesis study. Cancer Res. **56:** 3451–3460.
49. KAO, Y.C. *et al.* 2000. Catalytic differences between porcine blastocyst and placental aromatase isozymes. Eur. J. Biochem. **267:** 6134–6139.
50. KAO, Y.C. *et al.* 2001. Evaluation of the mechanism of aromatase cytochrome P450. A site-directed mutagenesis study. Eur. J. Biochem. **268:** 243–251.
51. ZHAO, J. *et al.* 2001. Different catalytic properties and inhibitor responses of the goldfish brain and ovary aromatase isozymes. Gen. Comp. Endocrinol. **123:** 180–191.
52. FAVIA, A.D. *et al.* 2006. Three-dimensional model of the human aromatase enzyme and density functional parameterization of the iron-containing protoporphyrin IX for a molecular dynamics study of heme-cysteinato cytochromes. Proteins **62:** 1074–1087.
53. HONG, Y. *et al.* 2006. Molecular basis for the aromatization reaction and exemestane-mediated irreversible inhibition of human aromatase. Mol. Endocrinol. In press.
54. MA, C.X. *et al.* 2005. Human aromatase: gene resequencing and functional genomics. Cancer Res. **65:** 11071–11082.
55. ADLERCREUTZ, H. 1995. Phytoestrogens: epidemiology and a possible role in cancer protection. Environ. Health Perspect. **103**(Suppl 7): 103–112.
56. GLADE, M.J. 1999. Food, nutrition, and the prevention of cancer: a global perspective. American Institute for Cancer Research/World Cancer Research Fund, American Institute for Cancer Research, 1997. Nutrition **15:** 523–526.
57. GRUBE, B.J. *et al.* 2001. White button mushroom phytochemicals inhibit aromatase activity and breast cancer cell proliferation. J. Nutr. **131:** 3288–3293.
58. ENG, E.T. *et al.* 2003. Suppression of estrogen biosynthesis by procyanidin dimers in red wine and grape seeds. Cancer Res. **63:** 8516–8522.
59. KIJIMA, I. *et al.* 2006. Grape seed extract is an aromatase inhibitor and a suppressor of aromatase expression. Cancer Res. **66:** 5960–5967.
60. LEE, D. *et al.* 2001. Aromatase inhibitors from *Broussonetia papyrifera*. J. Nat. Prod. **64:** 1286–1293.
61. FILLEUR, F. *et al.* 2001. Antiproliferative, anti-aromatase, anti-17beta-HSD and antioxidant activities of lignans isolated from *Myristica argentea*. Planta Med. **67:** 700–704.
62. SANDERSON, J.T. *et al.* 2004. Induction and inhibition of aromatase (CYP19) activity by natural and synthetic flavonoid compounds in H295R human adrenocortical carcinoma cells. Toxicol. Sci. **82:** 70–79.
63. BRUEGGEMEIER, R.W. *et al.* 2001. Effects of phytoestrogens and synthetic combinatorial libraries on aromatase, estrogen biosynthesis, and metabolism. Ann. N. Y. Acad. Sci. **948:** 51–66.
64. KAO, Y.C. *et al.* 1998. Molecular basis of the inhibition of human aromatase (estrogen synthetase) by flavone and isoflavone phytoestrogens: a site-directed mutagenesis study. Environ. Health Perspect. **106:** 85–92.
65. PELISSERO, C. *et al.* 1996. Effects of flavonoids on aromatase activity, an *in vitro* study. J. Steroid. Biochem. Mol. Biol. **57:** 215–223.

66. CAMPBELL, D.R. & M.S. KURZER. 1993. Flavonoid inhibition of aromatase enzyme activity in human preadipocytes. J. Steroid. Biochem. Mol. Biol. **46:** 381–388.
67. CHEN, S., Y.C. KAO & C.A. LAUGHTON. 1997. Binding characteristics of aromatase inhibitors and phytoestrogens to human aromatase. J. Steroid. Biochem. Mol. Biol. **61:** 107–115.
68. KIM, Y.W., J.C. HACKETT & R.W. BRUEGGEMEIER. 2004. Synthesis and aromatase inhibitory activity of novel pyridine-containing isoflavones. J. Med. Chem. **47:** 4032–4040.
69. GOBBI, S. *et al.* 2006. Lead optimization providing a series of flavone derivatives as potent nonsteroidal inhibitors of the cytochrome P450 aromatase enzyme. J. Med. Chem. **49:** 4777–4780.
70. RECANATINI, M. *et al.* 2001. A new class of nonsteroidal aromatase inhibitors: design and synthesis of chromone and xanthone derivatives and inhibition of the P450 enzymes aromatase and 17 alpha-hydroxylase/C17,20-lyase. J. Med. Chem. **44:** 672–680.
71. CHEN, S. *et al.* 2004. Biochemical and biological characterization of a novel anti-aromatase coumarin derivative. J. Biol. Chem. **279:** 48071–48078.
72. BALUNAS, M.J. *et al.* 2006. Interference by naturally occurring fatty acids in a noncellular enzyme-based aromatase bioassay. J. Nat. Prod. **69:** 700–703.
73. ENG, E.T. *et al.* 2002. Anti-aromatase chemicals in red wine. Ann. N. Y. Acad. Sci. **963:** 239–246.
74. ENG, E.T. *et al.* 2001. Suppression of aromatase (estrogen synthetase) by red wine phytochemicals. Breast Cancer Res. Treat. **67:** 133–146.

Hormonal Treatment of Human Hepatocellular Carcinoma

MASSIMO DI MAIO,[a] ERMELINDA DE MAIO,[a]
ALESSANDRO MORABITO,[a] ROBERTA D'ANIELLO,[a]
GIANFRANCO DE FEO,[a] CIRO GALLO,[b]
AND FRANCESCO PERRONE[a]

[a]Clinical Trials Unit, National Cancer Institute, Napoli, Italy

[b]Department of Medicine and Public Health, Second University, Napoli, Italy

ABSTRACT: Animal models of experimental liver carcinogenesis and epidemiological studies in humans suggest a relationship between sex hormones and hepatocellular carcinoma (HCC). In 1997, a systematic review of the existing, small randomized trials evaluating the antiestrogen tamoxifen yielded a positive result, but the large randomized CLIP-1 trial showed no survival advantage from the addition of tamoxifen to best supportive care. A possible explanation for the negative results is the lack of patient selection, but the expression of estrogen (ER) and progesterone (PgR) receptors in HCC does not clearly affect the survival outcome of the patients treated with tamoxifen. In the last years, it has been proposed that negative results might be due to the fact that tamoxifen in HCC could act via an ER-independent pathway, which requires much higher doses than those usually administered, but a double-blind Asian randomized trial conducted to assess possible dose-response effect showed no efficacy for tamoxifen, with an inversely negative impact with increasing dose. According to the results of large trials and of the Cochrane systematic review, neither further trials are warranted with tamoxifen in HCC, nor should any use in clinical practice be considered. Interesting results have been obtained when the type of hormonal treatment (tamoxifen or megestrol) has been chosen according to the presence of wild-type or variant ER, but these results should be confirmed in large randomized trials. Negative results have been obtained with antiandrogen therapy. In conclusion, hormonal treatment should not be a part of the current management of HCC patients.

KEYWORDS: hepatocellular carcinoma; tamoxifen; hormonal treatment

Address for correspondence: Francesco Perrone, Clinical Trials Unit, National Cancer Institute, via Mariano Semmola, 80131 Napoli, Italy. Voice: +39-081-5903571; fax: +39-081-7702938.
e-mail: fr.perrone@agora.it

Ann. N.Y. Acad. Sci. 1089: 252–261 (2006). © 2006 New York Academy of Sciences.
doi: 10.1196/annals.1386.007

INTRODUCTION

Hepatocellular carcinoma (HCC) is the fifth most common cancer worldwide, with more than 500,000 new cases per year, and, in order of mortality, the third most prevalent cancer.[1] The treatment options and prognosis of these patients largely depend not only on the characteristics of the tumor, but also on the severity of the underlying chronic hepatic disease that affects most of the patients. Prognosis is relatively better for the subset of patients eligible for surgical treatment (tumor resection, orthotopic liver transplantation) or other potentially curative loco-regional treatments (radiofrequency ablation, percutaneous ethanol injection). A worse outcome is expected in those patients who can be treated only with palliative loco-regional treatments (e.g., transarterial embolization) or who are not suitable for any of the above options. Currently, there is no standard pharmacological anticancer treatment for HCC patients. A great number of cytotoxic agents have been tested in patients with advanced HCC; unfortunately, none of them has shown encouraging results.[2] Furthermore, treatment with these drugs is often associated with unacceptable toxicity on account of the compromised hepatic function of these patients.

Hormonal treatment plays an established role in several solid tumors, first of all in breast cancer, where in the last decades the antiestrogen tamoxifen has been the most commonly used treatment for patients with estrogen receptor-alpha (ER)–positive breast cancer. The target of tamoxifen *in vivo* is the ER, and levels of ER expression are the best predictor of benefit from tamoxifen.[3] Tamoxifen is characterized by a favorable toxicity profile, which, together with the easy oral administration, makes this drug an interesting candidate for treatment of other solid tumors potentially responding to hormonal manipulation. Animal models of experimental liver carcinogenesis and epidemiological studies in humans suggest a relationship between exposure to sex hormones and development of HCC, with some evidence that these hormones may play a role as inducer and promoter in the process of liver carcinogenesis.[4] Expression of ER and progesterone receptors (PgR) can be found in a variable proportion of cases of HCC. TABLE 1 shows the percentage of ER+ and PgR+ HCC in studies analyzing the expression of these receptors by enzyme immunoassay or by immunohistochemistry.[5–8] Although only a limited percentage (between 15% and 39%) of HCC are ER+, in the last decades there has been great interest in the potential usefulness of tamoxifen for patients with HCC, especially because of the encouraging results of the first clinical trials and the lack of efficacy of other systemic treatments.

THE 1997 META-ANALYSIS AND THE CLIP-1 TRIAL

In 1997 a systematic review of the existing randomized trials evaluating the efficacy of the antiestrogen tamoxifen yielded a positive result.[9] Seven

TABLE 1. Expression of ER and PgR in hepatocellular carcinoma

Study	Patients	Ethnicity	Determination technique	ER	PgR
Boix[5]	26	Western	Enzyme immunoassay	15%	0%
Ng[6]	71	Chinese	IHC	24%	14%
Jonas[7]	33	Western	Enzyme immunoassay	39%	18%
Liu[8]	66	Chinese	IHC	27%	30%

IHC = immunohistochemistry.

trials were identified: two of those trials evaluated the addition of tamoxifen to chemotherapy, and the other five trials were designed to compare tamoxifen versus no treatment or placebo. In these latter studies, pooled odds ratio of surviving at 1 year for patients receiving tamoxifen was 2.0, with 95% confidence intervals (CI) 1.1–3.6. However, it should be emphasized that the studies considered in the meta-analysis were characterized by several methodological drawbacks, and by a really small sample size (ranging between 22 and 120). The authors of the meta-analysis suggested a note of caution in considering these results conclusive and called for a large randomized trial to definitely address the question of the efficacy of tamoxifen in HCC.

Two years before, in 1995, the Cancer of the Liver Italian Program (CLIP) investigators had initiated the CLIP-1 study, designed to verify whether optimistic data on tamoxifen effect were confirmed in a large randomized trial.[10] A pragmatic approach was chosen for the conduction of this randomized trial: eligibility criteria were broad, overall survival was the only end point of the intent-to-treat analysis, no placebo was used in the control arm, and no additional follow-up rule was added to the usual clinical practice of participating centers. All HCC patients with a life expectancy longer than 3 months were eligible. Patients assigned to experimental arm received oral tamoxifen at 40 mg daily until death or inability to consume the drug. Overall, 496 patients were randomized. The main patients and tumor characteristics were well balanced between the two treatment arms. Patients were predominantly males, with underlying viral cirrhosis. About half of them had a well-compensated liver function. The first results of the trial, published in 1998, showed no overall survival advantage deriving from the addition of tamoxifen to best supportive care.[10] Estimated median survival was 15 and 16 months in the tamoxifen and the control arm, respectively. One-year survival probability was similar in the two arms, 55% and 56%, respectively. After adjustment for known prognostic factors, the relative hazard of death for patients receiving tamoxifen was equal to 1.07 (95% CI 0.83–1.39). Furthermore, updated results of the CLIP-1 trial, published in 2002, confirmed the original negative result, both in the subgroup of advanced patients and in those eligible for potentially curative loco-regional treatments.[11] The results of the CLIP-1 study changed the conclusion of the above cited meta-analysis, but this is not surprising, if we consider that the sample size of the trial was much higher than that of all the previous studies. The addition of the CLIP-1 data to the four previous trials comparing tamoxifen-alone versus no active treatment (the fifth was a comparison of tamoxifen combined with luteinizing hormone–releasing hormone (LHRH) analogue vs. no active treatment) produced a pooled odds ratio of being alive at 1 year for patients receiving tamoxifen of 1.19 (95% CI 0.88–1.61), and there was no more statistically significant advantage for tamoxifen.

Recently, this lack of a survival advantage for HCC patients treated with tamoxifen has been confirmed by a French trial with 420 HCC patients randomly assigned tamoxifen or supportive care alone.[12] This phase III trial adds relevant information to the body of evidence regarding tamoxifen in HCC, because tamoxifen was ineffective also in a HCC population with a prevalence of alcohol-related liver cirrhosis, while in all previous trials the HCC in most of the patients developed on the basis of a chronic liver disease of viral etiology. However, following a *post hoc* unplanned subgroup analysis, the French investigators suggested that tamoxifen might be effective in a population of patients without major hepatic insufficiency (i.e., those with Okuda stage I or II) and that new trials on tamoxifen are still warranted, at least in this subset of patients. Subgroup analyses carry a relevant risk of false positive results, and their results should be always considered with great caution. We tried to validate the hypothesis of Barbare *et al.* using the updated data of the CLIP-1 randomized trial, but tamoxifen was still not effective both in patients with Okuda stage I–II and in those with Okuda stage III disease or Okuda unknown.[13] We also tested the same hypothesis in subgroups defined according to the CLIP score. The CLIP score is actually the most widely accepted and validated prognostic score for HCC,[14,15] and it takes into account liver function measured by Child–Pugh category, portal vein thrombosis, level of alpha-fetoprotein, and tumor size. In the patients in the CLIP-1 study, results were negative again both in patients with good CLIP score (0–1) and in those with worse or unknown CLIP score.[13]

A PROBLEM OF SELECTION?

A possible explanation for the negative results obtained with the use of tamoxifen in HCC patients is the lack of selection of the patients. It should be noted that none of the above-cited randomized trials was based on a selection of patients according to hormonal receptor expression. This may represent a significant problem. In breast cancer, it is now well established that the efficacy of hormonal treatment is relevant, but it is limited to patients with tumors expressing hormonal receptors. As shown in TABLE 1, the expression of these receptors is not so frequent in HCC, and this might have diluted the positive effect of tamoxifen, potentially limited to a small subgroup of patients. Greater emphasis should be probably given, when planning a clinical trial and when interpreting its results, to the great impact that the molecular heterogeneity of tumors, affecting sensitivity to the experimental treatment, may have on the results of a clinical trial.[16] The only attempt to correlate the efficacy of hormonal treatment with target expression comes from a secondary analysis of a Chinese randomized trial comparing tamoxifen versus no treatment for patients with advanced and otherwise untreatable HCC.[8] Immunohistochemical tests for ER and PgR were performed on the tumor tissues obtained from the patients enrolled in the study. The expression of hormone receptors in the tumors did not affect the survival outcome of the patients treated with tamoxifen.[8] However, it should be noted that, in that trial, the patients were not selected according to hormonal receptor expression; immunohistochemical determinations were performed only on a subgroup of 66 patients with adequate tissue specimen of 119 enrolled patients; and that the prognosis of the patients enrolled in that study was really dismal, with a median survival of 44 versus 41 days, in tamoxifen and control group, respectively. Adequately powered prospective phase III trials assessing the efficacy of tamoxifen in patients selected for the expression of ER are lacking.

Another intriguing hypothesis about the possibility that tamoxifen could be effective only in a selected subgroup of patients with HCC is related to the presence of variant estrogen receptors (vER).[17] The liver presents ERs alpha and beta and, as in breast cancer, a variant form of ER alpha transcript has been described in HCC. This variant is derived by an exon 5-deleted transcript, which lacks the hormone-binding domain of the receptor but, being intact in the DNA-binding domain, maintains constitutive transcriptional activity. These tumors with vER, which are a significant percentage of HCCs, are characterized by a worse prognosis, with significantly faster doubling time and significantly shorter survival.[17] Tamoxifen could not be effective in tumors with vER because of tamoxifen's inability to bind the receptor. In a small experimental experience,[18] antihormonal therapy of HCC was tailored according to the presence of wild-type or exon 5-deleted vER transcripts, limiting the administration of tamoxifen (at daily dose of 80 mg) to patients with wild-type ER, and treating patients with vER with megestrol acetate, at the daily dose of 160 mg. Interestingly, tumor volume in all patients with wild-type ERs was halved after 9 months of tamoxifen treatment, and the authors concluded that choosing antihormonal treatment according to the presence of wild-type or variant ERs in the tumor definitely improves the response rate to tamoxifen.

Of course, before claiming the efficacy of tamoxifen in a selected subgroup of HCC patients, these interesting results should be confirmed in adequately powered trials, selecting patients according to the presence of wild-type ERs and randomizing patients to receive tamoxifen or no treatment.

A PROBLEM OF DOSE?

Some years ago, some authors proposed that the negative results obtained with tamoxifen in HCCs might be due to the fact that the activity of tamoxifen

TABLE 2. Main suggested ER-independent mechanisms of action of tamoxifen[19]

- Interaction of tamoxifen and 4hydroxy-tamoxifen with membrane phospholipids, with decrease in cell membrane fluidity and inhibition of adenylate cyclase
- Inhibition of protein kinase C activity
- Inhibition of calmodulin-dependent cAMP phosphodiesterase
- Increase in TGF1b levels (also in ER-cells)

TGF = tumor growth factor.

in HCC could be related to an ER-independent pathway.[19] TABLE 2 synthesizes the proposed mechanisms by which tamoxifen could act on HCC cells independently of the expression of ERs. Interestingly, these mechanisms require much higher doses of tamoxifen for activation than those used in the trials described so far. In fact, tamoxifen is known to have therapeutic actions independent of ER status at higher doses (4–8 times that used for ER-positive breast carcinoma).[19] Thus, high-dose tamoxifen would potentially have therapeutic actions on both ER-positive and ER-negative HCCs. Calling for a "paradigm shift" to dissociate the action of tamoxifen from the expression of ERs in HCC, Tan *et al.* suggested that future trials with tamoxifen in HCC should use higher doses of tamoxifen, at least four- to eightfold that of the dose intended to be efficacious in an ER-dependent mechanism.[19]

Moving from this intriguing hypothesis, a double-blind randomized controlled trial was conducted in the Asian Pacific region with 329 HCC patients, comparing tamoxifen versus placebo.[20] Tamoxifen was given at two distinct doses (120 mg daily and 60 mg daily) in order to assess possible dose–response effect. Quite disappointingly, rather than indicating a dose–response effect in favor of tamoxifen, the analysis showed a significant detrimental effect for the higher dose of tamoxifen. Three-month survival rates were 44%, 41%, and 35%, respectively, for the groups receiving placebo, tamoxifen at 60 mg, and tamoxifen at 120 mg, with a statistically significant trend difference in survival across the three arms. There was a significantly higher risk of death in the tamoxifen 120-mg-group compared with the placebo group (hazard ratio, 1.39; 95% CI 1.07–1.81). The detrimental effect of tamoxifen seemed not to be related to a higher toxicity of the higher dose. The trial, indeed, was unable to identify significant toxicity due to tamoxifen, and the rate of reported treatment toxicity (3%) was extremely low, without significant differences among the arms; however, the authors cautiously postulated that the general rapid decline of patients with inoperable HCC could make it difficult to identify treatment toxicities.

Although the mechanism by which higher doses of tamoxifen seem to have a negative impact on the prognosis of HCC patients, the unexpected findings of the Asian trial are confirmed by the results of the recent Cochrane meta-analysis on tamoxifen in HCC.[21] In fact, there was an overall survival trend favoring the arm without tamoxifen, with increasing dose of tamoxifen. Namely, the hazard ratio for overall survival was lowest for trials of tamoxifen given at 20 mg daily (HR 0.88; 95% CI 0.69 to 1.44; $P = 0.71$), higher in trials of tamoxifen given at 40 mg daily (hazard ratio 1.00; 95% CI 0.85 to 1.19; $P = 1.0$), even higher in trials of tamoxifen given at 60 mg daily (hazard ratio 1.03; 95% CI 0.81 to 1.31; $P = 0.8$), and highest in the single trial of tamoxifen given at 120 mg daily (hazard ratio 1.29; 95% CI 1.04 to 1.6; $P = 0.02$).

Main results of this Cochrane meta-analysis, which considered 10 randomized trials for a total of 1,709 patients, show that tamoxifen versus placebo/no intervention had no significant effect on overall survival (Hazard Ratio 1.05; 95% CI 0.94 to 1.16; $P = 0.4$), without statistical heterogeneity between the trials.

According to these results, which are concordant with the results of all the above cited large randomized trials,[10, 12,20] we believe that, unfortunately, no further trials are warranted with tamoxifen in HCC, nor should any use in clinical practice be considered because of its clear lack of efficacy.

OTHER HORMONAL TREATMENTS

Efficacy of megestrol acetate has been tested in HCC with vER, according to the hypothesis that in these patients, a progestin drug like megestrol (which exerts its action on ER pathways at postreceptorial level) might represent a better therapeutic option than tamoxifen.[18, 22,23] A prospective, randomized study assigned 45 patients with inoperable HCC characterized by variant liver ERs to receive megestrol or placebo.[23] Twenty-four patients were randomized to no treatment and 21 to megestrol at the daily dose of 160 mg. Median survival in untreated patients was 7 months (95% CI 3.01–10.99 months) versus 18 months (95% CI 13.47–22.53 months) in patients treated with megestrol ($P = 0.0090$). According to the opinion of the investigators who conducted this trial, in patients with HCC characterized by variant ERs, that is, those patients with rapidly progressive disease, megestrol is able to remarkably increase survival in this small population, making a trial with this drug more than warranted. We agree with this last observation, and believe that no firm conclusions on the effectiveness of megestrol acetate in that selected subgroup of HCC patients might be drawn until it is confirmed in adequately powered randomized trials. Such trials should select patients according to the presence of variant ERs, randomizing patients to receive megestrol or no treatment.

Similarly to estrogens, there are several pieces of evidence supporting a positive influence of androgens on HCC growth, with a potential role of treatment with antiandrogens for patients with HCC. In tumor cells, androgen receptors seem to be present more frequently and in greater concentrations than ERs.[24] Furthermore, experimental studies have suggested a promoter effect of androgens on tumor growth,[25] which may be suppressed via antiandrogen treatment[26] or castration.[27]

A randomized trial conducted in unresectable HCC by the European Organization for Research and Treatment of Cancer tested the efficacy of antiandrogen therapy.[28] The trial was conducted according to a factorial two-by-two design. Unfortunately, neither pure antiandrogen (nilutamide 300 mg daily for 1 month, then 150 mg daily) nor LHRH agonist (goserelin acetate at 3.6 mg or triptorelin at 3.75 mg administered monthly by subcutaneous injection) showed significant efficacy in terms of survival.

Another randomized phase III trial designed with the aim of assessing the effect of antiandrogens in patients with advanced HCC was conducted by the French collaborative group GRETCH.[29] Male patients with advanced HCC were randomized into two arms. Patients assigned to the experimental arm received leuprorelin (3.75 mg/month subcutaneously), flutamide (750 mg orally daily), and tamoxifen (30 mg orally daily). Patients assigned to the control arm received tamoxifen alone, considered as a standard treatment at the time of study planning. Between February 1994 and January 1998, 376 male patients were included. No baseline imbalance was found between the groups. Median survival time was estimated to be 135.5 days and 176 days in treated and control groups, respectively ($P = 0.21$). Crude and adjusted relative risks of death in the treated group were estimated at 1.14 (95% CI, 0.93–1.40) and 1.08 (95%CI, 0.87–1.33), respectively. In conclusion, no benefit in survival was found with antiandrogenic treatment in male patients with advanced HCC.

CONCLUSION

In conclusion, hormonal treatments should not be part of the current standard management of patients affected by HCC. New effective treatments are strongly needed, and research dedicated to this type of cancer, which in the past has been often neglected,[2] should be strongly supported.

ACKNOWLEDGMENTS

Massimo Di Maio is recipient of an AIRC (Associazione Italiana per la Ricerca sul Cancro) fellowship. Ciro Gallo and Francesco Perrone have been funded from AIRC for studies in HCC.

REFERENCES

1. PARKIN, D.M. 2001. Global cancer statistics in the year 2000. Lancet Oncol. **2**:533–543.
2. DI MAIO, M., E. DE MAIO, F. PERRONE, *et al.* 2002. Hepatocellular carcinoma: systemic treatments. J. Clin. Gastroenterol. **35**(5 Suppl 2): S109–S114.

3. EARLY BREAST CANCER TRIALISTS' COLLABORATIVE GROUP. 1998. Tamoxifen for early breast cancer: an overview of the randomised trials. Lancet **351:** 1451–1467.
4. DE MARIA, N., M. MANNO & E. VILLA. 2002. Sex hormones and liver cancer. Mol. Cell. Endocrinol. **193:** 59–63.
5. BOIX, L., J. BRUIX, A. CASTELLS, *et al.* 1993. Sex hormone receptors in hepatocellular carcinoma. Is there a rationale for hormonal treatment? J. Hepatol. **17:** 187–191.
6. NG, I.O., M. NG & S.T. FAN. 1997. Better survival in women with hepatocellular carcinoma is not related to tumor proliferation or expression of hormone receptors. Am. J. Gastroenterol. **92:** 1355–1358.
7. JONAS, S., W.O. BECHSTEIN, T. HEINZE, *et al.* 1997. Female sex hormone receptor status in advanced hepatocellular carcinoma and outcome after surgical resection. Surgery **121:** 456–461.
8. LIU, C.L., S.T. FAN, I.O. NG, *et al.* 2000. Treatment of advanced hepatocellular carcinoma with tamoxifen and the correlation with expression of hormone receptors: a prospective randomized study. Am. J. Gastroenterol. **95:** 218–222.
9. SIMONETTI, R.G., A. LIBERATI, C. ANGIOLINI & L. PAGLIARO. 1997. Treatment of hepatocellular carcinoma: a systematic review of randomized controlled trias. Ann. Oncol. **8:** 117–136.
10. CANCER OF THE LIVER ITALIAN PROGRAM (CLIP) GROUP. 1998. Tamoxifen in treatment of hepatocellular carcinoma: a randomized controlled trial. Lancet **352:** 17–20.
11. PERRONE, F., C. GALLO, B. DANIELE, *et al.* 2002. Cancer of the Liver Italian Program (CLIP) Investigators. Tamoxifen in the treatment of hepatocellular carcinoma: 5-year results of the CLIP-1 multicentre randomised controlled trial. Curr. Pharm. Des. **8:** 1013–1019.
12. BARBARE, J.C., O. BOUCHE, F. BONNETAIN, *et al.* 2005. Randomized controlled trial of tamoxifen in advanced hepatocellular carcinoma. J. Clin. Oncol. **23:** 4338–4346.
13. GALLO, C., E. DE MAIO, M. DI MAIO, *et al.* 2006. Tamoxifen is not effective in good prognosis patients with hepatocellular carcinoma. BMC Cancer **6:** 196.
14. CANCER OF THE LIVER ITALIAN PROGRAM (CLIP) INVESTIGATORS. 1998. A new prognostic system for hepatocellular carcinoma: a retrospective study of 435 patients. Hepatology **28:** 751–755.
15. CANCER OF THE LIVER ITALIAN PROGRAM (CLIP) INVESTIGATORS: 2000. Prospective validation of the CLIP score: a new prognostic system for patients with cirrhosis and hepatocellular carcinoma. Hepatology **31:** 840–845.
16. BETENSKY, R.A., D.N. LOUIS & J.G. CAIRNCROSS. 2002. Influence of unrecognized molecular heterogeneity on randomized clinical trials. J. Clin. Oncol. **20:** 2495–2499.
17. VILLA, E., A. COLANTONI, A. GROTTOLA, *et al.* 2002. Variant estrogen receptors and their role in liver disease. Mol. Cell. Endocrinol. **193:** 65–69.
18. VILLA, E., A. DUGANI, E. FANTONI, *et al.* 1996. Type of estrogen receptor determines response to antiestrogen therapy. Cancer Res. **56:** 3883–3885.
19. TAN, C.K., P.K. CHOW, M. FINDLAY, *et al.* 2001. Use of tamoxifen in hepatocellular carcinoma: a review and paradigm shift. J. Gastroenterol. Hepatol. **15:** 725–729.
20. CHOW, P.K., B.C. TAI, C.K. TAN, *et al.* 2002. High-dose tamoxifen in the treatment of inoperable hepatocellular carcinoma: a multicenter randomized controlled trial. Hepatology **36:** 1221–1226.

21. NOWAK, A., M. FINDLAY, G. CULJAK & M. STOCKLER. 2004. Tamoxifen for hepatocellular carcinoma. Cochrane Database Syst. Rev. **3:** CD001024.

22. VILLA, E., L. CAMELLINI, A. DUGANI, *et al.* 1996. Variant liver estrogen receptors and response to tamoxifen. Gastroenterology **111:** 271–272.

23. VILLA, E., I. FERRETTI, A. GROTTOLA, *et al.* 2001. Hormonal therapy with megestrol in inoperable hepatocellular carcinoma characterized by variant oestrogen receptors. Br. J. Cancer **84:** 881–885.

24. GRANATA, O., G. CARRUBA, G. MONTALTO, *et al.* 2002. Altered androgen metabolism eventually leads hepatocellular carcinoma to an impaired hormone responsiveness. Mol. Cell. Endocrinol. **193:** 51–58.

25. MATSUMOTO, T., H. TAKAGI & M. MORI. 2000. Androgen dependency of hepatocarcinogenesis in TGFalpha transgenic mice. Liver **20:** 228–233.

26. MARUYAMA, S., N. NAGASUE, D.K. DHAR, *et al.* 2001. Preventive effect of FK143, a 5alpha-reductase inhibitor, on chemical hepatocarcinogenesis in rats. Clin. Cancer Res. **7:** 2096–2104.

27. YU, L.Q., N. NAGASUE, M. YAMAGUCHI & Y.C. CHANG. 1996. Effects of castration and androgen replacement on tumour growth of human hepatocellular carcinoma in nude mice. J. Hepatol. **25:** 362–369.

28. GRIMALDI, C., H. BLEIBERG, F. GAY, *et al.* 1998. Evaluation of antiandrogen therapy in unresectable hepatocellular carcinoma: results of an European Organization for Research and Treatment of Cancer muticentric double-blind trial. J. Clin. Oncol. **16:** 411–417.

29. GROUPE D'ETUDE ET DE TRAITEMENT DU CARCINOME HEPATOCELLULAIRE (GRETCH). 2004. Randomized trial of leuprorelin and flutamide in male patients with hepatocellular carcinoma treated with tamoxifen. Hepatology **40:** 1361–1369.

Metabolic Profiles of Androgens in Malignant Human Liver Cell Lines

ORAZIA M. GRANATA, LETIZIA COCCIADIFERRO, VITALE MICELI,
LUCIA M. POLITO, ILDEGARDA CAMPISI, AND GIUSEPPE CARRUBA

*Experimental Oncology Unit, Department of Oncology, ARNAS-Civico,
Palermo, Italy*

ABSTRACT: In this study we have investigated androgen (testosterone and androstenedione) metabolism in malignant HepG2, Huh-7, and HA22T human liver cell lines. Following 72-h incubation with testosterone or androstenedione, estrogen formation through aromatase activity was consistently higher in HepG2 cells (being nearly 100%) and moderate in Huh7 cells (34%), while it was undetectable in HA22T cells. The produced estrogens are completely conjugated by estrogen sulphotransferase (EST) in HepG2 cells, while nearly 25% remains in the free form in Huh-7 cells. The HA22T and Huh-7 cells show a markedly different balance of 5α- versus 5β-reduced androgens (65.7% vs. 2.5% and 2.6% vs. 22.2%, respectively), while no detectable 5α/5β-reduced androgen is formed in HepG2 cells. These divergent metabolic profiles, coupling aromatase to EST, and to 5α/5β-reductase, hint at a differential regulation of androgen metabolic pathways that may ultimately lead to a distinct impact of biologically active metabolites on growth and function of human liver cancer cells.

KEYWORDS: aromatase; EST; 5α-androgens; 5β-androgens; HCC cells

INTRODUCTION

The potential role of sex steroids in the development and progression of human hepatocellular carcinoma (HCC) is still uncertain. In different cohort studies, higher testosterone-to-estradiol ratio, increased testosterone serum levels, metabolic activation of testosterone, and/or androgen receptor (AR)-mediated transcriptional activity were all positively associated with the HCC risk.[1,2]

There is evidence that high-affinity binding sites of androgen can be expressed at sufficient concentrations to induce a biological response in both normal and malignant liver cells, although malignant hepatocytes are

Address for correspondence: Giuseppe Carruba, M.D., Ph.D., Experimental Oncology Unit, Department of Oncology, P.O. M. Ascoli, ARNAS-Civico, Piazzale N. Leotta 2, 90127 Palermo, Italy. Voice: +39-091-666-4348; fax: +39-091-666-4352.
e-mail: lucashbl@unipa.it

Ann. N.Y. Acad. Sci. 1089: 262–267 (2006). © 2006 New York Academy of Sciences.
doi: 10.1196/annals.1386.028

characterized by variable receptor concentrations, and a rapid conversion of androgens to less-active 5β derivatives[3] and/or to estrone.

Estrogenic hormones may antagonize androgen action in normal rat liver. On the other hand, the increase in the hepatic sensitivity to androgen observed in androgen-treated normal rats is also associated with the induction of estrogen sulfotransferase (EST), which is responsible for estrogen inactivation.[4] The castration of male mice decreases the incidence of chemically induced HCC compared to that of intact males,[5] whereas chronic administration of testosterone to female or castrated male animals increases the risk of spontaneous or chemically induced HCC.[6]

The aromatase enzyme appears to be expressed at relatively low levels in the disease-free adult liver, while it attains markedly higher levels in HCC tissues and cells.[7] This eventually leads to elevated tissue estrone and to reduced levels of the circulating substrate, testosterone.[8]

In this study, we have investigated the activity of steroid enzymes, including aromatase, EST, 17β-hydroxy steroid dehydrogenase (17β-HSD), and 5α/5β-reductase governing metabolic pathways of androgens in a panel of malignant human liver cell lines.

MATERIALS AND METHODS

Cell Cultures

The HepG2, Huh-7, and HA22T human liver cancer cells were maintained in RPMI-1640 medium, supplemented with 10% heat-inactivated fetal calf serum in a humidified 5% CO_2 atmosphere at 37°C. Cells having a narrow range of passage number were used for all experiments.

Measurement of Steroid Enzyme Activities

The methods and procedures used to assess the metabolic pathways of steroids have previously been established and optimized in our laboratories.[9,10] Cells (0.5×10^6) were seeded into 60-mm cell culture dishes in routine medium. After 48 h, cell were washed twice with phosphate-buffered saline (PBS-A) and incubated in FCS-free, phenol red-free RPMI medium containing 1 nM tritiated testosterone (T) or androstenedione (adione) as precursor. After 24-h and 72-h incubations, the medium was transferred to plastic tubes and stored at −20°C until steroid extraction. Extraction of steroids was performed with SPE method in Vac-Elut (Analytichem, Harbor City, CA, USA) apparatus using C18 cartridges on 1-mL aliquots of medium, as previously described.[11] In brief: two fractions were collected: in the first, conjugate (sulfate and glycosylate) steroids were eluted using water-methanol solution (60:40, v/v); and in the second, the free steroids were eluted using water-methanol solution (15-85, v/v). The two fractions were dried in a SVC100H Speed Vac evaporator concentrator (Savant Instruments, Inc., Farmingdale, NY, USA) and conjugate steroids were hydrolyzed at 37°C for 18 h, in 1 mL of a solution consisting of 970 μL of 0.2 M acetate buffer (pH 5.0) and 30 μL of glusulase enzyme mixture (duPont, Wilmington, DE, USA). The hydrolyzed steroids were extracted again by the SPE method using ethyl acetate and evaporated to dryness, as described above. Both free and conjugate steroids were analyzed in RP-HPLC using a Beckman 324 model HPLC system equipped with an UV detector set at 280 nm, and an on-line Flo-One/beta (500TR series) three-channel flow scintillation analyzer (Packard Instrument Co., Meriden, CT, USA). Steroids were eluted under isocratic condition using an Ultrasphere ODS column (250 × 4.6 I.D. mm) and the optimized mobile phases consisting of acetonitrile:tetrahydrofuran:0.05 M citric acid (39:6:55, v/v/v) at a flow rate of 1 mL/min. Routine data integration was achieved by the Flo-One radio-HPLC workstation software package (Packard) and computed in net counts per minute (cpm), after correction for both residence time and background subtraction.

RESULTS AND COMMENTS

In this work we have assessed rates and direction of androgen metabolism in cultured human liver cancer cells. Major metabolic pathways of gonadal steroids are illustrated in FIGURE 1.

Overall, data from our studies reveal that activities of steroid enzymes, including aromatase, EST, 17β-HSD, 5α-, and 5β-reductases, are markedly

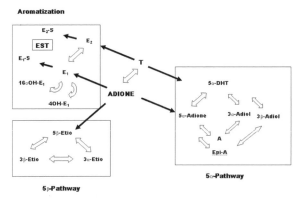

FIGURE 1. Metabolic pathways of sex steroids. T = testosterone; DHT = dihydrotestosterone; adione = androstenedione; 5α-adione = androstenedione; Epi-A = epiandrosterone; A = androsterone; 3α-Etio = etiocholan-3α-ol-17-one; 3β-Etio = etiocholan-3β-ol-17-one; 19OH-adione = 19-hydroxy androstenedione; E_2 = 17β-estradiol; E_1 = estrone; 16α-OH-E_1 = 16α-hydroxyestrone; 4OH-E_1 = 4-hydroxyestrone; S = sulfated form.

TABLE 1. Metabolic pathways of testosterone in malignant human liver cell lines

Steroid	HepG2		Huh-7		HA22T	
	24 h	72 h	24 h	72 h	24 h	72 h
T	4.0 ± 0.3	–	4.2 ± 0.2	–	3.3 ± 0.2	2.5 ± 0.1
Adione	27.6 ± 1.2	–	52.7 ± 2.0	9.6 ± 1.1	77.0 ± 2.6	29.3 ± 1.9
DHT	–	–	9.2 ± 0.8	1.4 ± 0.1	–	1.0 ± 0.1
5α-adione	–	–	–	–	14.7 ± 0.8	25.6 ± 1.5
A	–	–	1.3 ± 0.1	–	2.2 ± 0.3	27.7 ± 1.5
Epi-A	–	–	2.3 ± 0.1	1.6 ± 0.3	1.0 ± 0.1	11.4 ± 1.3
3α-etio	13.3 ± 0.3	–	16.3 ± 0.3	11.0 ± 0.3	–	–
3β-etio	–	–	–	–	1.8 ± 0.1	2.5 ± 0.4
3α-etio-S	–	–	1.2 ± 0.1	11.2 ± 0.9	–	–
19OH-adione	3.2 ± 0.2	–	7.3 ± 0.8	38.3 ± 1.3	–	–
E2	–	–	0.5 ± 0.1	4.7 ± 0.3	–	–
E1	–	–	1.0 ± 0.1	1.5 ± 0.1	–	–
E2-S	7.8 ± 0.4	13.4 ± 0.9	–	2.6 ± 0.2	–	–
E1-S	44.0 ± 1.9	85.9 ± 3.2	3.9 ± 0.3	18.1 ± 0.5	–	–

Values are expressed as average ($\pm$ SD) of two experiments performed in triplicate.

Abbreviations: T = testosterone; DHT = dihydrotestosterone; adione = androstenedione; 5α-adione = androstenedione; Epi-A = epiandrosterone; A = androsterone; 3α-Etio = etiocholan-3α-ol-17-one; 3β-Etio = etiocholan-3β-ol-17-one; 19OH-adione = 19-hydroxy androstenedione; E_2 = 17β-estradiol; E_1 = estrone; 16α-OH-E_1 = 16α-hydroxyestrone; 4OH-E_1 = 4-hydroxyestrone; S = sulfated form.

divergent in malignant HepG2, Huh-7, and HA22T human liver cell lines. Results of both 24-h and 72-h incubation of cells with the precursor testosterone (T) are reported in TABLE 1. After 24 h, all the three cell lines show a remarkable 17β-oxidation, with conversion rates to androstenedione (adione) of 28, 53, and 77% in HepG2, Huh-7, and HA22T cells, respectively. However, aromatization of T to estrogens (mostly as estrone sulfate) attains nearly 52% in HepG2 cells only, is much lower (5.4% as a whole) in Huh-7 cells, and absent in HA22T cells. In addition, 19-hydroxy androstenedione (19OH-adione), an intermediate product of aromatase activity, is found in both HepG2 (3.2%) and Huh-7 (7.3%) cells, but remains undetectable in HA22T cells.

The EST activity, which is responsible for estrogen sulfation, is strictly associated with aromatase activity in HepG2 cells, while in Huh-7 cells nearly 25% of formed estrogens remain in the free form. Once again, no detectable levels of EST are found in HA22T cells. Results after 72-h testosterone incubation are even more clear-cut (see TABLE 1). Aromatase activity rises up to nearly 100% in HepG2 cells and 27% in Huh-7 cells, while it remains under detection limits in HA22T cells. It is worth noting that HA22T cells show a predominant oxidative metabolism and a parallel prevalence of 5α-androgens over products of 5β-reductase activity (66% over 2.5%, respectively), while Huh-7 cells show a marked prevalence of less-active 5β-metabolites (22% as a sum) over 5α-androgens (3%) after 72 h.

Comparable results were obtained using adione as a tritiated precursor (see TABLE 2). Data obtained after 72-h incubation clearly show that aromatase activity is elevated (around 99%) in HepG2 cells, intermediate (34%) in Huh-7

TABLE 2. Metabolic pathways of androstenedione in malignant human liver cell lines

	HepG2		Huh7		HA22T	
Steroid	24 h	72 h	24 h	72 h	24 h	72 h
T	2.3 ± 0.1	–	4.4 ± 0.2	–	–	–
Adione	31.7 ± 0.9	–	55.3 ± 1.7	12.8 ± 0.8	81.5 ± 2.3	31.0 ± 1.0
DHT	–	–	8.8 ± 0.3	1.7 ± 0.1	–	–
5α-adione	–	–	–	–	15.7 ± 0.7	28.9 ± 0.9
A	–	–	–	–	1.7 ± 0.3	29.9 ± 1.3
Epi-A	–	–	1.5 ± 0.1	2.7 ± 0.1	1.1 ± 0.1	10.2 ± 0.5
3α-etio	15.6 ± 0.4	–	17.2 ± 0.8	12.2 ± 0.4	–	–
3β-etio	–	–	–	–	–	–
3α-etio-S	–	–	1.4 ± 0.1	24.5 ± 1.3	–	–
19OH-adione	3.0 ± 0.2	–	–	12.2 ± 0.7	–	–
E2	–	–	–	–	–	–
E1	–	–	–	1.5 ± 0.1	–	–
E2-S	2.9 ± 0.2	4.6 ± 0.7	0.7 ± 0.1	5.3 ± 0.2	–	–
E1-S	44.5 ± 1.5	94.9 ± 2.2	10.8 ± 0.3	27.1 ± 0.9	–	–

NOTE: Values are expressed as average (±SD) of two experiments performed in triplicate.

Abbreviations: T = testosterone; DHT = dihydrotestosterone; adione = androstenedione; 5α-adione = androstenedione; Epi-A = epiandrosterone; A = androsterone; 3α-Etio = etiocholan-3α-ol-17-one; 3β-Etio = etiocholan-3β-ol-17-one; 19OH-adione = 19-hydroxy androstenedione; E$_2$ = 17β-estradiol; E$_1$ = estrone; 16α-OH-E$_1$ = 16α-hydroxyestrone; 4OH-E$_1$ = 4-hydroxyestrone; S = sulfated form.

cells, and not detectable in HA22T cells. Again, the balance of 5α- and 5β-androgens is dramatically shifted toward 5α-compounds (69% vs. 0%) in HA22T cells and toward 5β-metabolites (37% vs. 4.4%) in Huh-7 cells.

The overall metabolic profiles of androgens in liver cancer cells are reported in FIGURE 2. It is immediately evident that while aromatase represents a highly prominent enzyme activity in HepG2 cells, while Huh-7 cells and HA22T cells exhibit opposing metabolic profiles, with Huh-7 cells having elevated aromatase activity and low 5α/5β ratio, and HA22T cells having no aromatase activity and very high 5α/5β ratio.

These divergent pathways of androgen metabolism appear to be strictly regulated and consistent over different incubation times and precursor used. This

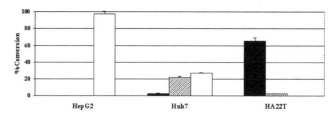

FIGURE 2. Metabolic profiles of androgens in human HCC cells. Cultured cells were incubated for 72 h with testosterone used as precursor. For methodological details see text. Values represent average (±SD) conversion rates from two experiments performed in triplicate. Pathways: ■, 5α-reduction; ■, 5β-reduction; □, aromatization.

evidence is relevant to better distinguish the potential role of gonadal steroids in development and/or progression of human HCC. A distinct expression/activity of key steroid enzymes may, in fact, ultimately point to a different impact of biologically active androgens and/or estrogens on growth and function of human liver cancer cells.

REFERENCES

1. TANAKA, K., H. SAKAI, *et al.* 2000. Serum testosterone:estradiol ratio and the development of hepatocellular carcinoma among male cirrhotic patients. Cancer Res. **60:** 5106–5110.
2. MING-WHEI Y., Y. YU-CHING, *et al.* 2001. Hormonal markers and hepatitis B virus-related hepatocellular carcinoma risk: a nested case-control study among men. J. Natl. Cancer Inst. **93:** 1644–1651.
3. GRANATA, O.M., G. CARRUBA, *et al.* 2002. Altered androgen metabolism eventually leads hepatocellular carcinoma to an impaired hormone responsiveness. Mol. Cell. Endocrinol. **193:** 51–58.
4. DEMYAN, W.F., C.S. SONG, *et al.* 1992. Estrogen sulfotransferase in the rat liver: complementary DNA cloning and age- and sex-specific regulation of messenger RNA. Endocrinology **6:** 589–597.
5. VESSELINOVITCH, S.D., L. ITZE, *et al.* 1980. Modifying role of partial hepatectomy and gonadectomy in ethylnitrosurea-induced hepatocarcinogenesis. Cancer Res. **40:** 1538–1542.
6. KEMP, C.J., C.N. LEARY & N.R. DRINKWATER. 1989. Promotion of murine hepatocarcinogenesis by testosterone is androgen receptor-dependent but not cell autonomous. Proc. Natl. Acad. Sci. USA **86:** 7505–7509.
7. CASTAGNETTA, L.A.M., B. AGOSTARA, *et al.* 2003. Local estrogen formation by nontumoral, cirrhotic, and malignant human liver tissues and cells. Cancer Res. **63:** 5041–5045.
8. AGARWAL, V.R., K. TAKAYAMA, *et al.* 1998. Molecular basis of severe gynecomastia associated with aromatase expression in a fibrolamellar hepatocellular carcinoma. J. Clin. Endocrinol Metab. **83:** 1797–1800.
9. CASTAGNETTA, L., O.M. GRANATA, *et al.* 1991. A simple approach to measure metabolic pathways of steroids in living cells. J. Chromatogr. **572:** 25–39.
10. CASTAGNETTA, L., O.M. GRANATA, *et al.* 1997. Product of aromatase activity in intact LNCaP and MCF-7 human cancer cells. J. Steroid Biochem. Mol. Biol. **61:** 287–292.
11. CASTAGNETTA, L., G. CARRUBA, *et al.* 2003. Increased estrogen formation and estrogen to androgen ratio in the synovial fluid of patients with rheumatoid arthritis. J. Rheumatol. **30:** 2597–2605.

Significance of Autologous Interleukin-6 Production in the HA22T/VGH Cell Model of Hepatocellular Carcinoma

MANUELA LABBOZZETTA,[a] MONICA NOTARBARTOLO,[a]
PAOLA POMA,[a] LYDIA GIANNITRAPANI,[b] MELCHIORRE CERVELLO,[c]
GIUSEPPE MONTALTO,[b] AND NATALE D'ALESSANDRO[a]

[a]Dipartimento di Scienze Farmacologiche, Università di Palermo, 90127 Palermo, Italy

[b]Dipartimento di Medicina Clinica e delle Patologie Emergenti, Università di Palermo, 90127 Palermo, Italy

[c]IBIM "A. Monroy," CNR, Palermo, Italy

ABSTRACT: Cancer cells may often support their own growth, survival, and drug resistance by autocrine/paracrine loops based on the production of different factors; results from us and others have shown that similar interleukin-6 (IL-6)-related loops are operative in multiple myeloma and prostate or renal cancer. Because this aspect has not been investigated in detail for hepatocellular carcinoma (HCC), we have examined it in HA22T/VGH cells. These differ from other primary liver cancer cell lines (that is, HepG2, HuH-6, and HuH-7) in that enzyme-linked immunosorbent assay (ELISA) showed the HA22T/VGH cells to secrete remarkable amounts of IL-6 (16.8 ng /10^6 cells/24 h); this production, due to constitutive activation of NF-κB, is inhibited by agents like curcumin and dehydroxymethylepoxyquinomicin (DHMEQ), which interfere with the transcription factor. Flow cytometry, ELISA, mRNA, and Western blotting analyses were performed to characterize the status of the IL-6 receptor in HA22T/VGH cells. Two transmembrane glycoproteins that form the functional IL-6 receptor have been identified: the ligand-binding gp80 and the signal-transducer gp130. Soluble forms of gp80 also trigger membrane gp130 signaling when complexed with IL-6, while soluble forms of gp130 inhibit the same process. Our results showed that HA22T/VGH cells express gp130 at their surface, but release only traces of its soluble form. For gp80, the cells produced the mRNAs of both its membrane and soluble form. However, in immunoblotting they exhibited a very faint content of the same subunit, which, in addition, was neither expressed at the cell surface nor secreted. In MTT assays, incubation with a neutralizing anti-IL-6

Address for correspondence: Prof. Natale D'Alessandro, Dipartimento di Scienze Farmacologiche, Università di Palermo, Via del Vespro 129, 90127 Palermo, Italy. Voice: +39-091-6553258; fax: +39-091-6553220.

e-mail: dalessan@unipa.it

Ann. N.Y. Acad. Sci. 1089: 268–275 (2006). © 2006 New York Academy of Sciences.
doi: 10.1196/annals.1386.014

antibody for up to 7 days did not affect the growth of HA22T/VGH cells. Also, other specific anti-IL-6 approaches (siRNA or AODN) failed to produce this result. In conclusion, autostimulatory loops mediated by IL-6 are less likely to occur in HCC than in other kinds of cancer. However, since release of IL-6 is frequent in HCC, especially in its more advanced stages, the use of agents like curcumin or DHMEQ might be beneficial to counteract its adverse systemic effects (e.g., cachexia).

KEYWORDS: hepatocellular carcinoma; interleukin-6; autocrine cell growth stimulatory loop; NF-κB

INTRODUCTION

Interleukin-6 (IL-6) is an inflammatory cytokine that induces a variety of biologic responses and influences the growth of several target cells. It may be an exogenous or autocrine growth factor for various tumors, including multiple myeloma and prostate or renal cancer,[1–4] but may also exert inhibitory effects on other tumor types.[5–8] In addition, in situations like melanoma, IL-6 can undergo transition from paracrine growth inhibitor to autocrine stimulator during malignant progression.[9]

Primary hepatocellular carcinoma (HCC) is a frequent tumor characterized by a very aggressive clinical course and lack of efficient drug therapies for the advanced stages.[10] While earlier reports had suggested that IL-6 inhibits the growth of both normal and malignant hepatocytes, more recent data have indicated that the cytokine may support hepatocyte proliferation and play a major role in liver regeneration after partial hepatectomy or toxic insults.[11–13] It may also favor the development of liver adenomas.[13] Nevertheless, it is not clear whether IL-6, apart from host-mediated effects, may exert direct influences on the growth of established hepatic tumors. We[14] and others[15] have reported that treatment with IL-6 exerts definite, though limited, growth-inhibitory influences on the human HCC cell line HepG2; similar effects have been documented in rat HCC models.[16,17] HCC cell growth inhibition from IL-6 can result from modifications of the expression of beta-catenin[14] and of the cyclin-dependent kinase inhibitors p21 and p27.[15] On the other hand, IL-6 release from tumor cells is frequent in HCC,[18] but it is not known whether, similar to other cancer types, the cytokine may support autocrine/paracrine growth regulatory loops in this tumor. To our knowledge, only one paper has addressed such a question, showing inhibition of cell growth by anti-IL-6 antisense strategy in the IL-6-producer cell line HCC-M.[19] Here, we have examined the same aspect in the HCC HA22T/VGH cells.

MATERIALS AND METHODS

Cell Culture

HA22T/VGH is a poorly differentiated hepatoma cell line that contains HBV integrants. It was kindly provided by Professor M. Levrero (Laboratory of Gene Expression, Fondazione Andrea Cesalpino, University of Rome "La Sapienza," Rome, Italy) and cultured in RPMI 1640 medium (Hy-Clone Europe Ltd., Cramlington, UK) supplemented with 10% heat-inactivated fetal calf serum (FCS), 2 mM L-glutamine, 1 mM sodium pyruvate, 100 units/mL penicillin, and 100 μg/mL streptomycin (all reagents were from HyClone Europe) in a humidified atmosphere at 37°C in 5% CO_2. Cells having a narrow range of passage number were used for all experiments.

Enzyme-Linked Immunosorbent Assays (ELISA)

Release of human IL-6 protein, soluble gp 80 and soluble gp130, was determined using highly sensitive commercially available ELISA kits (from Amersham, Little Chalfont, UK for IL-6 and from R & D Systems Inc., Minneapolis, MN, USA for soluble gp80 or gp130). In brief: 5×10^5 cells were incubated in complete medium. After 48 h of incubation, the culture medium of HA22T/VGH cells was collected to measure the extracellular content of the factors.

Assay of Cell Surface gp80 and gp130 by Flow Cytometry

Cell suspensions were washed with PBS containing 1% BSA and incubated on ice for 40 min with anti-human gp130 (AM64, PE-conjugated, Pharmingen, San Diego, CA, USA) or anti-human gp80 (B-N12, Biosource, Camarillo, CA, USA) mAbs. The reactivity of the anti-gp80 mAbs was detected with FITC-conjugated goat antibodies to mouse immunoglobulin (Pharmingen). Washes with PBS/BSA were performed after each incubation. Fluorescence was analyzed by flow cytometry using a FACSort instrument (Becton Dickinson, Mountain View, CA, USA). The results were analyzed using CellQuest™ software by subtracting the cells stained with the FITC-conjugated goat antibodies to mouse immunoglobulin alone or negative isotype-matched PE-conjugated immunoglobulins (Pharmingen) from the cell population stained with the antibodies recognizing gp80 or gp130, respectively.

RT-PCR and Immunoblotting Analyses

Total RNA was isolated from 1×10^6 HA22T/VGH cells using Trizol reagent (Invitrogen, Carlsbad, CA, USA). RT-PCR was then performed using the Superscript One-Step method (Invitrogen). All PCR products (10 μL) were analyzed by electrophoresis on 1.5% (w/v) agarose gel and photographed. The sequence of primers used was as follows:

gp 80: 5'- ACGCCTTGGACAGAATCCA-3' (sense) and 5'-TGGCTCGAG GTATTGTCAGA-3' (antisense);

gp130: 5′-GAGGTGTGAGTGGGATGGTGG-3′ (sense) and 5′-GCTGCA TCTGATTTGCCAAC-3′ (antisense);

β-actin: 5′-TCACCCACACTGTGCCCATCTACGA-3′ (sense) and 5′-CAG CGGAACCGCTCATTGCCAATGG-3′ (antisense).

For Western blot analyses, polyclonal rabbit antibody (C-20) against human gp 80 was obtained from Santa Cruz Biotechnology Inc. (Santa Cruz, CA, USA). Monoclonal mouse antibody against β-actin (AC-15) was from Sigma–Aldrich Srl (Milan, Italy). Aliquots of the whole cell lysates were subjected to SDS-PAGE. Proteins were electrophoresed onto nitrocellulose membrane (Amersham) using a semi-dry fast blot apparatus (Bio-Rad, Milan, Italy). Membranes were blocked with 3% (w/v) BSA in PBS-0.1% (v/v) Tween 20 for 1 h and then probed with the C-20 (1:500) or AC-15 (1:5,000) antibodies. Hybridization was visualized using an enhanced chemiluminescence detection kit (Amersham).

Effect of Anti-IL-6 Antibody or siRNA on HA22T/VGH Cell Growth and Proliferation

Cells were transfected with anti-IL-6 specific siRNA (5′-CUCAC CUCUUCAGAACGAATT-3′) or nonspecific control siRNA (5′-AGGUA GUGUAAUCGCCUUGTT-3′), both synthesized by MWG-Biothec AG, Martinsried, Germany, and LipofectAMINE 2000 (Invitrogen) diluted in OptiMEM (Invitrogen) for 6 h.

The ability of the siRNAs to inhibit DNA synthesis was determined by estimating the amount of bromodeoxyuridine (BrdU) incorporation into DNA by a colorimetric immunoassay (Roche Diagnostics GmbH, Mannheim, Germany). In brief: the transfected cells were incubated for 24 h in 96-well plates (2.5 × 10^3) with BrdU (10 μM final concentration) and either in the presence or absence of FCS 10%.

The effects of transfection with siRNAs or of incubation with an anti-IL-6-neutralizing antibody (MQ2-13A5, Pharmingen) on cell growth were assayed by examining bioreduction of 3-(4, 5-dimethylthiazol-2-yl)-5-(3-carboxymethoxyphenyl)-2-(4-sulphophenyl)-2H-tetrazolium dye (MTS, obtained from Promega Corporation, Madison, WI, USA).

RESULTS AND DISCUSSION

In a screening on the primary liver cancer cell lines present in our laboratory, the HA22T/VGH cells, but not the HepG2, HuH-6 or HuH-7, were shown to constitutively produce IL-6. In ELISA, the amount of IL-6 released by HA22T/VGH was 16.8 ng /10^6 cells/24 h. We have previously shown that this production, due to constitutive activation of NF-κB in the cells, is inhibited by agents like curcumin or dehydroxymethylepoxyquinomicin (DHMEQ), which interfere with the transcription factor.[20]

Different analyses were therefore performed to characterize the status of the IL-6 receptor in HA22T/VGH cells. Two transmembrane glycoproteins that form the functional IL-6 receptor have been identified and cloned: the ligand-binding receptor IL-6 receptor-α (gp80) and the signal-transducer gp130. IL-6 promotes the sequential assembling of a multisubunit receptor complex by binding first to gp80 with relatively low affinity. The high-affinity binding of the IL-6/gp80 complex to gp130 is then crucial for signal transduction, which may proceed through activation of the JAK tyrosine kinase and of different pathways, which include STAT, Ras-MAPK, and PI3-K/Akt.[21] Soluble forms of gp80 also trigger membrane gp130 signaling when complexed with IL-6, while soluble forms of gp130 inhibit the same process.[22]

Our results showed that HA22T/VGH cells express gp130 at their surface (FIG. 1A), but release only traces of its soluble form (in ELISA, data not shown). For gp80, the cells produced the mRNAs of both its membrane (398 bp) and soluble (304 bp) form (FIG. 1B). However, in immunoblotting (FIG. 1C), they exhibited only a very faint content of the same subunit, which, in addition, was neither expressed at the cell surface (FIG. 1A) nor secreted (in ELISA, data not shown).

As expected from the lack of membrane or soluble gp80, in MTS assays, incubation with a neutralizing anti-IL-6 antibody for up to 7 days did not affect the growth of HA22T/VGH cells (data not shown). However, to check the remaining possibility that the IL-6 produced might be still at the basis of an intracrine growth regulatory loop,[23] we tested the effects of a specific anti-IL-6 siRNA in the same cells. Transfection with this siRNA efficiently reduced IL-6 production by the cells (FIG. 2). Nevertheless, it did not affect cell growth and proliferation in MTS and BrdU incorporation (whether stimulated by FCS or not) assays (FIG. 3). The same results were observed when treating the cells with specific anti-IL-6 antisense oligodeoxynucleotides (data not shown).

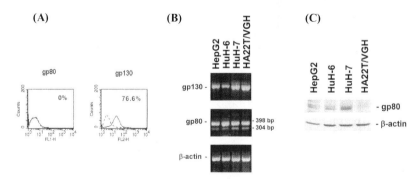

FIGURE 1. (**A**) Flow cytometry analysis of gp 80 and gp130 expression on the surface of HA22T/VGH cells. The percentages of positive cells are indicated in the panels; (**B**) RT-PCR analysis of gp130 and gp80 mRNA expression in HA22T/VGH cells. For a comparison, the results for HepG2, HuH-6, and HuH-7 cells are also shown; (**C**) Western blot analysis of gp80 expression in the cells.

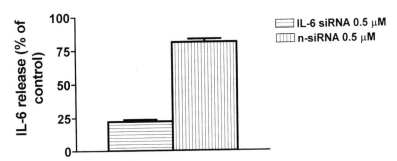

FIGURE 2. Effects of anti-IL-6 siRNA or nonspecific control siRNA on IL-6 release by HA22T/VGH cells. IL-6 release was evaluated by ELISA 48 h after transfection.

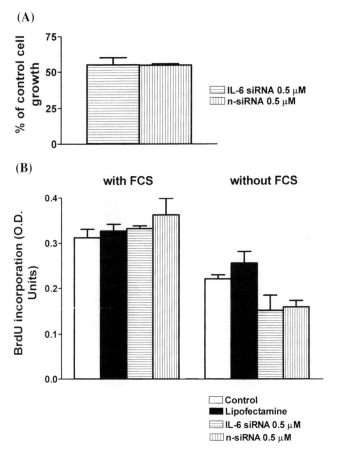

FIGURE 3. (A) Effects of anti-IL-6 siRNA or nonspecific control siRNA on HA22T/VGH cell growth evaluated by MTS assay 48 h after transfection; **(B)** effects of anti-IL-6 siRNA or nonspecific control siRNA on BrdU incorporation into DNA of HA22T/VGH cells evaluated 24 h after transfection.

On the basis of our observations on the HA22T/VGH and other HCC cell lines,[14] we can propose that cell growth stimulation processes mediated by autologous IL-6 are less likely to occur in HCC compared to other types of cancer. Nevertheless, since release of IL-6 by tumor cells is frequent in the more advanced stages of HCC,[18] the use of agents like curcumin or DHMEQ, which inhibit this process, might be beneficial to counteract the adverse systemic effects (e.g., cachexia) of the cytokine.

ACKNOWLEDGMENTS

This study was supported by PRIN MIUR 2005 "Sviluppo e progressione del carcinoma epatocellulare: meccanismi molecolari ed implicazioni terapeutiche."

REFERENCES

1. KAWANO, M., T. HIRANO, T. MATSUDA, et al. 1988. Autocrine generation and requirement of BSF/IL-6 for human multiple myelomas. Nature 332: 83–85.
2. MIKI, S., M. IWANO, Y. MIKI, et al. 1989. Interleukin-6 (IL-6) functions as an autocrine growth factor in renal cell carcinoma. FEBS Lett. 250: 607–610.
3. SIEGALL, C.B., G. SCHWAB, R.P. NORDAN, et al. 1990. Expression of the interleukin-6 receptor and interleukin-6 in prostate carcinoma cells. Cancer Res. 50: 7786–7788.
4. BORSELLINO, N., B. BONAVIDA, G. CILIBERTO, et al. 1999. Blocking signalling through the gp130 receptor chain by interleukin-6 and oncostatin M inhibits PC-3 cell growth and sensitizes the tumor cells to VP-16 and CDDP-mediated cytotoxicity. Cancer 85: 134–144.
5. ONOZAKI, K., Y. AKIYAMA, A. OKANO, et al. 1989. Synergistic regulatory effect of interleukin 6 and interleukin 1 on the growth and differentiation of human and mouse myeloid leukemic cell lines. Cancer Res. 49: 3602–3607.
6. MAEKAWA, T., D. METCALF & D.P. GEARING. 1990. Enhanced suppression of human myeloid leukemic cell lines by combinations of IL-6, LIF, GM-CSF and G-CSF. Int. J. Cancer 45: 353–358.
7. CHEN, L., L.M. SHULMAN & M. REVEL. 1991. IL-6 receptors and sensitivity to growth inhibition by IL-6 in clones of human breast carcinoma cells. J. Biol. Regul. Homeost. Agents 5: 125–136.
8. TAKIZAWA, H., T. OHTOSHI, K. OHTA, et al. 1993. Growth inhibition of human lung cancer cell lines by interleukin 6 in vitro: a possible role in tumor growth via an autocrine mechanism. Cancer Res. 53: 4175–4181.
9. LU, C. & R.S. KERBEL. 1993. Interleukin 6 undergoes transition from paracrine growth inhibitor to autocrine stimulator during human melanoma progression. J. Cell. Biol. 120: 1281–1288.
10. FALKSON, G., J.M. MACINTYRE & C.G. MOERTEL. 1994. Primary liver cancer. Cancer 54: 977–980.

11. HUGGETT, A.C., C.P. FORD & S.S. THORGEIRSSON. 1989. Effects of interleukin 6 on the growth of normal and transformed rat liver cells in culture. Growth Factors **2:** 83–89.

12. CRESSMANN, D.E., L.E. GREENBAUM, R.A. DEANGELIS, *et al.* 1996. Liver failure and defective hepatocyte regeneration in interleukin-6-deficient mice. Science **274:** 1379–1383.

13. MAIONE, D., E. DI CARLO, W. LI, *et al.* 1998. Coexpression of IL-6 and soluble IL-6R causes nodular regenerative hyperplasia and adenomas of the liver. EMBO J. **17:** 5588–5597.

14. CERVELLO, M., M. NOTARBARTOLO, M. LANDINO, *et al.* 2001. Downregulation of wild-type beta-catenin expression by interleukin 6 in human hepatocarcinoma HepG2 cells: a possible role in the growth-regulatory effects of the cytokine? Eur. J. Cancer **37:** 512–519.

15. KLAUSEN, P., L. PEDERSEN, J. JURLANDER & H. BAUMANN. 2000. Oncostatin M and interleukin 6 inhibit cell cycle progression by prevention of p27kip1 degradation in HepG2 cells. Oncogene **19:** 3675–3683.

16. KIM, H. & H. BAUMANN. 1999. Dual signaling role of the protein tyrosine phosphatase SHP-2 in regulating expression of acute-phase plasma proteins by interleukin-6 cytokine receptors in hepatic cells. Mol. Cell. Biol. **19:** 5326–5338.

17. MORAN, D.M., N. MAYES, L.G. KONIARIS, *et al.* 2005. Interleukin-6 inhibits cell proliferation in a rat model of hepatocellular carcinoma. Liver Int. **25:** 445–457.

18. GIANNITRAPANI, L., M. CERVELLO, M. SORESI, *et al.* 2002. Circulating IL-6 and sIL-6R in patients with hepatocellular carcinoma. Ann. N.Y. Acad. Sci. **963:** 46–52.

19. KUMAGAI, N., K. TSUCHIMOTO, S. TSUNEMATSU, *et al.* 2002. Inhibition of growth of human hepatoma cells by dual-function antisense IL-6 oligonucleotides. Hepatol. Res. **22:** 119–126.

20. POMA, P., M. NOTARBARTOLO, M. LABBOZZETTA, *et al.* 2006. Antitumor effects of the novel NF-kappaB inhibitor dehydroxymethyl-epoxyquinomicin on human hepatic cancer cells: analysis of synergy with cisplatin and of possible correlation with inhibition of pro-survival genes and IL-6 production. Int. J. Oncol. **28:** 923–930.

21. HIRANO, T., K. NAKAJIMA & M. HIBI. 1997. Signaling mechanisms through gp130: a model of the cytokine system. Cytokine Growth Factor Rev. **8:** 241–252.

22. JOHSTOCK, T., J. MULLBERG, S. OZBEK, *et al.* 2001. Soluble gp130 is the natural inhibitor of soluble interleukin-6 receptor transsignaling responses. Eur. J. Biochem. **268:** 160–167.

23. ALBERTI, L., M.C. THOMACHOT, T. BACHELOT, *et al.* 2004. IL-6 as an intracrine growth factor for renal carcinoma cell lines. Int. J. Cancer **111:** 653–661.

Anti-inflammatory and Neuroprotective Effect of a Phytoestrogen Compound on Rat Microglia

F. MAROTTA,[a,c] G.S. MAO,[b] T. LIU,[b] D.H. CHUI,[b] A. LORENZETTI,[a] Y. XIAO,[b] AND P. MARANDOLA[c]

[a]Hepato-Gastroenterology Unit, S. Giuseppe Hospital, Milan, Italy

[b]Neuroscience Research Institute, Peking University, Beijing, China

[c]G.A.I.A. Age-Management Foundation, Pavia, Italy

ABSTRACT: Ovariectomized Wistar rats received orally 15 mg/kg of a phytoestrogen compound (genistein, daidzein, glycitein, black cohosh, angelica sin., licorice, vitex agnus) for 2 weeks to test its ability to modulate inflammatory microglia response. Microglial proliferation was tested by trypan blue and by absorbance. Serial supernatant sampling was performed for 24 h to check TNF-α, IL-β, IL-6, and TGF-β. LPS caused a time course increase of all cytokines, with IL-β and TNF-α peaking at the 12th hour, whereas IL-6 and TGF-β peaked at the 24 h observation. Rats fed with the phytoestrogen displayed a significantly lower level of proinflammatory cytokines and a higher level of TGF-β, as shown also by Western blot analysis. This finding may offer promise in the field of nutraceutical intervention.

KEYWORDS: phytoestrogen; rat microglia; neuroprotection; cytokines

INTRODUCTION

There are a number of studies suggesting that glial cells, such as astrocytes, oligodendrocytes, and microglia, play a beneficial role in neural cell viability and survival. This phenomenon takes place through a fine regulation by cytokines and neurotrophins and the removal of potentially toxic cellular debris from degenerating neurons.[1] In particular, microglial cells, which constitute between 10% and 15% of cells within the central nervous system (CNS), belong to the monocyte/macrophage family releasing short-lived cytotoxic factors, including nitric oxide, hydrogen peroxide, and superoxide radical; they are considered to be the primary immune effector cells resident within the brain.[2]

Address for correspondence: Prof. F. Marotta, M.D., Ph.D., Piazza Firenze, 12, 20154 Milan, Italy. Voice/fax: +39-024077243.
e-mail: fmarchimede@libero.it

Ann. N.Y. Acad. Sci. 1089: 276–281 (2006). © 2006 New York Academy of Sciences.
doi: 10.1196/annals.1386.033

However, these cells may be triggered by several stimuli to become activated and secrete a large variety of inflammatory mediators, such as cytokines, nitric oxide, arachidonic acid derivatives, and proteases. Increased levels of these inflammatory components and microglia activation have been localized at the sites of neurodegeneration in several disorders such as Alzheimer's disease, multiple sclerosis, AIDS-associated dementia, and posttraumatic lesions. One of the main hypotheses for such conditions is that chronic inflammatory reaction, driven mainly by reactive microglia, may contribute to the process of neuronal loss and matrix destruction observed in chronic disorders.[3] Recently, it has been reported that microglia, by possessing specific estrogen receptors, may be an important target of estrogen, as increasing clinical and epidemiological evidence indicates that estrogens modulate the immune system. On clinical grounds, several studies have reported that estrogen replacement therapy delays the onset of neurodegenerative disorders, including AD.[4] In the present study we studied the effect of quality-controlled phytoestrogen compound (genistein, daidzein, glycitein, black cohosh, angelica sin., licorice, vitex agnus, Natural Estrogen®; LEF, Ft. Lauderdale, FL, USA) on the release of inflammatory cytokines induced by lipopolysaccharide (LPS) from primary cultured microglia.

MATERIALS AND METHODS

Preparation of Phytotherapeutic Compound

Natural estrogen, which is produced under quality-controlled procedures, was purchased from the Life Extension Foundation, Ft. Lauderdale, USA. It was then powdered at room temperature and filtered through a 0.45-mM filter.

Animals

Female Wistar neonatal rats were bred under conventional conditions and supplied food and water *ad libitum*. Two weeks after ovariectomy, the animals were fed a diet supplemented with 15 mg/kg of the phytoestrogen compound till sacrifice at 2 weeks (A). Ovariectomized rats fed normal chow represented the control group (B).

Microglial Culture

Cerebral cortices were isolated and dissociated in 1 mg of DNase. Then the tissue was homogenized in Dulbecco's modified Eagle's medium (DMEM) with 10% fetal calf serum (FCS) and the mixed cell suspension was plated in a flask. Mother cultures were incubated at 37°C, 95% humidity, and 5% CO_2 for 2 weeks. Microglia growing on the top of the confluent cell monolayer were removed by shaking gently under microscopic observation. Floating cells in the supernatant were collected, centrifuged, and plated onto a 96-well culture plate. The cells were washed twice with DMEM to remove nonadherent cells. The remaining microglia were left to stabilize for 1 week in DMEM with 10% FBS. The purity of microglia was above 97%, as determined by immunostaining with lectin GSA-I-B4.

Microglial Proliferation Assay

LPS (1μL/mL, LPS derived from *Salmonella enteritidis*; Sigma, St. Louis, MO, USA)-stimulated microglia from groups A and B were counted at 24 h as follows: (1) The microglia (2×10^4 cells/well) were stimulated by LPS, incubated in DMEM for 24 h, and then trypsinized at 37°C for 1 h. Then trypan blue was added into the supernatants, and cells were counted by means of a counting chamber microscope. (2) The number of cells was also estimated by a cell proliferation assay system using an absorbance indicator (450-nm wave length) with an established standard absorption curve 24 h after LPS stimulation.

Cytokine Assay

The concentrations of TNFα, IL-1β, and IL-6 in the supernatant of the microglia culture under LPS stimulation were determined by enzyme-linked immunosorbent assay (ELISA). The detection limits of TNF-α, IL-1β, and IL-6 were 7.5 pg/mL, 4.5 pg/mL, and 7 pg/mL, respectively. Each value was standardized by the cultured microglia numbers (2×10^4 cells/well). The amount of TGF-β1 was assessed by specific enzyme-linked immunosorbent assay. In brief: 96-well plates were coated with monoclonal TGF-β1 antibodies, which bind soluble TGF-β1 from the solution. Captured TGF-β1 was bound by a polyclonal antibody specific for TGF-β1 and detected by anti-rabbit IgG conjugated to horseradish peroxidase. Absorbance of samples was read at 450 nm using a plate reader. The sensitivity was 24 pg/mL and data are expressed as picograms per milliliter. Western blotting of cytokines was also performed as follows. Forty micrograms of microglial proteins were separated by SDS-PAGE gel electrophoresis and transferred to nitrocellulose membrane. The membrane was blocked with 5% skim milk in 10 mM Tris–HCl containing 150 mM NaCl and 0.5% Tween-20 and then incubated with primary antibody (1:1000) recognizing TNF-α, IL-1β, IL-6, and TGF-β1 protein. Then horseradish peroxidase-conjugated antibody was applied and the blot was developed by a chemiluminescence detection kit.

Statistical Evaluation

Statistical analysis was performed using Student's *t*-test and one-way analysis of variance (one-way ANOVA). The accepted level of significance was preset as *P* value <0.05. Data are represented as means and SEM.

RESULTS

Microglia Proliferation

Supplementation with phytoestrogen did not affect microglia counting at 24 h after LPS stimulation (1633 ± 26 vs. 1702 ± 43). No main electron microscopic differences were noted among the different groups (data not shown).

Cytokine Release from Stimulated Microglia and Protein Expression

As shown in FIGURE 1, in ovariectomized rats fed normal chow, the stimulation by LPS of microglia determined a time-course-significant increase of all tested proinflammatory cytokines ($P < 0.01$). Such a phenomenon was significantly mitigated in the microglia derived from rats pretreated with the

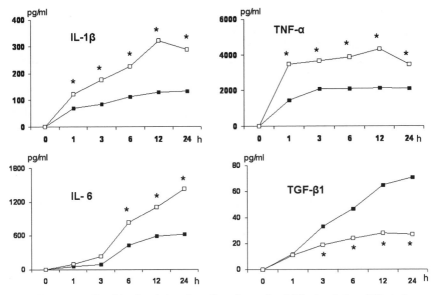

FIGURE 1. Cytokine levels in microglia culture after LPS stimulation: Effect of pretreatment with phytoestrogen.*: $P<0.05$ difference between rats fed phytoestrogen (*black squares*) and normal chow (*white squares*).

phytocompound ($P < 0.05$). Moreover, this group displayed a significant increase of TGF-β1 ($P < 0.05$). Such data were in accord with findings on Western blot analysis, where expression of pro-inflammatory cytokines was significantly suppressed, while TGFβ1 expression was significantly increased (data not shown).

CONCLUSION

Microglia are the immunocompetent, macrophage-like cells that reside in the CNS. However, the overactivation of microglial cells and their release of neurotoxic inflammatory mediators can also contribute to neuronal cell death in many neurodegenerative diseases. Upon their activation, microglial cells release a number of proinflammatory cytokines, which are considered to be important mediators of the inflammatory response. The expression of these cytokines depends on the activation of the transcriptional factor, nuclear factor κB, which is a critical intracelluar mediator of the inflammatory reaction. Therefore, agents that protect microglia from activation by proinflammatory signals may have therapeutic potential in cerebral inflammatory states caused by bacterial infection and neurodegenerative diseases. Although data suggest that estrogen replacement therapy can decrease the prevalence and the severity of age-related neurodegenerative disorders such as Alzheimer's disease, the mechanism involved in the estrogen-protective effects on neurodegeneration is still poorly understood. Estrogen is known to affect specific intracellular receptors which are hormone-regulated transcription factors modulating gene transcription by several mechanisms.[5-7] Although a specific analysis of the mechanism of action of complex phytocompound mixtures was beyond the aim of the study, most of its content was represented by isoflavone phytoestrogens, whose beneficial hormonal-like and antioxidant/anti-inflammatory properties have been shown in recent experimental studies.[8-11] Even though activated glial cells are probably a key factor in the development of brain disease, so far there have been few reports on the effects of estrogen on microglial cells. It was worth noting that microglial cultures from rats fed the phytoestrogen, when stimulated by LPS, exhibited a significantly higher expression of TGF-β1. This holds interest when considering that TGF-β1 has been demonstrated to protect neurons from a variety of insults in cell culture and *in vivo* through a number of possible mechanisms, such as by contributing to the inactivation of Bad, a pro-apoptotic member of the Bcl-2 family, by activating the Erk/MAP kinase pathway,[12] by repressing overactivation of microglial cells via inhibition of PI3K and its downstream signaling molecules,[13] inhibiting NO biosynthesis[14] and decreasing expression of Mac-1 integrins.[15] While current pharmacological treatments are under scrutiny in order to selectively limit their hormonal burden as well as long-term cancer risk, nutraceutical interventions with phytocompounds pose an interesting option to pursue in an overall therapeutic strategy aimed at reducing the detrimental effects of microglial activation in neurodegenerative disease.

REFERENCES

1. BRUCE-KELLER, A.J., J.L. KEELING, J.N. KELLER, *et al.* 2000. Antiinflammatory effects of estrogen on microglial activation. Endocrinology **141:** 3646–3656.
2. RAIVICH, G., M. BOHATSCHEK, C.U. KLOSS, *et al.* 1999. Neuroglial activation repertoire in the injured brain: graded response, molecular mechanisms and cues to physiological function. Brain Res. Rev. **30:** 77–82.
3. GONZALEZ-SCARANO. F. & G. BALTUCH. 1999. Microglia as mediators of inflammatory and degenerative diseases. Annu. Rev. Neurosci. **22:** 219–240.
4. KAWAS, C., S. RESNICK, A. MORRISON, *et al.* 1997. A prospective study of estrogen replacement therapy and the risk of developing Alzheimer's disease: the Baltimore Longitudinal Study of Aging. Neurology. **48:** 1517–1521.
5. GOODMAN, Y., A.J. BRUCE, B. CHENG & M.P. MATTSON. 1996. Estrogens attenuate and cortocosterone exasperates excitotoxicity, oxidative injury, and amyloid β-peptide toxicity in hippocampal neurons. J. Neurochem. **66:** 1836–1844.
6. WEBB, P., P. NGUYEN, C. VALENTINE, *et al.* 1999. The estrogen receptor enhances AP-1 activity by two distinct mechanisms with different requirements for receptor transactivation functions. Mol. Endocrinol. **13:** 1672–1685.
7. SINGH S.M., G. SETALO, X. GUAN, *et al.* 1999. Estrogen-induced activation of mitogen-activated protein kinase in cerebral cortical explants: convergence of estrogen and neurotrophin signaling pathways. J. Neurosci. **19:** 1179–1188.
8. GUTIERREZ-ZEPEDA A., R. SANTELL, Z. WU, *et al.* 2005. Soy isoflavone glycitein protects against beta amyloid-induced toxicity and oxidative stress in transgenic *Caenorhabditis elegans*. BMC Neurosci. **25:** 54–58.
9. GELINAS, S. & M.G. MARTINOLI. 2002. Neuroprotective effect of estradiol and phytoestrogens on MPP+-induced cytotoxicity in neuronal PC12 cells. J. Neurosci. Res. **1:** 90–96.
10. AZCOITIA, I., A. MORENO, P.. CARRERO, *et al.*. 2006. Neuroprotective effects of soy phytoestrogens in the rat brain. Gynecol. Endocrinol. **22:** 63–69.
11. SEIDLOVA-WUTTKE D., O. HESSE, H. JARRY, *et al.* 2003. Evidence for selective estrogen receptor modulator activity in a black cohosh (*Cimicifuga racemosa*) extract: comparison with estradiol-17beta. Eur. J. Endocrinol. **149:** 351–362.
12. ZHU, Y., G-Y. YANG, B. AHLEMEYER, *et al.* 2002. Transforming growth factor-beta1 increases bad phosphorylation and protects neurons against damage. J. Neurosci. **22:** 3898–3909.
13. KIM W.K., S.Y. HWANG, E.S. OH, *et al.* 2004. TGF-β1 represses activation and resultant death of microglia via inhibition of phosphatidylinositol 3-kinase activity. J. Immunol. **172:** 7015–7023.
14. LIEB, K., S. ENGELS & B.L. FIEBICH. 2003. Inhibition of LPS-induced iNOS and NO synthesis in primary rat microglial cells. Neurochem. Int. **42:** 131.
15. MILNER, R. & I.L. CAMPBELL. 2003. The extracellular matrix and cytokines regulate microglial integrin expression and activation. J. Immunol. **170:** 3850–3858.

Activation of NF-κB in Association with Prostate Carcinogenesis in Noble Rats

EMRAH YATKIN, JENNI BERNOULLI, AND RISTO SANTTI

Department of Anatomy, Institute of Biomedicine, University of Turku, Kiinamyllynkatu 10, 20520 Turku, Finland

ABSTRACT: There is an increasing interest in the role of chronic non-bacterial prostatitis in the development of prostate cancer. The aim of the study was to explore the role of NF-κB in the prostate of Noble rats treated with testosterone (T) and 17β-estradiol (E₂), a widely used model for prostate carcinogenesis. NF-κB-positive epithelial cells appeared in both inflamed and noninflamed glands and ducts at 13 weeks after hormone implantation in hypoandrogenemic, hyperestrogenemic rats. Both nuclear and cytoplasmic staining were observed. When daily dose of T was increased to give serum concentration above the level of control animals, dysplastic lesions and ductal carcinomas with NF-κB-positive cells were induced at 13 weeks and 26 weeks. The number of acini with NF-κB-positive cells decreased and no nuclear staining was observed. Surprisingly, no inflammation was seen in the periurethral region where ductal carcinomas developed. In conclusion, no unequivocal evidence was obtained to support the idea that NF-κB would be activated in association with inflammation in the development of ductal carcinomas. The hormonal control of NF-κB in the prostate warrants further studies.

KEYWORDS: inflammation; Noble rat; NF-κB; prostate carcinogenesis

BACKGROUND

The nuclear transcription factor (NF-κB) is well known for its involvement in inflammatory responses. Accumulating evidence shows that NF-κB and the signaling pathways involved in its activation may also play an important role in tumor development. In inflammation-associated models of liver cancer, in which tumor development progresses from chronic liver inflammation to dysplasia, carcinoma, and metastasis, NF-κB was shown to be crucial for malignant conversion.[1] In another model (colitis-associated cancer), selective

Address for correspondence: Emrah Yatkin, Department of Anatomy, Institute of Biomedicine, University of Turku, Kiinamyllynkatu 10, 20520 Turku, Finland. Voice: +358-2-3337438; fax: +358-2-3337352.

e-mail: emrah.yatkin@utu.fi

Ann. N.Y. Acad. Sci. 1089: 282–285 (2006). © 2006 New York Academy of Sciences.
doi: 10.1196/annals.1386.016

deletion of IKK-β—a key intermediary of NF-κB—in cells of the intestinal lining did not decrease intestinal inflammation, but did reduce the subsequent development of, intestinal tumors.[2] Data from these two studies indicated that NF-κB pathway did not affect initiation, but had a dual action: (1) prevention of the death of cells with malignant potential; and (2) stimulation of the production of proinflammatory cytokines by inflammatory cells in the tumor mass.[3] There is an increasing interest in the role of chronic nonbacterial prostatitis in the development of prostate cancer. Overexpression of p65 (active subunit of NF-κB) has been reported in the prostatic intraepithelial neoplasia and prostate cancer.[4-6] However, the findings of nuclear and cytoplasmic staining are inconsistent. NF-κB has been studied in the TRAMP model of prostate carcinogenesis[5] but to the best of our knowledge, not in the prostate of Noble rats treated with testosterone (T) and 17 estradiol (E_2), another widely used model for prostate carcinogenesis.

MATERIALS AND METHODS

Intact adult Noble rats were treated subcutaneously (s.c.) with hormone-releasing implants (Innovative Research of America, Florida, USA) for 13–26 weeks. Each animal received both T (either 240 μg/day or 800 μg/day) and estradiol (E_2) (70 μg/day) implants. Rats were kept on soy-free diet (SDS, Witham, Essex, UK). NF-κB/p65 (Novus Biologicals, Littleton, CO) primary antibody was used to detect activated NF-κB in the prostate. T and E_2 concentrations were measured in serum by using enzyme-linked immunosorbent assay (ELISA) (IBL, Hamburg, Germany) method.

RESULTS

Cotreatment of Noble rats with the doses of T and E_2, which resulted in "low" T (below control level) and "high" E_2 (above control level) in serum, induced a gradual development of perivascular, stromal, and glandular inflammation in the lateral lobe of the prostate. This estrogen-related inflammation developed within 6 weeks (Bernoulli *et al.*, unpublished data). NF-κB-positive epithelial cells appeared both in inflamed and noninflamed glands and ducts at 13 weeks. Both nuclear and cytoplasmic staining were observed for NF-κB (FIG. 1b, c). No dysplastic changes or carcinomas were observed within 26 weeks. When daily dose of T was increased to get "high" T (above control level) and "high" E_2 concentrations in serum, dysplastic lesions and ductal carcinomas with NF-κB-positive cells were induced within 13 and 26 weeks. Dysplastic lesions and ductal carcinomas showed cytoplasmic but not nuclear staining for NF-κB (FIG. 1e, f). The number of acini with NF-κB-positive epithelial cells with cytoplasmic staining decreased (FIG. 1d). Surprisingly, no

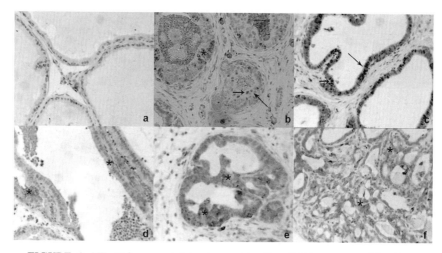

FIGURE 1. NF-κB immunostaining in prostates from Noble rats treated for 13 or 26 weeks. (**a**) placebo-treated rat; (**b** and **c**) 13-week treatment with T (240 μg/day) and E$_2$ (70 μg/day). Note the cytoplasmic as well as nuclear staining in the epithelium of both inflamed and noninflamed acini. (**d**) weaker staining in T (800 μg/day) and E$_2$ (70 μg/day) treatment for 13 weeks. Cytoplasmic staining in a dysplastic lesion in lateral prostate (**e**) and in a cancer in periductal area (**f**) in rat treated for 26 weeks. *Arrows:* nuclear staining; *stars:* cytoplasmic staining.

inflammation was seen in the periurethral region (inside the rhabdosphincter) where ductal carcinomas developed.

CONCLUSIONS

Data show that an increased ratio between the estradiol and testosterone concentrations in serum induced inflammation and NF-κB expression in the prostate. Intense nuclear as well as cytoplasmic staining was found in hypoandrogenemic, hyperestrogenemic animals. This is in agreement with the inverse correlation between androgen receptor status and NF-κB activity (reviewed in Ref. 7). Concordantly, the number of activated (nuclear) NF-κB-positive cells decreased when T concentration was increased above the control level in serum. This suggests an androgenic control of NF-κB expression in the prostate. Ductal carcinoma and dysplastic lesions showed only cytoplasmic staining. Although nuclear localization of p65 indicates the activated status of NF-κB, both nuclear and cytoplasmic staining have been found in human carcinoma samples.[6,4] In conclusion, no unequivocal evidence was obtained to support the idea that NF-κB would be activated in association with the development of ductal carcinomas. The role of cytoplasmic staining of NF-κB remains open. The hormonal control of NF-κB in the prostate warrants further studies.

ACKNOWLEDGMENT

Dr. Maarten Bosland is gratefully acknowledged for his kind professional support during the study. The financial support was provided by the National Technology Agency of Finland (TEKES, project No. 41006/04), Hormos Medical Corporation, and Orion Corporation Orion Pharma.

REFERENCES

1. PIKARSKY, E., M.P. RINNAT, I. STEIN, *et al.* 2004. NF-kB functions as a tumour promoter in inflammation-associated cancer. Nature **431:** 461–466.
2. GRETEN, F.R., L. ECKMANN, T.F. GRETEN, *et al.* 2004. IKKbeta links inflammation and tumorigenesis in a mouse model of colitis-associated cancer. Cell **118:** 285–296.
3. BALKWILL, F. & L.M. COUSSENS. 2004. An inflammatory link. Nature **431:**405–406.
4. DOMINGO-DOMENECH, J. *et al.* 2005. Activation of nuclear factor-kappaB in human prostate carcinogenesis and association to biochemical relapse. Br. J. Cancer **93:** 1285–1294.
5. NARAYANAN, B.A., N.K. NARAYANAN, B. PITTMAN & B. REDDY. 2006. Adenocarcinoma of the mouse prostate growth inhibition by colecoxib: downregulation of transcription factors involved in COX-2 inhibition. Prostate **66:** 257–265.
6. SHUKLA, S., G.T. MACLENNAN, P. FU, *et al.* 2004. Nuclear factor-kappaB/p65 (Rel A) is constitutively activated in human prostate adenocarcinoma and correlates with disease progression. Neoplasia **6:** 390–400.
7. SUH, J. & A.B. RABSON. 2004. NF-κB activation in human prostate cancer: important mediator of epiphenomenon. J. Cell. Biochem. **91:** 100–117.

Catechol Quinones of Estrogens in the Initiation of Breast, Prostate, and Other Human Cancers

Keynote Lecture

ERCOLE CAVALIERI AND ELEANOR ROGAN

Eppley Institute for Research in Cancer and Allied Diseases, University of Nebraska Medical Center, Omaha, Nebraska 8198-6805, USA

ABSTRACT: Estrogens can be converted to electrophilic metabolites, particularly the catechol estrogen-3,4-quinones, estrone(estradiol)-3,4-quinone [$E_1(E_2)$-3,4-Q], which react with DNA to form depurinating adducts. These adducts are released from DNA to generate apurinic sites. Error-prone repair of this damage leads to the mutations that initiate breast, prostate, and other types of cancer. The reaction of $E_1(E_2)$-3,4-Q with DNA forms the depurinating adducts 4-hydroxy$E_1(E_2)$-1-N3adenine [4-OHE$_1(E_2)$-1-N3Ade] and 4-OHE$_1(E_2)$-1-N7guanine(Gua). These two adducts constitute >99% of the total DNA adducts formed. The $E_1(E_2)$-2,3-Q forms small amounts of the depurinating 2-OHE$_1(E_2)$-6-N3Ade adducts. Reaction of the quinones with DNA occurs more abundantly when estrogen metabolism is unbalanced. Such an imbalance is the result of overexpression of estrogen-activating enzymes and/or deficient expression of deactivating (protective) enzymes. Excessive formation of $E_1(E_2)$-3,4-Q is the result of this imbalance. Oxidation of catechols to semiquinones and quinones is a mechanism of tumor initiation not only for endogenous estrogens, but also for synthetic estrogens such as hexestrol and diethylstilbestrol, a human carcinogen. This mechanism is also involved in the initiation of leukemia by benzene, rat olfactory tumors by naphthalene, and neurodegenerative diseases such as Parkinson's disease by dopamine. In fact, dopamine quinone reacts with DNA similarly to the $E_1(E_2)$-3,4-Q, forming analogous depurinating N3Ade and N7Gua adducts. The depurinating adducts that migrate from cells and can be found in body fluids can also serve as biomarkers of cancer risk. In fact, a higher level of estrogen-DNA adducts has been found in the urine of men with prostate cancer and in women with breast cancer compared to healthy controls. This unifying mechanism of the origin of cancer and other diseases suggests preventive

Address for correspondence: Ercole Cavalieri, Eppley Institute for Research in Cancer and Allied Diseases, University of Nebraska Medical Center, 986805 Nebraska Medical Center, Omaha, NE 68198-6805. Voice: 402-559-7237; fax: 402-559-8068.

e-mail: ecavalie@unmc.edu

Ann. N.Y. Acad. Sci. 1089: 286–301 (2006). © 2006 New York Academy of Sciences.
doi: 10.1196/annals.1386.042

strategies based on the level of depurinating DNA adducts that generate the first critical step in the initiation of diseases.

KEYWORDS: metabolism of estrogens; catechol quinones; genotoxicity of estrogens; depurinating DNA adducts; mutagenicity of estrogens; unifying mechanism of cancer initiation; biomarkers of cancer risk

ESTROGENS AND CANCER

One of the major obstacles to the advancement of cancer research is related to cancer's being defined as a problem of 200 diseases. This concept has hindered researchers from examining the etiology of cancer because the study would be extremely complex. The above definition is dictated by the different ways in which various types of cancer are expressed. Thus, the etiology of breast, prostate, and other kinds of cancer in humans is still virtually unknown.

A second obstacle to progress in cancer research is related to the reluctance of the scientific community to recognize that natural estrogens, estrone (E_1), estradiol (E_2), and their specific metabolites, are true carcinogens that induce tumors in hormone-dependent and -independent organs.[1-4] A third obstacle is related to the initial failure to demonstrate that estrogens induce mutations in bacterial and mammalian systems,[2,5-9] resulting in the classification of E_1 and E_2 as epigenetic carcinogens that function mainly by stimulating abnormal cell proliferation via estrogen receptor–mediated processes.[6,10-14] The stimulated cell proliferation would result in more opportunities for genetic damage leading to carcinogenesis.[10,14,15]

There is widespread agreement in the scientific community that cancer is basically a genetic disease, not in the sense that most cancers are inherited (they are not), but in the sense that cancer is triggered by genetic mutations. Thus, cancer can be considered a disease of mutated critical regulatory genes, resulting in abnormal DNA repair and replication, cell proliferation, differentiation and cell death.[16]

Exposure to estrogens has been strongly associated in epidemiological studies with an increase in breast cancer risk, with evidence of a dose–response relationship.[17,18] Induction of prostate adenocarcinomas in 100% of Noble rats implanted with E_2 plus testosterone compared to 40% of rats implanted only with testosterone led to the hypothesis that E_2 initiates and testosterone promotes the development of prostate tumors (see below).[19]

GENOTOXICITY OF ESTROGENS

Substantial evidence has resulted in a novel paradigm for the initiation of cancer. Discovery that specific oxidative metabolites of estrogens can react

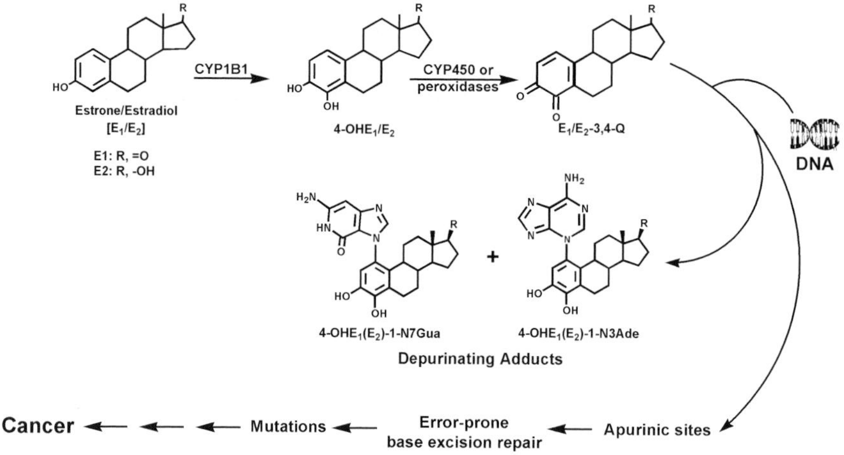

FIGURE 1. Major pathway leading to initiation of cancer.

with DNA led to the hypothesis that ultimately estrogen metabolites can become endogenous chemical carcinogens by generating the mutations that result in the initiation of cancer (FIG. 1).[20–28] Catechol estrogens are among the major metabolites of E_1 and E_2. If these metabolites are oxidized to the electrophilic catechol estrogen quinones, the latter may react with DNA. Specifically, the carcinogenic 4-hydroxy$E_1(E_2)$ [4-OHE$_1(E_2)$][2–4] are oxidized to $E_1(E_2)$-3,4-quinones [$E_1(E_2)$-3,4-Q], which react with DNA to form the depurinating adducts 4-OHE$_1(E_2)$-1-N3Ade and 4-OHE$_1(E_2)$-1-N7Gua.[20,22,25] The depurination of these adducts generates apurinic sites in the DNA. Error-prone base excision repair of these apurinic sites may lead to cancer-initiating mutations[26–28] that transform cells,[29–32] thereby initiating breast, prostate, and other types of human cancer (FIG. 1). The borderline carcinogenic 2-OHE$_2$[4] is oxidized to E_2-2,3-Q, which also forms depurinating DNA adducts, but to a much lesser extent than E_2-3,4-Q.[23]

This initiating mechanism can occur in both hormone-dependent and -independent tissues. Elimination of the initiating step should enable us to prevent a variety of human cancers, including those of the breast and prostate.

METABOLISM OF ESTROGENS AND FORMATION OF ESTROGEN-DNA ADDUCTS

E_1 and E_2 are obtained by aromatization of androstenedione and testosterone, respectively, catalyzed by cytochrome P450 (CYP) 19, aromatase. E_1 and E_2 are biochemically interconvertible by the enzyme 17β-estradiol dehydrogenase. They are metabolized by two major pathways: formation of

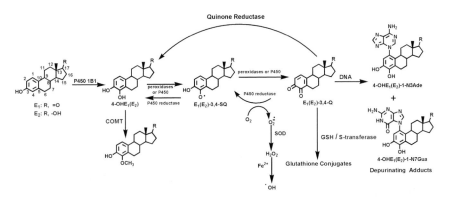

FIGURE 2. Formation, metabolism, and DNA adducts of 4-OHE$_1$(E$_2$).

catechol estrogens and 16α-hydroxylation. The catechol estrogens formed are the 2-OHE$_1$(E$_2$) and 4-OHE$_1$(E$_2$). These two catechol estrogens are generally inactivated by conjugating reactions such as glucuronidation and sulfation, especially in the liver. The most common pathway of conjugation in extra-hepatic tissues occurs, however, by *O*-methylation catalyzed by the ubiquitous catechol-*O*-methyltransferase (COMT),[33] as shown for 4-OHE$_1$(E$_2$) in FIGURE 2.

The level and/or induction of CYP1B1 and other 4-hydroxylases could render 4-OHE$_1$(E$_2$) as one of the major catechol estrogens. If conjugation of 4-OHE$_1$(E$_2$) via methylation in extrahepatic tissues becomes insufficient, the competitive catalytic oxidation of 4-OHE$_1$(E$_2$) to E$_1$(E$_2$)-3,4-Q can increase (FIG. 2).

Redox cycling generated by reduction of E$_1$(E$_2$)-3,4-Q to the semiquinones, catalyzed by CYP reductase, and subsequent oxidation back to E$_1$(E$_2$)-3,4-Q by O$_2$ generates superoxide anion radicals and subsequently H$_2$O$_2$ (FIG. 2). In the presence of Fe^{2+}, H$_2$O$_2$ generates hydroxyl radicals. In turn, hydroxyl radicals can produce lipid hydroperoxides.[34,35] In contrast to NADPH, the lipid hydroperoxides can act as unregulated cofactors of CYP, which give rise to an abnormal increase in the oxidation of 4-OHE$_1$(E$_2$) to E$_1$(E$_2$)-3,4-Q. This can represent one of the major contributions to the formation of E$_1$(E$_2$)-3,4-Q, which are the ultimate carcinogenic metabolites of estrogens.

The 4-OHE$_1$(E$_2$) have greater carcinogenic potency than the 2-OHE$_1$(E$_2$).[2-4] It is difficult to attribute the greater potency of 4-OHE$_1$(E$_2$) to the formation of hydroxyl radicals obtained by redox cycling of E$_1$(E$_2$)-3,4-semiquinones and E$_1$(E$_2$)-3,4-Q, because 2-OHE$_1$(E$_2$) and 4-OHE$_1$(E$_2$) have similar redox potentials.[36,37] Instead, one can relate the greater carcinogenic potency of the 4-OHE$_1$(E$_2$) to the much higher levels of depurinating DNA adducts formed by E$_1$(E$_2$)-3,4-Q compared to E$_1$(E$_2$)-2,3-Q (FIG. 3).[23] In summary, we think that cancer initiation by E$_1$(E$_2$)-3,4-Q occurs via formation of depurinating DNA

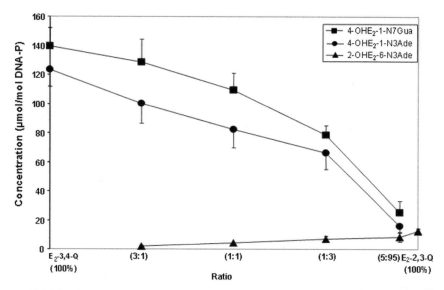

FIGURE 3. Depurinating adducts formed by mixtures of E_2-3,4-Q and E_2-2,3-Q at different ratios after 10 h of reaction with DNA. The level of stable adducts formed in the mixtures ranged from 0.1% to 1% of total adducts. Mixtures containing 0.87 mM E_2-3,4-Q and 3 mM DNA in 0.067 M sodium potassium phosphate, pH 7.0, were incubated at $37°C$. At the indicated times, DNA was precipitated with 2 volumes of ethanol and the depurinating adducts in the supernatant were analyzed.

adducts in which the role of hydroxyl radicals is related to increased formation of $E_1(E_2)$-3,4-Q. In fact, formation of lipid hydroperoxides, the unregulated cofactors of CYPs, by hydroxyl radicals renders oxidative stress more severe.

$E_1(E_2)$-3,4-Q can be neutralized by conjugation with glutathione (GSH, FIG. 2). A second inactivation pathway for $E_1(E_2)$-3,4-Q is their reduction to 4-$OHE_1(E_2)$ by quinone reductase and/or CYP reductase.[38,39] If these two inactivating processes are insufficient, $E_1(E_2)$-3,4-Q may react with DNA to form predominantly the depurinating adducts 4-$OHE_1(E_2)$-1-N3Ade and 4-$OHE_1(E_2)$-1-N7Gua.

IMBALANCES IN ESTROGEN HOMEOSTASIS

Cancer initiation by estrogens is based on estrogen metabolism that involves a disrupted homeostatic balance between activating and deactivating pathways. Several factors can unbalance estrogen homeostasis, namely the equilibrium between estrogen-activating and -deactivating pathways with the scope of averting oxidation of catechol estrogens to quinones and their reaction with DNA. These factors include higher levels of 4-$OHE_1(E_2)$ due to over-expression of CYP1B1, which converts $E_1(E_2)$ predominantly to 4-$OHE_1(E_2)$

(FIG. 2).[40,41] This could result in relatively large amounts of 4-OHE$_1$(E$_2$) and, subsequently, more extensive oxidation to their E$_1$(E$_2$)-3,4-Q. A second factor could be a low level or lack of COMT activity due to polymorphic variations. If this enzyme activity is insufficient, 4-OHE$_1$(E$_2$) will not be effectively methylated, but could be oxidized to the ultimate metabolite E$_1$(E$_2$)-3,4-Q (FIG. 2). Third, the formation of lipid hydroperoxides by hydroxyl radicals, generated by redox cycling of 4-OHE$_1$(E$_2$), semiquinones and E$_1$(E$_2$)-3,4-Q (FIG. 2), can produce an imbalance because lipid hydroperoxides, which are unregulated cofactors in the oxidation of estrogens to 4-OHE$_1$(E$_2$) and 4-OHE$_1$(E$_2$) to their semiquinones and quinones, can substitute for NADPH. This generates a progressive oxidative stress that results in excessive production of E$_1$(E$_2$)-3,4-Q. Fourth, a low level of GSH and/or low levels of quinone reductase and/or CYP reductase can leave available higher levels of E$_1$(E$_2$)-3,4-Q that may react with DNA (FIG. 2). We think that unbalanced estrogen homeostasis represents the critical factor in the initiation of cancer by estrogens.

The effects of some of these factors have already been observed in several animal models for estrogen carcinogenesis and in the human breast. Imbalances in estrogen homeostasis leading to substantial formation of GSH conjugates and depurinating DNA adducts have been seen in the kidney of male Syrian golden hamsters,[42] the prostate of Noble rats,[43] and the mammary gland of female estrogen receptor-α knockout ERKO)/Wnt-1 mice.[44]

Relative imbalances in estrogen homeostasis were also observed in women with breast carcinoma.[45] Levels of 4-OHE$_1$(E$_2$) ($P < 0.01$) and E$_1$(E$_2$)-Q-GSH conjugates ($P < 0.003$) appeared to be highly significant predictors of breast cancer.[45] Therefore, it appears that the oxidative stress that leads to the formation of semiquinones and quinones of catechol estrogens is the result of unbalancing one or more factors in estrogen homeostasis.

MUTAGENICITY OF ESTROGENS

4-OHE$_2$ and E$_2$-3,4-Q have been found to be mutagenic both *in vitro* and *in vivo* under appropriate assay conditions. The Big Blue® embryonic rat2 cell line was used to detect mutagenesis *in vitro*. When these cells were treated six times with 200 nM 4-OHE$_2$, the increase in mutant fraction (number of mutants/10^5 plaque-forming units) compared to untreated controls was statistically significant.[27] The major difference in the mutational spectra from the 4-OHE$_2$-treated cells and untreated control cells was a higher percentage of mutations at A:T base pairs in the treated cells than in the controls (ca. 24% vs. 6%). This is the first demonstration of mutagenic activity by 4-OHE$_2$.

E$_2$-3,4-Q has been shown to induce mutations in the skin of SENCAR mice[26] and the mammary gland of ACI rats (TABLE 1).[28] Although equal amounts of 4-OHE$_2$-1-N3Ade and 4-OHE$_2$-1-N7Gua adducts were formed in both models, the vast majority of mutations were A:T to G:C transitions. These results

TABLE 1. Mutagenesis by E$_2$-3,4-quinone

Tissue	Depurinating adducts μmole/mol DNA-P		Stable adducts μmol/mol DNA-P	H-*ras* mutations	
	4-OHE$_2$-1-N3Ade	4-OHE$_2$1-N7Gua		A →G Total clones	Other Total clones
SENCAR mouse skin[a]	12.5	12.1	0.004		
6 h				5/29	2/29
12 h				4/30	2/30
1 d				7/50	4/50
3 d				3/40	1/40
ACI rat mammary gland[b]	81	90	0.017		
6 h				16/29	3/29
12 h				14/34	6/34

[a]Ref. 26.
[b]Ref. 28.

suggest that the rapid depurination of the N3Ade adducts and slower depurination of the N7Gua adducts result predominantly in mutations at A:T base pairs. The rapid appearance of mutations in 6–12 h (TABLE 1) is consistent only with the mutations arising via error-prone base excision repair of the apurinic sites generated by the loss of the depurinating adducts.[25,26,28]

In summary, the estrogen metabolites 4-OHE$_2$ and E$_2$-3,4-Q have been shown to be mutagenic in cultured cells and in two animal models.[26-28] The pattern of mutations and their rapid appearance *in vivo* indicate that the mutations arise by error-prone base excision repair of the apurinic sites generated by the loss of 4-OHE$_2$-1-N3Ade adducts.

UNIFYING MECHANISM OF TUMOR INITIATION BY NATURAL AND SYNTHETIC ESTROGENS

Oxidation of catechol estrogens to semiquinones and quinones is a pathway that can initiate cancer by endogenous estrogens, as well as synthetic estrogens such as the human carcinogen, diethylstilbestrol (DES)[46] and its hydrogenated derivative, hexestrol (HES). These compounds, similar to the natural estrogens, are carcinogenic in the kidney of Syrian golden hamsters;[1,47] the major metabolites are their catechols.[47-50] These catechols are easily oxidized to catechol quinones. The catechol quinone of HES has chemical and biochemical properties similar to those of E$_1$(E$_2$)-3,4-Q; namely, it forms N3Ade and N7Gua adducts after reaction with DNA (FIG. 4), and the depurination of the N7Gua adduct occurs rather slowly, analogously to the respective adducts of the natural $E_1(E_2)$-3,4-Q.[51-53] As expected, the catechol of DES, when oxidized to its quinone in the presence of DNA, produces the depurinating 3'-OHDES-6'-N3Ade and 3'-OHDES-6'-N7Gua adducts (FIG. 4).[54]

Therefore, the catechol quinones of HES and DES appear to be the critical initiators of cancer by these synthetic estrogens. In turn, these results support the hypothesis that $E_1(E_2)$-3,4-Q may be endogenous tumor initiators because they react with DNA to form specifically N3Ade and N7Gua adducts. In summary, the catechol quinones of natural and synthetic estrogens can be initiators of a variety of human cancers, including those of breast and prostate.

UNIFYING MECHANISM OF INITIATION OF CANCER AND OTHER DISEASES BY CATECHOL QUINONES

Oxidation of catechols to semiquinones and quinones is not only a mechanism of tumor initiation for natural and synthetic estrogens, but could also be the mechanism of tumor initiation for the leukemogen benzene. It has long been known that benzene causes acute myelogenous leukemia in humans.[55-57] Metabolites of benzene include catechol (1,2-dihydroxybenzene, CAT) and hydroquinone (1,4-dihydroxybenzene).[58-60] CAT and hydroquinone can accumulate in bone marrow,[61,62] where they can be oxidized by peroxidases, including myeloperoxidase and prostaglandin H synthase.[63] The resulting CAT quinone can yield DNA adducts. In fact, oxidation of CAT by horseradish peroxidase, tyrosinase, or phenobarbital-induced rat liver microsomes in the presence of DNA yields the CAT-4-N7Gua adduct, while the CAT-4-N3Ade is obtained only with tyrosinase (FIG. 4).[64] Thus, formation of depurinating adducts specifically at the N-7 position of Gua and N-3 position of Ade by 1,4-Michael addition of benzene-1,2-quinone to DNA and the slow depurination of the N7Gua adduct[65] suggest that oxidation of the metabolite CAT may play a major role in tumor initiation by benzene.

Inhalation of naphthalene has been found to induce olfactory epithelial neuroblastomas in 5–10% of male and female rats chronically exposed to naphthalene for 2 years.[66] The only logical mechanism of activation of naphthalene is analogous to the one described above for natural and synthetic estrogens and benzene. In fact, naphthalene-1,2-quinone reacts with DNA to form analogous depurinating N3Ade and N7Gua adducts (FIG. 4).[67]

The catecholamine neurotransmitter dopamine produces semiquinones and quinones via metal ion oxidation, peroxidative enzyme, or CYP oxidation.[68-70] The oxidative process is similar to the one described above for the benzene metabolite CAT and the catechols of naphthalene and the natural and synthetic estrogens. In fact, reaction of dopamine quinone with DNA forms depurinating N7Gua and N3Ade adducts (FIG. 4).[64] The same adducts are obtained by enzymatic oxidation of dopamine in the presence of DNA.[64] Once again, the

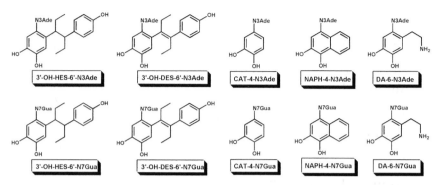

FIGURE 4. Structures of the depurinating adducts N3Ade and N7Gua formed by the quinones of the HES and DES catechols, benzene catechol, naphthalene catechol, and dopamine.

N7Gua depurinates slowly compared to the N3Ade adduct.[71] The mutations generated by this DNA damage may be at the origin of Parkinson's and other neurodegenerative diseases.

In conclusion, the catechol quinones of natural and synthetic estrogens, benzene, naphthalene, and dopamine can react with DNA to form specific depurinating adducts bonded at the N-7 of Gua or N-3 of Ade. The apurinic sites formed by these adducts, particularly the N3Ade adducts, may be converted by error-prone base excision repair into mutations that can initiate cancer and neurodegenerative diseases. This proposed unifying mechanism of the initiation of these diseases lays the groundwork for strategies to assess risk and prevent disease.

BIOMARKERS OF SUSCEPTIBILITY TO BREAST AND PROSTATE CANCER

We have hypothesized that the reaction of catechol estrogen quinones, in particular $E_1(E_2)$-3,4-Q, with DNA to form specific adducts is the first critical step in the process leading to cancer initiation. This suggests that imbalances in estrogen homeostasis result in higher levels of these adducts being formed in tissues in which cancer initiates. Since these adducts depurinate from DNA, they migrate from the cells and can be expected to be in body fluids and to serve as biomarkers of cancer risk.

We have determined the levels of adducts in urine from men with and without prostate cancer.[24] In this study, the 4-OHE$_1$(E$_2$)-1-N3Ade adduct was partially purified from urine and concentrated by using immuno-affinity chromatography with a monoclonal antibody specific for this adduct. The partially purified adduct was then identified and quantified by three different analytical

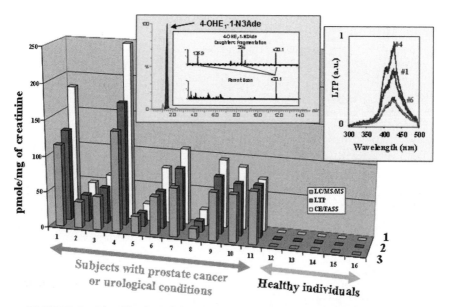

FIGURE 5. Identification of the 4-OHE₁-1-N3Ade adduct in human urine samples from men with prostate cancer or urological conditions and healthy men as controls. Right inset: The spectra labeled 1, 4, and 6 refer to individual samples 1, 4, and 6, respectively; the red spectrum is that of the standard adduct. Left inset: Identification of 4-OHE₁-1-N3Ade by LC/MS/MS. The m/z 420.1 corresponds to the molecular weight of the parent compound and m/z 135.9 and 296 are the fragmentation daughters selected for the unequivocal identification of the adduct.

methods: capillary electrophoresis with field-amplified sample stacking (CE-FASS), low-temperature phosphorescence (LTP), and ultraperformance liquid chromatography/tandem mass spectrometry (LC/MS/MS) (FIG. 5). The samples from men with prostate cancer or other urological conditions contained higher levels of 4-OHE₁(E₂)-1-N3Ade adduct (10–240 pmol/mg creatinine) compared to the samples from healthy control men (background levels). These results provide initial evidence that the N3Ade adduct is a potential biomarker for prostate cancer.

We have begun a similar study of the level of adducts in urine from women with and without breast cancer. In this study, the levels of both 4-OHE₁(E₂)-1-N3Ade and 4-OHE₁(E₂)-1-N7Gua adducts, as well as 30 estrogen metabolites and conjugates, are detected by LC/MS/MS (TABLE 2), after solid-phase extraction of the estrogen compounds from 2-mL aliquots of urine. The sum of the N3Ade and N7Gua adducts in women with breast cancer ranged from 49 to 822, whereas the sum of the adducts in urine from healthy control women was less than 4. These results provide initial evidence that the N3Ade and N7Gua adducts can serve as potential biomarkers for breast cancer.

TABLE 2. Excretion of estrogen-DNA adducts in urine by women with and without breast cancer[a]

Controls[c]	$\dfrac{\text{4-hydroxy estrogen-DNA adducts}}{\text{4-hydroxy estrogen compounds}^b} \times 10^3$						
	N3Ade	N7Gua	Total	Cases	N3Ade	N7Gua	Total
1 – 1	0.5	1.4	1.9	1[d]	131	167	298
1 – 2	0.6	0.9	1.5	2	47	120	167
2 – 1	1.0	2.9	3.9	3	38	174	212
2 – 2	0.5	2.4	2.9	4[e]	706	116	822
3 – 1	0.6	1.2	1.8	5	28	21	49
3 – 2	0.9	0.9	1.8				
4 – 1	0.8	0.8	1.6				

[a]In 2-mL aliquots of urine, 30 estrogen metabolites and estrogen conjugates plus 6 depurinating estrogen-DNA adducts were analyzed by ultraperformance liquid chromatography/tandem mass spectrometry.
[b]These are the 4-catechol estrogens + 4-methoxycatechol estrogens + 4-catechol estrogen-GSH conjugates.
[c]Control subjects provided 2 urine samples 1 week apart, except for no. 4.
[d]Possible recurrent breast cancer.
[e]Recurrent breast cancer.

CONCLUSIONS

We have acquired evidence for a unifying mechanism of initiation of cancer and other diseases. This mechanism predominantly entails formation of endogenous catechol estrogen-3,4-quinones that can react with DNA and yield depurinating adducts. E_2-3,4-Q induces depurinating adducts in mouse skin and rat mammary gland that generate apurinic sites in the DNA. The fast-depurinating N3Ade adducts induce DNA lesions that are important for mutagenesis. In fact, a majority of mutations in the reporter Harvey-*ras* gene are A.T to G.C transitions. Similar A.T to G.C mutations are observed in the *lac*I reporter gene in Big Blue embryonic rat2 cells. Such mutations are thought to be critical in leading to the initiation of cancer.

The human carcinogen DES-3′,4′-quinone, its hydrogenated derivative HES-3′,4′-quinone, the catechol quinone of benzene, the naphthalene-1,2-quinone, and dopamine quinone react with DNA to form N3Ade and N7Gua adducts analogous to those of the natural estrogen-3,4-quinones. In a further similarity, for all of these depurinating adducts, the Ade adducts depurinate quickly, whereas the N7Gua adducts depurinate with a half-life of a few hours. From these similarities, we foresee a common unifying mechanism of disease initiation by these compounds.

The higher levels of depurinating estrogen-DNA adducts observed in urine from subjects with breast or prostate cancer suggest that these adducts could serve as biomarkers of susceptibility that can potentially be used to monitor the risk of breast and prostate cancer. This unifying mechanism of cancer initiation provides knowledge of the factors involved in this first critical step. Furthermore, this mechanism of the origin of cancer and other diseases suggests preventive strategies based on the level of depurinating DNA adducts that constitute the first critical step in the initiation of disease.

ACKNOWLEDGMENTS

This research was supported by U.S. Public Health Service Grant P01 CA49210 from the National Cancer Institute and the Department of Defense Grant DAMD 17-00-1-0247 from the U.S. Army Breast Cancer Research Program. Core support at the Eppley Institute was provided by Grant P30 CA36727 from the National Cancer Institute.

REFERENCES

1. LI, J.J. *et al.* 1983. Relative carcinogenic activity of various synthetic and natural estrogens in the Syrian hamster kidney. Cancer Res. **43:** 5200–5204.
2. LIEHR, J.G. *et al.* 1986. Carcinogenicity of catechol estrogens in Syrian hamsters. J. Steroid Biochem. **24:** 353–356.
3. LI, J.J. & S.A. LI. 1987. Estrogen carcinogenesis in Syrian hamster tissues: role of metabolism. Fed. Proc. **46:** 1858–1863.
4. NEWBOLD, R.R. & J.G. LIEHR. 2000. Induction of uterine adenocarcinoma in CD-1 mice by catechol estrogens. Cancer Res. **60:** 235–237.
5. NANDI, S. 1978. Role of hormones in mammary neoplasia. Cancer Res. **38:** 4046–4049.
6. LI, J.J. 1993. Estrogen carcinogenesis in hamster tissues: update. Endocr. Rev. **14:** 94–95.
7. LANG, R. & U. REDMANN. 1979. Non-mutagenicity of some sex hormones in the Ames *Salmonella*/microsome mutagenicity test. Mutat. Res. **67:** 361–365.
8. LANG, R. & R. REIMANN. 1993. Studies for a genotoxic potential of some endogenous and exogenous sex steroids. I. Communication: examination for the induction of gene mutations using the Ames *Salmonella*/microsome test and the HGPRT test in V79 cells. Environ. Mol. Mutagen. **21:** 272–304.
9. DREVON, C. *et al.* 1981. Mutagenicity assays of estrogenic hormones in mammalian cells. Mut. Res. **89:** 83–90.
10. FEIGELSON, H.S. *et al.* 1996. Estrogens and breast cancer. Carcinogenesis **17:** 2279–2284.
11. DICKSON, R.B. *et al.* 2000. Estrogen receptor mediated processes in normal and cancer calls. *In* Estrogens as Endogenous Carcinogens in the Breast and Prostate, JNCI Monograph 27. E. Cavalieri & E. Rogan, Eds.: 135–145. Oxford University Press.
12. FURTH, J. 1982. Hormones as etiological agents in neoplasia. *In* Cancer. A Comprehensive Treatise. 1. Etiology: Chemical and Physical Carcinogenesis, chapt. 4. F.F. Becker, Ed.: 89–134. Plenum Press. New York.

13. LI, J.J. *et al.* 1990. Estrogen carcinogenesis in hamster tissue: a critical review. Endocr. Rev. **11:** 524–531.
14. NANDI, S. *et al.* 1995. Hormones and mammary carcinogenesis in mice, rats and humans: a unifying hypothesis. Proc. Natl. Acad. Sci. USA **92:** 3650–3657.
15. HAHN, W.C. & R.A. WEINBERG. 2002. Rules for making tumor cells. N. Engl. J. Med. **347:** 1593–1603.
16. WEINBERG, R.A. 1996. How cancer arises. Sci. Am. **275:** 62–77.
17. ENDOGENOUS HORMONES AND BREAST CANCER COLLABORATIVE GROUP. 2002. Endogenous sex hormones and breast cancer in postmenopausal women: reanalysis of nine prospective studies. J. Natl. Cancer Inst. **94:** 606–616.
18. KAAKS, R. *et al.* 2005. Serum sex steroids in premenopausal women and breast cancer risk within the European Prospective Investigation into Cancer and Nutrition (EPIC). J. Natl. Cancer Inst. **97:** 755–765.
19. BOSLAND, M.C. *et al.* 1995. Induction of a high incidence of ductal prostate adenocarcinomas in NBL/Cr and Sprague–Dawley Hsd:SD rats treated with a combination of testosterone and estradiol-17β or diethylstilbestrol. Carcinogenesis **16:** 1311–1317.
20. CAVALIERI, E.L. *et al.* 1997. Molecular origin of cancer: catechol estrogen-3,4-quinones as endogenous tumor initiators. Proc. Natl. Acad. Sci. USA **99:** 10937–10942.
21. MARKUSHIN, Y. *et al.* 2003. Spectral characterization of catechol estrogen quinone (CEQ)-derived DNA adducts and their identification in human breast tissue extract. Chem. Res. Toxicol. **16:** 1107–1117.
22. LI, K.M. *et al.* 2004. Metabolism and DNA binding studies of 4-hydroxyestradiol and estradiol-3,4-quinone *in vitro* and in female ACI rat mammary gland *in vivo*. Carcinogenesis **25:** 289–297.
23. ZAHID, M. *et al.* 2006. The greater reactivity of estradiol-3,4-quinone vs estradiol-2,3-quinone with DNA in the formation of depurinating adducts: implications for tumor-initiating activity. Chem. Res. Toxicol. **19:** 164–172.
24. MARKUSHIN, Y. *et al.* 2006. Potential biomarker for early risk assessment of prostate cancer. Prostate **66:** 1565–1571.
25. CAVALIERI, E. *et al.* 2006. Catechol estrogen quinones as initiators of breast and other human cancers: implications for biomarkers of susceptibility and cancer prevention. BBA-Rev. Cancer **1766:** 63–78.
26. CHAKRAVARTI, D. *et al.* 2001. Evidence that a burst of DNA depurination in SENCAR mouse skin induces error-prone repair and forms mutations in the H-*ras* gene. Oncogene **20:** 7945–7953.
27. ZHAO, Z. *et al.* 2006. Mutagenic activity of 4-hydroxyestradiol, but not 2-hydroxyestradiol, in BB rat2 embryonic cells, and the mutational spectrum of 4-hydroxyestradiol. Chem. Res. Toxicol. **19:** 475–479.
28. MAILANDER, P. *et al.* 2006. Induction of A.T to G.C mutations by erroneous repair of depurinated DNA following estrogen treatment of the mammary gland of ACI rats. J. Steroid Biochem. Mol. Biol. **101:** 204–215.
29. RUSSO, J. *et al.* 2002. 17Beta-estradiol is carcinogenic in human breast epithelial cells. J. Steroid Biochem. Mol. Biol. **80:** 149–162.
30. RUSSO, J. *et al.* 2003. Estrogen and its metabolites are carcinogenic agents in human breast epithelial cells. J. Steroid Biochem. Mol. Biol. **87:** 1–25.
31. LAREEF, M.H. *et al.* 2005. The estrogen antagonist ICI-182–780 does not inhibit the transformation phenotypes induced by 17beta-estradiol and 4-OH estradiol in human breast epithelial cells. Int. J. Oncol. **26:** 423–429.

32. FERNANDEZ, S.V., I.H. RUSSO & J. RUSSO. 2006. Estradiol and its metabolites 4-hydroxyestradiol and 2-hydroxyestradiol induce mutations in human breast epithelial cells. Int. J. Cancer **118:** 1862–1868.
33. MÄNNISTÖ, P.T. & S. KAAKKOLA. 1999. Catechol-*O*-methyltransferase (COMT): biochemistry, molecular biology, pharmacology, and clinical efficacy of the new selective COMT inhibitors. Pharmacol. Rev. **51:** 593–628.
34. KAPPUS, H. 1985. Lipid peroxidation: mechanisms, analysis, enzymology and biological relevance. *In* Oxidative Stress. H. Seis, Ed.: 273–310. Academic Press. New York.
35. LIEHR, J.G. 1997. Hormone-associated cancer: mechanistic similarities between human breast cancer and estrogen-induced kidney carcinogenesis in hamsters. Environ. Health Perspect. **105**(Suppl 3): 565–569.
36. MOBLEY, J.A., A.S. BHAT & R.W. BRUEGGEMEIER. 1999. Measurement of oxidative DNA damage by catechol estrogens and analogues in vitro. Chem. Res. Toxicol. **12:** 270–277.
37. CAVALIERI, E. 1994. Minisymposium on endogenous carcinogens: The catechol estrogen pathway. An introduction. Polycyclic Aromat. Compd. **6:** 223–228.
38. GAIKWAD, N.W. *et al.* 2006 NQO1-catalyzed reduction of estradiol-3,4-quinone. Implications for tumor initiation by estrogens. Proc. Am. Assoc. Cancer Res. **47:** 445.
39. ROY, D. & J.G. LIEHR. 1988. Temporary decrease in renal quinone reductase activity induced by chronic administration of estradiol to male Syrian hamsters. Increased superoxide formation by redox cycling of estrogen. J. Biol. Chem. **263:** 3646–3651.
40. HAYES, C.L. *et al.* 1996. 17 Beta-estradiol hydroxylation catalyzed by human cytochrome P450 1B1. Proc. Natl. Acad. Sci. USA. **93:** 9776–9781.
41. SPINK, D.C. *et al.* 1998. Differential expression of CYP1A1 and CYP1B1 in human breast epithelial cells and breast tumor cells. Carcinogenesis **19:** 291–298.
42. CAVALIERI, E.L. *et al.* 2001. Imbalance of estrogen homeostasis in kidney and liver of hamsters treated with estradiol: implications for estrogen-induced initiation of renal tumors. Chem. Res. Toxicol. **14:** 1041–1050.
43. CAVALIERI, E.L. *et al.* 2002. Catechol estrogen metabolites and conjugates in different regions of the prostate of Noble rats treated with 4-hydroxyestradiol: implications for estrogen-induced initiation of prostate cancer. Carcinogenesis **23:** 329–333.
44. DEVANESAN, P. *et al.* 2001. Catechol estrogen metabolites and conjugates in mammary tumors and hyperplastic tissue from estrogen receptor-alpha knock-out (ERKO)/Wnt-1 mice: implications for initiation of mammary tumors. Carcinogenesis **22:** 1573–1576.
45. ROGAN, E.G. *et al.* 2003. Relative imbalances in estrogen metabolism and conjugation in breast tissue of women with carcinoma: potential biomarkers of susceptibility to cancer. Carcinogenesis **24:** 697–702.
46. HERBST, A.L., H. ULFELDER & D.C. POSKANZER. 1971. Adenocarcinoma of the vagina. Association of maternal stilbestrol therapy with tumor appearance in young women. N. Engl. J. Med. **284:** 878–881.
47. LIEHR, J.G. *et al.* 1985. Carcinogenicity and metabolic activation of hexestrol. Chem. Biol. Interact. **55:** 157–176.
48. HAAF, H. & M. METZLER. 1985. *In vitro* metabolism of diethylstilbestrol by hepatic, renal and uterine microsomes of rats and hamsters. Effects of different inducers. Biochem. Pharmacol. **34:** 3107–3115.

49. BLAICH, G. *et al.* 1990. Effects of various inducers on diethylstilbestrol metabolism, drug-metabolizing enzyme activities and the aromatic hydrocarbon (Ah) receptor in male Syrian golden hamster liver. J. Steroid. Biochem. **35:** 201–204.
50. METZLER, M. & J.A. MCLACHLAN. 1981. Oxidative metabolism of the synthetic estrogens hexestrol and dienestrol indicates reactive intermediates. Adv. Exp. Med. Biol. **136**(Pt A): 829–837.
51. JAN, S.T. *et al.* 1998. Metabolic activation and formation of DNA adducts of hexestrol, a synthetic nonsteroidal carcinogenic estrogen. Chem. Res. Toxicol. **11:** 412–419.
52. SAEED, M. *et al.* 2005. Slow loss of deoxyribose from the N7deoxyguanosine adducts of estradiol-3,4-quinone and hexestrol-3′,4′-quinone. Implications for mutagenic activity. Steroids **70:** 29–35.
53. SAEED, M. *et al.* 2005. Formation of the depurinating N3adenine and N7guanine adducts by reaction of DNA with hexestrol-3′,4′-quinone or enzyme-activated 3′-hydroxyhexestrol. Implications for a unifying mechanism of tumor initiation by natural and synthetic estrogens. Steroids **70:** 37–45.
54. SAEED, M. *et al.* 2005. Mechanism of tumor initiation by the human carcinogen diethylstilbestrol. The defining link to natural estrogens. Proc. Amer. Assoc. Cancer Res. **46:** 2129.
55. RINSKY, R.A. *et al.* 1987. Benzene and leukemia. An epidemiologic risk assessment. N. Engl. J. Med. **316:** 1044–1050.
56. PAXTON, M.B. 1996. Leukemia risk associated with benzene exposure in the Pliofilm cohort. Environ. Health Perspect. **104**(Suppl 6): 1431–1436.
57. RINSKY, R.A. *et al.* 2002. Benzene exposure and hematopoietic mortality: a long-term epidemiologic risk assessment. Am. J. Ind. Med. **42:** 474–480.
58. SNYDER, R. & G.F. KALF. 1994. A perspective on benzene leukemogenesis. Crit. Rev. Toxicol. **24:** 177–209.
59. SABOURIN, P.J. *et al.* 1989. Effect of exposure concentration, exposure rate, and route of administration on metabolism of benzene by F344 rats and B6C3F1 mice. Toxicol. Appl. Pharmacol. **99:** 421–444.
60. SCHLOSSER, P.M., J.A. BOND & M.A. MEDINSKY 1993. Benzene and phenol metabolism by mouse and rat liver microsomes. Carcinogenesis **14:** 2477–2486.
61. RICKERT, D.E. *et al.* 1979. Benzene disposition in the rat after exposure by inhalation. Toxicol. Appl. Pharmacol. **49:** 417–423.
62. GREENLEE, W.F., E.A. GROSS & R.D. IRONS 1981. Relationship between benzene toxicity and the disposition of 14C-labelled benzene metabolites in the rat. Chem. Biol. Interact. **33:** 285–299.
63. SADLER, A., V.V. SUBRAHMANYAM & D. ROSS. 1988. Oxidation of catechol by horseradish peroxidase and human leukocyte peroxidase: reactions of o-benzoquinone and o-benzosemiquinone. Toxicol. Appl. Pharmacol. **93:** 62–71.
64. CAVALIERI, E.L. *et al.* 2002. Catechol ortho-quinones: the electrophilic compounds that form depurinating DNA adducts and could initiate cancer and other diseases. Carcinogenesis **23:** 1071–1077.
65. RAGHAVANPILLAI, A. *et al.* 2004. Slow loss of deoxyribose from N7deoxyguanosine adducts of catechol quinone: possible relevance for mutagenic activity. Proc. Amer. Assoc. Cancer Res. **45:** 1553.
66. NATIONAL TOXICOLOGY PROGRAM. 2000. Toxicology and Carcinogenesis Studies of Naphthalene (CAS No. 91-20-3) in F344/N Rats (Inhalation Studies) (NTP

Technical Report No. 500; NIH Publ. No. 01-4434). Research Triangle Park, NC.

67. SAEED, M. *et al.* 2006. Formation of depurinating N3Adenine and N7Guanine adducts after reaction of 1,2-naphthoquinone or enzyme-activated 1,2-dihydroxynaphthalene with DNA. Implications for the mechanism of tumor initiation by naphthalene. Submitted for publication.

68. MATTAMMAL, M.B. *et al.* 1995. Prostaglandin H synthetase-mediated metabolism of dopamine: implication for Parkinson's disease. J. Neurochem. **64:** 1645–1654.

69. KALYANARAMAN, B., C.C. FELIX & R.C. SEALY. 1985. Semiquinone anion radicals of catechol(amine)s, catechol estrogens, and their metal ion complexes. Environ. Health Perspect. **64:** 185–198.

70. KALYANARAMAN, B., C.C. FELIX & R.C. SEALY. 1984. Peroxidatic oxidation of catecholamines. A kinetic electron spin resonance investigation using the spin stabilization approach. J. Biol. Chem. **259:** 7584–7589.

71. KRISHNAMACHARI, V. *et al.* 2004. Reaction of dopamine *ortho*-quinone in the formation of depurinating adducts. Implications for neurodegenerative disorders. Proc. Amer. Assoc. Cancer Res. **45:** 1556.

Estrogen Action in Neuroprotection and Brain Inflammation

SILVIA POZZI, VALERIA BENEDUSI, ADRIANA MAGGI, AND
ELISABETTA VEGETO

*Center of Excellence on Neurodegenerative Diseases, Department of
Pharmacological Sciences, University of Milan, Via Balzaretti, 9,
20133 Milan, Italy*

ABSTRACT: The fertile period of women's life compared to menopause is
associated with a lower incidence of degenerative inflammatory diseases.
In brain, estrogens ameliorate brain performance and have positive effects on selected neural pathologies characterized by a strong inflammatory component. We thus hypothesized that the inflammatory response is
a target of estrogen action; several studies including ours provided strong
evidence to support this prediction. Microglia, the brain's inflammatory
cells, and circulating monocytes express the estrogen receptors ER-α and
ER-β and their responsiveness *in vivo* and *in vitro* to pro-inflammatory
agents, such as lipopolysaccharide (LPS), is controlled by 17β-estradiol
(E_2). Susceptibility of central nervous system (CNS) macrophage cells
to E_2 is also preserved in animal models of neuroinflammatory diseases,
in which ER-α seems to be specifically involved. At the molecular level,
induction of inflammatory gene expression is blocked by E_2. We recently
observed that, differently from conventional anti-inflammatory drugs,
E_2 stimulates a nongenomic event that interferes with the LPS signal
transduction from the plasma membrane to cytoskeleton and intracellular effectors, which results in the inhibition of the nuclear translocation
of NF-κB, a transcription factor of inflammatory genes. Interference
with NF-κB intracellular trafficking is selectively mediated by ER-α. In
summary, evidence from basic research strongly indicates that the use
of estrogenic drugs that can mimic the anti-inflammatory activity of E_2
might trigger beneficial effects against neurodegeneration in addition to
carrying out their specific therapeutic function.

KEYWORDS: estrogen receptors; inflammation; neurodegeneration

Address for correspondence: Elisabetta Vegeto, Ph.D., Center of Excellence on Neurodegenerative
Diseases, Department of Pharmacological Sciences, University of Milan, Via Balzaretti, 9, 20133
Milan, Italy. Voice: 0039-0250318263; fax: 0039-0250318284.
  e-mail: elisabetta.vegeto@unimi.it

Ann. N.Y. Acad. Sci. 1089: 302–323 (2006). © 2006 New York Academy of Sciences.
doi: 10.1196/annals.1386.035

INTRODUCTION

The steroid hormone 17β-estradiol (E_2) is commonly recognized as playing a pivotal role in female reproductive physiology. However, it is also involved in bone and lipid metabolism, in maintenance of the cardiovascular and neuronal systems, and in male reproductive development and physiology.

In particular, recent studies analyzed the involvement of E_2 and several of its metabolites in the central nervous system (CNS). It is established that the hormone is responsible for the differentiation of sex-specific brain nuclei and for the control of functions and behavior indispensable for reproduction. Recent results of experimental and clinical studies indicate that the hormone acts not only on hypothalamus and hypophysis, but also on other regions, influencing brain functions not related to reproductive activity. In these areas estrogens modulate memory mechanisms, cognition, postural stability, fine motor skills, mood, and affectivity and they exert a neuroprotective action in several brain disorders.

ESTROGEN TARGET CELLS IN BRAIN

The endogenous mediators of estrogen action in target cells are the two estrogen receptors (ERs), ER-α[1] and ER-β[2], encoded by separate genes and members of the superfamily of intracellular receptors. Upon binding the cognate ligand, ERs dimerize and bind to consensus sequences (estrogen-responsive elements [EREs]) in the promoter of target genes; through the interaction with coregulators, integrators, and other proteins of the transcription machinery, ERs regulate the synthesis of selected mRNAs. This genomic activity results in the control of gene expression and of the intracellular levels of estrogen target proteins.[3] In parallel, estrogens also exert their physiological effects through a nongenomic activity, which is characterized by very fast responses and mediated by cytoplasmic effectors such as Ca^+, cGMP, protein kinase (PK)-A, PK-B, PK-C, the Ca^{2+} calmodulin dependent kinase, MAP kinases, and PI-3 kinase.[4] Some groups suggest that these membrane receptors are different from ER-α and ER-β,[5,6] possibly coupled to G-proteins;[7,8] these novel receptors have not been cloned yet.

Localization studies provided a detailed map of neuronal expression of the ER-α and ER-β in rodent brain.[9,10] ER-β seems primarily localized to cell nuclei within selected regions of the brain including the olfactory bulb, cerebral cortex, septum, preoptic area, bed nucleus of the stria terminalis, amygdala, paraventricular hypothalamic nucleus, thalamus, ventral tegmental area, substantia nigra, dorsal raphe, locus coeruleus, and cerebellum. Extranuclear immunoreactivity is detected in several areas including fibers of the olfactory bulb, CA3 stratum lucidum, and CA1 stratum radiatum of the hippocampus and cerebellum. On the other hand, nuclear ER-α immunoreactivity is the predominant subtype in the hippocampus, preoptic area, and most of the hypothalamus, whereas it is sparse or absent from the cerebral cortex and cerebellum.

Recently, however, the presence of hormonally regulated ERs has also been found in glial cells,[11,12] in microglia,[13] and in neural stem cells.[14,15]

Expression of ERs has also been observed in other cell types within the CNS that participate in the inflammatory reaction, namely endothelial cells and circulating leukocytes.[16,17] The vascular activity of hormone has also been observed in the periphery and ascribed to a reduction in the expression of adhesion molecules in endothelial and leukocytic cells.[18,19]

ESTROGEN IN BRAIN PHYSIOLOGY AND HEALTH

Recently, the concept of estrogens and nonreproductive brain functions has largely been strengthened. Physiological fluctuations of estrogens or estrogen treatments are associated with dramatic changes in the plasticity of neurons in hippocampus.[20,21] Behavioral studies demonstrate sexual dimorphism[22] as well as estrogen-dependent alterations in the performance of cognitive and memory tests.[23,24] For example, acute rise of estradiol is associated with impaired learning on hippocampus-dependent tasks and avoidance memory tasks.[25] In contrast, long-term estradiol replacement alleviates deficits in performance of hippocampal tasks.[26,27] In addition, clinical studies have established that estrogens influence diverse aspects of memory and cognition, movements, and fine motor skills in healthy brain.[28] The availability of ER-α and ER-β selective knockout mice highlighted the importance of ER-β in sustaining learning tasks and social activities.[29,30] Also ER-α, which is essential for all sexually related functions, was shown to have a specific role in feeding and open field motility.[31,32]

Neuroprotection

In the last few years a clear and relevant protective role of estrogens against neural cell death has been delineated, as extensively illustrated by animal and cellular models of neurodegeneration.[33–35] This beneficial effect of estrogens can be explained by their neurotrophic and antiapoptotic functions and anti-inflammatory potential.

Neurotrophic Activity

Some studies propose that the trophic activities of estrogens during the maturation of the CNS may continue to exist in the adult brain and ensure that neurons maintain the synaptic connections indispensable for neural signaling and survival. Toran-Allerand demonstrated that estradiol treatment of explant cultures of cerebral cortex and hypothalamus stimulates extensive neurite outgrowth.[36] Since then, several studies in dissociated neurons in culture or in neuroblastoma cells showed that estradiol increases cell viability, differentiation, neurite outgrowth, and spine density and controls the ability of neurons to extend neurites and to form synaptic connections with other cells via dendritic spines.[4] Estrogens were shown to modulate the synthesis of growth factors, such as nerve growth factor (NGF), brain-derived neurotrophic factor (BDNF), insulin-like growth factor-1 (IGF-1), transforming growth factor-beta (TGF-β), and related receptors, TrkA and TrkB, in neurons and astroglia[37,38] and this *de novo* synthesis of growth factors is required for neurite formation.

Anti-Apoptotic Action

Estradiol protects neurons against cell apoptosis by regulating the expression of anti- and proapoptotic proteins, as observed in primary neuronal cell cultures, tumor-derived neuronal cell lines, mixed neuron/astrocyte cell culture, and organotypic explants. Several of the known antiapoptotic genes, such as Bcl-2 and BclXL, are transcriptionally activated by the hormone through the classic mechanism of transcriptional regulation, as EREs are present in the promoter sequence of these genes.[39–42] Accordingly, proapoptotic genes (bax, bad, bcl-Xs) are downmodulated by estrogens, thus indicating that the antiapoptotic activity of estradiol controls the balance between apoptotic and antiapoptotic genes.[33,42,43] In addition, estrogen acts on antiapoptotic protein activity by an indirect mechanism, as shown in the case of BNIP2, a protein that inactivates bcl-2 through protein–protein interaction,[44] which is negatively modulated by estrogens in different cellular systems.[45,46,33]

Anti-Inflammatory Potential

Recent data provided by *in vivo* and *in vitro* studies suggested that estrogens exert a protective effect against brain disorders by influencing the inflammatory response. This anti-inflammatory hypothesis also stemmed from the evidence that menopause, which is characterized by the drastic drop in estrogen levels, results in an increased incidence of inflammatory pathologies of brain and other tissues.

The anti-inflammatory properties of female steroid hormones have been observed *in vivo* in animal models of CNS inflammation, that is, experimental autoimmune encephalomyelitis (EAE, the animal model of MS), brain ischemia, globoid cell leukodistrophy, and experimental brain inflammation. Treatment with physiological doses of estrogen before the onset of disease downregulates the expression of inflammatory factors, including cytokines, chemokines, and their receptors,[47,48] apolipoprotein E,[49] and other modulators of leukocyte migration, such as matrix metalloproteinase-9, complement receptor-3, and scavenger receptor-A[50,51]; moreover, estradiol strongly opposes the influx of leukocytes into the CNS, which is a distinctive sign of ongoing inflammation in these pathologic conditions.[47,52–55]

Our laboratory has been involved in recent years in the study of estrogen action in microglia and brain inflammation. This study stemmed from our original observation that estrogen signaling pathway is active in monocyte/macrophages and that ERs are expressed in these cells.[56] On the basis of clinical data and on few preliminary experimental observations published at that time in the literature, we hypothesized that the protective effects of estrogens in neurodegenerative diseases occur by inhibiting the inflammatory response, whereas hormone withdrawal facilitates this event. Our goal was thus to demonstrate that the physiology of inflammatory cells is regulated by estrogens, that estrogen withdrawal/replacement affects the inflammatory response, and that specific intracellular effectors are involved in estrogen action. Using primary cultures of microglial cells we demonstrated that estrogen inhibits the synthesis of inflammatory mediators induced by a potent inducer of the innate immune response, namely lipopolysaccharide (LPS), a bacterial endotoxin.[56] Using an experimental model of brain inflammation, we then proved that the anti-inflammatory activity of estrogen also occurs *in vivo*. In particular, we injected LPS in the cerebral ventricles of rats and mice and analyzed microglial activation and cytokine expression following various hormonal, estrogenic replacement, and endotoxin settings.[50,51] Hormone action was also analyzed in the APP23 mice,[57] in which amyloid deposition is associated with reactive microglia;[58] we observed that hormone loss (induced by ovariectomy) facilitates, while E_2 replacement delays microglia activation,[51] showing that also chronic neuroinflammation can be regulated by the estrogenic status. In agreement with work by other groups that used different experimental systems of brain inflammation, we identified ER-α as the molecular player in hormone anti-inflammatory activity;[50] this is interesting information for future pharmacological research aimed at defining appropriate selective ER modulators. In addition, by using molecular tools and assays, we were able to show that estrogen anti-inflammatory activity interferes with the immediate early events stimulated by LPS in inflammatory cells.[59] In particular, we showed that estrogen-activated ER-α inhibits the cytoplasmic transport of NF-κB (a transcription factor for inflammatory genes) induced by inflammatory stimuli, thus inhibiting the induction of inflammatory gene transcription. This is a novel mechanism of action among anti-inflammatory drugs, which suggests the involvement of novel, cytoplasmic mediators of estrogen action in the control of inflammation, which may represent possible targets for therapeutic interventions in the control of neuroinflammation.

In summary and as further described in the following sections of this review, the inflammatory response gained the stage with a leading part in estrogen-regulated pathways and is actually receiving much attention from academic and industrial research operating in neuroscience as well as in several other fields of biomedical science on account of the widespread nature of the action field of estrogens and inflammation and of their relevance in human health.

ESTROGENS IN BRAIN PATHOLOGIES

Clinical and Epidemiological Observations

Both chronic or acute–traumatic brain diseases are known to be under estrogen control. These hormones may influence brain development dysfunctions (autism), neurotransporter impairments (depression, anorexia and bulimia), neurodegenerative diseases (Alzheimer's disease, Parkinson's disease, amyotrophic lateral sclerosis), traumatic episodes and injuries (epilepsy and skull trauma), immune system dysfunctions (multiple sclerosis), and ischemic damage (ictus).

The prominent role of estrogens in these CNS disorders has been hypothesized, and in some cases for a long time, based on the evidence that the incidence, course, and gravity of these disorders were strongly dependent on the plasma level fluctuations of these hormones, as it occurs during the menstrual phases, after parturition, or at menopause; additional indications arise from the comparison between age-matched males and females in the manifestation of disease. Several examples of these observations are present in the literature, relating to mood disorders,[52,60] psychotic episodes,[61] Alzheimer's disease (AD),[62] Parkinson's tremors,[63] amyotrophic lateral sclerosis (ALS),[64] or ischemic insults.[65]

ESTROGENS AND INFLAMMATORY-BASED CNS DISORDERS

It is now well established that estrogens are involved in the control of the inflammatory response. The following description summarizes some examples of brain diseases characterized by an inflammatory reaction state, in which estrogens were shown to be involved by molecular, cellular, and pathophysiological evidence. This summary is not meant to be comprehensive of all data reported in the literature on these issues; the evidence provided here helped to sustain both the role for inflammation in some brain pathologies and the involvement of estrogen as a neuroprotective agent through an anti-inflammatory activity.

Alzheimer's Disease

The inflammatory component plays a relevant role in this disease, in which there is a clear activation of the resident macrophage cell population. In human biopsies immunohistochemical analyses revealed a strong activation of microglia around senile plaques, the main pathologic feature of this disorder.[66] Other experiments showed the expression of some members of the α2-integrins family (CD11a, CD11b, CD11c), of LCA (leukocyte common antigen), and of immunoglobulins on the surface of microglia surrounding the plaques. This activated cell population also expresses some pro-inflammatory cytokines as IL-1, TNF-α , and their receptors.[67] Activation of microglia, increased levels of inflammatory mediators, and cells associated with amyloid deposition have also been observed in animal models of AD[58,68]; yet, the precise role of inflammation in AD progression is still debated. Clinical trials involving the use of nonsteroidal anti-inflammatory drugs reduced the incidence of AD.[69–72] On the other hand, many studies support the idea that microglia are beneficial to the diseased brain,[73] through the release of neurotrophic factors [74] and phagocytosis of amyloid deposits.[75,76]

The incidence of AD is higher in women than in men and the progression of this disease has different features in the two sexes.[77] Epidemiological evidences suggest protective effects of the hormone replacement therapy (HRT) on the onset of this pathology and some experimental analyses confirmed this evidence demonstrating the prevention of cerebral structure degeneration by estrogens.[78,79] Population studies on patients taking HRT revealed that there is a 29% reduction in developing the neurodegenerative pathology[80,81] and that cognitive faculties in symptomatic AD female patients can be maintained stably with this type of treatment.[78] Some studies do not show a difference in progression and symptoms in AD in female patients with or without HRT.[82,83] On the contrary, recent clinical trials on women taking progesterone–estrogen combination therapy suggested an increased risk of dementia.[84]

Recently, a model of brain estrogen-deficient AD mice was generated by crossing the aromatase knockout mice with an AD transgenic mouse line of AD.[85] Absence of the enzyme for the synthesis of estrogens specifically in brain areas resulted in the early onset of pathology and in increased β-amyloid peptide deposition.

Parkinson's Disease

Parkinson's disease (PD), a degenerative pathology of dopaminergic neurons localized in the substantia nigra pars compacta (SNc), is also characterized by the presence of activated microglia surrounding Lewy's bodies, α-synuclein accumulation elements. Some clinical studies suggested that this neuroinflammatory reaction can be a critical factor for the development of this disease.[86,87]

Immunological analyses of brain biopsies from PD patients showed the presence of activated microglia cells, with increased HLA-DR and CR3 receptor expression, without reactive astroglyosis[88,89]; in PD tissues, the levels of ROS, IL-1β, IL-6, and TNF-α are increased.[90,91]

Frequency of PD is high in men having a ratio of 1:5 or 3:7 (concerning the ethnic provenience) compared to that in women,[92] who show low symptom gravity and need lower doses of levodopa.[93] In women, pathological symptoms get worse with reduced estrogen levels during the menstrual cycle.[94] Furthermore, symptoms seem to increase in women, which interrupts their HRT.[95] Several retrospective clinical and epidemiological studies tried to connect estrogen treatment with onset and severity of the pathology. These results are discordant: some show indications of a late onset and a decrease in disease risk with estrogen,[96,97] whereas other observations show no difference in these parameters, but an amelioration in cognitive faculty.[98,99] Also, the prospective studies do not reach a definitive conclusion, as one shows that estrogens do not provide significant symptomatic variations,[100] while other studies indicate that hormone treatment reduces the levodopa dose after only 10 days of therapy[101] and that prolongs the follow-up period.[63] One recent clinical study demonstrated that estrogen therapy has a beneficial effect, establishing that women treated with estrogens have a low pathology risk than that of the not-treated ones.[102]

Amyotrophic Lateral Sclerosis

ALS is a neurodegenerative disease that involves primary cerebellar and spinal cord motorneurons. The man–woman ratio of ALS is 4:1 when age at onset is in the second decade, followed by a steady decline leading to a 1:1 ratio at ages above 60 years.[103] The average number of fertile years is significantly lower in women with ALS than in healthy controls, possibly indicating a lower cumulative estrogen exposure among women with ALS.[104] It has also been observed that women who develop ALS had a late menarche or a early menopause.[104] The relationship between sex and disease has been suggested also in mSOD1 transgenic mice (an animal model of ALS) in which it has been demonstrated that exercise leads both to more estrous cycles in female mice and to a delay in the onset of the disease. This is suggestive of a possible neuroprotective effect of female sex hormones in ALS.[105]

Recent studies provided evidence for the involvement of neuroinflammatory processes in this disease. Tissues from ALS patients show a widespread activation of microglia and astrocytes. In tissues, blood, or cerebrospinal fluid from ALS subjects there is an abundant expression of proinflammatory markers like TNF-α, IL-1β, IL-6, IL-2, IFN-γ, RANTES, and the COX enzyme. These data are confirmed also in animal models of mice and rats.[106–110]

The effect of E_2 on the occurrence or progression of ALS has not yet been studied prospectively nor has it been investigated by basic research. A recent study shows that astrocytes treated with E_2 can rescue primary cultures of spinal motorneurons undergoing degeneration induced by AMPA (this is an *in vitro* model of ALS neurodegeneration induced by excitotoxicity). This effect seems to involve soluble factors released by E_2 in astrocytes, among which is glial-derived neurotrophic factor (GDNF).[111] *In vitro* studies have also shown that E_2 protects motor neurons from glutamatergic–excitotoxic as well as from oxidative damage.[112,113]

Multiple Sclerosis

MS is an autoimmune disease in which the inflammatory component plays a crucial role. In the CNS, in particular spinal cord cerebellum and optical nerves, Th1 lymphocytes are stimulated against myelin and can enter the blood–brain barrier through adhesion molecules like integrins $\alpha4$, CD4, and VLA-4. The activated Th1 lymphocytes produce metalloproteinases that can destroy the extracellular matrix collagen type IV. In brain tissue they stimulate an inflammatory reaction, producing proinflammatory cytokines and chemokines like TNF-α, MCP1, MIP1-α, MIP1-β, and RANTES.[114] These molecules activate other lymphocytes, macrophages, plasma cells, and the resident microglia that can trigger a secondary inflammatory reaction. The MS neuroinflammation is triggered also by oligodendrocytes, a cell population that dies by apoptosis and releases other pro-inflammatory stimuli.

Immunopathologic evidence obtained in MS patients demonstrates this inflammatory state. Proinflammatory cytokines are found in MS plaques[115] and it has recently been shown that increased proinflammatory cytokine expression is consistently observed in the cerebrospinal fluid from patients.[116]

High estrogen levels during pregnancy[117] reduce the severity and ameliorate the pathological state of MS, which, instead, worsens after parturition.[118,53] Some MS female patients report a relationship between symptoms and the menstrual cycle, in that high levels of plasma estrogens are associated with remission of symptoms.[119,120]

Observations on the effects of menopause and HRT on disease progression or symptoms are still few. A study by Smith and Studd reported that symptoms get worse with menopause (54% of MS patients) and that HRT ameliorates the disease.[121] Another small study declares that estradiol therapy gives some beneficial effects on symptoms and decreases the TNF-α production.[122]

While clinical studies on estrogen's therapeutic potential in MS are certainly ongoing but results are still to come. Evidence on experimental autoimmune encephalomyelitis (EAE), an animal model of MS, show clearly that estrogen treatment delays onset of pathology and reduces symptom severity.[35,54,123,124]

Recently, it has been demonstrated that beneficial estrogen effects are due to an involvement of ER-α, possibly localized in inflammatory cells like microglia and endothelial cells.[125,126]

Schizophrenia

Studies on schizophrenia focused attention on the immune system after the observation of inflammatory events in schizophrenic patients.[127] These patients showed a correlation between neuroinflammation and the symptoms or severity of disease.[128-130] In tissues from schizophrenic patients an increase in the number of monocytes[131] and high levels of IL-6 expression have been observed. Additional evidence arises from immunohistochemical analyses of patients' tissue, where activated microglia have been observed in the hippocampus and cortical areas.[132]

The incidence of schizophrenia in men and women is approximately equal. Men and women, however, have been shown to differ in both the age of onset and course of illness. Women experience a later age of onset compared to that of men,[133,134] they seem to require less antipsychotic medication,[135] show a higher genetic loading for schizophrenia,[136] and have a second peak of illness onset after the menopause.[134]

The "estrogen theory" proposes that this female hormone allows women to be more protected from psychotic illnesses than men, especially during periods of high estrogen states. Women do not develop psychotic illness until later on in life or experience a less severe illness before menopause.[137] Women have been shown to be more vulnerable to psychotic breakdown at times of estrogen withdrawal, for example, after the delivery of their baby[138,139] and at menopause. The estrogen theory is not without controversy, as a causal link has not been proven. Results are, at the moment, unclear and there is no real evidence for or against the efficacy of adding estrogens to standard treatment for people with schizophrenia. A recent review attempts to present the current evidence for estrogens as a new adjunctive treatment for schizophrenia patients.[140]

Depression

In depressed patients activation of an acute inflammatory response associated with an increase of cytokines levels has been observed,[141] while cytokine levels in patients treated with anti-depressive drugs are in contrast.[142-144] The mechanisms by which cytokines can act in the depressive condition are not clear; it is known that some pro-inflammatory cytokines like IL-1 can influence serotonin signaling inducing synaptic reuptake,[145] prostaglandin expression or synthesis of reactive oxygen species. The inflammatory response that develops in pathological tissues can be related to microglial activation that is able to produce and release inflammatory factors. Unfortunately, there are few experimental observations for this activation. Only in one study conducted on tissue biopsies of patients with bipolar alteration and depression, a widespread microglial activation has been reported.[132]

Women may be more vulnerable than men to develop anxiety or depression disorders. There is a greater incidence of most types of anxiety disorders (i.e., social anxiety, phobias, posttraumatic stress disorder, general anxiety disorder) among women compared to men.[146–149] Women are twice as likely to experience major depression, particularly unipolar depression, compared to men.[150–152] Among depressive patients, pathologic episodes are more protracted and recur more frequently in women than in men.[150,152] Women's increased vulnerability to these mood disorders is especially apparent in major depression with anxiety disorders.[149] Women's increased vulnerability to mood disorders occurs postpubertally, with the beginning of cyclical changes in E_2 secretion from the ovaries.[153–155] Plasma E_2 levels are significantly lower among depressed women.[156] Thus, E_2 may precipitate the increased incidence and/or symptomology of mood disorders in women. Several data suggest that E_2 treatment lessens depressive symptoms among women with intact neuroendocrine feedback.[157–160]

Cerebral Ischemia

In ischemia, the local decrease of blood and oxygen supply to the brain, triggers the infiltration of leukocytes and the inflammatory response, which is a prominent component of the pathologic outcome.[161,162] Blood levels of TNF-α and IL-6 are higher in patients who underwent ischemic injury as compared to healthy individuals. Ictus patients also show increased levels of the adhesion protein ICAM-1 and a high number of leukocytes (monocytes/macrophages and polymorphonucleated cells) in the cerebrospinal fluid.[163] In rats, ischemia is associated with an increased expression of cytokines like IL-1, IL-6, TNF-α, and chemokines including MCP-1 and MIP-1.[161]

Ischemic injury affects women, in particular, when the estrogen levels are low (menopause phase). HRT has been considered a protective element against cardiovascular pathologies; in some clinical studies the administration of estrogens showed a 50% reduction of ictus risk[164] but some other analyses contradicted this observation. The HERS trial (Heart and Estrogen/Progestin Replacement Study) showed an increase in cardiovascular risk in the group of women with estroprogestinic therapy than in the placebo one;[165] the WEST (Woman Estrogen Stroke Trial) showed a complete absence of protection but not of risk; the WHI (Women's Health Initiative) study showed a 40% ictus risk in HRT in comparison with placebo group.[166]

On the other hand, basic research studies provided several evidences to support a critical, protective role for E_2 directly on the arterial wall. Estrogens induce the production and release of nitric oxygen (NO), relaxation of smooth muscle cells in the vascular wall, and the decrease of platelet aggregation.[167,168] The NO production in endothelial cells is mediated by the endothelial nitric oxygen synthase (eNOS). Some studies demonstrated that estrogen-activated

ER-α can activate eNOS by inducing the activity of the phosphoinositol-3 kinase (PI3K) and Akt, intracellular proteins directly connected to the activation of eNOS.[169,170] Other observations show that ER-α can bind directly with the promoter of the eNOS gene and induce its expression.[171] According to *in vitro* observations, animal models of ischemic injury showed beneficial effects of estrogens against neural cell loss through the activation of ER and the reduction of the inflammatory cascade.[55,172,173]

CONCLUSIONS

The data summarized here indicate that E_2 strongly influences the onset and course of selected brain disorders. Our studies on inflammatory model systems, in agreement with published data, underline the relevant anti-inflammatory role of E_2 in brain, which is specifically mediated by ER-α. Considering the relevance of inflammation in brain diseases, more studies are certainly needed to improve our understanding of the role of inflammatory cell activation in neurodegenerative diseases and to identify valid targets for chronic therapeutic settings. The availability of selective ER-α and ER-β ligands (SERMs) allows testing the possibility of selectively modulating inflammation and fostering our future commitment toward the identification of appropriate SERMs as drug candidates in the prevention of neuroinflammatory diseases.

ACKNOWLEDGMENTS

This work was supported by the European Programmes EWA (LSHM-CT-2005-518245), EMIL (LSHC-LT-2004-503569), DIMI (LSHB-CT-2005-512146); by NIH (RO1-AG027713-01); by Telethon Onlus Foundation (GP0127Y01) and by Ministero Italiano dell'Università e della Ricerca Scientifica (COFIN 2004057090_008).

REFERENCES

1. GREEN, S., P. WALTER, V. KUMAR, *et al.* 1986. Human oestrogen receptor cDNA: sequence, expression and homology to v-erb-A. Nature **320:** 134–139.
2. KUIPER, G.G., E. ENMARK, M. PELTO-HUIKKO, *et al.* 1996. Cloning of a novel receptor expressed in rat prostate and ovary. Proc. Natl. Acad. Sci. USA **93:** 5925–5930.
3. LEVIN, E.R. 2005. Integration of the extranuclear and nuclear actions of estrogen. Mol. Endocrinol. **19:** 1951–1959.
4. MAGGI, A., P. CIANA, S. BELCREDITO, *et al.* 2004. Estrogens in the nervous system: mechanisms and nonreproductive functions. Annu. Rev. Physiol. **66:** 291–313.

5. DAS, S.K., J.A. TAYLOR, *et al.* 1997. Estrogenic responses in estrogen receptor-alpha deficient mice reveal a distinct estrogen signaling pathway. Proc. Natl. Acad. Sci. USA **94:** 12786–12791.

6. NADAL, A., A.B. ROPERO, *et al.* 2000. Nongenomic actions of estrogens and xenoestrogens by binding at a plasma membrane receptor unrelated to estrogen receptor alpha and estrogen receptor beta. Proc. Natl. Acad. Sci. USA **97:** 11603–11608.

7. KELLY, M.J., J. QIU, *et al.* 2003. Estrogen modulation of G-protein-coupled receptor activation of potassium channels in the central nervous system. Ann. N. Y. Acad. Sci. **1007:** 6–16.

8. WYCKOFF, M.H., K.L. CHAMBLISS, *et al.* 2001. Plasma membrane estrogen receptors are coupled to endothelial nitric-oxide synthase through Galpha(i). J. Biol. Chem. **276:** 27071–27076.

9. COUSE, J.F., J. LINDZEY , K. GRANDIEN, *et al.* 1997. Tissue distribution and quantitative analysis of estrogen receptor-alpha (ERalpha) and estrogen receptor-beta (ERbeta) messenger ribonucleic acid in the wild-type and ERalpha-knockout mouse. Endocrinology **138:** 4613–4621.

10. SHUGHRUE, P.J. & I. MERCHENTHALER. 2001. Distribution of estrogen receptor beta immunoreactivity in the rat central nervous system. J. Comp. Neurol. **436:** 64–81.

11. JUNG-TESTAS, I., M. RENOIR, H. BUGNARD, *et al.* 1992. Demonstration of steroid hormone receptors and steroid action in primary cultures of rat glial cells. J. Steroid Biochem. Mol. Biol. **41:** 621–631.

12. SANTAGATI, S., R.C. MELCANGI, F. CELOTTI, *et al.* 1994. Estrogen receptor is expressed in different types of glial cells in culture. J. Neurochem. **63:** 2058–2064.

13. VEGETO, E., S. GHISLETTI, C. MEDA, *et al.* 2004. Regulation of the lipopolysaccharide signal transduction pathway by 17beta-estradiol in macrophage cells. J. Steroid Biochem. Mol. Biol. **91:** 59–66.

14. BRANNWALL, K., L. KORHONEN & D. LINDHOLM. 2002. Estrogen-receptor-dependent regulation of neural stem cell proliferation and differentiation. Mol. Cell. Neurosci. **21:** 512–520.

15. TANAPAT, P., N.B. HASTINGS, A.I. REEVES, *et al.* 1999. Estrogen stimulates a transient increase in the number of new neurons in the dentate gyrus of the adult female rat. J. Neurosci. **19:** 5792–5801.

16. GILMORE, W., I.P. WEINER & J. CORREALE. 1997. Effect of estradiol on cytokine secretion by proteolipid protein-specific T cell clones isolated from multiple sclerosis patients and normal control subjects. J. Immunol. **158:** 446–451.

17. CORREALE, J., M. ARIAS & W. GILMORE. 1998. Steroid hormone regulation of cytokine secretion by proteolipid protein-specific CD4C T cell clones isolated from multiple sclerosis patients and normal control subjects. J. Immunol. **161:** 3365–3374.

18. NATHAN, L., S. PERVIN, R. SINGH, *et al.* 1999. Estradiol inhibits leukocyte adhesion and transendothelial migration in rabbits in vivo: possible mechanisms for gender differences in atherosclerosis. Circ. Res. **85:** 377–385.

19. CAULIN-GLASER, T., W.J. FARRELL, S.E. PFAU, *et al.* 1998. Modulation of circulating cellular adhesion molecules in postmenopausal women with coronary artery disease. J. Am. Coll. Cardiol. **31:** 1555–1560.

20. Foy, M.R. & T.J. Teyler. 1983. 17-alphaestradiol and 17-beta-estradiol in hippocampus. Brain Res. Bull. **10:** 735–739.

21. Woolley, C.S., E. Gould, M. Frankfurt, *et al.* 1990. Naturally occurring fluctuation in dendritic spine density on adult hippocampal pyramidal neurons. J. Neurosci. **10:** 4035–4039.

22. Fugger, H.N., S.G. Cunningham, E.F. Rissman, *et al.* 1998. Sex differences in the activational effect of ERalpha on spatial learning. Horm. Behav. **34:** 163–170.

23. Luine, V. & M. Rodriguez. 1994. Effects of estradiol on radial arm maze performance of young and aged rats. Behav. Neural Biol. **62:** 230–236.

24. Packard, M.G. & L.A. Teather. 1997. Intrahippocampal estradiol infusion enhances memory in ovariectomized rats. Neuroreport **8:** 3009–3013.

25. Galea, L.A., M. Kavaliers, K.P. Ossenkopp, *et al.* 1995. Gonadal hormone levels and spatial learning performance in the Morris water maze in male and female meadow voles, *Microtus pennsylvanicus*. Horm. Behav. **29:** 106–125.

26. Fader, A.J., A.W. Hendricson & G.P. Dohanich. 1998. Estrogen improves performance of reinforced T-maze alternation and prevents the amnestic effects of scopolamine administered systemically or intrahippocampally. Neurobiol. Learn Mem. **69:** 225–240.

27. Gibbs, R.B. 1999. Estrogen replacement enhances acquisition of a spatial memory task and reduces deficits associated with hippocampal muscarinic receptor inhibition. Horm. Behav. **36:** 222–233.

28. Jarvik, L.F. 1975. Human intelligence: sex differences. Acta Genet. Med. Gamellol. **24:** 189–211.

29. Rissman, E.F., A.l. Heck, J.E. Leonard, *et al.* 2002. Disruption of estrogen receptor beta gene impairs spatial learning in female mice. Proc. Natl. Acad. Sci. USA **99:** 3996–4001.

30. Ogawa, S., D.B. Lubahn, K.S. Korach, *et al.* 1997. Behavioral effects of estrogen receptor gene disruption in male mice. Proc. Natl. Acad. Sci. USA **94:** 1476–1481.

31. Geary, N., l. Asarian, K.S. Korach, *et al.* 2001. Deficits in E2- dependent control of feeding, weight gain, and cholecystokinin satiation in ER-alpha null mice. Endocrinology **142:** 4751–4757.

32. Nomura, M., l. Durbak, J. Chan, *et al.* 2002. Genotype/age interactions on aggressive behaviour in gonadally intact estrogen receptor beta knockout (betaERKO) male mice. Horm. Behav. **41:** 288–296.

33. Meda, C., E. Vegeto, G. Pollio, *et al.* 2000. Oestrogen prevention of neural cell death correlates with decreased expression of mRNA for the pro-apoptotic protein nip-2. J. Neuroendocrinol. **12:** 1051–1059.

34. Behl, C., T. Skutella, F. Lezoualc'h, *et al.* 1997. Neuroprotection against oxidative stress by estrogens: structure-activity relationship. Mol. Pharmacol. **51:** 535–541.

35. Bebo, B.F. Jr, A. Fyfe-Johnson, K. Adlard, *et al.* 2001. Low-dose estrogen therapy ameliorates experimental autoimmune encephalomyelitis in two different inbred mouse strains. J. Immunol. **166:** 2080–2089.

36. Toran-Allerand, C.D., J. Gerlach & B. McEwen. 1980. Autoradiographic localization of [3H]estradiol related to steroid responsiveness in cultures of the newborn mouse hypothalamus and preoptic area. Brain Res. **184:** 517–522.

37. PEREZ-POLO, J.R., K. HALL, K. LIVINGSTON, et al. 1977. Steroid induction of nerve growth factor synthesis in cell culture. Life Sci. **21:** 1535–1544.
38. CARDONA-GOMEZ, G.P., J.A. CHOWEN & L.M. GARCIA-SEGURA. 2000. Estradiol and progesterone regulate the expression of insulin-like growth factor-I receptor and insulin-like growth factor binding protein- 2 in the hypothalamus of adult female rats. J. Neurobiol. **43:** 269–281.
39. DONG, L., W. WANG, F. WANG, et al. 1999. Mechanisms of transcriptional activation of bcl-2 gene expression by 17b-estradiol in breast cancer cells. J. Biol. Chem **274:** 32099–32107.
40. GOLLAPUDI, L. & M.M. OBLINGER. 1999. Estrogen and NFG synergically protect terminally differentiated, ERa-transfected PC-12 cells from apoptosis. J. Neurosci. Res. **56:** 471–481.
41. GARCIA-SEGURA, L.M., P. CARDONA-GOMEZ, F. NAFTOLIN, et al. 1998. Estradiol upregulates bcl-2 expression in adult brain neurons. Neuroreport **9:** 595–597.
42. PIKE, C.J. 1999. Estrogen modulates neuronal bcl-xL expression and β-amyloid-induced apoptosis: relevance to Alzheimer disease. J. Neurochem. **72:** 1552–1563.
43. PATRONE, C., S. ANDERSSON, L. KORHONEN, et al. 1999. Estrogen receptor dependent regulation of sensory neuron survival in developing dorsal root ganglion. Proc. Natl. Acad. Sci. USA **96:** 10905–10910.
44. BOYD. 1994. Adenovirus E1B 19 kDa and Bcl-2 proteins interact with a common set of cellular proteins. Cell. **79:** 341–351.
45. GARNIER, M., D. DI LORENZO, A. ALBERTINI, et al. 1997. Identification of estogen-responsive genes in neuroblastoma SK-ER3 cells. J. Neurosci. **17:** 4591–4599.
46. VEGETO, E., G. POLLIO, C. PELLICCIARI, et al. 1999. Estrogen and progesteron induction of survival of monoblastoid cells undergoing TNFa- induced apoptosis. FASEB J. **13:** 793–803.
47. MATSUDA, J., M.T. VANIER, Y. SAITO, et al. 2001. Dramatic phenotypic improvement during pregnancy in a genetic leukodystrophy: estrogen appears to be a critical factor. Hum. Mol. Genet. **10:** 2709–2715.
48. MATEJUK, A., K. ADLARD, et al. 2001. 17β-estradiol inhibits cytokine, chemochine and chemochine receptor mRNA expression in the central nervous system of female mice with experimental autoimmune encephalomyelitis. J. Neurosci. Res. **65:** 529–542.
49. HORSBURGH, K., I.M. MACRAE & H. CARSWELL. 2002. Estrogen is neuroprotective via an apolipoprotein E-dependent mechanism in a mouse model of global ischemia. J. Cereb. Blood Flow Metab. **22:** 1189–1195.
50. VEGETO, E., S. BELCREDITO, S. ETTERI, et al. 2003. Estrogen receptor-alpha mediates the brain antiinflammatory activity of estradiol. Proc. Natl. Acad. Sci. USA **100:** 9614–9619.
51. VEGETO, E., S. BELCREDITO, S. GHISLETTI, et al. 2006. The endogenous estrogen status regulates microglia reactivity in animal models of neuroinflammation. Endocrinology **147:** 2263–2272.
52. WEISSMAN, M.M., R. BLAND, R.P. JOYCE, et al. 1993. Sex differences in rates of depression: cross-national perspectives. J. Affect. Disord. **29:** 77–84.
53. JANSSON, L. & R. HOLMDAHL. 1998. Estrogen mediated immunosuppression in autoimmune diseases. Inflamm. Res. **47:** 290–301.

54. ITO, A., B.F. BEBO JR, A. MATEJUK, *et al.* 2001. Estrogen treatment down-regulates TNF-alpha production and reduces the severity of experimental autoimmune encephalomyelitis in cytokine knockout mice. J. Immunol. **167:** 542–552.
55. SANTINO, R.A., S. ANDERSON, *et al.* 2000. Effects of estrogen on leukocyte adhesion after transient forebrain ischemia. Stroke **31:** 2231–2235.
56. VEGETO, E., C. BONINCONTRO, *et al.* 2001. Estrogen prevents the lipopolysaccharide-induced inflammatory response in microglia. J. Neurosci. **21:** 1809–1818.
57. STURCHLER-PIERRAT, C., D. ABRAMOWSKI, M. DUKE, *et al.* 1997. Two amyloid precursor protein transgenic mouse models with Alzheimer disease-like pathology. Proc. Natl. Acad. Sci. USA **94:** 13287–13292.
58. BOMEMANN, K.D., K.H. WIEDERHOLD, C. PAULI, *et al.* 2001. Abeta-induced inflammatory processes in microglia cells of APP23 transgenic mice. Am. J. Pathol. **158:** 63–73.
59. GHISLETTI, S., C. MEDA, A. MAGGI, *et al.* 2005. 17beta-estradiol inhibits inflammatory gene expression by controlling NF-kappaB intracellular localization. Mol. Cell. Biol. **25:** 2957–2968.
60. GREGOIRE, A. & R. DRAHMOUNE. 2000. Clinical case of the month. Case report of adrenal metastases from lung adenocarcinoma Rev. Med. Liege **55:** 8–10.
61. HUBER, T.J., J. ROLLNIK, J. WILHELMS, *et al.* 2001. Estradiol levels in psychotic disorders. Psychoneuroendocrinology **26:** 27–35.
62. HENDERSON, V.W. 1997. Estrogen replacement therapy for the prevention and treatment of Alzheimer's disease. CNS Drugs **8:** 343–351.
63. TSANG, K.L., S.L. HO & S.K. LO. 2000. Estrogen improves motor disability in Parkinsonian postmenopausal women with motor fluctuations. Neurology **54:** 2292–2298.
64. VELDINK, J.K., P.R. BAR̆, E.A. JOOSTEN, *et al.* 2003. Sexual differences in onset of disease and response to exercise in a transgenic model of ALS. Neuromuscul. Disord. **13:** 737–743.
65. PAGANINI-HILL, A. 1995. Estrogen replacement therapy and stroke. Prog. Cardiovasc. Dis. **38:** 223–242.
66. KALARIA, R.N. & G. PERRY. 1993. Amyloid P component and other acute-phase proteins associated with cerebellar A beta deposits in Alzheimer's disease. Brain Res. **631:** 151–155.
67. TUPPO, E.E. & H.R. ARIAS. 2005. The role of inflammation in Alzheimer's disease. IJBCB **37:** 289–305.
68. SIMARD, A.R., D. SOULET, G. GOWING, *et al.* 2006. Bone marrow-derived microglia play a critical role in restricting senile plaque formation in Alzheimer's disease. Neuron **49:** 489–502.
69. STEWART, W.F., C. KAWAS, M. CORRADA, *et al.* 1997. Risk of Alzheimer's disease and duration of NSAID use. Neurology **48:** 626–632.
70. ANTHONY, J.C., J.C. BREITNER, P.P. ZANDI, *et al.* 2000. Reduced prevalence of AD in users of NSAIDs and H2 receptor antagonists: the Cache County study. Neurology **54:** 2066–2071.
71. IN T' VELD, B.A., A. RUITENBERG, A. HOFMAN, *et al.* 2001. Nonsteroidal antiinflammatory drugs and the risk of Alzheimer's disease. N. Engl. J. Med. **345:** 1515–1521.
72. YIP, A.G., R.C. GREEN, M. HUYCK, *et al.* 2005. Nonsteroidal anti-inflammatory drug use and Alzheimer's disease risk: the MIRAGE Study. BMC Geriatr. **5:** 2.

73. TURRIN, N.P. & S. RIVEST. 2006. Tumor necrosis factor alpha but not interleukin 1beta mediates neuroprotection in response to acute nitric oxide excitotoxicity. J. Neurosci. **26:** 143–151.
74. NGUYEN, M.D. & J.P. JULIEN& S. RIVEST. 2002. Innate immunity: the missing link in neuroprotection and neurodegeneration? Nat. Rev. Neurosci. **3:** 216–227.
75. ROGERS, J. & L.F. LUE. 2001. Microglial chemotaxis, activation, and phagocytosis of amyloid beta-peptide as linked phenomena in Alzheimer's disease. Neurochem. Int. **39:** 333–340.
76. LIU, Y., S. WALTER, M. STAGI, et al. 2005. LPS receptor (CD14): a receptor for phagocytosis of Alzheimer's amyloid peptide. Brain **128:** 1778–1789.
77. BARNES, L.L., R.S. WILSON, et al. 2005. Sex differences in the clinical manifestations of Alzheimer disease pathology. Arch. Gen. Psychiatry **62:** 685–691.
78. HENDERSON, V.W., A. PAGANINI-HILL, C.K. EMANUEL, et al. 1994. Estrogen replacement therapy in older women. Comparison between Alzheimer's disease cases and non-demented control subjects. Arch. Neurol. **51:** 896–900.
79. HENDERSON, V.W. 1997. The epidemiology of estrogen replacement therapy and Alzheimer's disease. Neurology **48:** S27–S35.
80. YAFFE, K., G. SAWAYA, et al. 1998. Estrogen therapy in postmenopausal women: effects on cognitive function and dementia. JAMA **279:** 688–695.
81. ZANDI, E. & M. KARIN. 1999. Bridging the gap: composition, regulation, and physiological function of the IkappaB kinase complex. Mol. Cell. Biol. **19:** 4547–4551.
82. HENDERSON, V.W., A. PAGANINI-HILL, B.L. MILLER, et al. 2000. Estrogen for Alzheimer's disease in women: randomised, double-blind, placebo controlled trial. Neurology **54:** 295–301.
83. MULNARD, R.A., C.W. COOMAN, C. KAWAS, et al. 2002. Estrogen replacement therapy for treatment of mild to moderate Alzheimer's disease: a randomised controlled trial. Alzheimer's Disease Cooperative Study. JAMA **23:** 1007–1015.
84. YAFFE, K. 2003. Hormone therapy and the brain. Am. Med. Assoc. **289:** 2717–2718.
85. YUE, X., M. LU, T. LANCASTER, et al. 2005. Brain estrogen deficiency accelerates Abeta plaques formation in an Alzheimer's disease animal model. Proc. Natl. Acad. Sci. USA **102:** 19198–19203.
86. CASALS, J., T.S. ELIZAN, et al. 1998. Postencephalic parkinsonism—a review. J. Neural Transm. **105:** 645–676.
87. LING, Z., D.A. GAYLE, et al. 2002. In utero bacterial endotoxin exposure causes loss of tyrosine hydroxylase neurons in the postnatal rat midbrain. Mov. Disord. **17:** 116–124.
88. MIRZA, B., H. HADBERG, et al. 2000. The absence of reactive astrocytosis is indicative of a unique inflammatory process in Parkinson's disease. Neuroscience **95:** 425–432.
89. BANATI, R.B., S.E. DANIEL, et al. 1998. Glial pathology but absence of apoptotic nigral neurons in long-standing Parkinson's disease. Mov. Disord. **13:** 221–227.
90. JENNER, P. & C.W. OLANOW. 1998. Understanding cell death in Parkinson's disease. Ann. Neurol. **44:** S72–S84.
91. HIRSCHE, E.C. 2000. Glial cells and Parkinson's disease. J. Neurol. **247:** 1158–1162.

92. RAJPUT, A.H., P. OFFORD, *et al.* 1984. Epidemiology of parkinsonism: incidence, classification, and mortality. Ann. Neurol. **16:** 278–282.
93. LYONS, K.E., J.P. HUBBLE, *et al.* 1998. Gender differences in Parkinson's disease. Clin. Neuropharmacol. **21:** 118–121.
94. QUINN, N.P. & C.D. MARDEN. 1986. Menstrual-related fluctuation in Parkinson's disease. Mov. Disord. **1:** 85–87.
95. SANDIK, R. 1989. Estrogens and the pathophysiology of Parkinson's disease. Int. J. Neurosci. **45:** 119–122.
96. SAUDERS-PULLMAN, R., J. GORDON-ELLIOTT, *et al.* 1999. The effect of estrogen in replacement on early Parkinson's disease. Neurology **52:** 1417–1421.
97. BENEDETTI, M.D., D.M. MARAGORE, *et al.* 2001. Hysterectomy, menopause, and estrogen use preceding Parkinson's disease: an exploratory case-control study. Mov. Disord. **16:** 830–837.
98. MARDER, K., M.X. TANG, B. ALFARO, *et al.* 1998. Postmenopausal estrogen use and Parkinson's disease with and without dementia. Neurology **50:** 1141–1143.
99. THULIN, P.C., W.R. WOODWARD, *et al.* 1998. Levodopa in human breast milk: clinical implication. Neurology **50:** 1920–1921.
100. STRIJKS, E., J.A. KREMER, *et al.* 1999. Effects of female sex steroids on Parkinson's disease in postmenopausal women. Clin. Neuropharmacol. **22:** 93–97.
101. BLANCHET, P.J., J. FANG, *et al.* 1999. Short-term effects of high-dose 17beta-estradiol in postmenopause PD patients: a crossover study. Neurology **53:** 91–95.
102. CURRIE, L.J., M.B. HARRISON, *et al.* 2004. Postmenopausal estrogen use effects risk for Parkinson's disease. Arch. Neurol. **61:** 886–888.
103. HAVERKAMP, L.J., V. APPEL & S.H. APPEL. 1995. Natural history of amyotrophic lateral sclerosis in a database population. Validation of a scoring system and a model for survival prediction. Brain **118:** 707–719.
104. CHIÒ, A., P. MEINERI, *et al.* 1991. Risk factors in motor neuron disease: a case control study. Neuroepidemiology **10:** 174–184.
105. VELDINK, J.H., P.R. BAR, E.A.J. JOOSTEN, *et al.* 2003. Sexual differences in onset of disease and response to exercise in a transgenic model of ALS. Neuromusc. Disord. **13:** 737–743.
106. HENSLEY, K., R.A. FLOYD, *et al.* 2002. Temporal patterns of cytokine and apoptosis-related gene expression in spinal cords of the G93A-SOD1 mouse model of amyotrophic lateral sclerosis. J. Neurochem. **82:** 365–374.
107. CHEN, Y.Z., C.L. BENNETT, *et al.* 2004. DNA/RNA helicase gene mutations in a form of juvenile amyotrophic lateral sclerosis (ALS4). Am. J. Hum. Genet. **74:** 1128–1135.
108. MALASPINA, A. & J. DE BELLEROCHE. 2004. Spinal cord molecular profiling provides a better understanding of amyotrophic lateral sclerosis pathogenesis. Brain. Res. Brain Res. Rev. **45:** 213–229.
109. OLSEN, M.K., S.L. ROBERDS, *et al.* 2001. Disease mechanisms revealed by transcription profiling in SOD1-G93A transgenic mouse spinal cord. Ann. Neurol. **50:** 730–740.
110. XIE, Y., P. WEYDT, *et al.* 2004. Inflammatory mediators and growth factors in the spinal cord of G93A SOD1 rats. Neuroreport **15:** 2513–2516.
111. PLATANIA, P., G. SEMINARA, *et al.* 2005. 17b-estradiol rescues spinal motoneurones from AMPA-induced toxicity: A role for glial cells. Neurobiol. Dis. **20:** 461–470.

112. KRUMAN, I.I., W.A. PEDERSEN, J.E. SPRINGER, *et al.* 1999. ALS-linked Cu/Zn-SOD mutation increases vulnerability of motor neurons by a mechanism involving increased oxidative stress and a perturbed calcium homeostasis. Exp. Neurol. **160:** 28–39.

113. NAKAMIZO, T., M. URUSHITANI, R. INOUE, *et al.* 2000. Protection of cultured spinal motor neurons by estradiol. Neuroreport **11:** 3493–3497.

114. MARTINO, G.V., P.L. POLIANI, R. FURLAN, *et al.* 2000. Cytokine therapy in immune-mediated demyelination disease of he central nervous system: a novel gene therapy approach. J. Neuroimmunol. **107:** 184–190.

115. BROSNAN, C.F., B. CANNELLA, L. BATTISTINI, *et al.* 1997. Cytokine localization in multiple sclerosis lesions: correlation with adhesion molecule expression and reactive nitrogen species. Neurology **45,** S16–S21.

116. CALABRESI, P.A., L.R. TRANQUILL, H.F. MAFARLAND, *et al.* 1998. Cytokine gene expression in cells derived from CSF of multiple sclerosis patients. J. Neuroimmunol. **89:** 198–205.

117. THOMPSON, D.S., L.M. NELSON, *et al.* 1986. The effects of pregnancy in multiple sclerosis: a retrospective study. Neurology **36:** 1097–1099.

118. DAMEK, D.M. & E.A. SHUSTER. 1997. Pregnancy and multiple sclerosis. Mayo. Clin. Proc. **72:** 977–989.

119. ZORGDRAGER, A. & J. DE KEYSER. 1997. Menstrually related worsening of symptoms in multiple sclerosis. J. Neurol. Sci. **149:** 95–98.

120. POZZILLI, C., P. FALASCHI, *et al.* 1999. MRI in multiple sclerosis during the menstrual cycle: relationship with sex hormone patterns. Neurology **53:** 622–624.

121. SMITH, R. & J.W. STUDD. 1992. A pilot study of the effect upon multiple sclerosis of the menopause, hormone replacement therapy and the menstrual cycle. J. R. Soc. Med **85:** 612–613.

122. SOLDAN, S.S., N.J. RETUERTO, R.R. SICOTTE, *et al.* 2002. Immune modulation in MS patients treated with pregnancy hormone estriol. J. Immunol. **171:** 6267–6270.

123. JANSSON, L., T. OLSSON, *et al.* 1994. Estrogen induces a potent suppression of experimental autoimmune encephalomyelitis and collagen-induced arthritis in mice. J. Neuroimmunol. **53:** 203–207.

124. MATEJUK, A., K. ADLARD, A. ZAMORA, *et al.* 2001. 17 beta-estradiol inhibits cytokine, chemokine, and chemokine receptor mRNA expression in the central nervous system of female mice with experimental autoimmune encephalomyelitis. J. Neurosci. Res. **65:** 529–542.

125. POLANCZYK, M., A. ZAMORA, *et al.* 2003. The protective effect of 17beta-estradiol on experimental autoimmune encephalomyelitis is mediated through estrogen receptor-alpha. Am. J. Pathol. **163:** 1599–1605.

126. GARIDOU, L., S. LAFFONT, V. DOUIN-ECHINARD, *et al.* 2004. Estrogen receptor alpha signaling in inflammatory leukocytes is dispensable for 17beta-estradiol-mediated inhibition of experimental autoimmune encephalomyelitis. J. Immunol. **173:** 2435–2442.

127. KORSCHENHAUSEN, D., H. HAMPEL, M. ACKENHEIL, *et al.* 1996. Fibrin degradation products in post mortem brain tissue of schizophrenics: a possible marker for underlying inflammatory processes. Schizophr. Res. **19:** 103–109.

128. CAZZULLO, C.L., S. SCARONE, B. GRASSI, *et al.* 1998. Cytokine production in chronic schizophrenia patients with or without paranoid behaviour. Prog. Neuropsychopharmacol. Biol. Psychiatry **22:** 947–957.

129. MULLER, N. & M.M. ACKENHEIL. 1995. Immunoglobulin and albumin content of cerebrospinal fluid in schizophrenic patients: relationship to negative symptomatology. Shizophr. Res. **14:** 223–228.
130. MAES, M., E. BOSMANS, J. CALABRESE, *et al.* 1995. Interleukin-2 and interleukin-6 in schizophrenia and mania: effects of neuroleptics and mood stabilizers. J. Psychiatr. Res. **29:** 141–152.
131. WILKE, I., V. AROLT, M. ROTHERMUD, *et al.* 1996. Investigations of cytokine production in whole blood cultures of paranoid and residual schizophrenic patients. Arch. Psychiatry Clin. Neurosci. **246:** 279–284.
132. BAYER, T.A., R. BESLEI, L. HAVAS, *et al.* 1999. Evidence for activation of microglia in patients with psychiatric illnesses. Neurosci. Lett. **271:** 126–128.
133. ANGERMEYER, M.C. & I. KUH. 1998. Gender differences in age at onset of schizophrenia. An overview. Eur. Arch. Psychiatry Neurol. Sci. **237:** 351–364.
134. HAFNER, H. & W. AN DER HEIDEN. 1997. Epidemiology of schizophrenia. Can. J. Psychiatry **42:** 139–151.
135. SEEMAN, M.W. 1983. Report on a survey of Canadian Friends of Schizophrenics. Am. J. Psychiatry **140:** 1648.
136. GOLDSTEIN, M.J. & J.A. DOANE. 1982. Family factors in the onset, course, and treatment of schizophrenic spectrum disorders: an update on current research. J. Nerv. Ment. Dis. **170:** 692–700.
137. RIECHER-ROSSLER, A. & H. HAFNER. 1993. Schizophrenia and oestrogens—is there an association? Eur. Arch. Psychiatry Clin. Neurosci. **242:** 323–328.
138. KENDELL, R.E., J.C. CHALMERS & C. PLATZ. 1987. Epidemiology of puerperal psychoses. Br. J. Psychiatry **150:** 662–673. Erratum in: Br. J. Psychiatry 1987 **151:**135.
139. MAHE, V. & A. DUMAINE. 2001. Oestrogen withdrawal associated psychoses. Acta Psychiatr. Scand. **104:** 323–331.
140. CHUA, W.L., A. IZQUIERDO DE SANTIAGO, J. KULKARNI, *et al.* 2006. Estrogen for schizophrenia [review]. The Cochrane Library Issue 3.
141. MAES, M. 1999. Major depression and activation of the inflammatory response system. Adv. Exp. Med. Biol. **461:** 25–46.
142. SLUZEWSKA, A., J.K. RYBAKOWSKI, M. LACIAK, *et al.* 1995. Interleukin-6 serum levels in depressed patients before and after treatment with fluoxetine. Ann. N. Y. Acad. Sci. **762:** 474–476.
143. MAES, M., C. SONG & A.H. LIN. 1999. Negative immunoregulatory effects of antidepressive inhibition of IFN-γ and stimulation of interleukin-10 secretion. Neuropsycopharmacology **20:** 370–379.
144. ANISMAN, H., A.V. RAVINDRAN, J. GRIFFITHS, *et al.* 1999. Endocrine and cytokine correlates of major depression and disthymia with typical or atypical features. Mol. Psychiatry **4:** 182–188.
145. RAMAMOORTHY, S., J.D. RAMAMOORTHY, P. PRADAD, *et al.* 1995. Regulation of the human serotonin transporter by interleukin-1 beta. Biochem. Biophys. Res. Commun. **216:** 560–567.
146. BRESLAU, N., l. SCHULTZ & E. PETERSON. 1995. Sex differences in depression: a role for preexisting anxiety. Psychiatr. Res. **58:** 1–12.
147. KESSLER, R.C., K.A. MCGONAGLE, S. ZHAO, *et al.* 1994. Lifetime and 12-month prevalence of DSM-III-R psychiatric disorders in the United States. Results from the National Comorbidity Survey. Arch. Gen. Psychiatry **51:** 8–19.

148. SCHNEIER, F.R., J. JOHNSON, C.D. HORNIG, *et al.* 1992. Social phobia. Comorbidity and morbidity in an epidemiologic sample. Arch. Gen. Psychiatry. **49:** 282–288.
149. SEEMAN, M.V. 1997. Psychopathology in women and men: focus on female hormones. Am. J. Psychiatry **154:** 1641–1647.
150. EARLS, F. 1987. Sex differences in psychiatric disorders: origins and developmental influences. Psychiatry. Dev. **5:** 1–23.
151. KESSLER, R.C., K.A. MCGONAGLE, M. SWARTZ, *et al.* 1993. Sex and depression in the National Comorbidity Survey. I: Lifetime prevalence, chronicity and recurrence. J. Affect. Disord. **29:** 85–96.
152. NOLEN-HOEKSEMA, S. 1987. Sex differences in unipolar depression: evidence and theory. Psychol. Bull. **101:** 259–282.
153. HAYWARD, C. & K. SANBORN. 2002. Puberty and the emergence of gender differences in psychopathology. J. Adolesc. Health **30:** 49–58.
154. KESSLER, R.C. & E.E. WALTERS. 1998. Epidemiology of DSM-III-R major depression and minor depression among adolescents and young adults in the National Comorbidity Survey. Depress. Anxiety **7:** 3–14.
155. LEWINSHON, P.M., P. ROHDE, J.R. SEELEY, *et al.* 1998. Major depressive disorder in older adolescents: prevalence, risk factors, and clinical implications. Clin. Psychol. Rev. **18:** 765–794.
156. YOUNG, E.A., A.R. MIDGLEY, N.E. CARLSON, *et al.* 2000. Alteration in the hypothalamic-pituitary-ovarian axis in depressed women. Arch. Gen. Psychiatry. **57:** 1157–1162.
157. SMITH, R.N., J.W. STUDD, D. ZAMBLERA, *et al.* 1995. A randomised comparison over 8 months of 100 micrograms and 200 micrograms twice weekly doses of transdermal oestradiol in the treatment of severe premenstrual syndrome. Br. J. Obstet. Gynaecol. **102:** 475–484.
158. AHOKAS, A., J. KAUKORANTA, K. WAHLBECK, *et al.* 2001. Estrogen deficiency in severe postpartum depression: successful treatment with sublingual physiologic 17beta-estradiol: a preliminary study. J. Clin. Psychiatr. **62:** 332–336.
159. GREGOIRE, A.J., R. KUMAR, B. EVERITT, *et al.* 1996. Transdermal oestrogen for treatment of severe postnatal depression. Lancet **347:** 930–933.
160. KLAIBER, E.L., D.M. BROVERMAN, W. VOGEL, *et al.* 1979. Estrogen therapy for severe persistent depressions in women. Arch. Gen. Psychiatr. **36:** 550–554.
161. PANTONI, L., C. SARTI, *et al.* 1998. Cytokines and cell adhesion molecules in cerebral ischemia. Arterioscler. Thromb. Vasc. Biol. **18:** 503–513.
162. ROSS, R. 1993. The pathogenesis of atheriosclerosis: a perspective for the 1990s. Nature **362:** 801–809.
163. HUANG, J., U.M. UPADHYAY & R.J. TAMARGO. 2006. Inflammation in stroke and focal cerebral ischemia. Surg. Neurol. **66:** 232–245.
164. PAGANINI-HILL, A., R.K. ROSS, *et al.* 1988. Postmenopausal oestrogen treatment and stroke: a prospective study. BMJ **297:** 519–522.
165. HULLEY, S., D. GRADY, *et al.* 1998. Randomized trial of estrogen plus progestin for secondary prevention of coronary heart disease in postmenopausal women. JAMA **280:** 605–613.
166. WRITING GROUP FOR THE WOMEN'S HEALTH INITIATIVE INVESTIGATORS. 2002. Risks and benefits of estrogen plus progestin in healthy postmenopausal women. JAMA-Express **288:** 321–333.
167. DARKOW, D.J., L. LU, *et al.* 1997. Estrogen relaxation of coronary artery smooth muscle is mediated by nitric oxide and cGMP. Am. J. Physiol. **272:** 2765–2773.

168. MONCADA, S. & A. HIGGS. 1993. The L-arginine-nitric oxide pathway. N. Engl. J. Med. **329:** 1002–1012.
169. HAYNES, M.P., L. LI, *et al.* 2001. Rapid vascular cell responses to estrogen and membrane receptors. Vascular Pharmacology **38:** 99–108.
170. HAYNES, M.P., L. LI, *et al.* 2003. Src kinase mediates phosphatidylinositol 3-kinase/Akt-dependent rapid endothelial nitric-oxide synthase activation by estrogen. J. Biol. Chem. **278:** 2118–2123.
171. MAC RITCHIE, A.N., S.S. JUN, *et al.* 1997. Estrogen upregulates endothelial nitric oxide synthase gene expression in fetal pulmonary artery endothelium. Circ. Res. **81:** 355–362.
172. DUBAL, D.B., H. ZHU, *et al.* 2001. Estrogen receptor alpha, not beta, is a critical link in estradiol-mediated protection against brain injury. Proc. Natl. Acad. Sci. USA **98:** 1952–1957.
173. WEN, Y., I. YANG, R. LIU, *et al.* 2004. Estrogen attenuates nuclear factor-kappa B activation induced by transient cerebral ischemia. Brain Res. **1008:** 147–154.

Estrogen, β-Amyloid Metabolism/ Trafficking, and Alzheimer's Disease

HUAXI XU,[a,b] RUISHAN WANG,[b] YUN-WU ZHANG,[a] AND XUE ZHANG[a]

[a]Center for Neuroscience and Aging, Burnham Institute for Medical Research, La Jolla, California 92037, USA

[b]Laboratory of Molecular and Cellular Neuroscience, School of Life Sciences and Institute for Biomedical Research, Xiamen University, Xiamen, China

ABSTRACT: Estrogen plays key regulatory roles in a variety of biological actions besides its classic function as a sex hormone. Recently, estrogen has been linked to neurodegenerative diseases including Alzheimer's disease (AD) and Parkinson's disease (PD). Several lines of evidence support the notion that brain estrogen exerts neuroprotective effects against various types of neurotoxicity in different cellular and animal models. Despite some controversies, estrogen replacement therapy (ERT) at an early stage, especially when given prior to menopause, has been shown to reduce the risk of AD in postmenopausal women. In addition, multiple lines of evidence have proven the neuroprotective effects of estrogen, such as enhancing neurotrophin signaling and synaptic activities pertinent to memory functions and protecting neurons against oxidative injuries and β-amyloid toxicity; the latter is widely accepted as the prime culprit known to trigger the pathogenesis of AD. Here we will summarize our findings that estrogen decreased generation and secretion of β-amyloid peptides in cultured cells and primary neurons and that administration of estrogen in estrogen-deprived mice reversed the elevated levels of brain Aβ. We will also discuss the molecular and cellular mechanisms underlying estrogen's effects on Aβ metabolism, which is highlighted by our demonstration that estrogen increases intracellular trafficking of β-amyloid precursor protein (βAPP) and hence reduces maximal Aβ generation within the *trans*-Golgi network (TGN), a subcellular compartment in which APP is known to be cleaved by the secretase enzymes to generate Aβ.

KEYWORDS: estrogen; Alzheimer's disease; β-amyloid; post-TGN trafficking.

Address for correspondence: Huaxi Xu, Ph.D., Center for Neurosciences and Aging, Burnham Institute for Medical Research, 10901 N. Torrey Pines Road, La Jolla, CA 92037. Voice: 858-795-5246; fax: 858-795-5273.

e-mail: xuh@burnham.org

Ann. N.Y. Acad. Sci. 1089: 324–342 (2006). © 2006 New York Academy of Sciences.
doi: 10.1196/annals.1386.036

INTRODUCTION

Alzheimer's disease (AD) is one of the most common and devastating neurodegenerative disorders in the elderly. Clinically, AD is featured by extracellular neuritic plaques, intracellular neurofibrillary tangles (NFTs),[1,2] synaptic dysfunctions, and neural degeneration in vulnerable brain regions including frontotemporal cortex and hippocampus that are essential for cognition, learning, and memory. Neuritic plaques are composed of aggregates of heterogeneous β-amyloid (Aβ) peptides, which are produced through sequential proteolysis of the β-amyloid precursor protein (βAPP). The neurotoxic Aβ peptides have been shown to accelerate the formation of intracellular NFTs[3,4] and to trigger a cascade of pathogenic events, such as calcium influx involving excitoactivation of glutamate/NMDA receptors and dystrophy of neuritis, culminating in neuronal apoptosis/death.[5–7]

βAPP belongs to the type I transmembrane protein family. Although its physiological functions have not been fully determined, βAPP has been suggested to play a role in transmembrane signal transduction, calcium metabolism, neurite outgrowth, neuronal protein trafficking through the axon, etc.[8–12] The route of βAPP to Aβ has been well defined. βAPP can be first cleaved by β-secretase to expose the N terminus of Aβ, resulting in the generation of APP C-terminal fragment β (CTFβ). APP CTFβ then can be cleaved by γ-secretase, a high molecular complex including at least four components, presenilin (PS), nicastrin, Pen-2, and APH-1, to release the highly hydrophobic amyloidogenic Aβ40/42 peptides. Both β-secretase and γ-secretase have been proposed as potential pharmacological targets to prevent Aβ aggregation. On the other hand, βAPP can be proteolized by α-secretase within Aβ domain to release the nonamloidogenic soluble APPα (sAPPα) fragment. The neuroprotective effects of sAPPα have been proposed and supported by a number of studies.[13,14]

Estrogen belongs to a family of sex hormones that function as sex steroids.[15,16] Besides its classic function, estrogen plays a variety of other roles in interacting with intracellular signaling transduction,[17–20] modulating transmembrane receptor activity,[21,22] regulating the transcription of various genes, and the process of synaptic morphogenesis and function.[23] In addition, estrogen's neuroprotective effects have been widely demonstrated in different neuronal cellular models against a variety of kinds of neuronal toxicity, such as Aβ toxicity,[24–26] oxidative stress,[27] bioenergetic deficiency,[28,29] mitochondrial failure,[30] and excitotoxicity.[31] Moreover, estrogen has been associated with neurodegenerative diseases including Parkinson's disease (PD)[32] and AD.[33] The first clue that estrogen may play a protective role in AD pathogenesis came from the observation that elderly women with reduced levels of circulating estrogen have an increased incidence of AD. The notion has been supported by a number of epidemiological studies showing decreased risks of AD onset in postmenopausal women who received estrogen replacement therapy (ERT).[33–37] Although the Women's Health Initiative (WHI)'s studies concluded that ERT was not an efficacious cure for AD (shown by little improvement on specific cognitive tasks following 2–15 months of trials of estrogen in women with clinically diagnosed AD),[38] prolactin included in the ERT could compromise estrogen's effect and ERT may be applied to delay the progression of AD pathogenesis but not to recover the lost functions. More recent studies indicated that early postmenopausal hormone therapy protects cognition later in life.[39–41]

It is still not clear how estrogen can protect from AD pathogenesis although a number of mechanisms have been proposed. First, estrogen's phenolic structure may contribute to its antioxidant effects observed in different types of neuronal cells and in adult, middle-aged, and reproductively senescent female rats.[42] Second, estrogen may play a role in anti-inflammation through acting on IL-6, a cytokine that is related to the formation of neuritic plaques.[43] Third, estrogen has been shown to be able to reduce the levels of apolipoprotein E (ApoE) in rodent tissues,[44] which is a risk factor for AD development. In addition, estrogen may reduce levels of Aβ by affecting βAPP metabolism, that is, stimulation of the α-secretory pathway of APP and inhibition of Aβ generation. Here, we will focus on and summarize the results of estrogen's effect on Aβ peptide metabolism in cellular and mouse models.[45,46] We will also discuss our finding that estrogen stimulated formation of vesicles containing βAPP from the *trans*-Golgi network (TGN) in the cell-free systems derived from both neuroblastoma cells and primary neurons, which precludes the maximum generation of Aβ.[47]

17β-ESTRADIOL REDUCES THE GENERATION OF Aβ IN CULTURED NEUROBLASTOMA CELLS AND PRIMARY NEURONS

To clarify the molecular mechanisms underlying estrogen's protective effects on AD pathogenesis, we studied the role of estrogen in Aβ generation using an estrogen analogue, 17β-estradiol (E_2), in both cultured mouse neuroblastoma (N2a) cells and rat cortical primary neurons. Treatment of N2a cells overexpressing human βAPP695 with 17β-E_2 stimulated the release of sAPPα and inhibited Aβ40 production in a dose-dependent manner (data not shown). Since Aβ42 is crucial in initiating Aβ deposition and formation of neuritic plaques, we determined specifically whether Aβ42 production was affected by the estrogen analogue. We used N2a cells expressing human βAPP695 and the familial AD-linked PS1 variant that lacks the amino acids encoded by exon-10 of PS1 gene (PS1E10), in which Aβ42 is readily detectable. Following exposure to 17β-E_2, the levels of secreted Aβ40/42 peptides were significantly decreased up to 50% accompanied by the increase of secreted sAPPα in the double transgenic N2a cells at the tested E_2 concentrations shown by autoradiographic analysis (FIGS. 1A and B). We also performed immunoprecipitation-mass

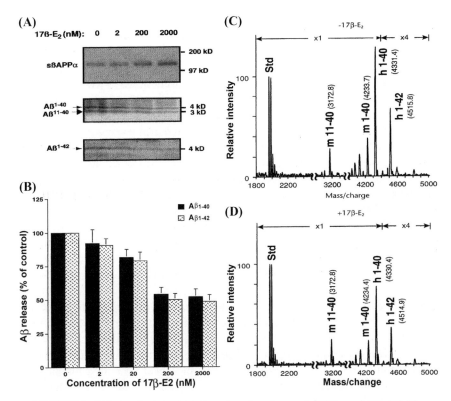

FIGURE 1. Effects of estrogen treatment on the release of sAPPα and Aβ. (**A**) Mouse N2a neuroblastoma cells coexpressing human βAPP695 and human PS1 mutant (PS1E10) were treated for 7–10 days with the indicated concentrations of 17β-E₂. After metabolic labeling with [³⁵S]methionine, conditioned media were sequentially immunoprecipitated with antibodies FCA3542 (*lower panel*), FCA3340 (*middle panel*), and 6E10 (*top panel*). The immunoprecipitated proteins were subjected to SDS-PAGE and autoradiography. (**B**) Quantification of released Aβ1–40 and Aβ1–42 in (**C**) as a function of estrogen concentration. Data were normalized to the amount of Aβ1–40 or Aβ1–42 from untreated samples, respectively, and represent mean ± SD. (**D**) Conditioned media from 17β-E₂-treated or -untreated cells were incubated with 4G8 antibody overnight and the immunoprecipitated proteins were subjected to Mass-spec analysis for Aβ release.

spectrometry (IP-MS) to quantify the released Aβ peptide species in conditional media with or without the presence of 17β-E₂. The IP-MS results confirmed that the levels of mouse and human Aβ40/42 peptides were decreased by 17β-E₂ (FIGS. 1C and D).

Only the basis of the observations in the cultured cells, we deepened our studies using rodent and human embryonic primary neurons. In rat cerebral cortical primary neurons, autoradiographic analysis after metabolic labeling and IP-MS demonstrated a significant decrease of Aβ40 accompanied by an increase of sAPPα (data not shown). The effect of estrogen on Aβ42 generation was assessed using mouse primary neurons in which Aβ42 is readily detectable. The levels of Aβ40/42 peptides were significantly decreased by about 50%, correlated with the increase of secreted sAPPα by 55% in the 17β-E$_2$-treated mouse neurons (data not shown). In addition, we tested the effect of estrogen on Aβ generation within physiological range (2–10 nM) using fetal human cerebrocortical neurons. The Aβ generation was decreased by about 40% when the neurons were treated with estrogen (data not shown). These data, together with the results in the cultured N2a cells, indicated that physiological concentrations of estrogen can affect βAPP metabolism to reduce Aβ generation, provided evidence in cellular models to support the notion that estrogen may protect against AD pathogenesis, and suggested a lead for understanding the basis of AD.

ESTROGEN MODULATES Aβ PEPTIDES IN TRANSGENIC MOUSE MODELS OF AD

To further establish the link between deprivation of estrogen and AD pathogenesis and to investigate the effects of estrogen on Aβ generation *in vivo*, we evaluated Aβ generation and formation of senile plaques in two AD mouse models with or without estrogen treatment. We used the mice overexpressing a mutant human βAPP (Tg2576)[48] and the mice bearing both a mutant human βAPP and PS1 (PS/βAPP) transgenes.[49,50] We first quantified the levels of both soluble and insoluble brain Aβ peptides in such mice with or without depletion of estrogen by ovariectomy (TABLE 1). After ovariectomy, there was a significant increase in the level of Aβ40 in Tg2576 mice and a robust (more than twofold) elevation of Aβ42 in the double transgenic mice. These results may explain the clinical observation of higher risk of AD pathogenesis in postmenopausal women, indicating that such transgenic mice can be used as models for *in vivo* studies on the relationship between AD pathogenesis and estrogen.

We then treated the ovariectomized AD mice with 17β-E$_2$ and found that the administration of the estrogen analogue reversed the increase of Aβ40 in both transgenic mice. The level of Aβ42 in the treated Tg2576 mice was decreased around border level, partially because of its relatively low basal level. Although the level of Aβ42 in the treated double transgenic mice was still significantly higher than that in sham-operated controls, the level was reduced more than 50% compared to that in vehicle-treated ovariectomized controls (TABLE 1). Recently, Yue *et al.* also reported early onset and increase of Aβ deposition in an AD transgenic mouse model with greatly reduced brain estrogen.[51] These data not only correspond to the *in vitro* studies supporting that ERT may reduce the risk of AD incidence, but also provide a model system allowing the estrogen-based therapeutics to be tested *in vivo*. In addition, the more

TABLE 1. Effect of ovariectomy and estrogen replacement on Aβ levels in APP and PS/APP mice

Effect of ovariectomy and estrogen replacement on Aβ levels in APP mice	Number	Aβ40 (pmol/g protein, mean ± SEM)	Aβ42 (pmol/g protein, mean ± SEM)
APP sham	7	70 ± 20	11 ± 2
APP OVX	10	85 ± 10[a]	14 ± 10
APP OVX + 1.7 mg E_2	6	70 ± 10	3 ± 1[b]
APP OVX + 5 mg E_2	7	50 ± 8[b]	Below limit of detection
Effect of ovariectomy and estrogen replacement on Aβ levels in PS/APP mice			
APP sham	5	224 ± 42	149 ± 42
APP OVX	8	337 ± 41	345 ± 53[a]
APP OVX + vehicle	3	350 ± 65	491 ± 14
APP OVX + estradiol	3	278 ± 33	237 ± 53[a]

The levels of Aβ were measured by ELISA or immunoprecipitation/mass spectrometry.

[a]$P < 0.05$, [b]$P < 0.01$.

SEM = standard error; ovx = ovariectomized; sham = sham-operated; ovx +1.7 mg (5 mg) E_2: ovariectomized and implanted with 1.7 mg (or 5 mg) estradiol pellet.

significant response of Aβ42 relative to Aβ40 upon estrogen treatment suggested that the mechanisms involved in the metabolism of Aβ42 are the preferential target for estradiol action. Moreover, the significant but partial recovery of the level of Aβ42 in estrogen-treated ovariectomized mice compared to sham-operated controls indicated that estrogen's effect was limited on high Aβ42 burden and implied that the treatment of estrogen at late stages of clinically defined AD may not be effective. This notion may provide an explanation on the limited cognitive improvement of AD female patients receiving estrogen treatment.

ESTROGEN LOWERS Aβ GENERATION BY STIMULATING TGN VESICLE BIOGENESIS

Although estrogen treatment had a dramatic effect on Aβ generation in both cellular and mouse models, estrogen showed little effect on the expression levels of βAPP or PS1, leaving the molecular mechanisms underlying how estrogen reduces Aβ generation an open question. Aβ is generated through the intracellular trafficking pathway of βAPP. Although a portion of Aβ can be found in the endoplasmic reticulum (ER) of both primary neurons and cultured human NT2N cells and in the endosomes, the majority of the secreted Aβ peptides is generated within the TGN,[52–54] a major site in which βAPP resides at steady state in neurons. On the other hand, it is believed that βAPP is cleaved by α-secretase on the plasma membrane to generate sAPPα. Thus, the biogenesis of the secretory vesicles and trafficking of βAPP from TGN to plasma membrane have direct influence on the relative generation of sAPPα versus Aβ.

Steroids such as glucocorticoids can stimulate protein trafficking from TGN to plasma membrane. It has been suggested that estrogen has a similar function in regulating late secretory pathway vesicle formation. Electron microscopy (EM) revealed an increase in proliferation of secretory vesicle in neuroendocrine cells in the presence of estrogen.[55] Although the direct link between estrogen and the mechanisms underlying TGN vesicle formation remains to be elucidated, several studies have provided clues for further exploring the pathway leading to the upregulation of secretory TGN vesicle trafficking by estrogen.[56–58] For instance, transcriptions of methylating enzymes functioning in the conversion of phospholipids and Rab11, a small GTPase that plays various roles in endocytosis and TGN trafficking, have been found to be upregulated in response to estrogen.

Using cell-free systems derived from both neuroblastoma cells and primary neurons, we demonstrated that 17β–E$_2$ stimulated formation of vesicles containing βAPP from the TGN. Subsequently, the accelerated βAPP trafficking precludes maximal Aβ generation within the TGN and leads to a significant decrease of Aβ secretion. A cell-free reconstitution system was derived from N2a cells overexpressing human βAPP, which has been characterized and widely used as a model to study βAPP trafficking and Aβ generation.[52, 54] Following estrogen treatment, the cell-free system containing nascent vesicles separated from donor membranes was reconstituted, and the [^{35}S] labeled βAPP in the vesicles was solubilized and assayed by immunoprecipitation followed by autoradiography. Twice the amount of βAPP was recovered from TGN-derived vesicles treated with 17β-E$_2$ compared with that in control (FIGS. 2A and B) during the 2-h chase, suggesting that 17β-E$_2$ exposure alters cellular trafficking machinery to accelerate the formation of βAPP-containing vesicles from the TGN. The same results were found from studies on the trafficking of other proteins within the same subcellular distribution including βAPP-like protein 2 (APLP2) and TrkB, an unrelated integral membrane molecule (data not shown). The similar observation of the enhanced TGN budding was also found in cell-free systems derived from rat, mouse, and human estrogen-primed primary neurons (data not shown). These data supported the notion that estrogen treatment can lead to a consistent and nonspecific increase in the formation of TGN vesicles. The increased formation of TGN-derived vesicles was expected to cause accumulation of βAPP molecules on the plasma membrane, which was confirmed by the increase of biotin-labeled βAPP at the membrane following estrogen exposure (FIG. 2C). Since the majority of secreted Aβ is generated within the TGN, these findings raised the possibility that the stimulated βAPP trafficking from TGN to plasma membrane may contribute to the decrease of Aβ generation/secretion by estrogen. However, since a population of Aβ is also produced from βAPP that is internalized from the cell surface, the estrogen's role in endocytosis still needs to be identified.

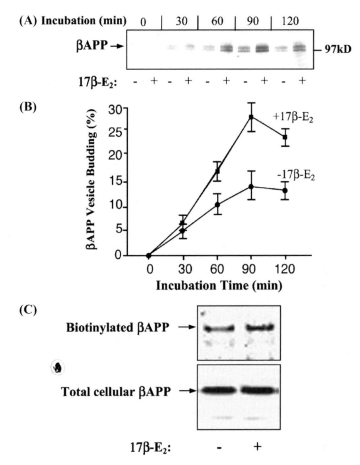

FIGURE 2. Estrogen stimulates cell-free formation of post-TGN vesicles containing APP. (**A**) 17β-E$_2$-treated or -untreated cells were labeled with [^{35}S]methionine at 37°C for 15 min followed by a 2-h chase at 20°C to accumulate βAPP in the TGN. Cells were permeabilized and incubated at 37°C for the indicated time. After centrifugation to separate TGN membranes and vesicles, the supernatant (containing vesicles) was subjected to immunoprecipitation with βAPP antibody 369, SDS-PAGE, and autoradiography. (**B**) Quantitation of (**A**) to show % βAPP budding after 0–120 min from TGN membranes derived from cells with or without prior estrogen exposure. Values are mean ± SD from three replications. (**C**) Biotinylation of N2a cells incubated either in the absence or presence of estrogen prior to the experiment. Biotinylated (*top panel*) and total cellular βAPP (*bottom panel*) was analyzed by Western blot using 369 antibody.

How does estrogen stimulate budding of TGN vesicles? Rab11, a cytosolic GTPase, which is important for both the formation of TGN-derived vesicles and for vesicle formation during endocytosis,[59,60] has been suggested to be induced in response to estrogen.[58] In the estrogen-treated N2a cells and human

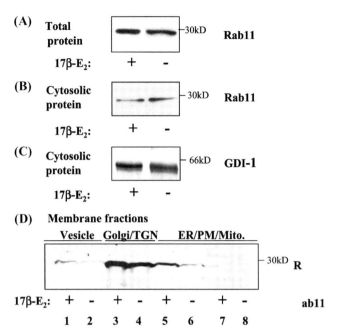

FIGURE 3. Rab11 is recruited to TGN membranes in response to 17β-E_2. N2a cells were incubated in the absence or presence of 17β-E_2 for 1 week. Cells were lysed and analyzed by Western blot for total Rab11 (**A**), cytosolic Rab11 (**B**), or cytosolic GDP dissociation inhibitor-1 (*GDI-1*) (**C**). Additional cells, prepared identically, were subjected to subcellular fractionation. Samples representing vesicle fractions (*lanes 1* and *2*) Golgi/TGN (*lanes 3* and *4*), and ER/PM/mitochondria (*lanes 5–8*) were analyzed for Rab11 by Western blot (**D**).

primary neurons, some Rab11 was translocated from cytosol to the membranes of ER, TGN, TGN-derived vesicles and mitochondria, demonstrated by a decrease in the levels of cytosolic Rab11 and an increase in the membrane fractions (FIG. 3). Combined with estrogen's effect on the change of βAPP localization, the translocation of Rab11 suggested a possible link between the trafficking factor and the transport of βAPP. This hypothesis was tested using a C-terminally truncated Rab11 mutant that cannot interact with membranes. Overexpression of the mutant Rab11 in the N2a cells significantly increased TGN Aβ generation and Aβ secretion (data not shown), suggesting that the recruitment of Rab11 to the membrane when stimulated by estrogen may be responsible for the changed localization of βAPP in response to estrogen.

The change of the lipid composition in the membrane is another important molecular event which is believed to initiate the formation of secretory vesicles besides the recruitment of cytosolic proteins to the plasma membranes.[61] In the presence of estrogen, a slight loss of phosphatidylethanolamine, phosphatidylserine, and phosphatidylcholine in TGN membranes was found to

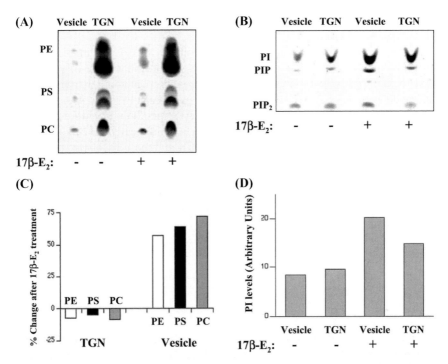

FIGURE 4. Phosphatidylinositol is redistributed from TGN to post-TGN vesicles in response to 17β-E₂. (**A**) Vesicle and TGN fractions were prepared using subcellular fractionation of N2a cells incubated in either the absence or the presence of 17β-E₂. Phospholipids were extracted from these fractions and analyzed using TLC. (**B**) Quantification of TLC represented as % change in TGN or vesicle fractions after 17β-E₂ treatment. (**C**) Vesicle and TGN fractions were prepared as described above, except that N2a cells were labeled first with tritiated inositol. Phosphatidylinositols were extracted from these fractions and analyzed using TLC. (**D**) Quantification of tritiated phosphatidylinositols before and after 17β-E₂ treatment in vesicle and TGN fractions. PE = phosphatidylethanolamine; PS = phosphatidylserine; PC = phosphatidylcholine; PI = phosphatidylinositol; PIP = phosphatidylinositol phosphate; PIP₂ = phosphatidylinositol bisphosphate.

correlate with an increase of these lipids in the post-TGN vesicles (FIGS. 4A and B). In addition, because phosphatidylinositol (PI) is essential for membrane vesiculation, we examined the levels of PI in TGN and post-TGN vesicles with or without estrogen treatment. The levels of PI in both TGN and post-TGN vesicles were nearly doubled by estrogen treatment (FIGS. 4C and D). More importantly, estrogen treatment caused a shift of PI from TGN membranes to the vesicle fraction, implying an increase of vesicle number. These data, together with the altered subcellular localization of Rab11, suggested molecular mechanisms by which estrogen enhances vesicle biogenesis and subsequent βAPP trafficking.

Summary

Estrogen has long been known for its neuroprotective effects in addition to its roles in regulating cellular functions as a sex hormone. The observation that postmenopausal women who receive estrogen replacement therapy (ERT) have a delayed onset and reduced risk for AD pathogenesis raised speculations on the mechanisms by which estrogen affects APP metabolism and Aβ generation. The findings that have been summarized here delineated the link between the estrogen-stimulated vesicle budding of TGN and the subsequent reduction of APP available for production of Aβ. However, it is plausible that estrogen may exert its protective effects through its additional activities, including modulation of basal forebrain cholinergic activity and integrity, dendritic plasticity, NMDA receptor density, and neurotrophin signaling, as well as prevention of oxidative toxicity of glutamate, free radicals, and Aβ.

METHODS AND MATERIALS

Cell Lines

Mouse neuroblastoma (N2a) cells doubly transfected with human APP695 and human mutant PS1 that lacks the amino acids encoded by exon-10 of PS1 gene (PS1E10) were maintained in medium containing 50% Dulbecco's modified Eagle's medium, 50% Opti-MEM, supplemented with 5% fetal bovine serum, antibiotics, and 200 μg/mL G418 (Invitrogen, Carlsbad, CA, USA). Cells were maintained in the absence or presence of 200 nM 17β-E_2 (Sigma, St. Louis, MO, USA) for 7days. In some experiments, cells were treated with various concentrations of 17β-E_2 (Sigma, St. Louis, MO, USA).

Antibodies

Monoclonal antibodies 4G8 and 6E10 were purchased from Senetek (Napa, CA, USA). FCA3340 recognizing Aβ40 but not Aβ42 and FCA3542 recognizing Aβ42 but not Aβ40 were kindly provided by F. Checler.[45] Polyclonal Rab11 antibody and polyclonal GDP dissociation inhibitor antibody were purchased from Zymed Laboratories Inc. (South San Francisco, CA, USA). Polyclonal antibody 369 against βAPP C terminus was developed in our laboratory.[52,62]

Aβ Immunoprecipitation

Conditioned media from 17β-E_2-treated cells were sequentially treated with antibody to immunoprecipitate Aβ1-42 (FCA3542), Aβ1-40/11-40

(FCA3340), and sβAPPα (6E10). Immunoprecipitated proteins were subjected to SDS-PAGE using 10-20% Tricine gels (for Aβ species) or 4–12% Tris glycine gels (for sβAPPα) and to autoradiography. Band intensities were analyzed and quantified using NIH ImageQuant software, version 1.52.

Immunoprecipitation/Mass Spectrometry

Following treatments, serum-free media were conditioned by cells for 24 h in the continued presence or absence of 17β-E$_2$. Secreted Aβ species in conditioned media were immunoprecipitated by antibody 4G8. The molecular masses and concentrations of immunoprecipitated Aβ species were analyzed by a matrix-assisted laser desorption/ionization time-of-flight mass spectrometer (MALDI-TOF-MS) (Voyager-DE STR BioSpectrometry Workstation, PerSeptive Biosystem, Framingham, MA, USA). Synthetic Aβ 12–28 peptide (20 nm, Sigma, St. Louis, MO, USA) was added as internal standard. Aβ peptides terminating at amino acids 40 and 42 were identified by molecular mass and quantified using relative peak intensities. Each mass spectrum was averaged from 256 measurements and calibrated using bovine insulin as an internal mass calibrant. Relative peak intensities of Aβ peptides to internal standard were used for quantitative analysis.

Preparation of Permeabilized N2a Cells

It has been well established that incubation of cells at 20°C leads to an accumulation of membrane and secretory proteins in the TGN.[52,54] To assay the budding of βAPP-containing vesicles from TGN, estrogen-treated or untreated N2a cells were pulse-labeled with [^{35}S]methionine (500 μCi/mL) for 15 min at 37°C, washed with phosphate-buffered solution (PBS; prewarmed to 20°C), and chased for 2 h at 20°C in complete media prewarmed to 20°C. Cells were then incubated at 4°C in "swelling buffer" (10 mM KCl, 10 mM Hepes, pH 7.2) for 10 min. The buffer was aspirated and replaced with 1 mL of "breaking buffer" (90 mM KCl, 10 mM Hepes, pH 7.2), after which the cells were broken by scraping with a rubber policeman. The cells were centrifuged at 800 × g for 5 min, washed in 3–5 mL of breaking buffer, and resuspended in 5 volumes of breaking buffer. This procedure resulted in >95% cell breakage evaluated by staining with trypan blue. Broken cells (~2 × 10^6 cells) were incubated in a final volume of 300 μL containing 2.5 mM MgCl$_2$, 0.5 mM CaCl$_2$, 110 mM KCl, and an energy-regenerating system (ERS) consisting of 1 mM ATP, 0.02 mM GTP, 10 mM creatine phosphate, 80 μg/mL creatine phosphokinase, and a protease inhibitor mixture. Incubations were carried out at 37°C for the indicated time. Each experiment was performed at least three times.

Formation of Nascent Secretory Vesicles in Permeabilized Cells

Following incubation of broken cells, vesicle and membrane fractions were separated by centrifugation at 14,000 rpm for 15 s at 4°C in a Brinkman centrifuge. Vesicle (supernatant) and membrane (pellet) fractions were extracted with a cell lysis buffer containing 0.5% Nonidet P-40 and 0.5% deoxylcholate.

Immunoprecipitation

Extracted proteins from the various fractions were brought to 0.5% SDS and heated for 3 min at 75°C. Samples were treated with IP buffer (10 mM sodium phosphate, pH 7.4, 100 mM sodium chloride, 1% Triton X-100) and the appropriate antibody added. After incubating overnight, samples were treated with protein A-Sepharose, and immunoprecipitated materials were analyzed by SDS-PAGE using 4–12% Tris glycine gels.

Cell Surface Biotinylation

Biotinylation was performed on confluent monolayer N2a cells by using sulfo-NHS-LC-biotin (sulfosuccinimidyl-6-(biotinamido)-hexanoate; Pierce, Rockford, IL, USA). The reagent was dissolved in PBS with calcium and magnesium, pH 7.2, at 0.5 mg/mL and added twice to the cultures for 20 min at 4°C. After thorough washing, the cells were lysed and incubated with immobilized streptavidin (Pierce, Rockford, IL, USA) to pull down all biotinylated proteins. The samples were analyzed by Western blot. Biotinylated βAPP was detected by using 369 antibody.

Preparation of Mammalian Cytosol Fraction

Ten plates of cells were collected in their media and washed with TEA buffer (10 mM triethanolamine, 140 mM KOAc, pH 7.2) followed by a wash in homogenization buffer (25 mM Hepes-KOH, pH 7.2, 125mM KOAc, protease inhibitor mixture) and resuspension in 1 volume of pellet/5 volumes of homogenization buffer. Cells were broken in a Ballet homogenizer (clearance 18 μm) and a postnuclear supernatant created by centrifuging at 800 × g for 5 min at 4°C. The postnuclear supernatant was then centrifuged at 100,000 × g for 1 h at 4°C. About 50-μL aliquots were frozen in liquid nitrogen after protein was measured by the Bradford assay and stored at −80°C.

Lipid Extraction

Fractions from the sucrose gradients were diluted to 1-mL total volume if necessary, transferred to 13 × 100 borosilicate test tubes, and mixed with

3.25 mL of chloroform/methanol 1:2.2.[63] The samples were vortexed and centrifuged to pellet proteins. Supernatants were transferred to clean tubes and
phase-separated by adding 1 mL each of chloroform and 20 mM acetic acid.
After aspirating the upper phases, lower phases were reduced in volume by
evaporation under a nitrogen stream and dried in a Speed-Vac concentrator.

Phospholipid Analysis

For phospholipid analysis, samples were diluted with 30 μL of chloro-
form/methanol (2:1), and 10-μL aliquots from each were spotted onto a
TLC plate. Plates were developed in chloroform/ethanol/triethylamine/water
(30:35:35:7) and visualized by spraying with 3% copper (II) acetate in 8%
phosphoric acid followed by charring. Quantitation for phospholipids was performed on a Storm 860 PhosphorImager in the blue fluorescence mode.

Inositol Lipid Extraction and Analysis

The method of Pike and Eakes[64] was used with minor modifications. One-
milliliter fractions were transferred to 13 × 100-mm borosilicate tubes containing 1 mL of methanol/concentrated HCl (10:1, v/v) and vortexed with 2 mL of
chloroform. The phases were separated and the aqueous phase discarded. The
organic phase was reextracted with 1 mL of methanol, 1 M HCl (1:1), phase-
separated, and the upper phase discarded. The lower organic phase was evaporated under a nitrogen stream and then dried in a Speed-Vac concentrator. Samples were dissolved in a minimal amount of chloroform/methanol/water (5:5:1)
and spotted onto TLC plates, impregnated with 1% potassium oxalate and developed in chloroform/methanol/water/ammonium hydroxide (17:13.2:2.8:1).
Tritiated phosphatidylinositols were detected by autoradiography, and their
identity was determined by comigration with authentic standards.

Mouse Surgery and Analysis

Line Tg2576 overexpresses a mutant APP transgene and has elevated levels
of human Aβ40 and Aβ42 relative to mouse, but does not deposit amyloid
until 10–12 months of age.[48] Double transgenic progeny from a cross between
Tg2576 and a mutant PS1 line (Line PS1 5.1, M146L)[49] have elevated levels
of Aβ42 relative to the Tg2576 parent and form visible amyloid aggregates
at approximately 16 weeks of age.[50] Tg2576 mice (termed *APP*) were used
to study the effects of ovariectomy and estradiol supplementation on soluble Aβ40 and Aβ42 levels by enzyme-linked immunosorbent assay (ELISA).

Ovariectomy was performed at 13 weeks of age and sham surgery was performed on littermate animals to provide a control group. For estrogen replacement groups, ovariectomized animals were simultaneously implanted subcutaneously with 90-day-release form of 17β-estradiol pellet at either 1.7 mg or 5 mg per pellet (Innovative Research of America, Sarasota, FL, USA). Mice were killed at 7 months of age. Prior to perfusion, uteri were weighed and plasma was collected for estradiol measurements using a radioimmunoassay (RIA) kit provided by Diagnostic Systems Laboratories, Inc. (Webster, TX, USA) according to the manufacturer's suggested method. Double transgenic mice (termed *PS/APP*) were used to study the effect of ovariectomy on amyloid accumulation in the brain by ELISA. Ovariectomy was performed at 5 weeks of age and sham surgery was performed on littermate animals. The animals were killed at 18weeks of age, brains were removed for analysis and uterine weights were assessed. For estrogen supplementation, mice were ovariectomized at 5 weeks of age. At 11 weeks of age, estradiol was administered in the drinking water according to the method of M.N. Gordon.[65] In brief: estradiol (Sigma, St Louis, MO, USA) was dissolved in ethanol to a concentration of 5 mg/mL, then aliquoted into fresh drinking water at 5 μg/mL. The amount of water used was monitored twice weekly and fresh estradiol solution was administered. Four ovariectomized PS/APP mice received vehicle (water plus 0.1% ethanol), whereas three received estradiol in 0.1% ethanol. In all experiments, mice were maintained on a casein-based diet following ovariectomy to prevent the introduction of extraneous estrogen through soy-based mouse chow.

Aβ ELISA

Formic acid extraction was used to solubilize all Aβ peptides in mouse hemibrains according to a method described in Refolo *et al.*[66] A sandwich ELISA kit from BioSource International (Hopkinton, MA, USA) was used to measure Aβ40 and Aβ42 peptides according to the manufacturer's protocol in both PS/APP and APP mouse brain homogenates.

REFERENCES

1. GRUNDKE-IQBAL, I. *et al.* 1986. Abnormal phosphorylation of the microtubule-associated protein tau (tau) in Alzheimer cytoskeletal pathology. Proc. Natl. Acad. Sci. USA **83:** 4913–4917.
2. TROJANOWSKI, J.Q. & V.M. LEE. 2000. "Fatal attractions" of proteins. A comprehensive hypothetical mechanism underlying Alzheimer's disease and other neurodegenerative disorders. Ann. N. Y. Acad. Sci. **924:** 62–67.
3. GOTZ, J. *et al.* 2001. Formation of neurofibrillary tangles in P301l tau transgenic mice induced by Abeta 42 fibrils. Science **293:** 1491–1495.
4. LEWIS, J. *et al.* 2001. Enhanced neurofibrillary degeneration in transgenic mice expressing mutant tau and APP. Science **293:** 1487–1491.

5. HARKANY, T. *et al.* 2000. beta-amyloid neurotoxicity is mediated by a glutamate-triggered excitotoxic cascade in rat nucleus basalis. Eur. J. Neurosci. **12:** 2735–2745.

6. KAMENETZ, F. *et al.* 2003. APP processing and synaptic function. Neuron **37:** 925–937.

7. HAN, P. *et al.* 2005. Suppression of cyclin-dependent kinase 5 activation by amyloid precursor protein: a novel excitoprotective mechanism involving modulation of tau phosphorylation. J. Neurosci. **25:** 11542–11552.

8. MUCKE, L., C.R. ABRAHAM & E. MASLIAH. 1996. Neurotrophic and neuroprotective effects of hAPP in transgenic mice. Ann. N. Y. Acad. Sci. **777:** 82–88.

9. MATTSON, M.P. & Q. GUO. 1997. Cell and molecular neurobiology of presenilins: a role for the endoplasmic reticulum in the pathogenesis of Alzheimer's disease? J. Neurosci. Res. **50:** 505–513.

10. NEVE, R.L., D.L. MCPHIE & Y. CHEN. 2000. Alzheimer's disease: a dysfunction of the amyloid precursor protein(1). Brain Res. **886:** 54–66.

11. KOO, E.H. 2002. The beta-amyloid precursor protein (APP) and Alzheimer's disease: does the tail wag the dog? Traffic **3:** 763–770.

12. ZHENG, H. & E.H. KOO. 2006. The amyloid precursor protein: beyond amyloid. Mol. Neurodegeneration **1:** 5–16.

13. FURUKAWA, K. *et al.* 1996. Increased activity-regulating and neuroprotective efficacy of alpha-secretase-derived secreted amyloid precursor protein conferred by a C-terminal heparin-binding domain. J. Neurochem. **67:** 1882–1896.

14. MEZIANE, H. *et al.* 1998. Memory-enhancing effects of secreted forms of the beta-amyloid precursor protein in normal and amnestic mice. Proc. Natl. Acad. Sci. USA **95:** 12683–12688.

15. EVANS, M.I., R. SILVA & J.B. BURCH. 1988. Isolation of chicken vitellogenin I and III cDNAs and the developmental regulation of five estrogen-responsive genes in the embryonic liver. Genes Dev. **2:** 116–124.

16. BEATO, M. 1989. Gene regulation by steroid hormones. Cell **56:** 335–344.

17. CURTIS, S.W. *et al.* 1996. Physiological coupling of growth factor and steroid receptor signaling pathways: estrogen receptor knockout mice lack estrogen-like response to epidermal growth factor. Proc. Natl. Acad. Sci. USA **93:** 12626–12630.

18. MIGLIACCIO, A. *et al.* 1996. Tyrosine kinase/p21ras/MAP-kinase pathway activation by estradiol-receptor complex in MCF-7 cells. EMBO J. **15:** 1292–1300.

19. MARINO, M., V. PALLOTTINI & A. TRENTALANCE. 1998. Estrogens cause rapid activation of IP3-PKC-alpha signal transduction pathway in HEPG2 cells. Biochem. Biophys. Res. Commun. **245:** 254–258.

20. WATTERS, J.J. & D.M. DORSA. 1998. Transcriptional effects of estrogen on neuronal neurotensin gene expression involve cAMP/protein kinase A-dependent signaling mechanisms. J. Neurosci. **18:** 6672–6680.

21. WETZEL, C.H. *et al.* 1998. Functional antagonism of gonadal steroids at the 5-hydroxytryptamine type 3 receptor. Mol. Endocrinol. **12:** 1441–1451.

22. GU, Q., K.S. KORACH & R.L. MOSS. 1999. Rapid action of 17beta-estradiol on kainate-induced currents in hippocampal neurons lacking intracellular estrogen receptors. Endocrinology **140:** 660–666.

23. MATSUMOTO, A. 1991. Synaptogenic action of sex steroids in developing and adult neuroendocrine brain. Psychoneuroendocrinology **16:** 25–40.

24. BEHL, C. *et al.* 1995. 17-beta estradiol protects neurons from oxidative stress-induced cell death in vitro. Biochem. Biophys. Res. Commun. **216:** 473–482.

25. GREEN, P.S., K.E. GRIDLEY & J.W. SIMPKINS. 1996. Estradiol protects against beta-amyloid (25-35)-induced toxicity in SK-N-SH human neuroblastoma cells. Neurosci. Lett. **218:** 165–168.
26. PIKE, C.J. 1999. Estrogen modulates neuronal Bcl-xL expression and beta-amyloid-induced apoptosis: relevance to Alzheimer's disease. J. Neurochem. **72:** 1552–1563.
27. WANG, X. *et al.* 2006. Neuroprotective effects of 17beta-estradiol and nonfeminizing estrogens against H2O2 toxicity in human neuroblastoma SK-N-SH cells. Mol. Pharmacol. **70:** 395–404.
28. REGAN, R.F. & Y. GUO. 1997. Estrogens attenuate neuronal injury due to hemoglobin, chemical hypoxia, and excitatory amino acids in murine cortical cultures. Brain Res. **764:** 133–410.
29. WILSON, M.E., D.B. DUBAL & P.M. WISE. 2000. Estradiol protects against injury-induced cell death in cortical explant cultures: a role for estrogen receptors. Brain Res. **873:** 235–242.
30. WANG, J., P.S. GREEN & J.W. SIMPKINS. 2001. Estradiol protects against ATP depletion, mitochondrial membrane potential decline and the generation of reactive oxygen species induced by 3-nitroproprionic acid in SK-N-SH human neuroblastoma cells. J. Neurochem. **77:** 804–811.
31. GOODMAN, Y. *et al.* 1996. Estrogens attenuate and corticosterone exacerbates excitotoxicity, oxidative injury, and amyloid beta-peptide toxicity in hippocampal neurons. J. Neurochem. **66:** 1836–1844.
32. MARDER, K. *et al.* 1998. Postmenopausal estrogen use and Parkinson's disease with and without dementia. Neurology **50:** 1141–1143.
33. TANG, M.X. *et al.* 1996. Effect of oestrogen during menopause on risk and age at onset of Alzheimer's disease. Lancet **348:** 429–432.
34. BALDERESCHI, M. *et al.* 1998. Estrogen-replacement therapy and Alzheimer's disease in the Italian Longitudinal Study on Aging. Neurology **50:** 996–1002.
35. ASTHANA, S. *et al.* 2001. High-dose estradiol improves cognition for women with AD: results of a randomized study. Neurology **57:** 605–612.
36. SLOOTER, A.J. *et al.* 1999. Estrogen use and early onset Alzheimer's disease: a population-based study. J. Neurol. Neurosurg. Psychiatry **67:** 779–781.
37. WARING, S.C. *et al.* 1999. Postmenopausal estrogen replacement therapy and risk of AD: a population-based study. Neurology **52:** 965–970.
38. MULNARD, R.A. *et al.* 2000. Estrogen replacement therapy for treatment of mild to moderate Alzheimer disease: a randomized controlled trial. Alzheimer's Disease Cooperative Study. JAMA **283:** 1007–1015.
39. MARKOU, A., T. DUKA & G.M. PRELEVIC. 2005. Estrogens and brain function. Hormones (Athens) **4:** 9–17.
40. MAKI, P.M. 2006. Potential importance of early initiation of hormone therapy for cognitive benefit. Menopause **13:** 6–7.
41. MAKI, P.M. 2006. Hormone therapy and cognitive function: is there a critical period for benefit? Neuroscience **138:** 1027–1030.
42. WISE, P.M. *et al.* 2001. Estradiol is a protective factor in the adult and aging brain: understanding of mechanisms derived from in vivo and in vitro studies. Brain Res. Brain Res. Rev. **37:** 313–319.
43. PAGANINI-HILL, A. 1998. Estrogen replacement therapy—something to smile about. Compend. Contin. Educ. Dent. (Suppl):S4–S8.
44. COLTON, C.A., C.M. BROWN & M.P. VITEK. 2005. Sex steroids, APOE genotype and the innate immune system. Neurobiol Aging **26:** 363–372.

45. XU, H. *et al.* 1998. Estrogen reduces neuronal generation of Alzheimer beta-amyloid peptides. Nat. Med. **4:** 447–451.

46. ZHENG, H. *et al.* 2002. Modulation of A(beta) peptides by estrogen in mouse models. J. Neurochem. **80:** 191–196.

47. GREENFIELD, J.P. *et al.* 2002. Estrogen lowers Alzheimer beta-amyloid generation by stimulating trans-Golgi network vesicle biogenesis. J. Biol. Chem. **277:** 12128–12136.

48. HSIAO, K. *et al.* 1996. Correlative memory deficits, Abeta elevation, and amyloid plaques in transgenic mice. Science **274:** 99–102.

49. DUFF, K. *et al.* 1996. Increased amyloid-beta42(43) in brains of mice expressing mutant presenilin 1. Nature **383:** 710–713.

50. HOLCOMB, L. *et al.* 1998. Accelerated Alzheimer-type phenotype in transgenic mice carrying both mutant amyloid precursor protein and presenilin 1 transgenes. Nat. Med. **4:** 97–100.

51. YUE, X. *et al.* 2005. Brain estrogen deficiency accelerates Abeta plaque formation in an Alzheimer's disease animal model. Proc. Natl. Acad. Sci. USA **102:** 19198–19203.

52. XU, H. *et al.* 1997. Generation of Alzheimer beta-amyloid protein in the trans-Golgi network in the apparent absence of vesicle formation. Proc. Natl. Acad. Sci. USA **94:** 3748–3752.

53. HARTMANN, T. *et al.* 1997. Distinct sites of intracellular production for Alzheimer's disease A beta40/42 amyloid peptides. Nat. Med. **3:** 1016–1020.

54. GREENFIELD, J.P. *et al.* 1999. Endoplasmic reticulum and trans-Golgi network generate distinct populations of Alzheimer beta-amyloid peptides. Proc. Natl. Acad. Sci. USA **96:** 742–747.

55. SCAMMELL, J.G., T.G. BURRAGE & P.S. DANNIES. 1986. Hormonal induction of secretory granules in a pituitary tumor cell line. Endocrinology **119:** 1543–1548.

56. DROUVA, S.V. *et al.* 1986. Estradiol activates methylating enzyme(s) involved in the conversion of phosphatidylethanolamine to phosphatidylcholine in rat pituitary membranes. Endocrinology **119:** 2611–2622.

57. DROUVA, S.V. *et al.* 1987. Variations of phospholipid methyltransferase(s) activity in the rat pituitary: estrous cycle and sex differences. Endocrinology **121:** 569–574.

58. CHEN, D. *et al.* 1999. Potential regulation of membrane trafficking by estrogen receptor alpha via induction of rab11 in uterine glands during implantation. Mol. Endocrinol. **13:** 993–1004.

59. CHAVRIER, P. & B. GOUD. 1999. The role of ARF and Rab GTPases in membrane transport. Curr. Opin. Cell. Biol. **11:** 466–475.

60. SCHLIERF, B. *et al.* 2000. Rab11b is essential for recycling of transferrin to the plasma membrane. Exp. Cell Res. **259:** 257–265.

61. HUTTNER, W.B. & A. SCHMIDT. 2000. Lipids, lipid modification and lipid-protein interaction in membrane budding and fission–insights from the roles of endophilin A1 and synaptophysin in synaptic vesicle endocytosis. Curr. Opin. Neurobiol. **10:** 543–551.

62. BUXBAUM, J.D. *et al.* 1990. Processing of Alzheimer beta/A4 amyloid precursor protein: modulation by agents that regulate protein phosphorylation. Proc. Natl. Acad. Sci. USA **87:** 6003–6006.

63. BLIGH, E.G. & W.J. DYER. 1959. A rapid method of total lipid extraction and purification. Can. J. Biochem. Physiol. **37:** 911–917.

64. PIKE, L.J. & A.T. EAKES. 1987. Epidermal growth factor stimulates the production of phosphatidylinositol monophosphate and the breakdown of polyphosphoinositides in A431 cells. J. Biol. Chem. **262:** 1644–1651.
65. GORDON, M.N. *et al.* 1986. Effective oral administration of 17 beta-estradiol to female C57BL/6J mice through the drinking water. Biol. Reprod. **35:** 1088–1095.
66. REFOLO, L.M. *et al.* 2000. Hypercholesterolemia accelerates the Alzheimer's amyloid pathology in a transgenic mouse model. Neurobiol. Dis. **7:** 321–331.

A Potential Role for Estrogen in Experimental Autoimmune Encephalomyelitis and Multiple Sclerosis

HALINA OFFNER[a,b,c] AND MAGDALENA POLANCZYK[a,c]

[a]Neuroimmunology Research, Veterans Affairs Medical Center, Portland, Oregon 97239, USA

[b]Department of Neurology, Oregon Health and Science University, Portland, Oregon 97239, USA

[c]Department of Anesthesiology and Perioperative Medicine, Oregon Health and Science University, Portland, Oregon 97239, USA

ABSTRACT: The extensive literature and the work from our laboratory illustrate the large number of complex processes affected by estrogen that might contribute to the striking ability of 17-β estradiol (E2) and its derivatives to inhibit clinical and histological signs of experimental autoimmune encephalomyelitis (EAE) in mice. These effects require sustained exposure to relatively low doses of exogenous hormone and offer better protection when initiated prior to induction of EAE. The E2 mediates inhibition of encephalitogenic T cells, inhibition of cell migration into central nervous system tissue, and neuroprotective effects that promote axon and myelin survival. E2 effects on EAE are mediated through *Esr-1* (α receptor for E2) but not *Esr-2* (β receptor for E2), as are its anti-inflammatory and neuroprotective effects. A novel finding is that E2 upregulated the expression of *FoxP3* that contributes to the activity of CD4 + CD25 + T regulatory cells (Treg). The protective effects of E2 in EAE suggest its use as a therapy for multiple sclerosis (MS). Possible risks may be minimized by using sub-pregnancy levels of exogenous E2 that produced synergistic effects when used in combination with another immunoregulatory therapy. Alternatively, one might envision using E2 derivatives alone or in combination therapies in both male and female MS patients.

KEYWORDS: estrogen; estrogen receptors; Treg; *FoxP3*; immunoregulation; neuroprotection; EAE; multiple sclerosis

Address for correspondence: Dr. Halina Offner, Neuroimmunology Research R&D-31, Portland VA Medical Center, 3710 SW U.S. Veterans Hospital Rd., Portland, OR 97239. Voice: 503-721-7893; fax: 503-721-7975.
e-mail: offnerva@ohsu.edu

Ann. N.Y. Acad. Sci. 1089: 343–372 (2006). © 2006 New York Academy of Sciences.
doi: 10.1196/annals.1386.021

INTRODUCTION

We demonstrated previously that relatively low doses of sex steroids, including estrogen (E2) confer protection against experimental autoimmune encephalomyelitis (EAE), an animal model for the human disease multiple sclerosis (MS). E2 may contribute to EAE resistance by influencing the development and function of potentially pathogenic T cells specific for myelin antigens, as well as regulatory T cells, including the newly described CD4 + CD25 + Treg cells that might modify the course of disease. Alternatively, E2 might affect the function of phagocytic macrophages, dendritic cells, or microglia, or nonimmune cells such as central nervous system (CNS) astrocytes, oligodendrocytes, or neurons. Previously, we reported that low doses of E2 can reduce the severity of EAE by inhibiting activation, production of cytokines (particularly TNF-α) and chemokines, and encephalitogenicity of murine T cells specific for myelin oligodendrocyte glycoprotein (MOG), proteolipid protein (PLP), or myelin basic protein (MBP),[2–4] and by inhibiting the recruitment of inflammatory cells into the CNS.[5] Recently, we demonstrated that ESR1$^{-/-}$ (ERKO) mice lacking *Esr-1* but not ESR2$^{-/-}$ (BERKO) mice lacking *Esr-2* were refractory to E2-mediated inhibition of chronic progressive EAE, thus implicating *Esr-1* in E2-mediated protection.[6] Overall, the effects of E2 on EAE involve immune regulation, inhibition of cell migration, and CNS neuroprotection, which all appear to be mediated through *Esr-1* expressed by both immune and nonimmune cells.

A distinct female predominance exists for a variety of human autoimmune disorders including rheumatoid arthritis (RA) 2–4:1, systemic lupus erythematosis (SLE) 5–13:1, scleroderma 3–4:1, Sjögren's syndrome 9:1, Grave's disease 4–8:1, and MS 2:1.[7] This differential gender susceptibility has also been observed in many experimental animal models of autoimmune disease[7] including lupus, insulin-dependent diabetes mellitus (IDDM), chronic thyroiditis (EAT), myasthenia gravis (MG), collagen- or adjuvant-induced arthritis (CIA or AA), and encephalomyelitis (EAE).[8,9] Recent evidence suggests that sex hormones play a central role in gender dimorphism. Gender differences in the immune response and susceptibility to autoimmune diseases usually become apparent after sexual maturity.[10] Furthermore, the increased levels of sex hormones (FIG. 1) produced during pregnancy are reported to reduce the clinical symptoms of MS and RA, but exacerbate symptoms of SLE.[11–13] Interestingly, the clinical symptoms of RA and MS worsen post partum, which is marked by reduced sex hormone levels.[12,14] The importance of sex steroids on pathogenic autoimmune disease has been demonstrated in experimental animal models by altering hormone levels. Androgens inhibit and estrogens enhance the incidence and severity of experimental murine lupus.[15] Oral contraceptives have been associated with disease exacerbation, and androgen analogues have shown some benefit in human SLE.[16] Orchidectomy increases and androgens decrease susceptibility of male rats to autoimmune

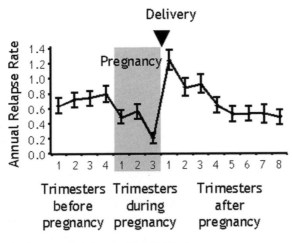

Confavreux, et al. *NEJM.* **339**, 285 (1998).
Vukusic, et al. *Brain.* **127**, 1353 (2004).

FIGURE 1. Relapse rates in MS patients before, during, and after pregnancy.

thyroiditis,[17] whereas E2 increases the production of anti-thyroglobulin anti-bodies.[18] Androgens have also been shown to reduce the incidence of experimental hemolytic anemia in mice[19] and rats,[20] and to decrease the severity of experimental Sjögren's syndrome–like lesions in mice.[21] E2 has been shown to suppress CIA and AA in rats,[22,23] and E2 or synthetic E2 analogues have also been shown to suppress EAE in both mice and rats.[24,25] In summary, females have a stronger immune response than males, which is likely responsible for their increased incidence of autoimmune disease. In males, decreased levels of circulating androgens after orchidectomy increases disease susceptibility, which is reversed by androgen replacement. In contrast, in females, E2 can enhance autoantibody production, resulting in increased severity of antibody-mediated diseases such as lupus, but at higher concentrations, E2 has also been shown to suppress experimental diseases mediated by T cells.

Gender differences in susceptibility to and severity of EAE have been known for many years, and for that reason, previous studies have used animals of the same sex. Although the precise mechanisms for this gender dimorphism remain elusive, there may be a regulatory role for sex hormones. Pregnancy has been shown to protect animals from EAE.[26–28] E2, administered at levels found during pregnancy (100-fold higher than basal levels), has been shown to suppress clinical EAE in mice and rats.[24,25] In addition, castration of female mice was shown to advance, and E2 treatment delay, the onset of EAE.[25] Recently, gender differences have been described in adoptively transferred EAE. Transfer of female MBP-sensitized lymph node cells (LNCs) into female mice resulted in typical severe EAE, while transfer into males produced attenuated disease symptoms.[29] Severe disease could be induced in male mice by transferring more cells or by castration. Furthermore, when MBP-specific LNCs from male and female mice were compared, the transfer of EAE with female cells resulted in more severe disease than with male cells.[29] Thus, gender differences in susceptibility to EAE are clearly multifactorial, with contributions from both the host and donor immune cells.

Although sex hormones are clearly involved in regulating the immune response, the mechanisms involved are complex and poorly understood. In some studies, females demonstrated stronger immune responses to vaccination, possibly due to an absolute increase in the number of CD4 + T cells. A number of studies have demonstrated the direct effects of sex hormones on immunocompetent cells. *In vitro* studies have shown that high doses of E2 can suppress mitogen- and antigen-induced proliferation of T cells, and depress suppressor T cell activity.[30,31] E2s have also been shown to inhibit delayed-type hypersensitivity (DTH) reactions.[32,33] Androgens have been shown to inhibit mitogen-induced proliferation, and enhance T suppressor activity.[34,35] Sex hormones have also been shown to influence the production of a number of inflammatory Th1 cytokines, including IFN-γ, TNF-α, IL-1, and IL-6, as well as anti-inflammatory Th2 cytokines IL-4, IL-5, and TGF-β.[7]

In addition to its well-characterized role in sexual differentiation and regulation of reproductive neuroendocrine function, E2 also has important neuroprotective effects in the central nervous system.[36,37] E2 promotes the growth and differentiation of neurons in the developing forebrain through high-affinity interactions with E2 receptors,[38] but generally is not active in the adult brain unless damage occurs, which stimulates neural regeneration. E2 appears to act in concert with neurotrophins (e.g., nerve growth factor, NGF; brain-derived neurotrophic factor, BDNF; and neurotrophins 3 and 4/5) that also have well-documented effects on the development, survival, plasticity, and aging of neurons that contribute to the reproductive and cognitive functions in the mammalian forebrain.[38] Neurons in the forebrain co-express E2 and neurotrophin receptors,[39] and also are abundant producers of E2[40] and neurotrophin. E2 and neurotrophins appear to reciprocally regulate each other's actions by cross-coupling of their signaling pathways, which ultimately lead to the induction of the same set of genes involved in neurite outgrowth and differentiation. Recently, Arvanitis demonstrated the presence of membrane-associated estrogen receptor (mER) in the oligodendrocyte plasma membrane and within the myelin sheath.[41] These data suggest the possibility that estrogen could act directly on myelin and contribute to its preservation and function. We have recently shown that E2 can prevent axonal loss in mice with EAE (Fig. 2).

In the last few years, there has been a renewed interest in regulatory CD4 + T cells that inhibit autoimmune diseases (see reviews by Mason,[1] Maloy and Powrie,[42] and Roncarolo[43]). Neonatal thymectomy of mice leads to the development of a spectrum of autoimmune diseases, including gastritis, oorphoritis, orchitis, and thyroiditis, all of which can be prevented by transferring CD4 +

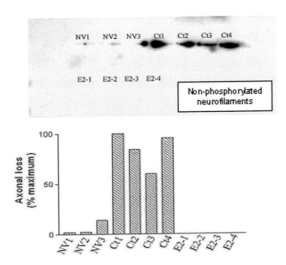

FIGURE 2. Estrogen prevents axonal loss in B6 mice with EAE.

T cells from normal mice.[44,45] These same diseases can be induced by CD4 + T cells that have been depleted of CD4 + CD25 + T cells, and transfer of CD4 + CD25 + T cells prevents the onset of disease induced by CD4 + CD25− T cells.[46,47] Similarly, in the experimental model of inflammatory bowel disease (IBD), cells capable of inhibiting IBD are found predominantly in the CD4 + CD45RB[lo]CD25 + subpopulation. [48] More recent studies demonstrate that CD4 + CD25 + T cells can inhibit EAE [49] and control type 1 diabetes in rats[50] and mice,[51] but these T cells can also suppress the ability of CD4 + CD25- effector T cells to eliminate the *Leishmania major* parasite from mouse skin lesions.[52] Taken together, these findings document the importance of the Treg subpopulation in regulating autoreactive as well as protective T effector cells *in vivo*.

The defining feature of Treg cells in both mice and humans is their ability to inhibit proliferation of other cell populations *in vitro*[53–60] through a cell–cell contact mechanism that may involve glucocorticoid-activated TNF receptor (GITR).[61,62] The suppressive activity requires T cell receptor (TCR) activation of Treg cells, but there are discrepant results as to whether co-stimulation through CTLA-4 is involved.[48,63,64] Ligation of CTLA-4 by B7.1 (CD80) and B7.2 (CD86) on APC strongly inhibits T cell activation,[65] and blockade of the CTLA-4 pathway reversed Treg suppression of allograft rejection.[66] Co-stimulation through CTLA-4 may enhance the production of membrane-bound TGF-β, which possibly contributes to the observed suppression.[67] However, in another study, Treg induction of anergy in the indicator cell population was not abrogated by blocking the B7-CTLA-4 pathway.[68] Both TGF-β and IL-10 have been implicated as possible players in the suppressive mechanism, although again there is not consensus. Oral antigen administration enhanced suppressive activity of CD4 + CD25 + T cells, which was partially dependent on both TGF-β and IL-10 in OVA/OVA-TCR transgenic mice.[69] Results from this model may be consistent with the ability of TGF-β to induce CD25 − T cells to become Th3 suppressor cells that secrete inhibitory levels of TGF-β, as well as regulatory cells that do not inhibit through TGF-β.[70] On the other hand, activation of Treg cells anergized indicator cells through a TGF-β-independent mechanism, but led to "infectious tolerance" through the indicator cells, which was partially mediated by soluble TGF-β.[71] IL-10 produced by Treg cells has been implicated in regulating the expansion of peripheral CD4 + T cells,[72] inhibiting the production of inflammatory cytokines,[73] and suppression of allograft rejection.[66] However, these effects could be mediated by co-isolated CD4 + (Tr1) type 1 regulatory T cells cells, which can produce suppressive levels of secreted IL-10 that can inhibit target cells through a cell contact–independent mechanism.[74] Thus, it seems likely that cell contact–dependent effects of Treg cells may be augmented *in vitro* by soluble TGF-β and IL-10 that may be secreted in limited quantities by the Treg cells themselves or in larger quantities by other regulatory subtypes present in the isolated CD4 + CD25 + fraction.

One difficulty in studying regulatory CD4 + CD25 + T cells has been the lack of a marker. Recently, the forkhead/winged helix transcription factor gene, *FoxP3*, has been strongly linked to the regulatory function of Treg cells.[75–77] *FoxP3* is defective in the mutant mouse strain, scurfy, which develops a lethal CD4 + T cell–mediated lymphoproliferative disease, and in humans with a similar lethal disease. *Scurfy* mice completely lack T regulatory CD4 + CD25 + T cell, and transfer of these T cells into *FoxP3*-deficient mice rescues the mice from disease. Moreover, ectopic expression of *FoxP3* confers Treg-suppressive function on peripheral CD4 + CD25– T cells. *FoxP3* is highly expressed by Treg cells, and forced expression of *FoxP3* strongly up-regulated several molecules typically associated with Treg function, including CD25, GITR, CD103, and CTLA-4. Importantly, transfer of *FoxP3*-transduced T cells prevented IBD and autoimmune gastritis. These findings clearly identify *FoxP3* as a key regulatory gene important in the development and function of Treg cells.

EAE is an inflammatory demyelinating disease of the CNS that is induced by the immunization of susceptible mice with myelin proteins or peptides.[78–80] EAE is a useful experimental model, and has provided considerable insight into the pathogenesis of the human disease MS. Immunization with myelin proteins or peptides in complete Freund's adjuvant induces autoreactive CD4+, Th1 cells that home specifically to the CNS and regulate the accumulation of inflammatory mononuclear cells, including T cells and macrophages, resulting in demyelination and clinical disease.[81] Encephalitogenic T cell lines or clones can be stimulated *in vitro* with specific antigen and are capable of transferring relapsing disease to naive hosts.[82] Analysis of inbred mouse strains demonstrated that specific MHC haplotypes (H-2^{p,q,r,s,u}) confer susceptibility to EAE.[83,84] In addition, non-MHC genes that control vascular sensitivity to vasoactive agents (e.g., histamine receptor H1), sex hormones, and other sex-linked gene products have been implicated in susceptibility to EAE.[85–87]

EFFECTS OF ESTROGENS ON EAE

Because of the increased susceptibility of females to autoimmune diseases, some have assumed that female sex hormones, including estrogen, actively facilitate the disease process. In contrast to this view, our studies clearly demonstrate an important regulatory role of estrogen in EAE (FIGS. 3 and 4). Both estrogen and testosterone had inhibitory effects on immunity, and it may be that the enhanced susceptibility to autoimmune disease in females versus males is simply due to less potent natural inhibition by estrogen than by testosterone. The following published and preliminary studies outline our key findings regarding the role of estrogen in EAE. Endogenous ovarian hormones naturally limit EAE.[2] To evaluate the possible regulatory effects of ovarian hormones on EAE, mice were ovariectomized (OVX) 1 week prior to the induction of the disease. OVX mice had significantly earlier onset and greater severity of EAE than sham-operated mice, clearly demonstrating that basal levels of ovarian hormones, including E2, acted to regulate rather than facilitate EAE. TNF-α, MIP-1α, and MIP-2 are associated with increased severity of EAE in ovariectomized or cytokine knockout mice.[4,88] To evaluate the contribution of various cytokines and chemokines on the induction of EAE, we compared the severity of EAE induced in wild-type and OVX BV8S2 Tg mice, and in wild-type and cytokine knockout C57BL/6J mice. We demonstrated that the severity of EAE was greatly reduced in TNF-α-deficient mice (reduction in peak EAE score and cumulative disease index, $P < 0.0001$,[4]), but was not significantly altered in IFN-γ, IL-4, or IL-10 knockout mice. IFN-γ is widely thought to contribute to the pathogenesis of EAE, but has also been implicated as a regulatory cytokine, based in part on a worsening of EAE in

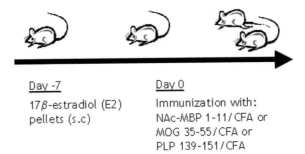

FIGURE 3. Experimental protocol for E2 protection.

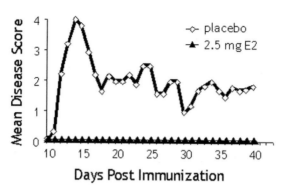

FIGURE 4. Estrogen suppresses EAE in SJL mice.

IFN-γ-deficient mice.[89,90] However, in our studies the loss of IFN-γ did not affect the course of EAE, failing to implicate this cytokine as being necessary for either the pathogenesis or regulation of EAE. Similarly, the loss of IL-4 or IL-10, cytokines known to possess immunomodulatory effects on EAE, did not affect the severity of EAE. Both MIP-1α and MIP-2 also appeared to be important contributors to EAE induction because the levels of expression of these two chemokines were markedly increased in CNS infiltrating cells from OVX mice that developed significantly worse EAE than did wild-type mice.[88] IL-12 also appears to be an important cytokine in EAE on account of the complete resistance to EAE of IL-12 knockout mice,[91] and our preliminary observation that the effects of E2 can be partially reversed by treatment with rIL-12 *in vivo* (data not shown).

E2 has a Marked Effect on the Expression of Cytokines and Chemokines in CNS, and Strongly Inhibits Recruitment of Inflammatory Cells

One major effect of E2 on EAE is to decrease inflammation in the CNS. As we have shown previously, E2-treated mice challenged to develop EAE had significantly lower histological scores, with >60% decrease in CNS infiltrating cells.[3,4,88,92] Recently, we found that E2 treatment strongly inhibited infiltration of total cells, macrophages, and T cells into the CNS, with a relative enrichment of microglial cells (Fig. 5).[4] This marked reduction in inflammatory cells was reflected in a strong reduction in the expression of chemokines RANTES, MIP-1α, MIP-2, IP-10, and MCP-1 (Fig. 6), chemokine receptors CCR1, 2, and 5 (not shown) in CNS of both intact and OVX mice, lymphokines LT-β, TNF-α, and IFN-γ in the CNS of intact mice (Fig. 6), and the expression of CCR1 and 5 in LNC (systemic effects).[88] Moreover, E2 inhibited intracellular staining of TNF-α in CNS macrophages, microglia, and T cells at the onset of EAE, and in macrophages at the peak of EAE (Fig. 7).[4]

(A)

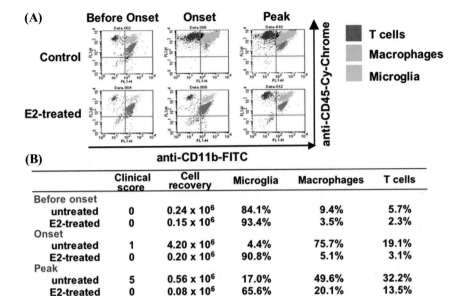

(B)

	Clinical score	Cell recovery	Microglia	Macrophages	T cells
Before onset					
untreated	0	0.24 x 10⁶	84.1%	9.4%	5.7%
E2-treated	0	0.15 x 10⁶	93.4%	3.5%	2.3%
Onset					
untreated	1	4.20 x 10⁶	4.4%	75.7%	19.1%
E2-treated	0	0.20 x 10⁶	90.8%	5.1%	3.1%
Peak					
untreated	5	0.56 x 10⁶	17.0%	49.6%	32.2%
E2-treated	0	0.08 x 10⁶	65.6%	20.1%	13.5%

FIGURE 5. E2 treatment suppresses the migration of inflammatory cells into CNS. C57BL/6J mice were treated with E2 (2.5 mg pellets) 1 week before induction of EAE with MOG-35-55/CFA + pertussogen. CNS mononuclear cells were isolated before onset (day 7), at onset (day 12), and at peak (day 19) of disease from perfused brains and spinal cords from 2 to 3 mice. The cells were cultured in the presence of GolgiPlug for 5 hr, and then double-stained with anti-CD45-Cy-chrome and anti-CD11b-FITC. **(A)** The plots show T cells (CD11b−, CD45^{high}) as red, macrophages (CD11b + , CD45^{high}) as green, and microglia (CD11b + , CD45^{low}) as blue dots. **(B)** Cell number of mononuclear cells recovered per CNS of 1 mouse. Cell number of each population is presented as a percentage of total cells. Note strong reduction of total cells, macrophages, and T cells in CNS tissue of E2-treated mice.

E2 Inhibits TNF-α Expression and Passive Transfer of EAE by Encephalitogenic T Cells

Our studies showed also that E2 treatment *in vivo* consistently inhibited EAE over a wide range of doses, and was active even at diestrous levels in some strains of mice. To investigate the mechanism of action, responses of encephalitogenic T cells were assessed in LN, spleen, and CNS cell cultures from E2-treated mice. Surprisingly, proliferation responses to encephalitogenic peptides were only modestly reduced, even in cultures from fully protected mice,[2-4] and there were no striking changes in the expression of cell surface markers from LN cells of E2-treated C57BL/6J mice, including VLA-4, CD44hi, CD69, FasL, CD25, CD40L, CD28, CD62lo.[4] However, PLP-139-151-activated LN cells from E2-treated SJL/J mice had a significantly reduced capacity to transfer EAE.[3] Moreover, MOG-35-55-stimulated CNS mononuclear cells from

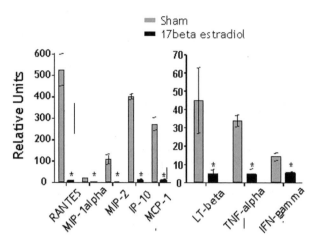

FIGURE 6. RPA analysis of cytokine and chemokine mRNA expression in the spinal cords of E2-treated and control TCR BV8S2 transgenic female mice with EAE. Quantification of individual RPA bands in comparison to the housekeeping gene L32 from spinal cord tissue at peak (day 17) of EAE induced by MBP-Ac1-11 peptide/CFA in BV8S2 Tg mice. Data are presented as the mean ± SD from four different experiments. Data quantified from RPA analysis revealed that gene expression in E2-treated versus control BV8S2 Tg female mice with EAE was significantly reduced for the chemokines RANTES, MIP-1alpha, MIP-2, IP-10, and MCP-1 ($P < 0.0001$); and lymphokines LT-β, TNF-α, and IFN-γ ($P = 0.019$, $P < 0.0001$ and $P < 0.01$, respectively).

E2-treated C57BL/6J mice exhibited (FIG. 7) a profound reduction in intracellular staining of TNF-α.[4] Furthermore, the addition of E2 to splenocyte cultures from wild-type or BV8S2 double transgenic mice stimulated with MBP-Ac1-11 or anti-CD3 mAb inhibited the percentage of TNF-α-stained T cells[4] and the secretion of IFN-γ, with no effect on proliferation responses or secretion of IL-10 or IL-12. The pronounced systemic effect of estrogen on TNF-α production was further verified among splenocytes from E2-treated and control mice, and, as indicated by microarray analysis, the expression of TNF-α was reduced >10-fold in splenocytes from E2-treated mice compared to control mice with EAE. [93] Thus, systemic E2 regulation of TNF-α production could account for much of the observed reduction in EAE severity by restricting the ability of encephalitogenic cells to enter the CNS, suppressing the recruitment and activation of other inflammatory cells, and/or inhibiting TNF-α-induced damage to myelin-producing oligodendrocytes. These novel observations, coupled with the established importance of TNF-α in the induction of EAE,[94] provide strong evidence that the inhibitory effects of estrogen on TNF-α production by T cells, macrophages, and microglial cells constitutes a major regulatory pathway.

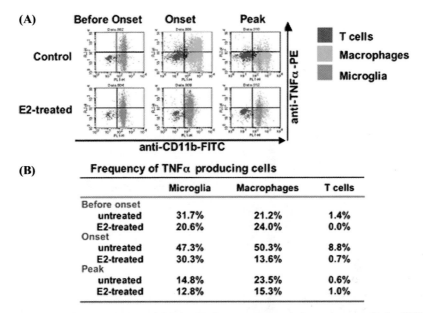

FIGURE 7. E2 treatment inhibits TNF-α producing inflammatory cells in CNS of mice with EAE. C57BL/6J mice were treated with E2 (2.5 mg pellets) 1 week before induction of EAE with MOG-35-55/CFA + pertussogen. CNS mononuclear cells were isolated before onset (day 7), at onset (day 12), and at peak (day 19) of disease from perfused brains and spinal cords from 2 to 3 mice. (**A**) The cells were triple-stained for expression of CD45, CD11b, and intracellular TNF-α. The plots were gated on CD45 + cells and show TNF-α+ (*upper quadrants*) T cells (CD11b−) as red, macrophages as green, and microglia as blue dots. The data are quantified in the table. (**B**) Note a strongly reduced percentage of TNF-α producing T cells and macrophages in E2-treated mice at disease onset.

E2 Alters APC Function of Macrophages and Dendritic Cells [95]

To further evaluate the effects of E2 on antigen-presenting cells, peritoneal macrophages from E2-treated or control mice were combined with T cells from E2-treated or control mice, and the mixtures stimulated with anti-CD3 mAb (FIG. 8). E2 treatment sharply reduced the number of macrophages obtained from the peritoneal cavity (FIG. 8A), and drastically altered the cytokine profile of the anti-CD3-stimulated mixture (FIG. 8B) by way of specific effects on macrophages but not T cells, causing a nearly complete reduction in the secretion of IL-12 and IFN-γ, and strongly upregulating the secretion of IL-10 (FIG. 8B). Moreover, E2 treatment *in vivo* reduced the percentage of CD11b+, CD11c+ dendritic cells (DCs) in the spleen and CNS at EAE onset and peak, and inhibited *in vitro* DC activation of MBP-Ac1-11–specific T cells from BV8S2 double Tg mice.[95] E2 treatment appears to have multiple effects on the DC population, which may contribute to a downregulation or block in the

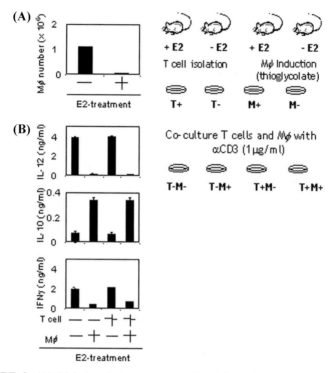

FIGURE 8. (A) E2-induced changes are mediated through antigen-presenting cells (APCs) rather than T cells. Peritoneal exudate cells were obtained 48 h after injection of thioglycolate from mice pretreated with or without E2, as shown in the cartoon. (B) E2 treatment inhibited recruitment of macrophages (Mφ) into the peritoneal cavity. Mφ (1×10^6 cells) obtained from the peritoneal cavity were used to stimulate T cells at a ratio of 1:1 in the presence of anti-mouse CD3 antibody (1 μg/mL) for 20 h. The activation of either E2-pretreated (T +) or untreated (T–) T cells in combination with E2-pretreated (Mφ +) macrophages resulted in a nearly complete reduction in secretion of IL-12 and IFN-γ and a pronounced increase in secreted IL-10. In contrast, T cells from E2-pretreated mice that were activated in the presence of untreated macrophages retained high levels of IL-12 and IFN-γ and low levels of IL-10.

activation of Th1 cells involved in the induction of EAE. In our recent studies we were able to identify E2-induced enhancement of programmed death-1 (PD-1) expression in DCs and macrophages but not in B cells. These novel findings indicate that E2-induced immunomodulation is mediated in part through potentiation in BM-DCs of the PD-1 co-stimulatory pathway.[96]

Estrogen Receptor Studies[6]

As mentioned above, there are two known classical intracellular estrogen receptors, *Esr-1* and *Esr-2*, which mediate their effects by transcription

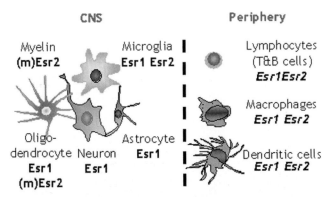

FIGURE 9. Expression of estrogen receptors in the CNS and periphery.

regulation, as well as a possibly distinct membrane-associated receptor (mER), which is associated with calcium flux and other signaling events (FIG. 9). One of our main goals was to determine which the estrogen receptor (ER) mediates various E2-related effects on EAE. To assess the role of intracytoplasmic estrogen receptors in mediating suppression of EAE, we studied ERKO and BERKO mice from the Taconic laboratory (Germantown, NY, USA). We demonstrated that the protective effect of E2 was abrogated in ERKO but not in BERKO mice.[6] The loss of E2-mediated protection from EAE in ERKO mice

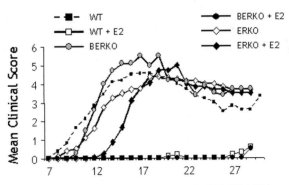

Days post-immunization with MOG35-55/CFA

FIGURE 10. E2 treatment suppressed actively induced EAE in C57BL/6 and BERKO but not in ERKO mice. Estrogen protection against EAE is mediated through *Esr-1*. Wild-type ERKO and BERKO female mice were implanted with 2.5 mg E2 or placebo pellets, respectively, 1 week before the induction of EAE. E2 treatment suppressed actively induced EAE in C57BL/6 and BERKO mice, while in ERKO mice this protective effect was lost. The data show mean clinical EAE scores for each day for C57BL/6 female mice treated with saline or E2 pellets; C57BL/6.129 ERKO females treated with saline or E2 pellets; and C57BL/6.129 BERKO females treated with saline or E2 pellets.

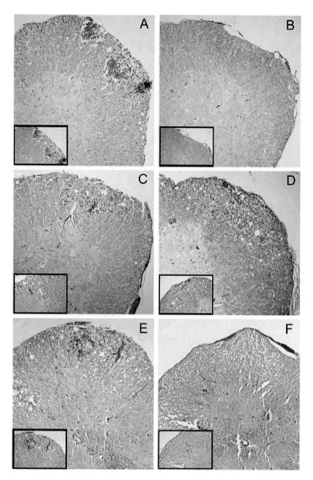

Histopathological examination of spinal cord sections from
C57BL/6, ERKO and BERKO mice reveals the lack of protection
against EAE in ERKO mice treated with 2.5 mg E2 pellet A)
C57BL/6 B) With E2 pellet C) ERKO D) With E2 pellet E) BERKO F)
With E2 pellet

FIGURE 11. Histopathological examination of spinal cord sections from C57BL/6 ERKO and BERKO mice reveals the lack of protection against EAE in ERKO mice treated with 2.5 mg E2 pellet. (**A**) C57BL/6 mice treated with placebo pellet with EAE (magnification × 50). (**B**) C57BL/6 mice treated with 2.5 mg E2 pellet, fully protected from EAE. No visible signs of inflammation were present within spinal cord tissue. (**C**) B6.129 ERKO mice treated with placebo pellet with EAE. (**D**) B6.129 ERKO mice treated with 2.5 mg E2 pellet with EAE. Several foci of inflammation are clearly evident within the spinal cord tissue. (**E**) B6.129 BERKO mice treated with placebo pellet with EAE. (**F**) B6.129 BERKO mice treated with 2.5 mg E2 pellet, fully protected from EAE. No visible signs of inflammation were present within spinal cord tissue. Histopathological sections for placebo- and E2-treated BERKO mice were essentially the same as in C57BL/6 mice.

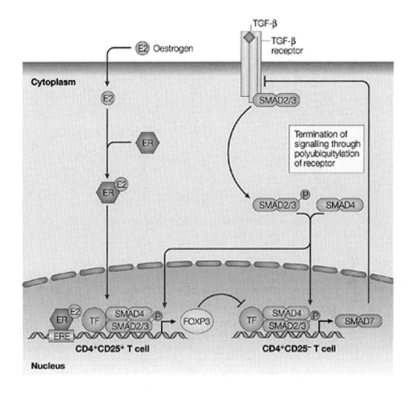

Coffer, PJ and Burgering, BM. *Nature Reviews Immunology* 4, 889-899 (2004)

FIGURE 12. *FoxP3* is a master regulator of regulatory T cells.

immunized with the encephalitogenic MOG-35-55 peptide was manifested phenotypically by the development of severe acute clinical signs (FIG. 10) and histopathologic lesions (FIG. 11), even in the presence of moderately high serum E2 levels. This is in contrast to C57BL/6 wild-type mice and BERKO mice in which E2 treatment resulted in comparable serum levels and markedly suppressed clinical signs of EAE and abolished inflammatory lesions in the CNS (FIG. 11). This pattern showing a lack of E2-dependent inhibition of EAE in ERKO mice was mirrored by an enhanced rather than a reduced secretion of TNF-α, IFN-γ, and IL-6 in MOG-specific splenocytes and a lack of inhibition of message for inflammatory cytokines, chemokines, and chemokine receptors in CNS tissue. These results indicate that the immunomodulatory effects of E2 in EAE are dependent on *Esr-1* and not *Esr-2* signaling. Our results have been independently confirmed[97] and are highly consistent with another recent report showing that *Esr-1* mediates anti-inflammatory effects of E2 in brain.[98]

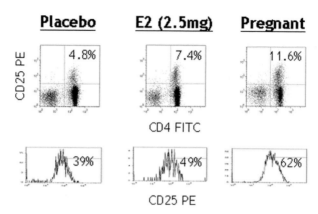

FIGURE 13. E2-induces an increase in CD4+CD25+ T cells in naïve mice. FACS analysis of sorted CD4 + CD25 + T cells isolated from placebo, E2-treated, and pregnant mice. FACS analysis was carried out on MACS-sorted CD4 + cells pooled from 8 to 10 mice per condition. The number in the upper right quadrant of the top figure in each panel indicates the percentage of CD25 + T cells present in the bead-sorted, CD4-enriched cell population. The number in the lower panel indicates the percentage of CD25[bright] cells (fluorescent intensity >100 U) found in the total CD4 + CD25 + subpopulation (upper right quadrant).

We also evaluated the lack of *Esr-1* and *Esr-2* on other E2 functions in placebo- or E2-treated female mice with EAE.[6] Quantification of serum E2 levels revealed a low but measurable concentration of endogenous E2 in ERKO placebo-treated mice, which was similar to that present in C57BL/6 wild-type littermate controls, but lower than in BERKO mice. Moreover, treatment with E2 pellets produced comparable levels of serum E2 in all three mouse strains, indicating that the lack of functional estrogen receptors did not effect E2 degradation. As expected, ERKO mice had no significant increase in uterine index (expressed as uterine weight [mg] divided by body weight [g]) compared to wild-type controls and BERKO mice. However, E2 treatment significantly increased the uterine index nearly threefold in WT and BERKO mice but not ERKO mice. In contrast, lack of either *Esr-1* or *Esr-2* resulted in a moderate decrease in thymic index compared to wild-type controls, and treatment with E2 strongly diminished thymus weight in all three mouse strains. Testosterone levels were low but detectable in WT and BERKO mice, but were markedly increased in ERKO mice, consistent with a previous report.[99] We have previously shown that testosterone can inhibit rather than promote encephalitogenic activity of myelin-specific T cells,[100] thus diminishing the possibility that increased testosterone levels enhanced EAE in ERKO mice. Taken together, these results are consistent with previous findings regarding the role of *Esr-1* and *Esr-2* signaling, and serve as internal controls for the observed effects on EAE.[101–105]

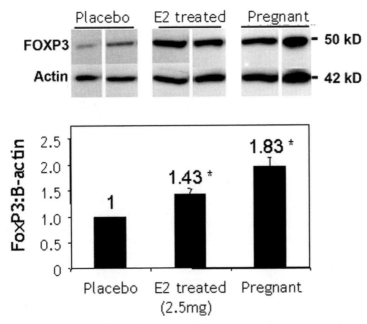

FIGURE 14. Enhanced FoxP3 expression in E2 treated naïve mice. *FoxP3* vs. β-actin Western blot analyses of FACS-sorted CD4 + CD25+ T cells isolated from the spleens of placebo, E2-treated, and pregnant mice. Cells were pooled from 8 to 10 mice before sorting. Figure shows blots from cells collected in two of eight separate experiments. Densitometry shows fold induction of *FoxP3*:β-actin ratio in E2-treated or pregnant mice relative to placebo mice. No *FoxP3* was detected in Western blots from sorted CD4 + CD25− T cells. *Significant difference in ratios determined by Student's t-test ($P < 0.05$).

Effects of E2 on Treg Activity and FoxP3 Expression[106]

CD4+CD25+ regulatory T cells are crucial to the maintenance of tolerance in normal individuals. However, the factors regulating this cell population and its function are largely unknown. Estrogen has been shown to protect against the development of autoimmune disease, yet the mechanism is not known. We demonstrated that E2 is capable of augmenting *FoxP3* expression *in vitro* and *in vivo* (FIG. 12). Treatment of naive mice with E2 increased both CD25+ cell frequency (FIG. 13) and *FoxP3* expression level (FIG. 14). Furthermore, the ability of E2 to protect against EAE correlated with its ability to upregulate *FoxP3* (FIG. 15), as both were reduced in E2 ESR1-deficient animals (FIGS. 15 and 16). Finally, E2 treatment and pregnancy induced *FoxP3* protein expression to a similar degree, suggesting that high estrogen levels during pregnancy may help to maintain fetal tolerance (FIG. 14). In summary, our data suggest that E2 promotes tolerance by expanding the regulatory T cell compartment. To

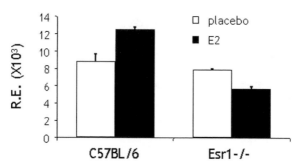

FIGURE 15. Induction of FoxP3 mRNA by E2 requires Esr1 *in vivo*. Real-time RT-PCR analysis of *FoxP3*. C57BL/6 and *Esr-1*$^{-/-}$ (ERKO) mice were implanted with placebo or 2.5 mg of E2 pellets and immunized 1 week later with 200 µg of MOG 35–55 peptide in CFA with pertussis toxin on days 0 and + 2. At the peak of clinical disease, mice were sacrificed and splenocytes sorted for CD4$^+$ cells. cDNA was prepared and analyzed by real-time PCR to determine *FoxP3* mRNA levels. Data are presented as *FoxP3* relative to housekeeping gene L32. Error bars are SD of triplicate samples.

evaluate E2 effects on Treg cell function, we studied Treg suppression in CD4 + CD25 + T cells from pregnant and E2-treated mice (FIG. 17), and overt Treg suppression in E2- versus placebo-pretreated mice with EAE (FIG. 18). The data clearly demonstrated that enhanced expression of *FoxP3*, which occurs in pregnant mice and in mice treated exogenously with E2 pellets, results in a concomitant increase in functional suppression within the CD4 + CD25 (bright) Treg fraction of splenocytes. The similarities in *FoxP3* expression and Treg cell function in E2-treated and pregnant mice implicate E2 as a major contributor for increasing Treg function during pregnancy.

Synergistic Effects of Estrogen Therapy and TCR Therapy in EAE [2]

Transgenic mice expressing the BV8S2 chain specific for myelin basic protein determinant Ac1-11 possess a naturally induced set of regulatory T cells directed against BV8S2.[107] Further activation of anti-BV8S2 T cells in male mice with recombinant BV8S2 protein can inhibit IFN-γ release by Ac1-11-specific T cells through a cytokine-driven mechanism and prevent induction of EAE.[108] In contrast, naive female mice possess fewer anti-BV8S2-reactive T cells, and treatment with BV8S2 delayed but did not prevent EAE. We demonstrated that combining TCR vaccination plus supplemental doses of E2 potentiated anti-BV8S2-reactive T cells to produce more IL-10 and deviated Ac1-11-specific T cells to produce IL-10 and TGF-β, resulting in full protection against EAE not observed with either therapy alone. These findings imply that supplemental E2 or E2 derivatives can enhance the efficacy of TCR-based immunotherapy for autoimmune diseases, which predominate in females.

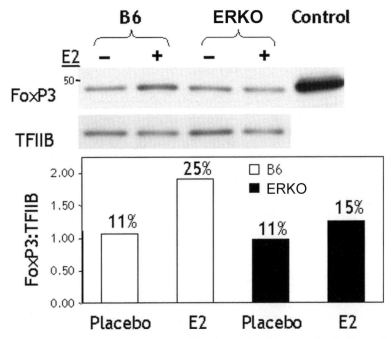

FIGURE 16. E2 treatment increases FoxP3 protein expression *in vivo* **by an Esr1-dependent mechanism.** Splenocytes were harvested from immunized WT C57BL/6 and (ERKO) female mice with EAE (peak of disease) implanted with placebo or E2 (2.5 mg pellets). The splenocytes were depleted of Thy1.2$^+$ cells by magnetic sorting on the autoMACS (Miltenyi Biotec). 5×10^4 T cell-depleted APCs and FACS-sorted CD4$^+$CD25$^-$ cells were plated in triplicate wells. Sorted CD4$^+$CD25$^+$ cells were added at ratios of 1:2 (10^5/well), 1:1 (5×10^4/well), 1:0.5 (2.5×10^4/well), 1:0 (no CD4 + CD25 + cells added) or 0:1 (5×10^4 CD4$^+$CD25$^+$, no CD4$^+$CD25$^-$), and stimulated with soluble anti-CD3 antibodies. Plates were pulsed with ^{3}H-thymidine after 48 h in culture and harvested after 72 h.

Summary and Proposed Mechanism of Action of E2 in EAE

The extensive literature and the work from our laboratory illustrate the large number of complex processes affected by E2 *in vivo* that might contribute to the striking ability of E2 to inhibit clinical and histological signs of EAE. The three main areas discussed above include direct and indirect inhibition of encephalitogenic T cells and APCs, inhibition of cell migration and infiltration into the CNS tissue, and neuroprotective effects that promote axon and myelin survival. Our work demonstrates that relatively low doses of E2 have strong inhibitory effects on the development of clinical and histological EAE. These effects require sustained exposure to constant levels of exogenous hormones and offer better protection when initiated prior to the induction of EAE. The E2 inhibition of EAE was clearly mediated through *Esr-1* and not *Esr-2*. It is

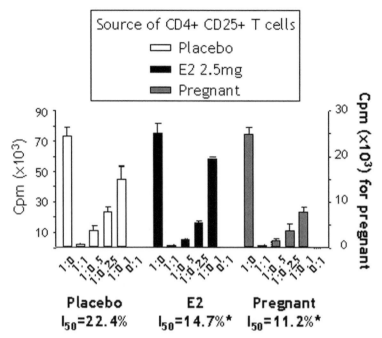

FIGURE 17. Enhanced suppressive activity of Treg cells in E2 treated and pregnant mice. The suppressive activity of Treg cells recovered from placebo, E2-treated and pregnant mice was measured by their ability to suppress the growth of CD4+ CD25− cells. The variable numbers of the suppressor populations were plated with (5×10^4/well) together with 10^5 APCs and 0.5 μg/mL anti-CD3 mAbs. In all conditions indicator cells originated from naïve donors. Each dilution was set in triplicate and culture was maintained for 3 d. All proliferations were monitored by the addition of [^{3}H]thymidine (1 μCi/well; for the last 12 h of culture), representative of three independent experiments. I_{50} = % of Treg cells that produced 50% suppression of indicator cells activated with CD3 Abs. Lower I_{50} indicates more suppression in E2-treated and pregnant mice.

of considerable interest to note that the anti-inflammatory and neuroprotective effects of E2 are also mediated through *Esr-1*.

The effects of E2 in preventing EAE appear to be mediated by both direct and indirect inhibition of encephalitogenic Th1 cells, macrophages, and dendritic cells. The most dramatic effect of E2 involved the strong inhibition of TNF-α by Th1 cells and APCs, and it is noteworthy that E2 also enhanced production of TGF-β3, which has been associated with EAE protection using other agents as well.[109] A novel finding is that E2 upregulated the expression of *FoxP3*, which contributes to the activity of Treg cells. These data provide an indirect mechanism by which E2 might enhance systemic immunoregulation. A consistent finding in our studies was the ability of E2 to inhibit infiltrating inflammatory cells during EAE. This effect was associated with the systemic

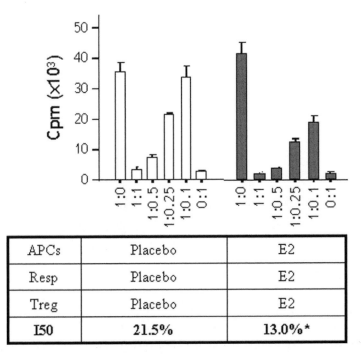

APCs	Placebo	E2
Resp	Placebo	E2
Treg	Placebo	E2
I50	21.5%	13.0%*

FIGURE 18. Treg function is strongly enhanced in E2-treated mice protected from EAE. Evaluation of Treg suppressive activity in E2-protected vs. placebo-treated mice with EAE. Female C57BL/6 mice were pretreated with E2 or placebo for 7 days prior to challenge with MOG-35–55 peptide/CFA/Ptx to induce EAE. At the peak of EAE in the placebo group (day 15 after induction), cells were harvested from both the placebo-treated mice (score = 4.5–5) and E2-treated mice (score = 0). Cell mixtures were combined within each treatment group. 5×10^4 CD4 + CD25− responder cells in combination with 5×10^4 APCs and the indicated ratios of CD4 + CD25 + suppressor cells were stimulated in triplicate wells with anti-CD3 mAbs for 3 days, with the addition of [^{3}H]-thymidine for the last 12 h of culture. Representative data from one of three independent experiments is shown. Treg cells from E2-pretreated donors showed greater suppressive activity than Treg cells from placebo controls, as determined by I_{50}. Significant differences ($P \leq 0.05$) were observed between groups at all ratios of indicator:Treg cells, as determined by Student's t-test.

reduction in the expression of the chemokine RANTES, and the upregulation of CCR3 thought to be expressed by Treg cells. We also found reduced expression of VLA-4 and LFA-1 in E2-treated mice that might prevent cell migration (unpublished studies). The reduction in inflammatory cell number likely accounts for the dramatic inhibition in the expression of cytokines, chemokines, and chemokine receptors within the CNS. However, E2 can easily cross the blood–brain barrier and is also locally synthesized within the damaged CNS, and it is probable that increased E2 levels afford some level of neuroprotection that also contributes to normal clinical function and the near absence of

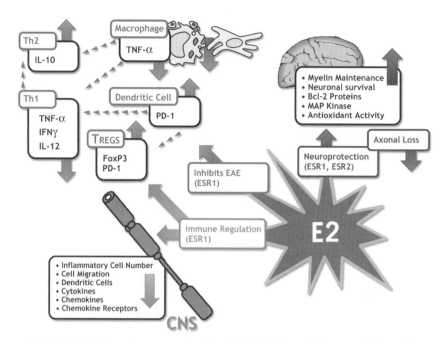

FIGURE 19. Neuroimmunoprotective effects of estrogen. E2 uses multiple pathways for inhibiting immune responses to encephalitogenic determinants and provides neuroprotection against axonal and myelin loss. E2 may enhance activity of Treg cells through upregulation of PD-1 and *FoxP3* expression, or directly inhibit production of TNF-α by encephalitogenic Th1 cells. E2 may also inhibit antigen presentation by dendritic cells (DCs) and macrophages. Moreover, E2 inhibits migration of inflammatory cells into the CNS through the inhibition of RANTES and upregulation of CCR3, thereby reducing the production of many cytokines, chemokines, and chemokine receptors within the CNS. Finally, E2 is known to have strong neuroprotective effects, including increasing production of Bcl-2 proteins and MAP kinase, which enhance neuronal and myelin survival and integral antioxidant properties.

histological disease in E2-treated mice. On a final note, the ability of E2 to potentiate Treg cells directed against TCR determinants underscores the potential of using E2 in combination with other therapeutic modalities.

THERAPEUTIC IMPLICATIONS FOR MS

The striking protective effects of E2 in EAE raise the possibility that some form of estrogen might be beneficial as a therapy for MS.[110,111] Moreover, the neuroprotective effects of estrogen might have a particular value in preserving the nerve viability and myelin function in the CNS that is gradually lost during the progression of MS.[112] As discussed above, MS patients experience a significant decrease in relapses, especially during the third trimester of pregnancy,[12] possibly implicating the effects of highly elevated sex hormones, 17-β-estradiol, and estriol. Rhonda Voskuhl and colleagues have now completed a phase I clinical trial of estriol to treat 10 female MS patients.[113] Their study demonstrated that at a dose of 8 mg/day given orally for 6 months (producing serum levels of about 4 ng/mL), the patients had decreased delayed-type hypersensitivity reactions to tetanus recall antigen, decreased IFN-γ levels in blood mononuclear cells, and reduced numbers and volumes of gadolinium-enhancing lesions. Moreover, there was a significant improvement in cognitive scores using the paced auditory serial addition (PASAT) test in women with relapsing–remitting MS, but not secondary progressive MS. These are encouraging results that suggest a role for sex hormones in the treatment of MS. It is of particular importance that the preclinical studies in EAE involved a treatment regimen in which estriol was given 10–14 days prior to the transfer of encephalitogenic T cells, resulting in disease reduction but not complete protection.[28] This treatment regime has some similarity to the fully protective regime we used routinely with low doses of E2 to prevent EAE and indicate that results obtained in our E2 pretreatment studies might also be translatable to MS patients.

ACKNOWLEDGMENTS

Dr. Offner wishes to thank collaborators and associates who contributed to the work described in this review, including Dr. Arthur A. Vandenbark, Dr. Agata Matejuk, Dr. Bruce Bebo, Dr. Cory Teuscher, Alex Zamora, Sandhya Subramanian, Corwyn Hopke, and Micah Tovey, as well as Eva Niehaus for assistance in preparing this review. This work was supported by Grants AI42376 and NS23444 from the National Institutes of Health, a grant from the National Multiple Sclerosis Society, the Nancy Davis MS Center without Walls, and the Biomedical Laboratory R&D Service, Department of Veterans' Affairs.

REFERENCES

1. MASON, D. & F. POWRIE. 1998. Control of immune pathology by regulatory T cells. Curr. Opin. Immunol. **10**: 649–655.
2. OFFNER, H. *et al*. 2000. Estrogen potentiates treatment with T-cell receptor protein of female mice with experimental encephalomyelitis. J. Clin. Invest. **105**: 1465–1472.
3. BEBO, B.F. *et al*. 2001. Low-dose estrogen therapy ameliorates experimental autoimmune encephalomyelitis in two different inbred mouse strains. J. Immunol. **166**: 2080–2089.
4. ITO, A. *et al*. 2001. Estrogen treatment down-regulates TNF-α production and reduces the severity of experimental autoimmune encephalomyelitis in cytokine knockout mice. J. Immunol. **167**: 542–552.

5. MATEJUK, A. *et al.* 2000. Reduced chemokine and chemokine receptor expression in spinal cords of TCR BV8S2 transgenic mice protected against experimental autoimmune encephalomyelitis with BV8S2 protein. J. Immunol. **164:** 3924–3931.

6. POLANCZYK, M. *et al.* 2003. The protective effect of 17B-estradiol on experimental autoimmune encephalomyelitis is mediated through estrogen receptor-α. Am. J. Pathol. **163:** 1599–1605.

7. WHITACRE, C.C.. 2001. Sex differences in autoimmune disease. Nature Immunol. **2:** 777–780.

8. BEBO, B.F., A.A. VANDENBARK & H. OFFNER. 1996. Male SJL mice do not relapse after induction of EAE with PLP 139–151. J. Neurosci. Res. **45:** 680–689.

9. VOSKUHL, R.R. *et al.* 1996. Gender differences in autoimmune demyelination in the mouse: Implications for multiple sclerosis. Ann. Neurol. **39:** 724–731.

10. BLAZKOVEC, A.A. & M.W. ORSINI. 1976. Ontogenetic aspects of sexual dimorphism and the primary immune response to sheep erythrocytes in hamster from prepuberty through senescence. Intl. Arch. Allergy Appl. Immunol. **50:** 55–60.

11. OKA, M. & U. VAINIO. 1966. Effect of pregnancy on the prognosis and serology of RA. Acta Rheumatol. Scand. **12:** 47–53.

12. CONFAVREUX, C. *et al.* 1998. Rate of pregnancy-related relapse in multiple sclerosis. New Engl. J. Med. **339:** 285–291.

13. GARSENSTEIN, M., V.E. POLLAK, & R.M. KARK. 1962. Systemic lupus erythematosus and pregnancy. New Engl. J. Med. **267:** 917–921.

14. OSTENSEN, M. & G.A. HUSBY. 1983. A prospective clinical study of the effect of pregnancy on rheumatoid arthritis and ankylosing spondylitis. Arthritis & Rheumatol. **25:** 1155–1160.

15. ROUBINIAN, J.R., R. PAPOIAN & N. TALAL. 1977. Androgenic hormones modulate autoantibody responses and improve survival in murine lupus. J. Clin. Inv. **59:** 1066–1071.

16. JUNGERS, P., M. DOUGADOS, C. PELISSIER, *et al.* 1982. Influence of oral contraceptive therapy on activity of systemic lupus erythematosus. Arthritis & Rheumatol. **125:** 618–625.

17. ANSAR, A.S. & W.J. PENHALE. 1982. The influence of testosterone on the development of autoimmune thyroiditis in thymectomized and irradiated rats. Clin. Exp. Immunol. **48:** 367–372.

18. OKAYASU, I., Y.M. KONG & N.R. ROSE. 1981. Effect of castration and sex hormones on experimental autoimmune thyroiditis. Clin. Immunol. Immunopathol. **20:** 240–246.

19. STERNBERG, A.D., P.A. SMATHERS & W.B. BOEGEL. 1980. Effects of sex hormones on autoantibody production of NZB mice and modification by environmental factors. Clin. Immunol. Immunopathol. **17:** 562–570.

20. MILCH, D.R. & M.E. GERSHWIN. 1981. Murine autoimmune hemolytic anemia via xenogeneic erythrocyte immunization. III. Differences in sex. Clin. Immunol. Immunopathol. **18:** 1–7.

21. ARIGA, H., J. EDWARDS & D.A. SULLIVAN. 1989. Androgen control of autoimmune expression in lacrimal gland of MRL-MP/lpr-lpr mice. Clin. Immunol. Immunopathol. **53:** 499–504.

22. LARSON, P. & R. HOLMDAHL. 1987. Estrogen-induced suppression of collagen arthritis. II. Treatment of rats suppresses development of arthritis but does not affect the anti-type II collagen humoral response. Scand. J. Immunol. **27:** 579–586.

23. TOIVANEN, P., H. SUKALA, P. LAIHO, & T. PAAVLIAINES. 1967. Suppression of adjuvant arthritis by estrone in adrenalectomized and ovarectomized rats. Experentia **23:** 560–568.

24. TROOSTER, W.J. *et al.* 1993. Suppression of acute experimental allergic encephalomyelitis by the synthetic sex hormone 17-alpha-ethinylestradiol: an immunological study in the Lewis rat. Intl. Arch. Allergy & Immunol. **102:** 133–140.

25. JANSSON, L., T. OLSSON & R. HOLMDAHL. 1994. Estrogen induces a potent suppression of experimental autoimmune encephalomyelitis and collagen-induced arthritis in mice. J. Neuroimmunol. **53:** 203–207.

26. EVRON, S., T. BRENNER & O. ABRAMSKY. 1984. Suppressive effect of pregnancy on the development of experimental allergic encephalomyelitis in rabbits. Am. J. Reprod. Immunol. **5:** 109–114.

27. MERTIN, L.A. & V.M. RUMJANEK. 1985. Pregnancy and susceptibility of Lewis rats to experimental allergic encephalomyelitis. J. Neurol. Sci. **68:** 15–21.

28. VOSKUHL, R.R. & K. PALASZYNSKI. 2001. Sex hormones in experimental autoimmune encephalomyelitis: implications for multiple sclerosis. Neuroscientist **7:** 258–270.

29. SMITH, M.E. & N.L. ELLER. 1996. Gender influences EAE both before and after sexual maturation. FASEB J. **10:** A1353.

30. STIMSON, W.H. & I.C. HUNTER. 1976. An investigation into the immunosuppressive properties of estrogen. J. Endocrinol. **69:** 42–50.

31. PAAVONEN, T., L.C. ANDERSON & H. ADLERCREUTZ. 1981. Sex hormone regulation of *in vitro* immune response. Estradiol enhances human B cell maturation via inhibition of suppressor T cells in pokeweed mitogen-stimulated cultures. J. Exp. Med. **154:** 1935–1941.

32. TAUBE, M., S. SVENSSON & H. CARLSTEN. 1998. T lymphocytes are not the target for estradiol-mediated suppression of DTH in reconstituted female severe combined immunodeficient (SCID) mice. Clin. Exp. Immunol. **114:** 147–153.

33. SALEM, M.L. *et al.* 2000. β-estradiol suppresses T cell-mediated delayed-type hypersensitivity through suppression of antigen-presenting cell function and Th1 induction. Int. Arch. Allergy. Immunol. **121:** 161–169.

34. WYLIE, F.A. & J.R. KENT. 1977. Immunosuppression by sex steroid hormones. I. The effect upon PHA and PPD stimulated lymphocytes. Clin. Exp. Immunol. **27:** 407–412.

35. HOLDSTOCK, G., B.F. CHASTENAY & E.L. KRAWITT. 1982. Effect of testosterone, oestradiol and progesterone on immune regulation. Clin. Exp. Immunol. **47:** 449–456.

36. MCEWEN, B.S.. 2001. Genome and hormones: gender differences in physiology. Invited review: estrogens effects on the brain: multiple sites and molecular mechanisms. J. Appl. Physiol. **91:** 2785–2801.

37. CZLONKOWSKA, A., A. CIESLELSKA & I. JONIEC. 2003. Influence of estrogens on neurodegenerative processes. Med. Sci. Monit. **9:** 247–256.

38. TORAN-ALLERAND, C.D., M. SINGH & G. SETALO. 1999. Novel mechanisms of estrogen action in the brain: new players in an old story. Frontiers Neuroendocrinol. **20:** 97–121.

39. MIRANDA, R.C. & C.D. TORAN-ALLERAND. 1993. Neuronal colocalization of mRNAs for neurotrophins and their receptors in the developing central nervous system suggests a potential for autocrine interactions. Proc. Natl. Acad. Sci. USA. **90:** 6439–6443.

40. ZWAIN, I.H. & S.S. YEN. 1999. Neurosteroidogenesis in astrocytes, oligodendro-cytes, and neurons of cerebral cortex of rat brain. Endocrinology **140:** 3843–3852.

41. ARVANITIS, D.N. *et al.* 2004. Membrane-associated estrogen receptor and caveolin-1 present in central nervous system myelin and oligodendrocyte plasma membranes. J. Neurosci. Res. **75:** 603–613.

42. MALOY, K.J. & F. POWRIE. 2001. Regulatory T cells in the control of immune pathology. Nature Immunol. **2:** 816–822.

43. RONCAROLO, M.G. & M.K. LEVINGS. 2000. The role of different subsets of T regulatory cells in controlling autoimmunity. Curr. Opin. Immunol. **12:** 676–683.

44. SHEVACH, E.M.. 2000. Regulatory T cells in autoimmunity. Annu. Rev. Immunol. **18:** 423–449.

45. SAKAGUCHI, S.. 2000. Animal models of autoimmunity and their relevance to human diseases. Curr. Opin Immunol. **12:** 684–690.

46. SAKAGUCHI, S. *et al.* 1995. Immunologic self-tolerance maintained by activated T cells expressing IL-2 receptor a-chains (CD25). Breakdown of a single mech-anism of self-tolerance causes various autoimmune diseases. J. Immunol. **155:** 1151–1164.

47. ASANO, M. *et al.* 1996. Autoimmune disease as a consequence of developmental abnormality of a T cell subpopulation. J. Exp. Med. **184:** 387–396.

48. READ, S., V. MALMSTROM & F. POWRIE. 2000. Cytotoxic T lymphocyte-associated antigen 4 plays an essential role in the function of CD25 + CD4 + regulatory cells that control intestinal inflammation. J. Exp. Med. **192:** 295–302.

49. KOHM, A.P. *et al.* 2002. CD4 + CD25 + regulatory T cells suppress antigen-specific autoreactive immune responses and central nervous system inflamma-tion during active experimental autoimmune encephalomyelitis. J. Immunol. **169:** 4712–4716.

50. STEVENS, L.A. & D. MASON. 2000. CD25 is a marker for CD4 + thymocytes that prevent autoimmune diabetes in rats, but peripheral T cells with this function are found in both CD25 + and CD25- subpopulations. J. Immunol. **165:** 3105–3110.

51. GREEN, E.A., Y. CHOI & R.A. FLAVELL. 2002. Pancreatic lymph node-derived CD4(+)CD25(+) Treg cells: highly potent regulators of diabetes that require TRANCE-RANK signals. Immunity **16:** 183–191.

52. BELKAID, Y. *et al.* 2002. CD4 + CD25 + regulatory T cells control *Leishmania major* persistence and immunity. Nature **420:** 502–507.

53. TAKAHASHI, T. *et al.* 1998. Immunologic self-tolerance maintained by CD25 + CD4 + naturally anergic and suppressive T cells: induction of autoimmune disease by breaking their anergic/suppressive state. Int. Immunol. **10:** 1969–1980.

54. THORNTON, A.M. & E.M. SHEVACH. 1998. CD4 + CD25 + immunoregulatory T cells suppress polyclonal T cell activation *in vitro* by inhibiting interleukin 2 production. J. Exp. Med. **188:** 287–296.

55. SURI-PAYER, E. *et al.* 1998. CD4 + CD25 + T cells inhibit both the induction and effector function of autoreactive T cells and represent a unique lineage of immunoregulatory cells. J. Immunol. **160:** 1212–1218.

56. STEVENS, L.A. *et al.* 2001. Human CD4 + CD25 + thymocytes and periph-eral T cells have immune suppressive activity. Eur. J. Immunol. **31:** 1247–1254.

57. TAAMS, L.S. *et al.* 2001. Human anergic/suppressive CD4 + CD25 + T cells: a highly differentiated and apoptosis-prone population. Eur. J. Immunol. **31:** 1122–1131.

58. DIECKMANN, D. *et al.* 2001. Ex vivo isolation and characterization of CD4 + CD25 + T cells with regulatory properties from human blood. J. Exp. Med. **193:** 1303–1310.

59. LEVINGS, M.K., R. SANGREGORIO & M.-G. RONCAROLO. 2001. Human CD25 + CD4 + T regulatory cells suppress naive and memory T cell proliferation and can be expanded in vitro without loss of function. J. Exp. Med. **193:** 1295–1301.

60. MURAKAMI, M. *et al.* 2002. CD25 + CD4 + T cells contribute to the control of memory CD8 + T cells. Proc. Natl. Acad. Sci. USA. **99:** 8832–8837.

61. MCHUGH, R.S. *et al.* 2002. CD4 + CD25 + immunoregulatory T cells: gene expression analysis reveals a functional role for glucocorticoid-induced TNF receptor. Immunity **16:** 311–323.

62. SHIMIZU, J. *et al.* 2002. Stimulation of CD25 + CD4 + regulatory T cells through GITR breaks immunological self-tolerance. Nature Immunol. **3:** 135–142.

63. SALOMON, B. *et al.* 2000. B7/CD28 costimulation is essential for the homeostasis of the CD4 + CD25 + immunoregulatory T cells that control autoimmune diabetes. Immunity **12:** 431–440.

64. TAKAHASHI, T. *et al.* 2000. Immunologic self-tolerance maintained by CD25 + CD4 + regulatory T cells constitutively expressing cytotoxic lymphocyte-associated antigen 4. J. Exp. Med. **192:** 303–309.

65. CHAMBERS, C.A. *et al.* 2001. CTLA-4-mediated inhibition in regulation of T cell responses: mechanisms and manipulation in tumor immunotherapy. Annu. Rev. Immunol. **19:** 565–594.

66. KINGSLEY, C.I. *et al.* 2002. CD25 + CD4 + regulatory T cells prevent graft rejection: CTLA-4- and IL-10-dependent immunogregulation of alloresponses. J. Immunol. **168:** 1080–1086.

67. NAKAMURA, K., A. KITANI & W. STROBER. 2001. Cell contact-dependent immunosuppression by CD4 (+) CD25 (+) regulatory T cells is mediated by cell surface-bound transforming growth factor beta. J. Exp. Med. **194:** 629–644.

68. ERMANN, J. *et al.* 2001. CD4(+)CD25(+) T cells facilitate the induction of T cell anergy. J. Immunol. **167:** 4271–4275.

69. ZHANG, X. *et al.* 2001. Activation of CD25(+)CD4(+) regulatory T cells by oral antigen administration. J. Immunol. **167:** 4245–4253.

70. ZHENG, S.G. *et al.* 2002. Generation ex vivo of TGF-beta-producing regulatory T cells from CD4 + CD25- precursors. J. Immunol. **169:** 4183–4189.

71. JONULEIT, H. *et al.* 2002. Infectious tolerance: human CD25(+) regulatory T cells convey suppressor activity to conventional CD4(+) T helper cells. J. Exp. Med. **196:** 255–260.

72. ANNACKER, O. *et al.* 2001. CD25 + CD4 + T cells regulate the expansion of peripheral CD4 T cells through the production of IL-10. J. Immunol. **166:** 3008–3018.

73. PONTOUX, C., A. BANZ & M. PAPIERNIK. 2002. Natural CD4 CD25(+) regulatory T cells control the burst of superantigen-induced cytokine production: the role of IL-10. Intl. Immunol. **14:** 233–239.

74. JONULEIT, H. & E. SCHMITT. 2003. The regulatory T cell family: distinct subsets and their interrelations. J. Immunol. 6323–6327.

75. KHATTRI, R. *et al.* 2003. An essential role for Scurfin in CD4 + CD25 + T regulatory cells. Nature Immunol. **4:** 337–342.

76. HORI, S., T. NOMURA & S. SAKAGUCHI. 2003. Control of regulatory T cell development by the transcription factor *Foxp3*. Science **299:** 1057–1061.

77. FONTENOT, J.D., M.A. GAVIN & A.Y. RUDENSKY. 2003. *Foxp3* programs the development and function of CD4 + CD25 + regulatory T cells. Nature Immunol. **4:** 330–336.

78. FRITZ, R.B., C.-H.J. CHOU & D.E. MCFARLIN. 1983. Induction of experimental allergic encephalomyelitis in PL/J and (SJL/JxPL/J)F1 mice by myelin basic protein and its peptides: Localization of a second encephalitogenic determinant. J. Immunol. **130:** 191–196.

79. TROTTER, J.L. *et al.* 1987. Myelin proteolipid protein induces demyelinating disease in mice. J. Neurol. Sci. **79:** 173–184.

80. MCRAE, B.L. *et al.* 1992. Induction of active and adoptive relapsing experimental autoimmune encephalomyelitis (EAE) using an encephalitogenic epitope of proteolipid protein. J. Neuroimmunol. **38:** 229–235.

81. PATERSON, P.Y. & R.H. SWANBORG. 1988. Demyelinating diseases of the central and peripheral nervous systems. *In* Immunological Diseases. M. Sampter, D.W. Talmage, M.M. Frank, K.F. Austen, & H.N. Claman, Eds.: 1877–1916. Little, Brown and Co. Boston.

82. KUCHROO, V.K. *et al.* 1992. Experimental allergic encephalomyelitis mediated by cloned T cells specific for a synthetic peptide of myelin proteolipid protein. Fine specificity and T cell receptor Vβ usage. J. Immunol. **148:** 3776–3782.

83. BERNARD, C.C.A.. 1976. Experimental autoimmune encephalitis in mice: Genetic control of susceptibility. J. Immunogenetics **3:** 263–270.

84. ARNON, R.. 1981. Experimental allergic encephalomyelitis-susceptibility and suppression. Immunol. Rev. **55:** 5–9.

85. LINTHICUM, D. & J. FRELLINGER. 1982. Acute autoimmune encephalomyelitis in mice. II. Susceptibility is controlled by the combination of H-2 and histamine sensitization genes. J. Exp. Med. **155:** 31–38.

86. MONTGOMERY, I.N. & H.C. RAUCH. 1982. Experimental autoimmune encephalomyelitis (EAE) in mice: primary control of EAE susceptibility is outside the H-2 complex. J. Immunol. **128:** 421–429.

87. MA, R.Z. *et al.* 2002. Identification of *Bphs*, and autoimmune disease locus, as histamine receptor H1. Science **297:** 620–623.

88. MATEJUK, A. *et al.* 2001. 17β-estradiol inhibits cytokine, chemokine, and chemokine receptor mRNA expression in the central nervous system of female mice with experimental encephalomyelitis. J. Neurosci. Res. **65:** 529–542.

89. KRAKOWSKI, M. & T. OWENS. 1996. Interferon-γ confers resistance to experimental allergic encephalomyelitis. Eur. J. Immunol. **26:** 1641–1646.

90. WILLENBORG, D.O. *et al.* 1996. IFN-γ plays a critical down-regulatory role in the induction and effector phase of myelin oligodendrocyte glycoprotein-induced autoimmune encephalomyelitis. J. Immunol. **157:** 3223–3227.

91. SEGAL, B.M., B.K. DWYER & E.M. SHEVACH. 1998. An interleukin (IL)-10/IL-12 immunoregulatory circuit controls susceptibility to autoimmune disease. J. Exp. Med. **187:** 537–546.

92. MATEJUK, A. *et al.* 2003. 17β-estradiol treatment profoundly down-regulates gene expression in spinal cord tissue in mice protected from experimental autoimmune encephalomyelitis. Archi. Immunol. Ther. Exp. **51:** 185–193.

93. MATEJUK, A. *et al.* 2002. Evaluation of the effects of 17B-estradiol (17B-E2) on gene expression in experimental autoimmune encephalomyelitis using DNA microarray. Endocrinology **143:** 313–319.
94. KLINKERT, W.E. *et al.* 1997. TNF-alpha receptor fusion protein prevents EAE and demyelination in Lewis rats: an overview. J. Neuroimmunol. **72:** 163–168.
95. LIU, H.Y., A. BUENAFE, A. MATEJUK, *et al.* 2002. Estrogen inhibition of EAE may involve differential effects on mature vs. immature dendritic cells. J. Neurosci. Res. **70:** 238–248.
96. POLANCZYK, M.J. *et al.* 2006. Estrogen-mediated immunomodulation involves reduced activation of effector T cells, potentiation of Treg cells, and enhanced expression of the PD-1 costimulatory pathway. J. Neurosci. Res. **84:** 370–378.
97. LIU, H. *et al.* 2003. Estrogen receptor α mediates estrogen's immune protection in autoimmune disease. J. Immunol. **171:** 6936–6940.
98. VEGETO, E. *et al.* 2003. Estrogen receptor-alpha mediates the brain antiinflammatory activity of estradiol. Proc. Natl. Acad. Sci. USA **100:** 9614–9619.
99. COUSE, J.F., M.M. YATES, V.R. WALKER & K.S. KORACH. 2003. Characterization of the hypothalamic-pituitary-gonadal (HPG) axis in estrogen receptor null mice reveals hypergonadism and endocrine sex-reversal in females lacking Era but not Erβ. Mol. Endocrinol. **17:** 1039–1053.
100. BEBO, B.F., J.C. SCHUSTER, A.A. VANDENBARK & H. OFFNER. 1999. Androgens alter the cytokine profile and reduce encephalitogenicity of myelin-reactive T cells. J. Immunol. **162:** 35–40.
101. LUBHAN, D.B., J.S. MOYER, T.S. GOLDING, *et al.* 1993. Alterations of reproductive function but not prenatal sexual development after insertional disruption of the mouse estrogen receptor gene. Proc. Natl. Acad. Sci. USA. **90:** 11162–11166.
102. KREGE, J.H., J.B. HODGIN, J.F. COUSE, *et al.* 1998. Generation and reproductive phenotypes of mice lacking estrogen receptor β. Proc. Natl. Acad. Sci. USA. **95:** 15677–15682.
103. ERLANDSSON, M.C., C. OHLSSON, J-A GUSTAFSSON H. CARLSTEN. 2001. Role of oestrogen receptors alpha and beta in immune organ development and in oestrogen-mediated effects on thymus. Immunology **103:** 17–25.
104. YELLAYI, S.T.C., C. TEUSCHER, J.A. WOODS, *et al.* 2000. Normal development of thymus in male and female mice requires estrogen/estrogen receptor-apha signaling pathway. Endocrine. **12:** 207–213.
105. STAPLES, J.E., T.A. GASIEWICZ, N.C. FIORE, *et al.* 1999. Estrogen receptor alpha is necessary in thymic development and estradiol-induced thymic alterations. J. Immunol. **163:** 4168–4174.
106. POLANCZYK, M.J. *et al.* 2004. Cutting edge: estrogen drives expansion of the CD4 + CD25 + regulatory T cell compartment. J. Immunol. **173:** 2227–2230.
107. OFFNER, H., G.A. HASHIM & A.A. VANDENBARK. 1991. T cell receptor peptide therapy triggers autoregulation of experimental encephalomyelitis. Science **251:** 430–432.
108. OFFNER, H. *et al.* 1998. Vaccination with BV8S2 protein amplifies TCR-specific regulation and protection against experimental autoimmune encephalomyelitis in TCR BV8S2 mice. J. Immunol. **161:** 2178–2186.
109. MATEJUK, A. *et al.* 2003. Differential expression of TGF-ß3 is associated with protection against experimental autoimmune encephalomyelitis. Cytokine **25:** 45–51.
110. JANSSON, L. & R. HOLMDAHL. 1998. Estrogen-mediated immunosuppression in autoimmune diseases. Inflamm. Res. **47:** 290–301.

111. POLMAN, C.H. & B.M.J. UITDEHAAG. 2003. New and emerging treatment options for multiple sclerosis. Lancet Neurol. **2:** 563–566.
112. BJARTMAR, C., J.R. WUJEK & B.D. TRAPP. 2003. Axonal loss in the pathology of MS: consequences for understanding the progressive phase of the disease. J. Neurol. Sci. **206:** 165–171.
113. SICOTTE, N.L. *et al.* 2002. Treatment of multiple sclerosis with pregnancy hormone estriol. Ann. Neurol. **52:** 421–428.

Implications for Estrogens in Parkinson's Disease

An Epidemiological Approach

PAOLO RAGONESE, MARCO D'AMELIO, AND GIOVANNI SAVETTIERI

Dipartimento Universitario di Neuroscienze Cliniche, Università di Palermo, Palermo, Italy

ABSTRACT: Evidence from experimental and epidemiological studies suggests a role of sex hormones in the pathogenic process leading to neurodegenerative diseases, (i.e., Alzheimer's and Parkinson's disease). The effects of sexual steroid hormones are complex and vary with the events of women's fertile life. Estrogens are supposed to influence dopamine synthesis, metabolism, and transport; however, there is no consensus regarding the direction, locus, and mechanism of the effect of estrogens on the dopaminergic system. A neuroprotective effect of estrogens has been demonstrated in 1-methyl-4-phenyl-1,2,3,6-tetrahydropyridine (MPTP)-animal models of Parkinson's disease (PD). Epidemiological studies indicate gender differences regarding the onset and the prognosis of PD. Most of the analytical studies explored the relationship between PD and exogenous estrogens. Only three studies investigated the role of endogenous estrogens in the risk of developing PD. These studies reported an increased risk of PD in conditions causing an early reduction in endogenous estrogens (early menopause, reduced fertile life length). Longer cumulative length of pregnancies has also been associated with an increased PD risk. A lack of consensus still exists on the effect of the type of menopause (surgical vs. natural) on PD risk. Finally, the effect of postmenopausal estrogen replacement therapy is still debated. Inconsistencies across studies are in part explained by the complexity of the mechanisms of action of sexual hormones and by the paucity of analytical studies.

KEYWORDS: Parkinson's disease; epidemiology; risk factors; fertile life; age at menopause; women

Address for correspondence: Giovanni Savettieri, M.D., Dipartimento Universitario di Neuroscienze Cliniche, Università di Palermo, Via Gaetano La Loggia 1-90129 Palermo, Italy. Voice: +39-091-6555146; fax: +39-091-6555147.
e-mail: gsavetti@tin.it

Ann. N.Y. Acad. Sci. 1089: 373–382 (2006). © 2006 New York Academy of Sciences.
doi: 10.1196/annals.1386.004

INTRODUCTION

Parkinson's disease (PD) is a neurodegenerative disorder characterized by progressive damage of mesencephalic dopaminergic (DA) neurons of the substantia nigra (SN) and the striatal projections. The clinical features of PD are represented by an insidious and progressive appearance of a resting tremor, bradykinesia, and rigidity. Impaired postural reflexes are often accessory symptoms, but their early onset may suggest a different diagnosis (i.e., multiple system atrophy or other kind of parkinsonism).[1]

Mechanisms leading to DA neuronal degeneration are still debated, but several pathogenic pathways are supposed to play a role in the cascade of this pathology: oxidative stress, protein misfolding, reduction of trophic factors, reduced tolerance to excitotoxicity, and inflammatory mechanisms.[1,2]

Although estrogen activity was originally believed to be restricted to the control of reproduction, increasing evidence suggests that estrogen's influences extend beyond systems, and its activity in the central nervous system (CNS) may determine, or influence, the susceptibility for the development of neurodegenerative diseases.[3–7]

Indication for an estrogenic involvement in PD etiology derives from several sources: experimental *in vitro* studies, descriptive epidemiological surveys, analytical case–control and prospective cohort studies and, although with conflicting results, from clinical trials.

Most of this research, however, was conducted exploring the influence of exogenous estrogens, focusing mainly on 17-β-estradiol, while scanty data exist at the moment on the indicators of the endogenous exposure. Moreover, 17-β-estradiol action has been assumed as a paradigm of the estrogenic mechanism of action without considering the emerging diversities of activity of the other sexual steroid hormones on the brain. In this article, we will focus on data supporting the possible role of sexual steroid hormones and PD emerging from experimental, descriptive, and analytical epidemiological studies, and from clinical trials.

In vitro *and Experimental Studies on Estrogens and PD*

One of the first reports to hint at a possible neuroprotective effect of sex steroids was published over a decade ago. In that study, female gerbils experienced a lower incidence and less severe brain damage following carotid artery occlusion than male gerbils did.[8–10] Many reports have shown that exogenous administration of 17β-E2 dramatically reduces infarct volume following MCAO (middle cerebral arterial occlusion) in ovariectomized female rats,[11–13] in male rats,[14] and in aged, reproductively senescent female rats,[15] which represent a model of female menopause. Particularly interesting is the fact that there is not a dose-dependent relationship between 17β-E2 and cerebral blood flow, thus suggesting that the neuroprotective effects are exerted directly on the brain.[13,16]

Recent reports indicate that conjugated equine estrogens, the most prescribed estrogen replacement hormone in the United States, are neuroprotective against neuronal cell death induced by β-amyloid,[17–27] hydrogen peroxide, and glutamate. In addition, conjugated equine estrogens induce neurite outgrowth in cortical, hippocampal, and basal forebrain neurons.[28,29]

In murine models, estrogens might enhance dopaminergic function by increasing dopamine synthesis,[5,30] downregulating enzymes that are involved in dopamine metabolism,[31] or by increasing dopamine receptor density.[32,33]

It has also been suggested that estrogens can exert their neuroprotective activity by inhibiting dopamine transporter function,[34] increasing mitochondrial activity, and acting as an antioxidant.[35] By contrast, estrogens might act directly to suppress dopaminergic function by shifting D2-dopamine receptors from high- to the low-affinity state[36] or indirectly via prolactin release, which has an inhibitory effect on the dopaminergic system.[37] Similarly, no consensus exists regarding the role of progesterone and progestin. Some evidence suggests that progesterone can also provide neuroprotection[38] and, depending on the method and the dose of infusion, enhances or inhibits dopaminergic activity.[39] The few studies exploring the effects of both estrogens and progesterone on the dopaminergic system indicated antagonist interaction or no interaction between these hormones.[40,41]

Recently, it has been postulated that hormones can act on glial response to inflammation and oxidative stress induced by MPTP.[42] According to this hypothesis, endogenous glucocorticoids and estradiol could inhibit the neuroinflammatory cascade, protecting astrocytes and microglia from programmed cell death.

These results are in line with those studies indicating an increased resistance of cultured dopaminergic neurons to the neurodegeneration induced by MPTP and in mouse models of parkinsonism.[43,44]

Descriptive and Analytical Epidemiologic Studies on Indicators of Estrogenic Activity and PD

Epidemiologic and experimental studies all suggest a relationship between estrogens and dopaminergic pathways. Incidence of PD is almost double in men compared to women,[45–49] suggesting a possible sex-related protective influence in predisposition to the disease.

Previous analytic studies explored the relationship between PD and exogenous estrogens.[50–53] Some recent studies also investigated the association between indicators of endogenous estrogen effects and PD risk.[54–56] TABLE 1 summarizes the main findings of the studies investigating the association between PD and risk factors related to exposure to estrogens. PD has been

TABLE 1. Summary of the analytical epidemiologic studies on the association between PD and women's fertile life

Authors	Study design	Age at menarche	Early menopause	Surgical menopause	Fertile life length	Pregnancy	HRT	HRT duration of use	Comments
Benedetti et al. (2000)[54]	Incidence of PD cases (1976–1995) identified by record linkage system; controls from the same population.	NR	DA	DA	NR	NR	NA	NR	Hypothesis generating study; large confidence intervals
Ragonese et al. (2004)[55]	PD cases from two hospitals; controls from the general population.	NA	DA	IA	IA	DA[a]	NA	NR	Included prevalent cases
Popat et al. (2005)[56]	Incidence of PD cases and controls (1994–1995) selected from computerized membership records.	NA	IA	NA	NR	NA[b]	NA	DA	Included proxy respondents: 19% among cases, 15% among controls

[a]Includes abortion and miscarriages and is calculated by months of pregnancies. [b]Calculated by a number of full-term pregnancies. HRT = hormone replacement therapy; NR = not reported; NA = no association; DA = direct association; IA = inverse association.

associated with a reduced fertile life and to an early menopause. These results, if taken all together, suggest a relationship between the progressive slope of estrogen rates during the perimenopausal transition (usually starting two or three years before menopause) and the pathologic process leading to PD. The stimulating observation of an association between a cumulative length of pregnancies above 30 months and PD risk need, of course, to be confirmed.

Surprisingly, Popat *et al.* reported a direct association between PD and estrogen replacement therapy in women who underwent hysterectomy.

While for some exposures (i.e., shorter length of fertile life and an early menopause) the association is definitively not hard to explain, as these are conditions associated with lowering estrogens' levels, whereas for others the relationship is more complex.

The association between PD and the type of menopause is inconsistent across studies. The most plausible explanation, apart from the methodological aspects, is that surgical menopause includes the sum of many events often related to each other. The type of menopause therefore, is a non-specific indicator, not sufficient *per se* to provide information about the type and the duration of the estrogenic release. The use of this parameter does not allow, moreover, establishing an accurate temporal relationship between the surgical procedure and the subsequent estrogenic slope unless the concomitant bilateral oophorectomy and the use of postmenopausal estrogen replacement therapy are well defined.

In a recent study, age at PD onset was found to be correlated with age at menopause and fertile life duration.[57]

These results, together with the others reported above, suggest that PD onset and age at menopause share a common process possibly related to the disease. These common processes could reside in the relationship between ovarian failure and the hypothalamic-pituitary axis activity. It is still not clear whether the relationship between the hypothalamic-pituitary axis and menopause is dependent on ovarian failure acting as a negative feedback on brain tissue inhibiting the hypothalamus, or if the hypothalamus itself rules the vascular and hormonal regulation of ovaries starting the menopausal transition.[58] It is consequently questionable whether a possible genetic background or other causes may independently determine both early menopause and striatal degeneration or if an early decrease of estrogens is the first step of a pathogenic process whose consequence is the acceleration of dopaminergic loss.

A recent investigation suggesting an association between polymorphisms of the estrogen receptor beta and an early age at onset of PD[59] gives strength to the first hypothesis, postulating that the association was due to a different brain sensitivity to estrogens modulated by genetic factors. The correlation of PD onset with age at menopause may therefore indicate that length of estrogen activity may modify also brain sensitivity to degeneration, influencing disease onset.

Potential Therapeutic Role of Estrogens

The potential therapeutic role of exogenous estrogens in the treatment of PD derives from observational studies and from clinical trials. These results have been conflicting. Some investigation showed an association between post-menopausal estrogen replacement therapy with a lower risk of PD,[54-56,60] while others did not observe any association with disease risk.[41,61] The effects of duration and timing of postmenopausal hormone therapy use (both estrogens alone and estrogen–progestin combination therapy) on PD risk have not been adequately examined.

Studies previously performed revealed that postmenopausal estrogen replacement therapy may lower the risk of dementia in parkinsonian patients, but did not prove a definite efficacy in preventing PD.[52] Furthermore, estrogens seem to have beneficial effects on cognitive performances, but improvement has not been confirmed on motor symptoms.[51,52]

CONCLUSIVE CONSIDERATION

The relationship between hormones and PD is complex. This association must not be considered by looking only at dose–effect phenomena. Estrogen effects differ in fact also by type of stimulation (estradiol, estriol, or estrone), and by duration of exposure (menses fluctuation, pregnancies). For example, estriol activity changes according to its concentration, and in general estrogen effects vary in relationship to other factors, such as hormone-binding globulin concentration.

Many data support these premises. Sex steroid hormone levels are lower in parous women compared to women with no previous pregnancies.[62-65] Hormone levels may be still in the normal ranges, but, by contrast, the bioavailability is reduced because of the higher levels of "sex hormone–binding globulin." This reduced bioavailability has been documented by the comparison between parous and nulliparous women.[66,67]

Estriol mechanism of action, the main estrogen during pregnancy, has been considered antiestrogenic for a long time.[68] This estriol effect was recently reconsidered as a partial agonist at the concentration of nonpregnant phases during menstrual cycles, while it should be antiestrogenic at the concentrations of pregnancies.[69]

The whole amount of these data indicates differentiated mechanisms of action for sexual steroid hormones in the different times of women's fertile life.

Inferences made in this review are based on few studies. Though the investigations we considered are those trying to transfer experimental data into clinical practice, many aspects still remain obscure and unproved. The mechanisms of action and the effects of estrogens during life are naturally changing (menstrual cycles, pregnancies, menopause), but are actually influenced by exogenous events (use of drugs, stress, life habits). For this reason, it is extremely difficult to extrapolate a single effect of estrogens on PD pathology.

REFERENCES

1. OLANOW, C.W. 2003. Neuroprotection for Parkinson's disease: prospects and promises. Ann. Neurol. **53**(Suppl 3): S1–S2.
2. JENNER, P. 2003. Oxidative stress in Parkinson's disease. Ann. Neurol. **53**(Suppl 3): S26–S38.
3. VAN HARTESVELDT, C. & J.N. JOYCE. 1986. Effects of estrogen on the basal ganglia. Neurosci. Biobehav. Rev. **10**: 1–14.
4. KOMPOLITI, K. 1999. Estrogen and movement disorders. Clin. Neuropharmacol. **22**: 318–326.
5. PASQUALINI, C., V. OLIVIER, B. GUIBERT, *et al.* 1995. Acute stimulatory effect of estradiol on striatal dopamine synthesis. J. Neurochem. **65**: 1651–1657.
6. XIE, T., S.L. HO & D. RAMSDEN. 1999. Characterization and implications of estrogenic down-regulation of human catechol-O-methyltransferase gene transcription. Mol. Pharmacol. **56**: 31–38.
7. DISSHON, K.A., J.W. BOJA & D.E. DLUZEN. 1998. Inhibition of striatal dopamine transporter activity by 17beta-estradiol. Eur. J. Pharmacol. **345**: 207–211.
8. ALKAYED, N.J., I. HARUKUNI, A.S. KIMES, *et al.* 1998. Gender-linked brain injury in experimental stroke. Stroke **29**: 159–166.
9. HALL, E.D., K.E. PAZARA & K.L. LINSEMAN. 1991. Sex differences in postischemic neuronal necrosis in gerbils. J. Cereb. Blood Flow Metab. **11**: 292–298.
10. DHANDAPANI, K.M. & D.W. BRANN. 2002. Protective effects of estrogen and selective estrogen receptor modulators in the brain. Biol. Rep. **67**: 1379–1385.
11. SIMPKINS, J.W., G. RAJAKUMAR, Y.Q. ZHANG, *et al.* 1997. Estrogens may reduce mortality and ischemic damage caused by middle cerebral artery occlusion in the female rat. J. Neurosurg. **87**: 724–730.
12. DUBAL, D.B., M.L. KASHON, L.C. PETTIGREW, *et al.* 1998. Estradiol protects against ischemic injury. J. Cereb. Blood Flow Metab. **18**: 1253–1258.
13. RUSA, R., N.J. ALKAYED, B.J. CRAIN, *et al.* 1999. 17b-Estradiol reduces stroke injury in estrogen-deficient animals. Stroke **30**: 1665–1670.
14. TOUNG, T.J.K., R.J. TRAYSTMAN & P.D. HURN. 1998. Estrogen-mediated neuroprotection after experimental stroke in males. Stroke **29**: 1666–1670.
15. ALKAYED, N.J., B.J. CRAIN, R.J. TRAYSTMAN & P.D. HURN. 1999. Estrogen-mediated neuroprotection in reproductively senescent rats [abstract]. Stroke **30**: 274.
16. DUBAL, D.B. & P.M. WISE. 2001. Neuroprotective effects of estradiol in middle aged female rats. Endocrinology **142**: 43–48.
17. WILSON, M.E., D.B. DUBAL & P.M. WISE. 2000. Estradiol protects against injury induced cell death in cortical explant cultures: a role for estrogen receptors. Brain Res. **873**: 235–242.
18. DUBAL, D.B., P.J. SHUGHRUE, M.E. WILSON, *et al.* 1999. Estradiol modulates bcl-2 in cerebral ischemia: a potential role for estrogen receptors. J. Neurosci. **19**: 6385–6393.

19. SINGER, C.A., K.L. ROGERS & D.M. DORSA. 1998. Modulation of Bcl-2 expression: a potential component of estrogen protection in NT2 neurons. Neuroreport **9:** 2565–2568.

20. ALKAYED, N.J., S. GOTO, N. SUGO, et al. 2001. Estrogen and Bcl-2: gene induction and effect of transgene in experimental stroke. J. Neurosci. **21:** 7543–7550.

21. KUIPER, G.G., E. ENMARK, M. PELTO-HUIKKO, et al. 1996. Cloning of a novel receptor expressed in rat prostate and ovary. Proc. Natl. Acad. Sci. USA **93:** 5925–5930.

22. TREUTER, E., M. WARNER & J. GUSTAFSSON. 2000. Mechanism of oestrogen signalling with particular reference to the role of ER beta in the central nervous system. Novartis Found. Symp. **230:** 7–14.

23. DUBAL, D.B., H. ZHU, J. YU, et al. 2001. Estrogen receptor alpha, not beta, is a critical link in estradiol-mediated protection against brain injury. Proc. Natl. Acad. Sci. USA **98:** 1952–1957.

24. SAMPEI, K., S. GOTO, N.J. ALKAYED, et al. 2000. Stroke in estrogen receptor-a-deficient mice. Stroke **31:** 738–744.

25. COUSE, J.F., S.W. CURTIS, T.F. WASHBURN, et al. 1995. Analysis of transcription and estrogen insensitivity in the female mouse after targeted disruption of the estrogen receptor gene. Mol. Endocrinol. **9:** 1441–1454.

26. WANG, L., S. ANDERSSON, M. WARNER & J.A. GUSTAFSSON. 2001. Morphological abnormalities in the brains of estrogen receptor beta knockout mice. Proc. Natl. Acad. Sci. USA **98:** 2792–2796.

27. KUROKI, Y., K. FUKUSHIMA, Y. KANDA, et al. 2001. Neuroprotection by estrogen via extracellular signal-regulated kinase against quinolinic acid-induced cell death in the rat hippocampus. Eur. J. Neurosci. **13:** 472–476.

28. DIAZ-BRINTON, R., S. CHEN, M. MONTOYA, et al. 2000. The Women's Health Initiative estrogen replacement therapy is neurotrophic and neuroprotective. Neurobiol. Aging **21:** 475–496.

29. BRINTON, R.D., S. CHEN, M. MONTOYA, et al. 2000. The estrogen replacement therapy of the Women's Health Initiative promotes the cellular mechanisms of memory and neuronal survival in neurons vulnerable to Alzheimer's disease. Maturitas **34**(Suppl 2): S35–S52.

30. DI PAOLO, T., C. ROUILLARD & P. BEDARD. 1985. 17 beta-estradiol at a physiological dose acutely increases dopamine turnover in rat brain. Eur. J. Pharmacol. **117:** 197–203.

31. XIE, T., S.L. HO & D. RAMSDEN. 1999. Characterization and implications of estrogenic down-regulation of human catechol-O-methyltransferase gene transcription. Mol. Pharmacol. **56:** 31–38.

32. HRUSKA, R.E. & E.K. SILBERGELD. 1980. Increased dopamine receptor sensitivity after estrogen treatment using the rat rotation model. Science **208:** 1466–1468.

33. ROY, E.J., D.R. BUYER & V.A. LICARI. 1990. Estradiol in the striatum: effects on behavior and dopamine receptors but no evidence for membrane steroid receptors. Brain Res. Bull. **25:** 221–227.

34. DISSHON, K.A., J.W. BOJA & D.E. DLUZEN. 1998. Inhibition of striatal dopamine transporter activity by 17beta-estradiol. Eur. J. Pharmacol. **345:** 207–211.

35. DISSHON, K.A. & D.E. DLUZEN. 1997. Estrogen as a neuromodulator of MPTP induced neurotoxicity: effects upon striatal dopamine release. Brain Res. **764:** 9–16.

36. LEVESQUE, D. & T. DI PAOLO. 1988. Rapid conversion of high into low striatal D2-dopamine receptor agonist binding states after an acute physiological dose of 17 beta-estradiol. Neurosci. Lett. **88:** 113–118.

37. DUPONT, A., T. DI PAOLO, B. GAGNE & N. BARDEN. 1981. Effects of chronic estrogen treatment on dopamine concentrations and turnover in discrete brain nuclei of ovariectomized rats. Neurosci. Lett. **22:** 69–74.

38. CALLIER, S., M. MORISSETTE, M. GRANDBOIS, *et al.* 2001. Neuroprotective properties of 17beta-estradiol, progesterone, and raloxifene in MPTP C57Bl/6 mice. Synapse **41:** 131–138.

39. DLUZEN, D.E. & V.D. RAMIREZ. 1987. Intermittent infusion of progesterone potentiates whereas continuous infusion reduces amphetamine-stimulated dopamine release from ovariectomized estrogen-primed rat striatal fragments superfused in vitro. Brain Res. **406:** 1–9.

40. FERNANDEZ-RUIZ, J.J., R. DE MIGUEL, M.L. HERNANDEZ & J.A. RAMOS. 1990. Time course of the effects of ovarian steroids on the activity of limbic and striatal dopaminergic neurons in female rat brain. Pharmacol. Biochem. Behav. **36:** 603–606.

41. KALIA, V., C. FENSKE, D.R. HOLE & C.A. WILSON. 1999. Effect of gonadal steroids and gamma-aminobutyric acid on LH release and dopamine expression and activity in the zona incerta in rats. J. Reprod. Fertil. **117:** 189–197.

42. MARCHETTI, B., P.A. SERRA, F. L'EPISCOPO, *et al.* 2005. Hormones are key actors in gene x environment interactions programming the vulnerability to Parkinson's disease: glia as a common final pathway. Ann. N.Y. Acad. Sci. **1057:** 296–318.

43. CALLIER, S., M. MORISSETTE, M. GRANDBOIS & T. DI PAOLO. 2000. Stereospecific prevention by 17beta-estradiol of MPTP-induced dopamine depletion in mice. Synapse. **7:** 245–51.

44. XU, K., Y. XU, D. BROWN-JERMYN, *et al.* 2006. Estrogen prevents neuroprotection by caffeine in the mouse 1-methyl-4-phenyl-1,2,3,6-tetrahydropyridine model of Parkinson's disease. J. Neurosci. **26:** 535–541.

45. MAYEUX, R., K. MARDER, L.J. COTE, *et al.* 1995. The frequency of idiopathic Parkinson's disease by age, ethnic group, and sex in northern Manhattan, 1988–1993. Am. J. Epidemiol. **142:** 820–827.

46. BOWER, J.H., D.M. MARAGANORE, S.K. MCDONNEL & W.A. ROCCA. 1999. Incidence and distribution of parkinsonism in Olmsted County, Minnesota, 1976–1990. Neurology **52:** 1214–1220.

47. BALDERESCHI, M., A. DI CARLO, W.A. ROCCA, *et al.* 2000. Parkinson's disease and parkinsonism in a longitudinal study: two-fold higher incidence in men. Neurology **55:** 1358–1363.

48. ELBAZ, A., J.H. BOWER, D.M. MARAGANORE, *et al.* 2002. Risk tables for parkinsonism and Parkinson's disease. J. Clin. Epidemiol. **55**(1): 25–31.

49. DE RIJK, M.C., L.J. LAUNER, K. BERGER, *et al.* 2000. Prevalence of Parkinson's disease in Europe: a collaborative study of population-based cohorts. Neurology **54:** S21–S23.

50. MORISSETTE, M. & T. DI PAOLO. 1993. Effect of chronic estradiol and progesterone treatments of ovariectomized rats on brain dopamine uptake sites. J. Neurochem. **60:** 1876–1883.

51. SAUNDERS-PULLMAN, R., J. GORDON-ELLIOTT, M. PARIDES, *et al.* 1999. The effect of estrogen replacement therapy on early Parkinson's disease. Neurology **52:** 1417–1421.

52. MARDER, K., M.-X. TANG, B. ALFARO, *et al.* 1998. Postmenopausal estrogen use and Parkinson's disease with and without dementia. Neurology **50:** 1141–1143.

53. DISSHON, K.A. & D.E. DLUZEN. 1997. Estrogen as a neuromodulator of MPTP-induced neurotoxicity: effects upon striatal dopamine release. Brain Res. **764:** 9–16.

54. BENEDETTI, M.D., D.M. MARAGANORE, J.H. BOWER, *et al.* 2001. Hysterectomy, menopause, and estrogen use preceding Parkinson's disease: an exploratory case-control study. Mov. Disord. **16:** 830–837.
55. RAGONESE, P., M. D'AMELIO, G. SALEMI, *et al.* 2004. Risk of Parkinson's disease in women: effect of fertile life characteristics. Neurology **62:** 2010–2014.
56. POPAT, R.A., S.K. VAN DEN EEDEN, C.M. TANNER, *et al.* 2005. Effect of reproductive factors and postmenopausal hormone use on the risk of Parkinson disease. Neurology **65:** 383–390.
57. HANKINSON, S.E., G.A. COLDITZ, D.J. HUNTER, *et al.* 1995. Reproductive factors and family history of breast cancer in relation to plasma estrogen and prolactin levels in postmenopausal women in the Nurses' Health Study (United States). Cancer Causes Control **6:** 217–224.
58. WINDHAM, G.C., E. ELKIN, L. FENSTER, *et al.* 2002. Ovarian hormones in premenopausal women: variation by demographic, reproductive and menstrual cycle characteristics. Epidemiology **13:** 675–684.
59. DORGAN, J.F., M.E. REICHMAN, J.T. JUDD, *et al.* 1995. Relationship of age and reproductive characteristics with plasma estrogens and androgens in premenopausal women. Cancer Epidemiol. Biomarkers Prev. **4:** 381–386.
60. BERNSTEIN, L., M.C. PIKE, R.K. ROSS, *et al.* 1985. Estrogen and sex hormone-binding globulin levels in nulliparous and parous women. J. Natl. Cancer Inst. **74:** 741–745.
61. MOORE, J.W., T.J. KEY, R.D. BULBROOK, *et al.* 1987. Sex hormone binding globulin and risk factors for breast cancer in a population of normal women who had never used exogenous sex hormones. Br. J. Cancer **56:** 661–666.
62. MOORE, J.W., T.J. KEY, G.M. CLARCK, *et al.* 1987. Sex-hormone-binding globulin and breast cancer risk. Anticancer Res. **7:** 1039–1047.
63. COLE, P. & B. MACMAHON. 1969. Oestrogen fractions during early reproductive life in the etiology of breast cancer. Lancet **1:** 604–609.
64. MELAMED, M., E. CASTAÑO, A.C. NOTIDES & S. SASSON. 1997. Molecular and kinetic basis for the mixed agonist/antagonist activity of estriol. Mol. Endocrinol. **11:** 1868–1878.
65. RAGONESE, P., M. D'AMELIO, G. CALLARI, *et al.* 2006. Age at menopause predicts age at onset of Parkinson's disease. Mov. Disord. In press.
66. WILDT, L. & T. SIR-PETERMANN. 1999. Oestrogen and age estimations of perimenopausal women. Lancet **354:** 224.
67. WESTBERG, L., A. HAKANSSON, J. MELKE, *et al.* 2004. Association between the estrogen receptor beta gene and age of onset of Parkinson's disease. Psychoneuroendocrinology **29:** 993–998.
68. CURRIE, L.J., M.B. HARRISON, J.M. TRUGMAN, *et al.* 2004. Postmenopausal estrogen use affects risk for Parkinson disease. Arch. Neurol. **61:** 886–888.
69. ASCHERIO, A., H. CHEN, M.A. SCHWARZSCHILD, *et al.* 2003. Caffeine, postmenopausal estrogen, and risk of Parkinson's disease. Neurology **60:** 790–795.

The Role of Flow Cytometric Immunophenotyping in Myelodysplastic Syndromes

GUIDO PAGNUCCO, CATERINA GIAMBANCO, AND FRANCESCO GERVASI

Division of Hematology, Department of Oncology, ARNAS Civico-Benfratelli, G. Di Cristina e M. Ascoli, 90100 Palermo, Italy

ABSTRACT: The myelodysplastic syndromes (MDSs) are a group of heterogeneous hematological disorders characterized by bilineage or trilineage dysplastic morphology, abnormal clonal populations, progressive bone marrow failure, and a high rate of transformation to acute myeloid leukemia. A combination of morphology, to detect multilineage dysplasia in the bone marrow and peripheral blood, and cytogenetics to detect characteristic clonal abnormalities, is used in establishing a diagnosis of MDS. Although diagnostic criteria are well established, a significant number of patients have blood and bone marrow findings that make diagnosis and classification difficult. Flow cytometric immunophenotyping is an accurate and highly sensitive method for quantitative and qualitative evaluation of hematopoietic cells in the different maturative compartments, and several groups have used flow cytometry in the study of MDSs. Findings of recent studies suggest that flow cytometry immunophenotyping might provide useful information in the diagnosis and the management of MDS patients.

KEYWORDS: myelodysplastic syndrome; flow cytometry; immunophenotyping

INTRODUCTION

Myelodysplastic syndromes (MDSs) are a group of heterogeneous hematological disorders characterized by bilineage or trilineage dysplastic morphology, abnormal clonal populations, progressive bone marrow (BM) failure, and a high rate of transformation to acute myeloid leukemia (AML). The basic mechanism of disease in MDS is largely unknown. No unifying testable hypothesis is yet available, but various cytogenetic abnormalities resulting in

Address for correspondence: Guido Pagnucco, M.D., Division of Hematology, Department of Oncology, ARNAS-Civico, Via Carmelo Lazzaro 2, 90127 Palermo, Italy. Voice: +39-091-666-4216; fax: +39-091-666-4222.

e-mail: gpagnucco@ospedalecivicopa.org

Ann. N.Y. Acad. Sci. 1089: 383–394 (2006). © 2006 New York Academy of Sciences.
doi: 10.1196/annals.1386.031

neoplastic clonal proliferation, coupled with the hyperactivity of cellular destruction via an increase of clearance or apoptosis, play important roles in the pathogenesis of these syndromes.[1,2] The emergence of immunologic factors and the evidence of abnormal function of the marrow microenvironment are also of major importance and emphasize the need for early detection.[3,4]

Patients usually present with peripheral blood cytopenias and hypercellular BM, although the BM is hypocellular in one-fifth of the cases.[5,6] The current diagnostic approach to MDS includes peripheral blood and BM morphology (to evaluate abnormalities of peripheral blood cells and hematopoietic precursors), BM biopsy (to assess marrow cellularity and topography), and cytogenetics (to identify nonrandom chromosomal abnormalities).[1] The pathologic hallmark of MDS is marrow dysplasia, which represents the basis of the World Health Organization (WHO)'s classification of these disorders.[7,8] The combination of overt marrow dysplasia and clonal cytogenetic abnormality allows a conclusive diagnosis of MDS, but this is found in only a portion of patients. In many instances, cytogenetics is not informative, and the diagnosis of MDS is based entirely and exclusively on morphological criteria. Moreover, morphological distinction between hypoplastic MDS and severe aplastic anemia can be especially difficult because both can present with hypocellular BMs and pancytopenia.[9]

Because morphologic evaluation is inherently subjective, and cytogenetics, while objective, identifies abnormalities in only 30–40% of cases of MDS, additional objective correlates of MDSs are needed. Flow cytometric immunophenotyping represents a highly sensitive and reproducible method for quantitative and qualitative evaluation of hematopoietic cells in the different maturative compartments during normal myelopoiesis,[10] and several groups have used flow cytometry (FC) in the study of MDS. MDS patients have been found to have abnormal expression of several single-surface antigens, as indicated by either the intensity of fluorescence or the percentage of positive cells.[11,12] A major advance in this field was achieved by the immunophenotypic definition of the normal and dysplastic patterns of myeloid and erythroid cell differentiation in BM using multiparameter FC, in which multiple antibody combinations were used together with sensitive data acquisition methods ("live gate") to assess the expression of multiple antigens on a single cell, allowing the discrimination between the healthy and neoplastic counterparts.[13,14] By comparing patterns of antigen expression on a given cell population with the patterns identified on normal cells of that type, one can potentially identify abnormalities that, if sufficiently great, might substitute for clonality studies in identifying malignancy. Similar to the concept that multiple rather than single dysplastic features (as described by the French-American-British [FAB] group[15]) in one or more cell lines have to be present to establish a diagnosis of MDS, single immunophenotypic abnormalities alone may not be sufficient to accurately diagnose MDS or to assess prognosis in these patients. Therefore multiparameter FC can be used diagnostically to exclude other causes of cytopenias, document the immunophenotypic manifestations of myeloid and erythroid dysplasia, and provide analysis of blast and CD34+ progenitor cells and of monocytic differentiation pathway.[16-25]

Treatment decisions in patients with MDS are generally based on disease status and the expected tempo of the disease process. Patients with advanced disease by the criteria of the FAB classification[15] and by the International Prognostic Scoring System (IPSS)[26] are often considered for early hematopoietic stem cell transplantation (SCT) if a suitable donor is identified, whereas patients with low risk factors initially may be observed or treated with less aggressive therapeutic modalities. Therefore, patient management relies heavily on accurate determination of disease status at the time of evaluation, and findings of recent studies suggest that FC immunophenotyping may be especially useful for evaluation of dysplasia and risk assessment of MDSs.

IMMUNOPHENOTYPIC EVALUATION OF DYSPLASIA

Many studies have shown a variety of immunophenotypic abnormalities as detected by FC in patients with MDS. A review of these immunophenotypic abnormalities in MDS has been presented by Elghetany[11] in 1998. Few, if any, single immunophenotypic abnormalities in MDS have been proven to be of prognostic significance. Furthermore, although these studies defined abnormalities in MDS, they did not address the potential contribution of flow cytometric evaluation to the diagnosis of MDS.

The diagnostic utility of flow cytometric immunophenotyping using the CD45/SSC gating strategy in MDSs was first examined by Stetler-Stevenson *et al.*[16] in 45 patients with straightforward MDS. The results were compared with those obtained in a series of patients with aplastic anemia, healthy donors, and patients with a history of nonmyeloid neoplasia in complete remission. A series of different double-staining combinations were used to detect immunophenotypic abnormalities associated with myeloid (CD11b/CD16, CD13/CD16), erythroid (CD71/glycophorin A), and megakaryocytic (CD41a/CD61) dysplasia of the different BM cell populations within the gates drawn on the dot-plot CD45/SSC. The most common myelomonocytic abnormalities detected were neutrophil hypogranulation (84%), abnormal CD13/CD16 (78%) or CD11b/CD16 (70%) patterns, and CD64 negativity (66%). Myeloid and erythroid dysplasia were detectable by FC in 98 and 77% of the patients, respectively. The authors showed that flow cytometric immunophenotyping was more sensitive than morphology for detection of myeloid, but less sensitive for detection of erythroid dysplasia. Because only quantitative flow cytometric findings were seen in the megakaryocytic lineage and morphologic evaluation was more sensitive, the authors concluded that flow cytometric evaluation of megakaryocytic lineage abnormalities is of limited use in MDS. Such an approach could also detect dual-lineage or trilineage immunophenotypic abnormalities in 15 (75%) of 20 challenging cases ultimately diagnosed with MDS when combined morphology and cytogenetics were nondiagnostic. In addition, flow cytometric analysis was informative even in cases in which the BM aspirates collected for morphology were inadequate and was very helpful in differentiating hypocellular MDS from aplastic anemia. In conclusion, as marrow morphology and cytogenetics allowed for the diagnosis of MDS in the majority of cases, these investigators recommended that flow cytometric immunophenotyping need not be part of the routine work-up of MDS, but might be of value in cases of inconclusive morphology and cytogenetics.

A 3-color FC assay based on the experience acquired in the diagnosis of acute leukemia was used by Maynadié et al.[12] to determine whether immunophenotypic abnormalities could be defined in MDSs and could correlate with the FAB classification and cytogenetics. The CD45 marker was tested in each combination to allow a primary gating of BM cell subsets based on CD45 antigen expression and side scatter (SS) laser light diffraction. Analysis was performed on 275 BM samples (207 MDS patients, 68 controls) and 25 control blood samples. Although the data were collected as multiparameters, the analysis treated each antigen separately and fluorescence labeling was expressed in a simplified numerical form, corresponding to the fluorescence ratio of the whole cell subset gated for each marker tested. The mean intensities of antigen expression in marrows were determined for blasts, monocytes, and granulocytes for 17 different antigens. Hierarchical clustering was performed to assess the similarities and differences between patient groups. No differences were observed for the antigens expressed on monocytes. The data obtained for granulocytes show that (1) the most discriminating markers were CD11b, CD13, CD33, CD36, CD38, CD71, and HLA-DR; (2) clusters related to increased mean intensity expression of CD38, CD13, and CD33 were associated with more advanced MDS stages (refractory anemia [RA] with excess blasts and RA with excess blasts in transformation), as might be expected from a shift to the left reflecting increases in myeloblasts and immature myeloid cells; (3) clusters related to high levels of CD36 expression were associated with a poor IPSS score; and (4) high levels of CD71 expression were associated with RA with ring sideroblasts (RA/RARS). These results show a close relationship between objective and quantitative immunophenotypic abnormalities and BM dysplasia, and suggest that FC could be a future tool for the diagnostic and prognostic characterization of MDSs.

Wells et al.[17] characterized by multidimensional FC mononuclear marrow cells from 115 patients with MDS, 104 patients with various disorders, and 25 healthy donors with the aim to identify immunophenotypic correlates of prognosis in MDSs. Based on phenotypic and scatter characteristics a scoring system was developed that allowed expression of complex flow cytometric abnormalities in a numerical score. This flow cytometric scoring system (FCSS) was based on the types of abnormalities in myeloid cells and monocytes, the assessment of blast counts, and the lymphoid-to-myeloid *ratio* as a reflection of the degree of impaired myelopoiesis. Additional weight was given to lineage infidelity (presence of lymphoid antigens on myeloid or monocytic cells) or marked maturational asynchrony, as shown by CD34 expression on maturing myeloid cells or monocytes. The flow cytometric scores were categorized as normal/mild (0–1), moderate (2–3), or severe (>4). Most flow cytometric abnormalities were significantly more frequent in patients with MDS than in the control cohort. Flow cytometric scores in MDS patients were then retrospectively compared with marrow blast counts assessed by morphology, cytogenetics, hematologic parameters, and IPSS risk categorization. The flow cytometric scores correlated inversely with leukocyte and absolute neutrophil counts and correlated directly with IPSS scores and with IPSS cytogenetic risk categories. In the 111 MDS patients who underwent allogeneic hematopoietic SCT, flow scores correlated with posttransplantation outcome. In multivariate analyses, there was a significant contribution of the flow score independent of the IPSS in predicting survival and relapse. The authors concluded that FCSS is useful in assessing marrows for diagnosis of MDS and in determining the prognostic outcome in patients with this disorder.

Del Canizo *et al.*[18] used 3-color FC to assess the usefulness of seven myeloid-associated antigens in identifying the immunophenotypic differences between patients with MDS and normal individuals, including changes in distribution in cell lineages, as well as blockades in cell maturation pathways and phenotypic aberrations. In addition to an abnormal distribution of the BM cell compartment, significant differences were demonstrated in CD34+ compartments, as well as in monocytic and neutrophil lineages, which may be useful for the detection of MDS. Surprisingly, with the combinations of monoclonal antibodies used, the authors observed an increased proportion of monocytic cells with a decreased percentage of cells of the neutrophil lineage, and maturational arrests in the monocytic but not in the neutrophil differentiation pathway, supporting the hypothesis that the monocytic component may be more relevant in the pathogenesis of MDS than previously suspected. In RA with excess blasts in transformation (RAEB-t) such blockades mainly occurred during the earliest stages of differentiation, but in the other MDS subtypes they occurred in later stages. Aberrant immunophenotypes occurred in 90% of the 101 patients with MDS who were studied, and a high proportion of cases showed ≥ 2 aberrations. Overexpression of CD33 on neutrophils and aberrant HLADR expression on mature granulocytes were found in 71 and 27% of the cases, respectively.

Kussick and Wood[19] retrospectively evaluated 4-color FC data from more than 400 BM aspirates obtained from patients suspected of having a nonchronic myeloid leukemia (CML), myeloproliferative disorder, or an MDS, to identify normal patterns of antigen expression during myeloid maturation and to determine whether flow cytometric evaluation of myeloid maturation represents an additional objective way to assess the likelihood of a stem cell neoplasm. Maturing erythrocytes and megakaryocytes were not evaluated because of methodological concerns, given the fewer antibodies available for study of the erythroid and megakaryocytic lineage and because platelet binding to the surfaces of nonmegakaryocytic cells may result in artifactual positivity for platelet-associated antigens. This data set has allowed demonstration of reproducible patterns of antigen expression in normal granulocytic and monocytic maturation, including changes seen in benign and reactive settings such as marrow regeneration and G-CSF therapy, and to distinguish benign from neoplastic abnormalities of antigen expression. In addition, these authors summarized data, presented in detail elsewhere, from a retrospective comparison of the sensitivity of FC with conventional cytogenetics for a large number of BMs on which both types of studies were performed. Their findings showed that more than 90% of MDS cases with a clonal cytogenetic abnormality can be identified as abnormal by 4-color FC. The same authors recently validated this approach for assisting in the diagnosis of MDS by showing strong concordance of the FC results with the morphologic and cytogenetic features in 124 BM aspirates from unselected patients (selected only to have adequate FC, cytogenetic, morphologic, and clinical data available) with unexplained cytopenias and/or monocytosis.[20] Given the large number of myeloid and nonmyeloid antigens evaluated, 4-color FC permitted the evaluation of more complex relationships among antigens during the course of the full range of myeloid maturation from blasts to maturing granulocytes and monocytes, and seemed to be of particular use when the myeloid blast count was low or morphologic features were equivocal. Of interest, this method showed high sensitivity and specificity in the evaluation of MDSs. With this assay, an abnormal 4-color FC result was 89% sensitive and 88% specific for identifying a BM aspirate satisfying gold-standard morphologic or cytogenetic criteria for the diagnosis of MDS. The overall sensitivity of 4-color FC for identifying any abnormality (indeterminate or definitively abnormal) in a gold-standard case of MDS was 95%, whereas the overall specificity was 67%.

Malcovati *et al.*[21] used a simple form of 4-color FC immunophenotyping that provides percentages of positive cells to develop a flow cytometric approach to the evaluation of erythroid and myeloid dysplasia in patients with MDS. They first studied a cohort of 103 MDS patients as well as 46 pathological and healthy controls. Analysis of erythroid cells showed higher proportions of immature cells and decreased levels of CD71 expression on nucleated red cells in MDS. Analysis of myeloid cells showed lower proportions of CD10+ and higher proportions of CD56+ granulocytes, and increased ratios of immature to mature cells. Because no single immunophenotype could accurately differentiate MDS from other conditions, they used discriminant analysis for generating erythroid and myeloid classification functions performed to identify the presence of erythroid and myeloid dysplasia, with the aim of differentiating MDS and pathologic controls, and of classifying, together with flow cytometric blast percentage, MDS into WHO subgroups. With this approach an accurate FC evaluation of marrow dysplasia was achieved using combinations of eight MoAbs, including MoAbs against CD45, CD10, CD16, CD33, CD34, CD56,

CD71, and GlyA-PE. This immunophenotypic approach allowed correct classification of more than 90% of MDSs with definitive morphological marrow
dysplasia in the learning cohort and was validated in the prospective analysis of a testing cohort of 69 MDS patients and 46 pathological controls. A
diagnosis of MDS was obtained in 60 of 69 cases (87%). No false-positive
results were noticed among controls. Significant correlations between values
of these functions and both degree of morphological dysplasia and the IPSS
were found. Finally, this FC approach for the evaluation of marrow dysplasia
using discriminant analysis to generate erythroid and myeloid classification
functions was proven to be sensitive in a high proportion of cases with indeterminate morphology, as well as repeatable and reproducible in an intralaboratory
setting.

Erythroid dysplasia is found in almost all patients with MDS and is the only
morphological abnormality in those with RA, that is, the pure erythroid disorders of the WHO classification. Evaluation of erythroid dysplasia represents
a challenge in the immunophenotypic analysis of myelodysplastic marrows,
mainly because of the limited availability of specific antibodies. To overcome
this limitation, Della Porta *et al.*[22] developed a 4-color FC approach largely
based on the evaluation of proteins of erythroid iron metabolism, using antibodies against cytosolic ferritin subunits (H-ferritin [HF] and L-ferritin [LF]), MtF,
transferrin receptor [CD71], and of the CD105 antigen (endoglin), an accessory receptor for members of the transforming growth factor beta superfamily,
which was previously found to be specifically expressed on proerythroblasts.
Their expression was evaluated in erythroblasts from 104 patients with cytolog-
ical diagnosis of MDS according to the WHO classification, 69 pathologic control patients, and 19 healthy subjects. Compared with pathologic and healthy
controls, MDS patients had higher expression of HF and CD105 and lower
expression of CD71. MtF was specifically detected in MDS with ringed sideroblasts, and there was a close relationship between its expression and Prussian
blue staining. *In vitro* cultures of myelodysplastic hematopoietic progenitors
showed that both HF and MtF were expressed at a very early stage of erythroid
differentiation, and that MtF expression is specifically related to mitochondrial iron loading. A classification function based on expression levels of HF,
CD71, and CD105 allowed correct classification of >95% of MDS patients.
This flow cytometry approach provides an accurate quantitative evaluation of
erythroid dysplasia and allows a reliable diagnosis of sideroblastic anemia, and
may therefore be a useful tool in the work-up of patients with MDS.

IMMUNOPHENOTYPIC ANALYSIS OF BLAST CELLS

Contrary to the case in *de novo* AML, few phenotypic data have been
compiled regarding MDS blasts.[10] One of the main reasons for this is that
MDS blasts are not predominant cells in the BM and peripheral blood (PB),

making reliable analysis of blasts difficult. CD45 is a hematopoietic lineage-restricted cell-surface marker that is expressed on all hematopoietic cells, from hematopoietic stem cells to mature blood cells, except for erythroid cells, platelets, and plasma cells, which lose this antigen during maturation. The characteristic intensity of CD45 expression in normal populations of BM (more intense in lymphocytes and monocytes, less intense in granulocytes and maturing myeloid cells, absent in erythroid precursors and platelets) made it possible to discriminate leukemic cells of any origin from normal mature cells, and to facilitate the analysis of leukemic blasts present at low frequencies by using the CD45/SSC gating, because leukemic blasts usually appear in a position where few healthy cells are located.[13,14] Lymphoblasts are typically CD45 low or negative with low SSC level; myeloid blasts have an intermediate CD45 expression and a higher SSC value.

In the study conducted by Maynadié et al.[12] phenotypic clustering of the blast cells showed correlation between antigens normally expressed on blasts (CD34, CD117, CD33, CD13, HLA-DR) as distinct from antigens expressed later during development (CD11b, CD14, CD15, CD16) and antigens not normally expressed on myeloid cells. Eight clusters of patients were identified based on intensity relationships among CD16, CD34, CD36, CD38, CD17, and HLA-DR on the blast cells. The eight groups exhibited differences in IPSS scores, cytogenetic risk factors, and percentage of blasts.

Using a new density centrifugation reagent for blast enrichment, Ogata et al.[23] studied immunophenotypic characteristics of marrow and peripheral blood blasts in 116 patients with MDS or secondary acute myelogenous leukemia (sAML). Immunophenotyping was performed by 3-color FCM, in which enriched blast cells and other cell populations were gated by a CD45 gating method. The majority of enriched blasts were shown to be committed myeloid precursors with a $CD34^+CD38^+HLADR^+CD13^+CD33^+$ immunophenotype, irrespective of the MDS subtype. Other antigens such as CD117, CD15, CD11b, or CD56 were expressed at various proportions (64, 64, 48, and 27% of the cases, respectively). The authors noted that the proportion of cases with myeloblasts expressing CD7, CD10, CD15, and CD117 differed significantly between early and advanced stages of MDS, whereas all other markers studied did not differ. Markers reflecting immaturity of myeloid cells such as CD7 and CD117 were more frequently expressed in advanced stages of MDS and sAML. In contrast, markers for maturity of myeloid cells (CD10 and CD15) were more prevalent in early stages of MDS. Most importantly, expression of CD7 on marrow cells, which was detected only in advanced stages of MDS, was found to be independently associated with a short overall and transformation-free survival in this series.

In the study conducted by Malcovati et al.[21] blast cells were identified as CD45lowSSClow cells on the CD45/SSC dot-plot and confirmed with a back-gating technique. Immature B-cell precursors were identified in the CD45lowSSClow region on the basis of CD10, CD19, and CD34 co-expression, and were excluded from the analysis. A strong positive linear correlation between the proportion of BM blast cells estimated by morphology and the proportion of blast cells gated on the dot-plot CD45/SSC was noticed. A positive linear correlation was also found between the proportion of blast cells estimated by FC and the proportion of both CD34+ and CD34+/CD33+ BM cells. Repeated measure analysis of variance showed that between-investigator and within-investigator variances did not significantly affect the results of such an analysis.

Other studies have focused on the quantification and characterization of CD34+ cells, because in the flow cytogram the cells isolated as CD34+ and CD45dull with a low side-scatter intensity are now known to represent immature stem/hematopoietic progenitor cells.[18,21,24,25]

In the study conducted by Del Canizo *et al.*[18] the proportion of BM CD34+ cells was greater in normal patients but the more immature progenitors (CD34+/CD34−) were less represented. By contrast the proportion of myeloid-committed (CD34+/CD33+) progenitors was greater in normal individuals, translating into a higher CD34+ CD33+ /CD34+ CD33− hematopoietic progenitor cell *ratio* and suggesting that in MDS the majority of CD34+ cells are already committed to the myeloid lineage. The most frequent phenotypic aberration in the CD34+ compartment was represented by CD34+CD15+HLADR− cell populations.

In the study conducted by Malcovati *et al.*[21] the percentages of CD34+ cells and CD34+/CD33+ cells were significantly higher in MDS patients than in controls. Linear regression analysis showed a close relationship between the degree of erythroid and myeloid dysplasia (morphological assessment) and the proportion of CD34+ cells. The ratio between the CD34+/CD33+ and CD34+/CD33− cells was significantly higher in MDS patients than in controls and positively correlated with both erythroid and myeloid dysplasia. The results of CD34 and CD34/CD33 count were not significantly affected by between- and within-investigator variability.

Fuchigami *et al.*[24] scored absolute numbers of circulating CD34-positive cells by a highly sensitive triple-color flow cytometric analysis using CD45 monoclonal antibody, CD34 monoclonal antibody, and propidium iodide. Forty-one patients with MDS, 12 patients with aplastic anemia (AA), and 36 age-adjusted normal subjects were studied. Total circulating CD34+ cells in peripheral blood were decreased in RA patients, but increased in patients with RA with excess of blasts (RAEB) and RAEB in transformation (RAEB-T) patients as compared to normal. The differences in these groups may be explained as a result of a decrease in normal CD34+ cells in RA patients as compared to healthy individuals, and the identification of circulating abnormal blasts in RAEB or RAEBT patients, because distinct light-scattering pattern differences were observed. The authors conclude that this method allows one to distinguish RA from other MDS subtypes more reliably than by morphology alone and provides early signs of progression to acute leukemia.

Granulocyte colony-stimulating factor (G-CSF) receptor (G-CSFR [CD 114]) on CD34+ cells was recently described by Sultana et al.[25] as more highly variable for patients with advanced stages of MDS as compared to normal controls. The expression of CD114 on the CD34+ cells in patients with lower grades of MDS were more like normal than they were in patients with more advanced stages of disease based on FAB classification. Although all patients with low expression of CD114 on the CD34+ cells developed neutropenia, many patients with normal as well as high CD114 expression also had decreased circulating neutrophils. The G-CSFR signal transduction pathway in the normal and high group was not deficient of messenger RNA for either janus kinases (Jaks) or signal transducers and activators of transcription (Stats). These findings suggest that the lowered expression of G-CSFR may cause neutropenia in MDS and MDS-AML patients and therefore may partially explain the neutropenia in myelodysplastic patients.

SUMMARY

Immunophenotyping has been used increasingly to establish diagnosis and assess prognosis in patients with MDS. From a diagnostic point of view, cytomorphologic examination of marrow aspirates or biopsies together with cytogenetic study has remained the mainstay of establishing a diagnosis of MDS. However, flow cytometric evaluation of marrow and peripheral blood can be helpful to distinguish MDS from other BM failure diseases or when results of tests of marrow morphology and cytogenetics are inconclusive. For the assessment of prognosis in patients with MDS, recent data suggest that FC adds important prognostic information. Further studies are needed to prospectively evaluate the prognostic value of immunophenotypic abnormalities in MDS patients with and without transplantation. Because interlaboratory variability has been demonstrated to be a problematic issue in flow cytometric immunophenotyping, technical standardization and consensus as to which markers or combination of markers might be most powerful in predicting prognosis would be a prerequisite for such studies.

REFERENCES

1. CAZZOLA, M. & L. MALCOVATI. 2005. Myelodysplastic syndromes—coping with ineffective hematopoiesis. N. Engl. J. Med. 352: 536–538.
2. PARKER, J.E., G.J. MUFTI, F. RASOOL, et al. 2000. The role of apoptosis, proliferation, and the Bcl-2-related proteins in the myelodysplastic syndromes and acute myeloid leukemia secondary to MDS. Blood 96: 3932–3938.
3. HAMBLIN, T.J. 2002. Immunology of the myelodysplastic syndromes. In The Myelodysplastic Syndromes. J.M. Bennet, Ed.: 65–87. Marcel Dekker. New York.

4. LINDBERG, E.H. 2005. Strategies for biology- and molecular-based treatment of myelodysplastic syndromes. Curr. Drug Targets **6:** 713–725.

5. JACOBS, A. 1985. Myelodysplastic syndromes: pathogenesis, functional abnormalities, and clinical implications. J. Clin. Pathol. **38:** 1201–1217.

6. ALESSANDRINO, E.P., S. AMADORI, M. CAZZOLA, *et al.* 2001. Myelodysplastic syndromes: recent advances. Haematologica **86:** 1124–1157.

7. VARDIMAN, J.W., N.L. HARRIS & R.D. BRUNNING. 2002. The World Health Organization (WHO) classification of the myeloid neoplasms. Blood **100:** 2292–2302.

8. MALCOVATI, L., M.G. DELLA PORTA, C. PASCUTTO, *et al.* 2005. Prognostic factors and life expectancy in myelodysplastic syndromes classified according to WHO criteria: a basis for clinical decision making. J. Clin. Oncol. **23:** 7594–7603.

9. BARRETT, J., Y. SAUNTHARARAJAH & J. MOLLDREM. 2000. Myelodysplastic syndrome and aplastic anemia: distinct entities or diseases linked by a common pathophysiology? Semin. Hematol. **37:** 15–29.

10. PAGNUCCO, G., L. VANELLI & F. GERVASI. 2002. Multidimensional flow cytometry immunophenotyping of hematologic malignancy. Ann. N.Y. Acad. Sci. **963:** 313–321.

11. ELGHETANY, M.T. 1998. Surface marker abnormalities in myelodysplastic syndromes. Haematologica **83:** 1104–1115.

12. MAYNADIÉ, M., F. PICARD, B. HUSSON, *et al.* 2002. Immunophenotypic clustering of myelodysplastic syndromes. Blood **100:** 2349–2356.

13. STELZER, G.T., K.E. SHULTS & M.R. LOKEN. 1993. CD45 gating for routine flow cytometric analysis of human bone marrow specimens. Ann. N.Y. Acad. Sci. **677:** 265–280.

14. BOROWITZ, M.J., K.L. GUENTER, K.E. SHULTS, *et al.* 1993. Immunophenotyping of acute leukemia by flow cytometric analysis: use of CD45 and right-angle light scatter to gate on leukemic blasts in three-color analysis. Am. J. Clin. Pathol. **100:** 534–540.

15. BENNETT, J.M., D. CATOVSKY, M.T. DANIEL, *et al.* 1982. Proposals for the classification of the myelodysplastic syndromes. Br. J. Haematol. **51:** 189-199.

16. STETLER-STEVENSON, M., D.C. ARTHUR, N. JABBOUR, *et al.* 2001. Diagnostic utility of flow cytometric immunophenotyping in myelodysplastic syndrome. Blood **98:** 979–987.

17. WELLS, D.A., M. BENESCH, M.R. LOKEN, *et al.* 2003. Myeloid and monocytic dyspoiesis as determined by cytometric scoring in myelodysplastic syndrome correlates with the IPSS and with outcome after hematopoietic stem cell transplantation. Blood **102:** 394–403.

18. DEL CANIZO, M.C., E. FERNANDEZ, A. LOPEZ, *et al.* 2003. Immunophenotypic analysis of myelodysplastic syndromes. Haematologica **88:** 402–407.

19. KUSSICK, S.J. & B.L. WOOD. 2003. Using 4-color flow cytometry to identify abnormal myeloid populations. Arch. Pathol. Lab. Med. **127:** 1140–1147.

20. KUSSICK, S.J., J.R. FROMM, A. ROSSINI, *et al.* 2005. Four-color flow cytometry shows strong concordance with bone marrow morphology and cytogenetics in the evaluation for myelodysplasia. Am. J. Clin. Pathol. **124:** 170–181.

21. MALCOVATI, L., M.G. DELLA PORTA, M. LUNGHI, *et al.* 2005. Flow cytometry evaluation of erythroid and myeloid dysplasia in patients with myelodysplastic syndrome. Leukemia **19:** 776–783.

22. DELLA PORTA, M.G., L. MALCOVATI, R. INVERNIZZI, *et al.* 2006. Flow cytometry evaluation of erythroid dysplasia in patients with myelodysplastic syndrome. Leukemia **20:** 549–555.

23. OGATA, K., K. NAKAMURA, N. YOKOSE, *et al*. 2002. Clinical significance of phenotypic features of blasts in patients with myelodysplastic syndromes. Blood **100:** 3887–3896.
24. FUCHIGAMI, K., H. MORI, T. MATSUO, *et al*. 2000. Absolute number of circulating CD34+ cells is abnormally low in refractory anemias and extremely high in RAEB and RAEB-t: novel pathologic features of myelodysplastic syndromes identified by highly sensitive flow cytometry. Leuk. Res. **24:** 163–174.
25. SULTANA, T.A., H. HARADA , K. ITO, *et al*. 2003. Expression and functional analysis of granulocyte colony-stimulating factor receptors on CD34++ cells in patients with myelodysplastic syndrome (MDS) and MDS-acute myeloid leukaemia. Br. J. Haematol. **121:** 63–75.
26. GREENBERG, P., C. COX, M.M. LEBEAU, *et al*. 1997. International scoring system for evaluating prognosis in myelodysplastic syndromes. Blood **89:** 2079–2088.

Clinical Relevance of Cytogenetics in Myelodysplastic Syndromes

PAOLO BERNASCONI, MARINA BONI, PAOLA MARIA CAVIGLIANO, SILVIA CALATRONI, ILARIA GIARDINI, BARBARA ROCCA, RITA ZAPPATORE, IRENE DAMBRUOSO, AND MARILENA CARESANA

Department of Blood, Heart and Lung Medical Sciences of the University of Pavia and Division of Hematology, Fondazione Policlinico San Matteo IRCCS, Pavia, Italy

ABSTRACT: Myelodysplastic syndromes (MDS) are a group of heterogeneous stem cell disorders with different clinical behaviors and outcomes. Conventional cytogenetics (CC) studies have demonstrated that the majority of MDS patients harbor clonal chromosome defects. The probability of discovering a chromosomal abnormality has been increased by fluorescence *in situ* hybridization (FISH), which has revealed that about 15% of patients with a normal chromosome pattern on CC may instead present cryptic defects. Cytogenetic abnormalities, except for the interstitial long-arm deletion of chromosome 5 (5q−), are not specific for any French-American-British (FAB)/World Health Organization (WHO) MDS subtypes, demonstrate the clonality of the disease, and identify peculiar morphological entities, thus confirming clinical diagnosis. In addition, chromosome abnormalities are independent prognostic factors predicting overall survival and the likelihood of progression in acute myeloid leukemia.

KEYWORDS: myelodysplastic syndromes; FAB subtype; chromosomal abnormalities; fluorescence *in situ* hybridization

INTRODUCTION

Myelodysplastic syndromes (MDS) are clonal stem cell disorders most frequently affecting the elderly.[1] They are characterized by a hypercellular marrow that exhibits a defective maturation of all marrow cell lineages, determining ineffective hemopoiesis and peripheral blood cytopenia. Apart from constitutional conditions (such as Fanconi's anemia and other congenital dyserythropoietic anemias), these oncohematological disorders are distinguished in *de novo* MDS, which arises without exposure to any well-known carcinogenic

Address for correspondence: Paolo Bernasconi, M.D., Division of Hematology, Fondazione IRCCS Policlinico San Matteo, University of Pavia, Piazzale Golgi 1, 27100 Pavia, Italy. Voice: +39-0382-503065; fax: +39-0382502250.
e-mail: p.bernasconi@smatteo.pv.it

Ann. N.Y. Acad. Sci. 1089: 395–410 (2006). © 2006 New York Academy of Sciences.
doi: 10.1196/annals.1386.034

agent, and secondary MDS, which develops after a previous exposure to carcinogenic agents or chemotherapeutic treatments performed for a preceding cancer. MDS clinical outcome is extremely variable with most patients surviving for several years and dying from frequent infections and hemorrhages due to a progressive worsening of peripheral blood cytopenia, and in 30–40% of patients acute myeloid leukemia (AML) evolves within few months.

In 1982 the French-American-British (FAB) group[2] proposed the first MDS classification that was based on morphological criteria. It recognized five distinct subtypes of the disease: refractory anemia (RA), refractory anemia with ringed sideroblast (RARS), RA with excess of blasts (RAEB), RAEB in transformation (RAEB-t), and chronic myelomonocytic leukemia (CMML). The FAB classification succeeded in overcoming the lack of a uniform nomenclature of previous classification systems and for more than 20 years it represented a solid basis for an accurate characterization of every MDS patient. However, despite all these merits, it has important limits. It does not recognize that RA and RARS with unilineage dysplasia have a clinical outcome significantly better than that of RA/RARS with multilineage dysplasia; that RAEB with 5–10% blast percentage has a clinical outcome significantly better than that of RAEB with 11–20% blast percentage; that RAEB-t is much more related to AML than to MDS; and that CMML, especially the form with hyperleukocytosis, is much more related to chronic myeloproliferative disorders than to MDS. All these problems lead to the development of a new classification system that was introduced by the World Health Organization (WHO).[3] This new classification considers the prognostic importance of multilineage dysplasia, fixes at $\geq 20\%$ the blast percentage required for an AML diagnosis, and no longer includes RAEB-t and CMML within MDS. It recognizes six MDS subtypes: RA, RARS, refractory cytopenia with multilineage dysplasia with and without ringed sideroblasts (RCMD/RCMDRS), RAEB (distinguished in RAEB-1 [blast percentage: 5–10%] and RAEB-2 [blast percentage: 11–20%]), MDS unclassifiable, and MDS with 5q−.

After the introduction of FAB classification, various studies demonstrated the diagnostic and prognostic power of CC. Subsequently, the clinical relevance of CC was further stressed by the WHO classification that recognized the 5q− syndrome as a new MDS subtype and by the International Prognostic Scoring System (IPSS), which demonstrated that cytogenetic abnormalities, number/type of peripheral cytopenia, and blast cell percentage are the main independent prognostic factors in MDS patients. Afterwards, most studies have showed that the chromosomal abnormality confirms the monoclonality of the disease, identifies peculiar biological and clinical entities, and provides fundamental help not only in making a differential diagnosis, but also in introducing patients to innovative therapeutic options. The added value of fluorescence *in situ* hybridization (FISH) relies on the possibility of analyzing interphase cells and correlating genotypic with phenotypic data.

INCIDENCE AND FEATURES

The incidence of recurrent chromosomal abnormalities is about 40–70% in *de novo* MDS and 95% in secondary MDS. The frequency of unrelated clones, one of which is marked by +8, is about 5%. These differences are due to technical and clinical factors. The most relevant technical factors are *in vitro* cell culture duration and the limited number of metaphases (20–30) examined by CC. In the past, the most important clinical factors were the use of different diagnostic and patients' selection criteria, the lack of a distinction between *de novo* and secondary MDS, and the fact that some patient series included a significant number of patients with advanced MDS which, having an increased blast cell percentage, present a high incidence of chromosomal abnormalities.

In MDS patients most chromosomal defects are not specific for the disease because they can be observed in other oncohematological disorders and, except for 5q−, none is specifically associated with any FAB/WHO subtype even if some abnormalities identify peculiar biological and clinical entities. Chromosomal deletions, being present in about 50% of patients, are the most common defects in either *de novo* or secondary MDS. The deletion is more often interstitial (with loss of chromosomal material between two different bands) than terminal (with loss of chromosomal material between a particular band and the telomere) and has a quite variable size. Despite these features, a chromosomal segment constantly lost, the so-called "common deleted region" (CDR), has been identified in most deletions. The most frequent deletions involve the long arms of chromosomes 5, 7, 20, 11, 13 and the short arms of chromosomes 12 and 17. The deletion is often present as a single defect in low-risk MDS, whereas it occurs along with other abnormalities in advanced MDS.

The loss of whole chromosomes is the second most frequent abnormality. The most common monosomies involve chromosomes 7 (−7), 5, and Y. Deletions and monosomies may cause MDS by acting through the same mechanism. These defects could determine the loss of one allele of a "tumor suppressor gene" (TSG) followed by the submicroscopic deletion of the other allele, mapped on the chromosome with a normal appearance on CC. So, the TSG, which normally behaves as a recessive gene and requires the normal function of both alleles, is inactivated and unable to control cell cycle, DNA repair mechanisms, and apoptosis.

Trisomies (gains of entire chromosomes) are the third most common cytogenetic defect and most frequently involve chromosomes 8, 11, and 21.

Balanced chromosomal translocations, so frequently discovered in AML, are very rare in MDS. The incidence of these defects has been further reduced by the WHO classification that considers as true AML t(8;21)/inv(16) patients having 20–30% blasts in the marrow. In contrast, unbalanced translocations (with loss of chromosomal material) are rather common in MDS, being present in about 15% of patients. The chromosomes most frequently involved are numbers 5 and 7.

FISH RELEVANCE

The need for mitotic cells is the major drawback of CC and is one of the factors making the incidence of chromosomal defects quite difficult to determine. FISH, which can be performed on mitotic as well as on interphase cells, overcomes this limitation and can be quickly performed with high specificity and sensitivity, and thus has acquired a more and more fundamental role in oncohematology.

In MDS this technique has been applied to establish which is the most primitive hemopoietic cell targeted by the neoplastic event. In order to achieve this goal many studies have analyzed FACS-sorted cells obtained from MDS patients who harbored a cytogenetic defect already demonstrated by CC on clinical diagnosis. Initially it was observed that +8 was confined to CD34+, CD33+ myeloid committed progenitors. Subsequently, the analysis of 5q− patients revealed that 94% of CD34+, CD38− cells, and 25–90% of CD34+, CD19+ cells presented with this chromosomal defect. Later on, it was shown that 5q− was constantly present in CD34+, CD38−, and Thy-1+ progenitors; in contrast +8 appeared in daughter cells only. More recently, FISH has documented that myeloblasts and CD45−, CD34−, CD38−, Lin− cells (which along with CD45+, CD34−, CD38−, Lin− cells are considered very immature hemopoietic cells) share the same cytogenetic defect. On the basis of this result it was suggested that in MDS the neoplastic event occurs in these very immature hemopoietic progenitor cells.

The other main application of FISH has been to clarify whether MDS patients with a normal cytogenetic pattern on CC can instead present cryptic defects. FISH has revealed that 15–18% of these patients may truly harbor clonal cryptic defects, which consist of submicroscopic deletions. However, in some patients the clonal cell population may escape CC detection because of either the poor quality of metaphases or the low mitotic index. An abnormal FISH pattern is associated with a shorter overall survival and a higher risk of AML evolution. In one study the presence of an abnormal FISH pattern worsened patients' IPSS cytogenetic category. Because the incidence of cryptic defects revealed by FISH varied in different reports, a recent study evaluated which is the minimum number of metaphases to be screened by CC studies in order to achieve the same sensitivity as FISH. It was showed that CC equals FISH when more than 20 metaphases are analyzed and nowadays 20 metaphases are mandatory to consider any CC analysis successful in MDS patients.

MOST FREQUENT ABNORMALITIES

5q— Syndrome and Monosomy 5

The 5q— syndrome, whose incidence is 10%, was described for the first time by van den Berghe in 1974.[4] It identifies a specific MDS subtype in the WHO classification. Initially, the criteria used for defining the 5q— syndrome were very ambiguous. Recently, various studies, including the WHO classification, have established that patients with this syndrome should have a marrow blast cell percentage ≤5% and should harbor the 5q—, always produced by an interstitial deletion, as a single karyotype defect. On the basis of these criteria the syndrome is much more common in female than in male patients (female:male ratio = 3:1) and has the highest incidence between 60 and 65 years of age. From a cytogenetic point of view, the most common proximal breakpoint is located at band 5q13 and the distal breakpoint at band 5q33. The mechanism leading to the development of the deletion that identifies the 5q— syndrome has been discussed for a long time. It has been suggested that during the ageing process and only in the female sex the deletion proximal breakpoint gets nearer and nearer to the centromere. The 5q— syndrome occurs only when such a breakpoint falls within band 5q13.

From a clinical point of view these patients present macrocytic anemia and sometimes a reduced white blood cell (WBC) count. Microscopically, bone marrow cellularity is more often normal or increased, and rarely reduced. The erythroid lineage shows dysplastic changes (megaloblastosis, multinuclearity, internuclear bridges), the granulopoietic lineage is predominantly represented by immature precursors, and the megakaryocytic lineage shows important dysplastic changes (hypolobulated megakaryocytes and micromegakaryocytes). Usually these patients have a high red blood cell transfusion requirement, which may cause iron overload. So, in these patients iron-chelating therapy is absolutely required in order to prevent organ damage. The clinical outcome of these patients is favorable and is not modified by the development of additional chromosomal abnormalities, among which the most common is trisomy 22. An AML evolution occurs in only 2% of patients. Other deletions, always interstitial [formally defined as del(5)(q12q31-33),del(5)(q12q23),del(5)(q23q32)], and monosomy 5 are more frequently associated with a blast cell percentage ≥5% and further chromosomal abnormalities, which more commonly consist of monosomy 7 or del(7q). So, most patients belong to the RAEB and RAEB-t subtypes. The incidence of 5q—/−5 is 10–20% in *de novo* and 40% in secondary MDS. Various studies have correlated these abnormalities with a previous exposure to benzene derivatives. This event seems to especially occur in patients presenting a polymorphism in genes that code for enzymes required for the degradation of these chemical compounds. In some patients a previous exposure to alkylating agents and immunosuppressive drugs has also been reported.

Numerous efforts have been undertaken to map a possible CDR within the deleted segment of chromosome 5 in order to identify any potential TSG. The 5q13-q33 region contains genes, coding for interleukin-4 (IL-4), IL-5, IRF-1, IL-9, IL-3, EGR-1, which have a significant role in normal hemopoiesis. It has been demonstrated that, in 90% of 5q− patients, the CDR corresponds to band 5q31. However, it is still debated whether the 5q− syndrome is determined by the loss of genes located within either the proximal/distal breakpoints or the deleted segment. The analysis of 3 patients with the 5q− syndrome has allowed us to establish that the CDR, corresponding to band 5q33, is 3.0 Mb in size and is located in between the ADRB2 and ILI2B genes. More recently, additional molecular and FISH studies have allowed further reduction of the size of this region to 1.5 Mb. This novel CDR is located in between the polymorphic site D5S413 and the "glycine receptor alpha 1" gene. It contains nine genes, each of which could behave as a TSG. In patients presenting with other 5q interstitial deletions it has been established that the CDR corresponds to band 5q31. This CDR, which is more proximal than that of patients with the 5q− syndrome, has an extent of 1.5 Mb and is located in between the D5S479 and D5S500 polymorphic sites. In conclusion, all these studies suggest the presence of two distinct CDRs. One, corresponding to band 5q33, contains a TSG the loss of which determines the 5q− syndrome and the other, corresponding to band 5q31, contains a TSG the loss of which causes other 5q deletions in *de novo* and secondary MDS.

Monosomy 7 and 7q Deletion

In *de novo* MDS these abnormalities occur as single chromosomal defects in about 1% of patients and along with further karyotype defects, among which the most common is the rearrangement of the long arm of chromosome 3, observed in 5–10% of patients. Because 50–60% of patients with secondary MDS show −7/7q plus other defects, it has been suggested that these defects might be targeted by various cytotoxic agents. However, the fact that myeloid disorders with −7 or 7q− as a single chromosomal defect share the same biological and clinical features has lead to the hypothesis that they might be induced by the loss of the same gene(s). In fact, a monosomy 7 syndrome predominantly affecting the male sex and with clinical characteristics (liver and spleen enlargement, high WBC counts, reduced platelet counts, and unfavorable outcomes) similar to those of juvenile CMML has been described in pediatric patients. Monosomy 7 is also the most common chromosomal defect discovered in the bone marrow of patients with constitutional syndromes (Fanconi's anemia, type I neurofibromatosis, severe congenital neutropenia) that predispose to myeloid disorders. Molecular analyses of these patients have demonstrated that −7 is a secondary event in the pathogenesis of the disease. In fact, the primary event might be an impairment in the phosphorylation and de-phosphorylation of kinetochore proteins, which are absolutely required for a normal mitotic segregation of chromosomes.

Monosomy 7 is present in all MDS subtypes, even if it is much more common in advanced forms. From a morphological point of view the marrow of all −7 patients shows the presence of trilineage dysplasia with micromegakaryocytes. During clinical outcome infective episodes are very frequent because of an impairment in neutrophil functions. Monosomy 7 determines an unfavorable prognosis. So its discovery is particularly important in patients who are at a low risk of developing MDS based only on clinical and hematological parameters. As far as 7q− is concerned, patients harboring a del(7)(q31-q36) have an inferior response to chemotherapy and a shorter survival than those with del(7)(q22).

FISH and molecular studies have tried to identify a CDR within the deleted segment on 7q. All these studies have documented that the extent of 7q deletion is very variable and the chromosomal segment constantly lost very often corresponds to band 7q22. In these last patients the proximal breakpoint resides in 7q11-22 and the distal breakpoint in 7q22-36. The CDR identified within this region has an extent of about 2.0 Mb and contains genes that play a crucial role in normal hemopoiesis. However, none seems to function as a TSG. Other studies have suggested the existence of a different, more distal CDR residing between bands 7q32 and 7q33.

del(17)(p13)

A loss of chromosomal material from the short arm of chromosome 17 is not only determined by simple deletions, but also by unbalanced translocations, iso(17q) and, more rarely, monosomies of the entire chromosome. A 17p deletion occurs in 7% of patients with advanced MDS, more often secondary. Despite their heterogeneity, these defects have been unified because all of them cause the loss of one p53 allele. In addition, during follow-up 70% of these patients develop either a mutation or a submicroscopic deletion of the other p53 allele, located on the other chromosome 17 with a normal appearance on CC investigation. The 17p deletion is always accompanied by other chromosomal defects and often participates in a complex karyotype (with ≥3 chromosomal abnormalities). Recently, it has been noted that 17p- is frequently associated with 5q− and duplication of the MLL gene, mapped at band 11q23. For all these reasons the assessment of the role of 17p- in the multistep process of MDS evolution has been a formidable task. However, because all 17p- patients, including those with p53 nullisomy, present a loss of large DNA regions, it has been proposed that this deletion is not a primary step in the pathogenesis of the disease; instead, it may play a crucial role in MDS evolution.

Morphologically, 70% of 17p- patients show dysplastic changes affecting the granulocytic lineage with ≥5% of neutrophils presenting pseudo-Pelger-Huet hypolobulations, small granules, and vacuoles in the cytoplasm. From a clinical point of view the deletion causes a poor response to chemotherapy and a short survival.

Loss of the Y Chromosome

The clinical significance of this cytogenetic defect is still undefined and the defect seems to be determined by the ageing process. In fact, −Y is not only discovered in 10% of MDS patients, but also in 7% of the elderly people without any haematological disorder. So, the IPSS has established that an MDS diagnosis cannot be based on the presence of −Y alone; instead, when biological and clinical parameters point to an MDS diagnosis, the loss of the Y chromosome identifies patients with a favorable clinical outcome. Despite these data, elderly people with a high percentage of −Y marrow cells are at risk of developing a hematological disorder and in MDS patients the abnormality is surely clonal because it is present at the onset of the disease and disappears upon achievement of complete remission.

Trisomy 8

This chromosomal abnormality is not specific to MDS because it can be discovered in other oncohematological disorders. The incidence of trisomy 8 varies between 5% and 20%; it occurs in 19% of chromosomally abnormal patients and in 10% of all MDS patients. It can be hypothesized that in half of the patients such a trisomy would be a secondary event, appearing during the clinical course. However, it is worth noting that the percentage of +8 cells varies during the follow-up independently of response to chemotherapy. This condition has been clarified by FISH, which has documented that some patients may present a constitutional mosaicism. In other patients +8 is surely an acquired clonal abnormality and FISH has demonstrated its presence in $CD33^+$, $CD34^+$ hemopoietic precursors.

The incidence of trisomy 8 varies among the different MDS subtypes. It is more often discovered in RARS and in RAEB. Some patients who harbor two cell populations, one marked by trisomy 8 and the other by tetrasomy 8, disease frequently evolves to AML and they develop extramedullary disease, often involving the skin. From a prognostic point of view +8 is associated with an intermediate outcome.

20q Deletion

20q deletion is a recurrent chromosomal abnormality observed in myeloproliferative disorders. It is discovered in 5% of patients with *de novo* MDS and in 7% of those with secondary MDS. The incidence of this karyotype defect might be underestimated because monosomy 20 and unbalanced translocations involving fragments of the q arm of the chromosome occur as frequently as 20q−. FISH has demonstrated that the deletion is rather large, has a variable extent, and involves most of 20q. FISH analyses in combination with molecular studies exploring heterozygosity have documented that the CDR on chromosome 20 is about 5.0-Mb long and corresponds to band 20q11.2-q12. This chromosomal region contains numerous genes, but none behaves as a TSG.

The deletion may be present as a single defect or may be associated with additional abnormalities and is rather common in RARS and RA. Morphologically, the erythroid and megakaryocytic lineages show evident dysplastic changes. FISH has demonstrated that neutrophils undergo apoptotic death within the marrow.

The IPSS has included 20q− within the low-risk cytogenetic category. Usually, these patients are classified as having RA, rarely evolve in AML, and their median overall survival is 45 months. In contrast patients presenting with 20q− as part of a complex karyotype (≥3 abnormalities) experience an unfavorable clinical outcome with a median survival of only 9.3 months.

Deletion (12)(p13)

Various oncohematological disorders harbor balanced translocations or interstitial deletions involving band 12p13. In MDS these karyotype defects are correlated with a RAEB and RAEB-t diagnosis. Band 12p13 contains the ETV6 gene, which functions as a negative transcription regulator. So it might behave as a TSG. Another gene mapped within the same band is KIP1, which codes for the p27 protein. This protein inhibits cyclin-dependent kinases. It blocks cellular proliferation by controlling the progression through the cell cycle. Therefore, it is the TSG whose loss may favor neoplastic transformation. It has been demonstrated that the smallest deleted region of band 12p13 is mapped in between the KIP1 gene in proximal position and the ETV6 gene in terminal position. Up to now no TSG has been discovered within this region and no ETV6 and KIP1 mutations have been detected.

From a prognostic point of view, the IPSS has included 12p13 deletion within the intermediate-risk cytogenetic category, but recent studies suggest that this defect determines a clinical outcome similar to that of patients included within the low-risk category.

Chromosome 3 Abnormalities

Chromosome 3 is involved in various rearrangements that share numerous clinical and prognostic features (have 2% and 5% incidence in *de novo* and secondary MDS), are frequently associated with −7/7q− and 5q−, and determine a short survival and a poor response to chemotherapy. Inv(3)(q21q26) and t(3;3)(q21;q26) are also observed in AML and in the blast crisis of chronic myeloid leukemia (CML). These chromosomal defects are more common in young female patients (age ≤55 years). The peripheral blood count commonly reveals a high platelet count and the morphological analysis of bone marrow cells shows trilineage dysplasia, especially involving the megakaryocytic cell compartment. This datum suggests that the target of the neoplastic event might be a pluripotent stem cell. The region involved in the defect contains various genes that play a crucial role in normal hematopoiesis: the transferrin gene, mapped at q21; the lactoferrin gene, mapped at q21-q23; the transferrin receptor gene, mapped at q26.2-qter; the CALLA-CD10 gene, mapped at q21-q27; and the EVI1 gene, mapped at q26. However, none seems to be responsible for the disease. Two hypotheses have been suggested to explain the dysplastic changes affecting the megakaryocytic cell lineage: one suggests a pluripotent stem cell functional defect caused by the juxtaposition of bands q21 and q26, and the other a functional abnormality of a not yet identified gene (s).

The t(3;5)(q25.1;q34) is discovered not only in MDS but also in AML. The rearrangement determines the fusion of the NPM gene (coding for the nucleophosmin gene), mapped in 3q25.1, with the MLF1 gene ("myelodysplasia/myeloid leukemia factor 1), mapped in 5q34. The NPM gene codes for a nucleo-cytoplasmic protein that functions as a chaperone between the nucleolus and the cytoplasm during the assembly of ribosomal proteins. The MLF1 gene codes for a protein that could have a role in DNA replication and cell cycle control. The NPM-MLF1 fusion protein alters DNA replication and mRNA processing and causes an impairment in cellular growth.

Iso dic(X)(q13)

This is a rare defect with the most common breakpoint in q13. Usually, this defect is observed in female patients older than 65 years of age. Probably, it develops in an early hemopoietic progenitor and morphologically it is associated with marrow iron overload. Patients' survival is variable.

t(11;16)(q23;p13.3)

This is a rare defect observed in secondary MDS and especially in the RAEB-t subtype. The involvement of band 11q23 indicates that most patients have been previously exposed to topo-isomerase II inhibitors, especially high-dose epipodophyllotoxin derivatives. The targets of the translocation are the MLL gene, mapped at band 11q23, and the CBP gene, mapped at 16p13.3. The rearrangement causes an impaired function of the MLL gene, which induces an altered expression of the "homeobox" genes. These last have a pivotal role in normal hemopoiesis and stem cell maturation. The CBP gene is a transcriptional co-activator, which cooperates with various transcription factors and is able to carry out histone acetylation, which determines an increased gene expression. In addition, the CBP gene controls cell cycle progression. Its mutation has been discovered in the constitutional Rubinstein–Taybi syndrome, which is associated with a high risk of cancer development. So, the CBP gene is thought to be a TSG. The MLL-CBP fusion gene is no more able to regulate the cell cycle and could favor a progression to a therapy-resistant AML.

Nucleoporins Abnormalities

The NUP98 gene, mapped at 11p15.1, codes for a nucleoporin that functions as a chaperone for proteins and RNA, which are transferred from the nucleus to the cytoplasm and *vice versa*. This gene is involved in various translocations detected in secondary MDS/AML patients. The transcript produced by these rearrangements contains the GLFG repeats, located at NUP98 amino-terminal, fused to the carboxy-terminal of the partner gene.

PROGNOSTIC SIGNIFICANCE

Beginning from the middle of the 1980s, various studies have analyzed the impact of biological factors on MDS clinical outcome. In 1985 Mufti[5] developed the first prognostic scoring system (the "Bournemouth score") based on blood cell count and bone marrow morphology. A second prognostic system was introduced by the Spanish group of Sanz *et al.*[6] and recognized age, blast cell percentage, and platelet count as the most important prognostic factors in MDS patients. Subsequently, Aul and co-workers[7] demonstrated that a marrow blast cell percentage $\geq 5\%$, a lactic dehydrogenase (LDH) value >200 international units, a hemoglobin value $\leq 9g/dL$, and a platelet count $\leq 100 \times 10^9/L$ were the only factors that accurately predicted MDS clinical outcome and the so-called "Dusseldorf score" was developed. This score presented two advantages over the Bournemouth score: the LDH value allowed an easier identification of CMML patients and the combination of the four parameters more precisely identified poor-risk RA/RARS. This is why the Dusseldorf score recognizes high-risk MDS patients more accurately than any other system. A recent study, carried out on 180 patients with MDS, showed that 32.2% were classified as high-risk patients when the Dusseldorf score was applied; in contrast only 13–20% of them were classified within this category when other scores were applied.

In 1993 the Lille group[8] developed a new scoring system that included karyotype as a novel prognostic variable. Based on the CC pattern, the study subdivided the 235 patients in the following groups: normal karyotypes, 5q— as a single defect, 5q— with further defects, +8 as a single defect, −7/7q— as single defects, 20q— as a single defect, −Y as a single defect, miscellaneous defects, −7/7q— with further defects, and complex karyotype. Multivariate analysis showed that overall survival was significantly influenced by marrow blast cell percentage, karyotype, and platelet count, whereas the risk of AML evolution was significantly influenced by marrow blast cell percentage and karyotype. The major drawback of this study was that the clinical relevance of CC was not fully determined because normal and complex karyotypes were the only cytogenetic categories that included a number of patients sufficient for statistical analyses.

In 1997 Greenberg and co-workers developed a new scoring system, the IPSS,[9] which recognized the karyotype along with number/type of peripheral cytopenia (hemoglobin $<10g/dL$, absolute neutrophil count $<1.8 \times 10^9/L$, and platelet count $<100 \times 10^9/L$) and marrow blast cell percentage as the most relevant parameters for predicting MDS clinical outcome. The 800 MDS patients analyzed were subdivided into three cytogenetic categories: a prognostically favorable category that included normal karyotypes, 5q— as a single defect, 20q— as a single defect, and −Y as a single defect; a prognostically intermediate category that included +8 and miscellaneous defects; and a prognostically unfavorable category that included −7/7q— and complex karyotypes (with ≥ 3 abnormalities). Patients of the favorable cytogenetic category had a median survival of 3.8 years; those of the intermediate category, 2.4 years; and those of the unfavorable category, 0.8 years. Twenty-five percent of patients belonging to each cytogenetic category developed AML 5.6, 1.6, and 0.9 years from diagnosis. A score was given to each of the three parameters: 0–0.5 to the amount of peripheral cytopenia, 0–1.0 to the cytogenetic category, and 0–2.0 to the marrow blast cell percentage. By combining these scores four prognostically different patients' categories were identified: low risk (score = 0), intermediate-1 risk (score = 0.5–1.0), intermediate-2 risk (score = 1.5–2.0), and high risk (score ≥ 2.5). The four categories showed different median survivals: 5.7, 3.5, 1.2, and 0.4 years. In addition, 25% of patients belonging to each category developed AML 9.4, 3.3, 1.1, and 0.2 years from diagnosis. IPSS strongly stressed the prognostic importance of karyotype: the lack of the cytogenetic data significantly affected the prognostic stratification of patients, especially those belonging to the intermediate-1 and intermediate-2 risk categories. Afterward, the effectiveness of IPSS in predicting MDS clinical outcome was confirmed by various studies that underlined the prognostic power of the cytogenetic pattern. In addition, it was observed that IPSS cytogenetic categories maintained their prognostic relevance, even in patients submitted to intensive treatments or allogeneic bone marrow transplantation. Only one study reported that the prognostic significance of the cytogenetic defect was strongly modified by sex. In this report male patients belonging to the IPSS low and intermediate cytogenetic categories experienced a survival shorter than that of female patients. Considering patients of the low-risk category such a difference was entirely due to the higher incidence of 5q− syndrome and low smoking habits in women, but for patients of the intermediate category no factor responsible for such a difference was identified. However, despite its efficacy in predicting clinical outcome, IPSS still presents some major drawbacks, which are an absolute requirement for the cytogenetic result and the inclusion of various defects with a still undetermined impact on OS and AML evolution within the intermediate cytogenetic category. The first attempt to overcome these limits was made by Solè and co-workers.[10] They reported that 12p- was associated with clinical outcome similar to that of the low-risk category; in contrast a trisomy 1q and +8 were associated with a survival worse than that of patients included within the intermediate cytogenetic category. Another study more precisely defined 5q− prognostic significance.[11] This report showed that after a median follow-up of 67 months, patients with 5q− alone presented a median survival significantly better than that of patients with 5q− plus additional karyotype defects (146 vs. 45 months). The survival of 5q− patients was unaffected by sex, interstitial breakpoints, and severity of dysplastic changes, but it was relevantly influenced by blast cell percentage. In fact, 5q− patients with >5% blasts presented a median survival of 24 months, significantly worse than that of 5q− patients with ≤5% blast cells. The risk of developing AML was 80% for the first group of patients and 9% for the second group. A more recent study[12] showed that patients with 3q rearrangements have a clinical outcome similar to that of the poor-risk cytogenetic category. In addition, del(7)(q31q35) patients presented a survival better than that of patients belonging to the poor-risk category, but when this cytogenetic defect was entered as a new entity, the prognostic power of IPSS was not improved. This report also underlined that the prognostic relevance of complex karyotypes is independent of blast cell percentage. Recently, Solè and co-workers[13] modified the IPSS cytogenetic categories in order to ameliorate their prognostic accuracy. This study included 11q and 12p deletions within the IPSS low-risk cytogenetic category, 3q21q26 rearrangements, +8, +9, 11q translocations and 17p deletion within the IPSS intermediate-risk category, rare defects within a novel poor-risk category, and complex karyotypes (≥3 abnormalities), −7/del(7q), iso(17q) within a novel very poor-risk category. In this series patients' survival was significantly influenced by age, hemoglobin value, number of cytopenia, FAB subtype, and new cytogenetic categories, whereas the likelihood of AML progression was statistically influenced by hemoglobin value, FAB subtypes, and new cytogenetic categories. By combining all these factors four patient groups having different clinical outcomes were identified. The authors concluded that the better prognostic stratification was entirely due to the improvement in the definition of patients belonging to the intermediate cytogenetic category. Another study showed that such a goal could also be achieved by combining IPSS and WHO classification.[14]

IMPACT ON TREATMENT

It has been reported that a specific cytogenetic defect identifies patients particularly sensitive to a specific clinical treatment. This association was for the first time demonstrated by a study[15] that analyzed erythropoietin response in low-risk MDS patients presenting with a mixture of chromosomally normal and abnormal cells on either CC or FISH studies. On clinical diagnosis responsive patients showed a higher percentage of chromosomally normal CD34[+] and erythroid cells than did unresponsive patients and during treatment they experienced a further progressive increase of such percentage. Because erythropoietin in combination with G-CSF induced a reduction in the apoptosis of CD34[+] cells, it was hypothesized that the mechanism underlying responses was an improvement in the balance between pro- and antiapoptotic proteins. However, the fact that telomere length remained unchanged before and after treatment suggested that erythropoietin and G-CSF induced the proliferation of CD34[+] which had already acquired a functional defect.

An investigational trial showed that 5q− is another defect that identifies patients particularly sensitive to lenalidomide.[16] This thalidomide derivative was able to induce an independence from transfusion support in 56% of the 43 patients studied. Response was associated with an improvement in marrow dysplasia, an effect especially evident for the erythroid and megacaryocytic cell lineages. Because erythroid cells showed a reduction in ringed sideroblasts, it was suggested that lenalidomide response was due to a selective suppression of the clonal cell population and a re-expansion of normal erythropoiesis. Median time to response was shorter in 5q− patients than in those with other defects or a normal karyotype. Considering the 20 patients with an abnormal karyotype a complete response was achieved in 9/10 5q− patients and a partial response in the remaining 11 patients. After a median follow-up of 81 weeks median duration from transfusion support was not yet achieved and median hemoglobin value was 13.2g/dL.

Patients with a complex karyotype (≥3 defects), which is included within the poor-risk cytogenetic category, seem to be particularly sensitive to 5-azacytidine and decytabine. These drugs are S-phase-specific antimetabolites which, once incorporated into the DNA, become potent inhibitors of the methylation process and form covalent compounds with DNA methyl transferase 1. A recent study[17] reported a complete or a major cytogenetic response, defined following the criteria already applied to CML patients, in 31% of the 61 patients studied. Any clinical response of 7.5 months' median duration (complete, partial remissions and minimal responses) was achieved after a median number of three courses of therapy. Considering the cytogenetic pattern any type of response was reached in 60% of low-risk patients, 20% of intermediate risk patients, and 38% of high-risk patients. The median survival of the three groups of patients was 30, 8, and 13 months, respectively. Patients who achieved a major cytogenetic response presented a mortality rate significantly better than that of nonresponders and their median survival was 24 months versus 11 months. However, such a treatment did not eradicate the disease because 10 of 19 responsive patients relapsed. A subsequent study showed that 5-azacytidine induced a higher percentage of response, and was able to delay AML progression, but it did not affect overall survival.[18]

REFERENCES

1. HEANY, M.L. *et al.* 1999. Myelodysplasia. N. Engl. J. Med. **340:** 1649–1653.
2. BENNET, J.M. *et al.* 1976. Proposals for the classification of the acute leukemias (FAB cooperative group). Br. J. Haematol. **33:** 451–458.
3. HARRIS, N.L. *et al.* 1999. World Health Organization classification of neoplastic diseases of the haematopoietic and lymphoid tissues: report of the Clinical Advisory Committee meeting – Airlie House, Virginia, November 1997. J. Clin. Oncol. **17:** 3835–3849.
4. VAN DEN BERGHE H. *et al.* 1974. Distinct haematological disorder with deletion of the long arm of no. 5 chromosome. Nature **251:** 437–438.
5. MUFTI, G.J. *et al.* 1985. Myelodysplastic syndromes: a scoring system with prognostic significance. Br. J. Haematol. **59:** 425–433.
6. SANZ, G.F. *et al.* 1989. Two regression models and a scoring system for predicting survival and planning treatment in myelodysplastic syndromes: a multivariate analysis of prognostic factors in 370 patients. Blood **74:** 395–408.
7. AUL, C. *et al.* 1992. Primary myelodysplastic syndromes: analysis of prognostic factors in 235 patients and proposal for an improved scoring system. Leukemia **6:** 52–59.
8. MOREL P. *et al.* 1993. Cytogenetic analysis has strong independent prognostic value in *de novo* myelodysplastic syndromes and can be incorporated in a new scoring system: a report on 408 cases. Leukemia **7:** 1315–1323.
9. GREENBERG, P. *et al.* 1997. International scoring system for evaluating prognosis in myelodysplastic syndromes. Blood **89:** 2079–2088.
10. SOLÈ, F. *et al.* 2000. Incidence, characterization and prognostic significance of chromosomal abnormalities in 640 patients with primary myelodysplastic syndromes. Br. J. Haematol. **108:** 346–356.
11. GIAGOUNIDIS, A.A.N. *et al.* 2004. Clinical, morphological, cytogenetic, and prognostic features of patients with myelodysplastic syndromes and del(5q) including band q31. Leukemia **18:** 113–119.
12. BERNASCONI, P. *et al.* 2005. Incidence and prognostic significance of karyotype abnormalities in de novo primary myelodysplastic syndromes: a study on 331 patients from a single institution. Leukemia **19:** 1424–1431.
13. SOLÈ, F. *et al.* 2005. Identification of novel cytogenetic markers with prognostic significance in a series of 968 patients with primary myelodysplastic syndromes. Haematologica **90:** 1168–1178.
14. MALCOVATI, L. *et al.* 2005. Prognostic factors and life expectancy in myelodysplastic syndromes classified according to WHO criteria: a basis for clinical decision making. J. Clin. Oncol. **23:** 7594–7603.
15. RIGOLIN, G.M. *et al.* 2004. In patients with myelodysplastic syndromes response to rHuEpo and G-CSF treatment is related to an increase of cytogenetically normal CD34+ cells. Br. J. Haematol. **126:** 501–507.

16. LIST, A. *et al*. 2005. Efficacy of lenalidomide in myelodysplastic syndromes. N. Engl. J. Med. **352:** 549–557.
17. LUBBERT, M. *et al*. 2001. Cytogenetic response in high-risk myelodysplastic syndrome following low-dose treatment with the DNA methylation inhibitor 5-aza-2'-deoxycytidine. Br. J. Haematol. **114:** 349–357.
18. SILVERMAN, L.R. *et al*. 2002. Randomized controlled trial of azacitidine in patients with the myelodysplastic syndrome: a study of the cancer and leukemia study group B. J. Clin. Oncol. **20:** 2429–2440.

Genetic Abnormalities as Targets for Molecular Therapies in Myelodysplastic Syndromes

DANIELA CILLONI, EMANUELA MESSA, FRANCESCA MESSA,
SONIA CARTURAN, ILARIA DEFILIPPI, FRANCESCA ARRUGA,
VALENTINA ROSSO, RENATA CATALANO, ENRICO BRACCO,
PAOLO NICOLI, AND GIUSEPPE SAGLIO

*Department of Clinical and Biological Sciences of the University of Turin,
S. Luigi Gonzaga Hospital, 10043, Orbassano-Turin, Italy*

ABSTRACT: Recent advances in molecular genetics have increased knowledge regarding the mechanisms leading to myelodysplastic syndrome (MDS), secondary acute myeloid leukemia (AML), and therapy-induced MDS. Many genetic defects underlying MDS and AML have been identified thereby allowing the development of new molecular-targeted therapies. Several new classes of drugs have shown promise in early clinical trials and may probably alter the standard of care of these patients in the near future. Among these new drugs are farnesyltransferase inhibitors and receptor tyrosine kinase inhibitors including FLT3 and VEGF inhibitors. These agents have been tested in patients with solid tumors and hematologic malignancies such as AML and MDS. Most of the studies in MDS are still in early stages of development. The DNA hypomethylating compounds azacytidine and decitabine may reduce hypermethylation and induce re-expression of key tumor suppressor genes in MDS. Biochemical compounds with histone deacetylase inhibitory activity, such as valproic acid (VPA), have been tested as antineoplastic agents. Finally, new vaccination strategies are developing in MDS patients based on the identification of MDS-associated antigens. Future therapies will attempt to resolve cytopenias in MDS, eliminate malignant clones, and allow differentiation by attacking specific mechanisms of the disease.

KEYWORDS: myelodysplastic syndromes; molecular therapy; WT1; EVI1; tyrosine kinase

Address for correspondence: Daniela Cilloni, M.D., Department of Clinical and Biological Sciences of the University of Turin, San Luigi Hospital, Gonzole 10, 10043 Orbassano-Torino, Italy. Voice: +39-011-9026610; fax: +39-11-9038636.
e-mail: daniela.cilloni@unito.it

Ann. N.Y. Acad. Sci. 1089: 411–423 (2006). © 2006 New York Academy of Sciences.
doi: 10.1196/annals.1386.030

MOLECULAR BIOLOGY
OF MYELODYSPLASTIC SYNDROMES

Myelodysplastic syndromes (MDS) constitute a heterogeneous group of clonal disorders of the hematopoietic stem cell (HSC), which exhibit ineffective hematopoiesis with an increased risk of transformation to acute myeloid leukemia (AML).[1,2] Expansion of the abnormal clone is characterized by morphological dysplasia, impaired differentiation, defective cellular functions, and genetic instability. The consequences of ineffective hematopoiesis are peripheral cytopenias that frequently involve all three blood cell lineages: erythroid, granulocytic, and megakaryocytic.[1,2]

MDS patients are at high risk for progression; approximately 30–40% of cases evolve to AML. Patients with MDS-associated leukemia are often refractory to chemotherapy and have a poor prognosis.[1,2] Clonal karyotypic abnormalities are observed in approximately 40–50% of primary MDS cases and 90% of secondary (therapy-related) MDS.[3]

Single or complex chromosomal abnormalities may be present initially and evolutionary changes may occur during the course of the disease. These genetic derangements reflect the multistep process believed to underlie the evolution of MDS.[4] Chromosomal aberrations vary from single numerical or structural changes to complex genomic lesions involving three or more different chromosomes.[3–5]

The loss of gene function may occur in a number of ways, including chromosomal loss or deletion, balanced translocations, point mutations, or by transcriptional silencing via methylation of the control elements of the gene.[6] Compared to AML, where a major part of the chromosomal changes are balanced translocations, deletion of a part of a chromosome or the entire chromosome loss are among the most frequently encountered genomic changes in MDS.[3] Deletions result in the loss of genes, mainly of tumor suppressor genes.[3] The most common abnormalities are partial or complete chromosome loss involving del(5q) or -5, del(7q) or -7, del(20q), del(11q), and -Y, while balanced translocations are rarely found.[7,8] Point mutations in *RAS* proto-oncogenes and the *p53* tumor suppressor gene have been previously reported.[9] *FLT3* duplications and *p15* promoter hypermethylation have been associated with disease progression to AML.[10,11] However, none of these alterations is specific for MDS and the underlying molecular causes of the disease remain poorly understood.

FARNESYL TRANSFERASE INHIBITORS

The most extensively studied gene family in MDS is the RAS family.[11–16] RAS proteins are a crucial component of the signaling transduction pathways and result in the control of cellular proliferation, differentiation, and cell death.[11–16] Under normal conditions, RAS activation is triggered by the binding of growth factors to plasma membrane receptors with tyrosine kinase activity.[14] The activation of these pathways is dependent on farnesylation. Once activated by a cell surface receptor, RAS proteins induce a cascade of kinase activity, resulting in the transduction of the signals to the nucleus. Mutant RAS proteins retain the active GTP-bound form, promoting constitutive activation. Oncogenic mutations in RAS have been found to occur at critical regulatory sites, constitutively activating mutant RAS and resulting in unregulated stimulation of cell proliferation.[17] Activating point mutations of N-RAS have been detected at high frequency in hematological malignancies. In MDS, N-RAS mutations have been detected in 10–40% of cases.[16] These mutations have been associated with poor prognosis, higher incidence of transformation to AML, and shorter survival. Patients with abnormal karyotypes and N-RAS mutations have the highest likelihood of transformation. Moreover, even in the absence of RAS mutations, alternative mechanisms of RAS dysfunction may be operative.

Farnesyl transferase inhibitors (FTIs) represent a novel class of chemotherapeutic agents originally developed to antagonize oncogenic RAS, but they have been shown to have activity against a wide range of transformed cells, regardless of RAS mutation. FTIs are also active inhibitors of other prenylation-dependent molecules and have been found to affect multiple signaling pathways, including p53, phosphoinositol-3-kinase, Rheb (a small G-protein), and centromere-associated protein.[17–19] FTIs have shown antiproliferative, antiangiogenic, and proapoptotic activity *in vitro* and in cancer-specific pathways.[19,20] Their diverse activity, minimal effect on normal cells, and oral bioavailability make FTIs attractive anticancer agents. There are various heterocyclic oral FTIs at different stages of development in clinical trials.[18] These include tipifarnib (R115777, Zarnestra), lonafarnib (SCH66336, Sarasare), and BMS214662. These agents have been used as single agents and in combination with radio- and chemotherapy in various solid tumors and hematological malignancies.[18] The FTI tipifarnib has been investigated in high-risk MDS and AML patients.[21]

Tipifarnib (R115777, Zarnestra), an orally active heterocyclic agent, has been found to downregulate the RAS-MAPK (mitogen-activated protein kinase) pathway[22] with activity in both wild-type and mutant RAS tumor cell lines.[23] Karp *et al.*[21] have tested this drug in patients with refractory and relapsed AML and MDS. In the initial phase I trial, tipifarnib was found to accumulate in the bone marrow, producing clinical responses in 29% of refractory or relapsed AML patients, including two complete remissions.[21] Trilineage responses were observed in some AML patients. Importantly, none of the patients enrolled in this study were found to harbor RAS mutations.

Lonafarnib (Sarasar, SCH6636), a tricyclic inhibitor of the CAAX binding motif, selectively inhibits chronic myeloid leukemia (CML) cells.[24] Like tipifarnib, lonafarnib has shown activity when combined with cytotoxic agents such as cyclophosphamide, 5-fluorouracil, and vincristine.[25] In a randomized phase II study in patients with advanced hematologic malignancies, which included high-risk MDS, refractory, and poor-risk AML and CML in blast crisis, the hematologic responses were observed in 3 of 15 MDS patients.[26] These promising data suggest that this agent merits further investigation.

Feldman et al.[27] have reported results from a Phase I/II study of lonafarnib in 32 patients with advanced MDS (RAEB, RAEB-t) and 35 patients with chronic myelomonocytic leukemia (CMML) with 31% responses including 2 complete responses and 11 cases of hematological improvement. Although the reported clinical responses observed in patients with myeloid malignancies to different FTIs would suggest the possibility of introducing these drugs to clinical practice, the optimal use of these agents in these disorders will require further exploration of dosing schedules and potential combinations of FTIs with other classes of biologically active agents.

RECEPTOR TYROSINE KINASE INHIBITORS

Angiogenesis and the proangiogenic VEGF are considered to play a significant role in the biology of MDS. Therefore, many VEGF inhibitors are in development, including small molecules, such as SU5416, SU11248, PTK787, AGL3736, which target the autophosphorylation of the VEGF receptor (VEGFR). These agents are classified as receptor tyrosine kinase (RTK) inhibitors, and have a structure similar to adenosine triphosphate, with a specificity extending from VEGFR-1, VEGFR-2 to other type III receptors such as FLT3, c-KIT, and PDGFβ.[28,29] AML and MDS precursors express these receptors specifically; they express VEGF, stem cell factor, and FLT3 ligand, leading to autocrine and paracrine stimulation. All these RTKs stimulate cell proliferation and may provide new therapeutic targets.[30]

SU5416 and SU11248 are small molecules that have been shown to effectively inhibit VEGF-mediated cell growth.[31] SU5416 is an RTK inhibitor of VEGFR-2, c-kit, and both wild-type and mutant FLT3. All these receptors are expressed on AML blasts. SU5416 has completed the phase II trials in MDS and AML. A multicenter phase II trial in 22 high-risk MDS and 33 refractory AML patients showed limited clinical activity (7% overall response).[32]

SU11248 is a third-generation agent with increased potency against both KDR and PDGF-R while maintaining c-kit activity. SU11248 inhibits phosphorylation of both wild-type and internal tandem duplication (ITD)-mutant FLT3 receptors. A phase I study was conducted with oral SU11248 in 29 AML patients. FLT3 phosphorylation was inhibited in 50% of FLT3-wild-type patients and in 100% of FLT3-mutant patients. Despite the limit that a single dose of drug be administered, 5 of 29 patients developed large decreases in peripheral blast counts, suggesting potential clinical activity of this signal transduction inhibitor.[33] Further evidence of the impact of VEGF on leukemic proliferation and survival comes from the data obtained by treating with the anti-VEGF antibody bevacizumab a subset of patients with relapsed and refractory AML. Bevacizumab has also been studied in MDS with preliminary positive results, supporting the further development of drugs that target VEGF and VEGF signaling in MDS and AML patients.[34]

Activating mutations of FMS-like tyrosine kinase 3 (FLT3) are present in approximately 30% of patients with *de novo* AML and are associated with lower cure rates from standard chemotherapy-based treatment.[35] These mutations, although not typical of MDS, could be detected in a number of therapy-related MDS. Targeting the mutation by inhibiting the tyrosine kinase activity of FLT3 is cytotoxic to cell lines and primary AML cells harboring FLT3 mutations. CEP-701 is an orally available, novel RTK inhibitor that selectively inhibits FLT3 autophosphorylation. A phase I/ II clinical trial to determine the *in vivo* hematologic effects of CEP-701 as a single agent, such as salvage treatment for patients with refractory, relapsed, or poor-risk AML expressing FLT3-activating mutations, has been completed.[36] Five of 14 heavily pretreated AML patients, treated with CEP-701 had clinical evidence of biologic activity and measurable clinical response, including significant reductions in bone marrow and peripheral blood blasts. Laboratory data confirmed that clinical responses correlated with sustained FLT3 inhibition to CEP-701. The data show that FLT3 inhibition is associated with clinical activity in AML patients harboring FLT3-activating mutations and indicate that CEP-701 holds promise as a novel, molecularly targeted therapy for this disease.

The t(5;12) (q33;p13) translocation has been reported in a small proportion of CMML patients, ranging, in different studies, from 1 to 5%. The gene encoding the beta chain of platelet-derived growth factor receptor (*PDGFRβ*) resides on chromosome 5. This translocation creates a fusion gene and fusion protein containing the 5′ portion of *TEL*, a transcriptional repressor involved in more than 40 translocations, and the 3′ portion of *PDGFRβ*.[37,38] The fusion proteins possess a constitutive PDGFRβ tyrosine kinase activity, leading to aberrant signaling and cellular transformation. Another PDGFRβ fusion protein associated with CMML, the t(5;7) (q33;q11.2), which gives origin to the fusion transcript *HIP-PDGFRβ*, has been detected in CMML patients.[39] Other PDGFRβ fusion proteins involving the fusion partners Rab5, H4, and CEV 14 have been described.[22–24] Other uncharacterized PDGFRβ fusion proteins exist, which may also affect the total frequency of PDGFRβ fusion proteins in CMML.

The bcr-abl tyrosine kinase inhibitor imatinib mesylate (Gleevec, STI571) can bind to the adenosine triphosphate-binding pocket of PDGFβ receptor inhibiting its kinase activity.[40] Imatinib monotherapy had no activity in patients with AML, MDS, or CMML that do not carry the *PDGFR* fusion genes.[41] However, promising activity of imatinib were observed in this subset of CMML patients presenting translocations involving the PDGFβ receptor. Treatment of four CMML patients with chromosomal translocations involving 5q33 with imatinib mesylate (400 mg daily) resulted in a sustained complete cytogenetic response in all four patients.[42] The inhibition of other mechanisms used in signal transduction at present show modest early results in AML and MDS.

EPIGENETIC ALTERATIONS

Epigenetic modulation of gene function is one of the cellular mechanism leading to silencing of gene expression.[43] Several recent reports suggest an association between methylation of many genes, such as the *p15ink4b* gene promoter, and risk for AML transformation in myelodysplastic patients.

DNA methylation is an epigenetic modification of DNA that has a role in the control of gene expression.[44] Aberrant DNA methylation of promoter-associated CpG islands is frequent in leukemias.[45,46] By inactivating genes important for cell function, aberrant DNA methylation is considered a functional equivalent to the genetic disruption of these genes. DNA hypermethylation has therefore been suggested as an attractive therapeutic target in this disorder. It is postulated that reversal of abnormal methylation patterns that characterize a significant subset of patients with leukemia[45,46] may result in the reactivation of aberrantly silenced genes and in suppression of the malignant leukemic clone. The DNA hypomethylating pyrimidine analogues 5-azacytidine and 5-aza-2-deoxycytidine (decitabine) may reduce hypermethylation and induce re-expression of key tumor suppressor genes in MDS. The effect of azacytidine has been recently evaluated in a randomized phase III trial.[47] Azacytidine-treated patients showed a better overall response compared to those treated only with supportive care (60% vs. 5%) and a longer time to progression to AML or death, but no overall survival advantage.[47]

Nucleosome-associated histone tails can undergo several changes in their biochemical composition, including acetylation. The biochemical composition of these tails is associated with specific gene activation.[48] For instance, acetylation of specific residues in histone H3 and H4 is associated with an open chromatin configuration and gene transcription. In contrast, deacetylation of these residues is associated with a repressive status.[48] These changes in histone acetylation are mediated by enzymes with histone acetylase and deacetylase activity,[49] and are therefore reversible. Inhibition of deacetylase activity results in accumulation of histone acetylation and a permissive gene expression state.[50] To exploit this phenomenon clinically, biochemical compounds with histone deacetylase inhibitory activity, of which valproic acid (VPA) is one, are being developed as antineoplastic agents.[50] VPA is a short-chained fatty acid used clinically as an antiepileptic and mood stabilizer.[51] VPA also inhibits histone deacetylase activity.[52] Differentiation therapy with VPA was of clinical benefit in approximately 30% of elderly patients with AML and MDS with unfavorable prognostic features.[53] The platelet transfusion-independence lasting several months may be obtained in some patients, reducing the burden of palliative cure and improving the quality of life.[53,54] DNA methylation of promoter-associated CpG island and modifications in the biochemical composition of nucleosome-associated histone tails cooperate in the control of gene expression.[55] It is not currently known which alteration is dominant, but much evidence demonstrated that the combination of a hypomethylating agent with a histone deacetylase inhibitor results in enhanced gene reactivation.[56] Recently, a phase I/II clinical trial to evaluate the safety, clinical efficacy, and molecular consequences of the combination of decitabine and VPA in patients with leukemia has been completed.[57] Twenty-two percent of the patients had objective response, including 19% of complete remissions (CRs) and 3% of CRs with incomplete platelet recovery (CRp). Among 10 elderly patients with acute myelogenous leukemia or MDS, 50% had a response (4CR, 1CRp).[57]

EVI-1 OVEREXPRESSION

Specific chromosomal abnormalities involving bands 3q21 and 3q26 have been observed in MDS.[58–61] The rearrangements encountered are the paracentric inversion inv(3)(q21;q26) and a reciprocal translocation t(3;3)(q21;q26).[62] A recurrent translocation or inversion between the regions of 3q21 and 3q26 gives rise to the so-called 3q21q26 syndrome, which is found in 0.5–2% of adult patients with MDS. The 3q26.2 chromosome band contains the *EVI1* proto-oncogene, which has been demonstrated to be involved in the pathogenesis of human AMLs and MDS.[58,59,61] Although these rearrangements are infrequent in MDS, they are of remarkable prognostic value. In normal tissues, *EVI-1* is also found in a longer isoform, named *MDS-EVI1*, which encodes a protein with an additional proximal extension of 188 amino acids, which results from the splicing from exon 2 of the MDS1 gene to the second exon of *EVI1*. *MDS1-EVI1* encodes a longer protein containing the entire EVI1 protein but with an additional, unique N-terminal extension. Although related, the two proteins EVI1 and MDS1-EVI1 may have opposite properties.[62] Several studies have shown that inappropriate expression of *EVI1* in immature hematopoietic cells interferes with erythroid and granulocytic development. Several studies showed that high *EVI1* expression occurs with high frequency in patients without 3q26 abnormalities,[58] suggesting other mechanisms of aberrant *EVI1* expression. It has been demonstrated that patients with 3q26 abnormality represent a minor subgroup of patients with high *EVI1* expression. In fact, only about 10% of the patients with high *EVI1* expression have been reported to carry a 3q26 abnormality. Moreover, it has been demonstrated that the expression of *EVI1* and not of *MDS1-EVI1* is associated with highly aggressive AML or MDS.[63] High *EVI1* expression is significantly correlated with the presence of unfavorable cytogenetic abnormalities. Favorable-risk karyotypes were not present among the *EVI1*-expressing groups. These data underline that *EVI1* rather than *MDS1-EVI1* is the transforming gene in MDS. Sporadic reports indicated an increased sensitivity to arsenic trioxide (ATO) in patients with high pretherapy EVI-1 expression.[64]

Recently, ATO has been demonstrated as an encouraging therapeutic agent in MDS. A phase II study to evaluate the efficacy and safety of ATO as monotherapy in patients with MDS has been completed with an acceptable profile of toxicity.[65] Among patients who received one or more doses or completed two or more cycles, the hematological improvement (HI) rates were 34% and 39% in lower-risk patients, and 6% and 9% in higher-risk patients, respectively; the overall major HI rates were 20% and 22%. One higher-risk patient achieved a complete remission (3%). Transfusion-independence or reduction of transfusions by 50% occurred in 33% of patients. The clinical data[65] showed that ATO monotherapy has moderate activity against MDS, with a manageable adverse effect profile. Therefore, further studies of ATO in MDS, particularly in combination with other agents, are warranted.

WT1 AS AN MDS-ASSOCIATED ANTIGEN FOR IMMUNOTHERAPY

There is growing evidence that WT1 is a highly interesting antigen to target in immunotherapy of cancer. *WT1* shows high expression in a wide range of malignant neoplasms, is absent or shows very low expression in normal tissues, and plays a key role in tumor cell proliferation.[66,67] *WT1* is a tumor-suppressor gene coding for a zinc-finger transcription factor located on chromosome 11p13, which was originally identified for its involvement in the pathogenesis of the Wilms' tumor.[68] Overexpression of *WT1* in leukemic blasts of acute and chronic leukemias, including AML, ALL, CML, and MDS, is well documented both on RNA and protein levels.[69–72] Physiologic hematopoietic stem cell compartments also express low levels of *WT1*. However, there is an agreement that a "malignant" *WT1* expression can be clearly distinguished from a physiologic expression based on quantitative detection methods such as semiquantitative reverse transcription polymerase chain reaction (RT-PCR), and real-time quantitative RT-PCR (qRT-PCR). We have clearly demonstrated that *WT1* expression is increased also in MDS.[72] In most MDS, including approximately two-thirds of cases of refractory anemia (RA), *WT1* is expressed above the range observed in normal controls in both bone marrow and peripheral blood samples. A good correlation of the *WT1* expression levels with the clinical subsets (WHO classification) and the IPSS (International Prognostic Scoring System), a frequently used risk-assessment system for MDS, could be shown. The WT1 protein can therefore be identified as a novel, overexpressed tumor antigen. Using qRT-PCR it was even possible to define a cutoff level, which in our experience is represented by 1,000 *WT1* copies/10^4 *ABL* copies to distinguish between the intermediate low-risk and the intermediate high-risk subgroups of MDS.[72] This distinction is of high clinical relevance regarding therapeutic decisions, because it determines whether a particular MDS patient is to receive more aggressive chemotherapy.

Several studies performed *in vitro* and in the animal model[72,73] demonstrated that stimulation *in vitro* of HLA-A2.1-positive or A24.2-positive peripheral blood mononuclear cells with 9-mer WT1 peptides containing major histocompatibility complex (MHC) class 1 binding anchor motifs elicited WT1-specific cytotoxic T lymphocytes (CTLs). These CTLs specifically killed WT1-expressing tumor cells in an HLA class 1–restricted manner and inhibited colony formation by transformed CD34+ progenitor cells isolated from patients with CML. Similarly, immunization *in vivo* of mice with a 9-mer WT1 peptide containing anchor motifs for binding to MHC class I molecules or with WT1 plasmid DNA-elicited WT1-specific CTLs. The immunized mice rejected challenges with *WT1*-expressing tumor cells.[73] These findings indicated that WT1 protein is an attractive, novel tumor antigen for cancer immunotherapy. *In vitro* and *in vivo* evidence of cellular immune responses against the WT1 protein led to the possibility that humoral immune responses against the WT1 protein could be elicited in patients with WT1-expressing hematopoietic malignancies.[74]

In animal models, a vigorous T-cell response can be elicited by vaccination with the WT1 epitope 126–134, which is homologous to the human epitope, resulting in rejection of *WT1*-expressing tumor cells. Phase I/II studies are ongoing in Germany and Japan to analyze the immunogenicity and toxicity of WT1 126–134 peptide vaccination in AML and MDS patients. The results in the first four AML patients treated within an ongoing phase I/II WT1 peptide vaccination studies are encouraging.[75,76] In the German study,[75] four patients have been enrolled in the first trial with one patient who achieved a complete remission, one who persisted in CR although at high risk of relapse, one patient who showed stable disease, and one who progressed. In the second trial carried out in Japan,[76] many clinical responses were observed. In a patient with overt leukemia from MDS, only a single dose of WT1 vaccination induced an increase in WT1-specific CTLs and a resultant rapid reduction in WT1 level and leukemic blast cells. A similar phenomenon was observed in a patient with MDS with myelofibrosis. Taken together, the findings from early clinical trials are very promising and show the efficacy of peptide-based vaccines to induce WT1-specific T cells associated with clinical efficacy.

REFERENCES

1. MUFTI, G.J. & D.A. GALDON. 1986. Myelodysplastic syndromes: natural history and features of prognostic importance. Clin. Haematol. **15:** 953–971.
2. HEANEY, M.L. & D.W. GOLDE. 1999. Myelodysplasia. N. Engl. J. Med. **340:** 1649–1660.
3. MECUCCI, C. *et al.* 1992. Cytogenetics. Hematol. Oncol. Clin. North Am. **6:** 523–541.

4. PIERRE, R.V. *et al.* 1989. Clinical-cytogenetic correlation in myelodysplasia (preleukemia). Cancer Genet. Cytogenet. **40:** 149–161.
5. MUFTI, G. 1992. Chromosomal deletions in the myelodysplastic syndromes. Leuk. Res. **40:** 35–41.
6. BIANCHI, E. 2003. Dissecting oncogenes and tyrosines kinases in AML cells. Med-GenMed. **21:** 10.
7. LE BEAU, M.M. *et al.* 2001. Cytogenetics of myelodysplastic syndromes. Best. Pract. Res. Clin. Haematol. **14:** 479–495.
8. THIRD MIC COOPERATIVE STUDY GROUP. 1987. Morphologic Immunologic and Cytogenetic (MIC) working classification of the primary myelodysplastic syndromes and therapy related myelodysplasias and leukemias. Cancer **32:** 1–10.
9. NEUBAUER, A. 1994. Mutations in the Ras proto-oncogenes in patients with myelodysplastic syndromes. Leukemia **8:** 638–641.
10. HORIIKE, S. *et al.* 1997. Tandem duplications of the FLT3 receptor gene are associated with leukemic transformation of myelodysplasia. Leukemia **11:** 1442–1446.
11. PADUA, R.A. *et al.* 1998. RAS, FMS and p53 mutations and poor clinical outcome in myelodysplasias: a 10 year follow-up. Leukemia **12:** 887–892.
12. PAQUETTE, R.L. *et al.* 1993. N-ras mutations are associated with poor prognosis and increased risk of leukaemia in myelodysplastic syndromes. Blood **82:** 590–599.
13. GALLAGHER, A. *et al.* 1997. Ras and the myelodysplastic syndromes. Pathol. Biol. **45:** 561–568.
14. BARBACID, M. 1987. Ras genes. Annu. Rev. Biochem. **56:** 779.
15. BOS, J.L. 1989. Ras oncogenes in human cancer. A review. Cancer Res. **49:** 4682.
16. NEUBAUER, A. *et al.* 1994. Prognostic importance of mutations in the ras proto-oncogenes in *de novo* acute myeloid leukaemia. Blood **83:** 1603–1611.
17. CLIPPERFIELD, R.G. *et al.* 1985. Activation of H-ras p21 by substitution, deletion, and insertion mutations. Mol. Cell. Biol. **5:** 1809–1813.
18. BRUNNER, T.B. *et al.* 2003. Farnesyltransferase inhibitors: an overview of the results of preclinical and clinical investigations. Cancer Res. **63:** 5656–5566.
19. ROWINSKY, E.K. *et al.* 1999. Ras protein farnesyltransferase: a strategic target for anticancer therapeutic development. J. Clin. Oncol. **17:** 3631–3652.
20. JIANG, K. *et al.* 2000. The phosphoinositide 3-OH kinase/AKT2 pathway as a critical target for farnesyltransferase inhibitor-induced apoptosis. Mol. Cell. Biol. **20:** 139–148.
21. KARP, J.E. *et al.* 2001. Clinical and biologic activity of the farnesyltransferase inhibitor R115777 in adults with refractory and relapsed acute leukemias: a phase 1 clinical-laboratory correlative trial. Blood **97:** 3361–3369.
22. ASHAR, H.R. *et al.* 2000. Farnesyl transferase inhibitors block the farnesylation of CENP-E and CENP-F and alter the association of CENP-E with the microtubules. J. Biol. Chem. **275:** 30451–30457.
23. END, D.W. *et al.* 2001. Characterization of the antitumor effects of the selective farnesyl protein transferase inhibitor R115777 *in vivo* and *in vitro*. Cancer Res. **61:** 131–137.
24. PETERS, D.G. *et al.* 2001. Activity of the farnesyl protein transferase inhibitor SCH66336 against BCR/ABL-induced murine leukemia and primary cells from patients with chronic myeloid leukemia. Blood **97:** 1404–1412.
25. NIELSEN, L.L. *et al.* 2000. Combination therapy with SCH58500 (p53 adenovirus) and cyclophosphamide in preclinical cancer models. Oncol. Rep. **7:** 1191–1196.

26. CORTES, J. *et al.* 2002. Continuous oral lonafarnib (Sarasar) for the treatment of patients with advanced hematological malignancies: a phase II study. Blood **100:** 793a.

27. FELDMAN, E.J. *et al.* 2003. Continuous oral lonafarnib (Sarasar) for the treatment of patients with myelodysplastic syndrome. Blood **102:** 421a.

28. SMOLICH, B.D. *et al.* 2001. The antiangiogenic protein kinase inhibitors SU5416 and SU6668 inhibit the SCF receptor (c-kit) in a human myeloid leukemia cell line and in acute myeloid leukemia blasts. Blood **97:** 1413–1421.

29. SPIEKERMENN, K. *et al.* 2003. The protein tyrosine kinase inhibitor SU5614 inhibits FLT3 and induces growth arrest and apoptosis in AML-derived cell lines expressing a constitutively activated FLT3. Blood **101:** 1494–1504.

30. LIN, B. *et al.* 2002. The vascular endothelial growth factor receptor tyrosine kinase inhibitor PTK787/ZK222584 inhibits growth and migration of multiple myeloma cells in the bone marrow microenvironment. Cancer Res. **62:** 5019–5026.

31. GLADE-BENDER, J. *et al.* 2003. VEGF blocking therapy in the treatment of cancer. Exp. Opin. Biol. Ther. **3:** 263–276.

32. GILES, F.J. *et al.* 2003. SU5416, a small molecule tyrosine kinase receptor inhibitor, has biologic activity in patients with refractory acute myeloid leukemia or myelodysplastic syndromes. Blood **102:** 795–801.

33. O'FARRELL, A.M. *et al.* 2003. An innovative phase I clinical study demonstrates inhibition of FLT3 phosphorylation by SU11248 in acute myeloid leukemia patients. Clin. Cancer Res. **9:** 5465–5476.

34. KARP, J.E. *et al.* 2004. Targeting vascular endothelial growth factor for relapsed and refractory adult acute myelogenous leukemias: therapy with sequential 1-beta-D-arabinofuranosylcytosine, mitoxantrone, and bevacizumab. Clin. Cancer Res. **10:** 3577–3585.

35. SMALL, D. *et al.* 1994. STK-1, the human homolog of Flk-2/Flt-3, is selectively expressed in CD34+ human bone marrow cells and is involved in the proliferation of early progenitor/stem cells. Proc. Natl. Acad. Sci. USA **91:** 459–463.

36. SMITH, B.D. *et al.* 2004. Single-agent CEP-701, a novel FLT3 inhibitor, shows biologic and clinical activity in patients with relapsed or refractory acute myeloid leukaemia. Blood **103:** 3669–3676.

37. GOLUB, T.R. *et al.* 1994. Fusion of PDGF receptor beta to a novel ets-like gene, tel, in chronic myelomonocytic leukaemia with t(5;12) chromosomal translocation. Cell **77:** 307–316.

38. SJOBLOM, T. *et al.* 1999. Characterization of the chronic myelomonocytic leukaemia associated TEL-PDGF beta R fusion protein. Oncogene **18:** 7055–7062.

39. ROSS, T.S. *et al.* 1998. Fusion of huntingtin interacting protein 1 to platelet-derived growth factor beta receptor (PDGFbetaR) in chronic myelomonocytic leukaemia with t(5;7) (q33;q11.2). Blood **91:** 4419–4426.

40. TOMASSON, M.H. *et al.* 1999. TEL/PDGF beta R induces hematologic malignancies in mice that respond to a specific tyrosine kinase inhibitor. Blood **93:** 1707–1714.

41. CORTES, J. *et al.* 2003. Results of imatinib mesylate therapy in patients with refractory or recurrent acute myeloid leukemia, high-risk myelodysplastic syndrome, and myeloproliferative disorder. Cancer **97:** 2760–2766.

42. APPERLEY, J.F. *et al.* 2002. Response to imatinib mesylate in patients with chronic myeloproliferative diseases with rearrangements of the platelet-derived growth factor receptor beta. N. Engl. J. Med. **347:** 481–487.

43. ISSA, J.P. 2004. CpG island methylator phenotype in cancer. Nat. Rev. Cancer **4:** 988–993.

44. ROBERTSON, K.D. & A.P. WOLFFE. 2000. DNA methylation in health and disease. Nat. Rev. Genet. **1:** 11–19.
45. TOYOTA, M. *et al*. 2001. Methylation profiling in acute myeloid leukemia. Blood **97:** 2823–2829.
46. GARCIA-MANERO, G. *et al*. 2002. DNA methylation of multiple promoter-associated CpG islands in adult acute lymphocytic leukemia. Clin. Cancer Res. **8:** 2217–2224.
47. SILVERMAN, L.R. *et al*. 2002. Randomized controlled trial of azacitidine in patients with the myelodysplastic syndrome: a study of the cancer and leukemia group B. J. Clin. Oncol. **20:** 2429–2440.
48. RICE, J.C. 2001. Code of silence. Nature **414:** 258–261.
49. MARKS, P.A. *et al*. 2003. Histone deacetylases. Curr. Opin. Pharmacol. **3:** 344–351.
50. RICHON, V.M. & J.P. O'BRIEN. 2002. Histone deacetylase inhibitors: a new class of potential therapeutic agents for cancer treatment. Clin. Cancer Res. **8:** 662–664.
51. JOHANNESSEN, C.U. *et al*. 2003. Valproate: past, present, and future. CNS Drug Rev. **9:** 199–216.
52. GOTTLICHER, M. *et al*. 2001. Valproic acid defines a novel class of HDAC inhibitors inducing differentiation of transformed cells. EMBO J. **20:** 6969–6978.
53. PILATRINO, C. *et al*. 2005. Increase in platelet count in older, poor risk patients with acute myeloid leukemia or myelodysplastic syndrome treated with valproic acid and all-trans retinoic acid. Cancer **104:** 101–109.
54. KUENDGEN, A. *et al*. 2004. Treatment of myelodysplastic syndromes with valproic acid alone or in combination with all-trans retinoic acid. Blood **104:** 1266–1269.
55. JONES, P.L. & A.P. WOLFFE. 1999. Relationships between chromatin organization and DNA methylation in determining gene expression. Semin. Cancer Biol. **9:** 339–347.
56. YANG, H. *et al*. 2005. Antileukemia activity of the combination of 5-aza-2′-deoxycytidine with valproic acid. Leuk. Res. **29:** 739–748.
57. GARCIA-MANERO, G. *et al*. 2006. Phase I/II study of the combination of 5-aza-2′-deoxycytidine with valproic acid in patients with leukaemia. Blood; DOI 10.1182.
58. RUSSELL, M. *et al*. 1994. Expression of EVI-1 in myelodysplastic syndromes and other haematological malignancies without 3q26 translocations. Blood **84:** 1243–1248.
59. DREYFUS, F. *et al*. 1995. Expression of EVI-1 gene in myelodysplastic syndromes. Leukemia **9:** 203–205.
60. JOLKOWSKA, J. *et al*. 2000. The EVI-1 gene-its role in pathogenesis of human leukemias. Leuk. Res. **24:** 553–558.
61. NUCIFORA, G. *et al*. 1997. The EVI-1 gene in myeloid leukaemia. Leukemia **11:** 2022–2031.
62. MORISHITA, K. *et al*. 1992. Activation of EVI-1 gene expression in human acute myelogenous leukemias by translocations spanning 300–400 kilobases on chromosome band 3q26. Proc. Natl. Acad. Sci. USA **89:** 3937–3941.
63. PINTADO, T. *et al*. 1985. Clinical correlation of he 3q21;q26 cytogenetic anomaly. A leukemic or myelodysplastic syndrome with preserved or increased platelet production and lack of response to cytotoxic drug therapy. Cancer **55:** 535–541.
64. RAZA, A. *et al*. 2004. Arsenic trioxide and thalidomide combination produces multi-lineage hematological responses in myelodysplastic syndromes patients, particularly in those with high pre-therapy EVI1 expression. Leuk. Res. **28:** 791–803.

65. SCHILLER, G.J. *et al.* 2006. Phase II multicenter study of arsenic trioxide in patients with myelodysplastic syndromes. J. Clin. Oncol. **24:** 2456–2464.

66. BAIRD, P.N. & P.J. SIMMONS. 1997. Expression of the Wilms' tumor gene (WT1) in normal hematopoiesis. Exp. Hematol. **25:** 312–320.

67. MENSSEN, H.D., H.J. RENKL, *et al.* 1995. Presence of Wilms' tumor gene (WT1) transcripts and the WT1 nuclear protein in the majority of human acute leukemias. Leukemia **9:** 1060–1067.

68. CALL, K.M. *et al.* 1990. Isolation and characterization of a zinc finger polypeptide gene at the human chromosome 11 Wilms' tumor locus. Cell **60:** 509–520.

69. MIWA, H. *et al.* 1992. Expression of the Wilms' tumor gene (WT1) in human leukemias. Leukemia **6:** 405–409.

70. INOUE, K. *et al.* 1997. Aberrant overexpression of the Wilms tumor gene (WT1) in human leukemia. Blood **89:** 1405–1412.

71. CILLONI, D. *et al.* 2002. Quantitative assessment of WT1 expression by real time Q-PCR may be a useful tool for monitoring minimal residual disease in acute leukemia patients. Leukemia **16:** 2115–2121.

72. CILLONI, D. *et al.* 2003. Very significant correlation between WT1 expression level and the IPSS score in patients with myelodysplastic syndromes. J. Clin. Oncol. **21:** 1988–1995.

73. GAIGER, A. *et al.* 2000. Immunity to WT1 in the animal model and in patients with acute myeloid leukemia. Blood **96:** 1480–1489.

74. OKA, Y. *et al.* 2000. Cancer immunotherapy targeting Wilms tumor gene WT1 product. J. Immunol. **164:** 1873–1880.

75. MAILAENDER, V. *et al.* 2004. Complete remission in a patient with recurrent acute myeloid leukemia induced by vaccination with WT1 peptide in the absence of hematological or renal toxicity. Leukemia **18:** 165–166.

76. OKA, Y. *et al.* 2003. Wilms tumor gene peptide-based immunotherapy for patients with overt leukemia from myelodysplastic syndrome or MDS with myelofibrosis. Int. J. Hematol. **78:** 56–61.

Rapid Estrogen Actions in the Cardiovascular System

TOMMASO SIMONCINI, PAOLO MANNELLA,
AND ANDREA RICCARDO GENAZZANI

*Molecular and Cellular Gynecological Endocrinology Laboratory (MCGEL),
Department of Reproductive Medicine and Child Development, Division of
Gynecology and Obstetrics, University of Pisa, 56100 Pisa, Italy*

ABSTRACT: In the last two decades, several studies have unveiled a series of original signaling mechanisms through which so-called "nuclear"
receptors can mediate rapid actions of steroid hormones. These rapid
signaling actions are independent of the synthesis of mRNA or protein,
and are therefore known as "nontranscriptional" or "nongenomic" as
opposed to the classical genomic mechanisms. Nongenomic signaling of
estrogens plays a prominent role in nonreproductive tissues, and between
these is the vascular wall. At this level, estrogen triggers rapid vasodilatation, exerts anti-inflammatory effects, stimulates endothelial growth and
migration, and protects the vessels from atherosclerotic degeneration.
Nongenomic signaling mechanisms have been involved in many of these
actions and are increasingly considered to be of importance for vascular
function in physiological and pathophysiological conditions. Rapid actions of steroid hormones have been implicated with vascular as well as
with myocardial protection in animal experimental models. Moreover,
the nongenomic signaling of estrogens is tightly interconnected with the
nuclear pathways, and there are several indications that, through nongenomic modulation of signaling cascades, estrogens are also able to modulate the expression of several relevant genes in endothelial cells. In conclusion, while we are still in an early phase of the investigations of the
nontranscriptional actions of steroid hormone receptors, it is clear that
this newly recognized category of signaling mechanisms is responsible
for critical steroid actions in nonreproductive tissues.

KEYWORDS: estrogen; estrogen receptors; nongenomic signaling; endothelial cells

Address for correspondence: Tommaso Simoncini, Molecular and Cellular Gynecological Endocrinology Laboratory (MCGEL), Department of Reproductive Medicine and Child Development,
Division of Gynecology and Obstetrics, University of Pisa, 56100 Pisa, Italy. Voice: +39-050-992690;
fax: +39-050-553410.
 e-mail: t.simoncini@obgyn.med.unipi.it

Ann. N.Y. Acad. Sci. 1089: 424–430 (2006). © 2006 New York Academy of Sciences.
doi: 10.1196/annals.1386.001

ESTROGEN RECEPTOR (ER) SIGNALING IN HUMAN CELLS

Estrogen receptors (ERs) are multifunctional regulators of a vast array of cellular functions. Basically all human cells contain and respond to ER activation with relevant functional modifications. Once bound by their steroidal ligand, ERs modulate the expression of target genes in the nucleus.[1] Indeed, the binding of estradiol with the ER ligand-binding domain (LBD) induces a conformational modification of the receptor, which allows homo/heterodimerization of the ligand-bound receptors, nuclear translocation, and their binding to estrogen response elements (EREs, i.e., nucleotide sequences specifically recognized by ERs) on the promoter regions of the target genes[1] (FIG. 1).

In addition to this, in the past few years, consistent evidence has been generated that shows that ERs also trigger actions that are determined outside of the nuclear compartment. These mechanisms lead to quicker modifications of cell function without requiring RNA or protein synthesis. To highlight this feature, this category of actions of ERs has been indicated as "nongenomic" or "nonnuclear,"[2] although a warm debate is still ongoing on what should be the proper labeling of these actions.

After many years of tight research, an agreement has been reached on the fact that the ERs that elicit rapid signaling events in different cells are structurally

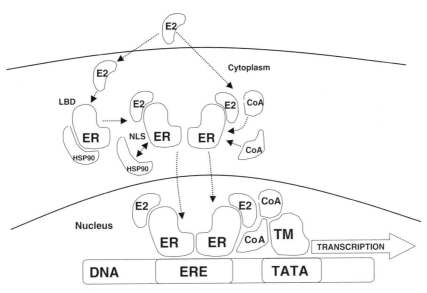

FIGURE 1. Nuclear modulation of gene expression by ERs. ERs act as transcription factors; once bound by estradiol, ERs detach from chaperone proteins and homo/heterodimerize. In these forms, ERs translocate to the nucleus and recognize specific DNA sequences in the promoter region of target genes, called EREs . The binding of ERs to these sequences allows for gene expression activation or repression by the ER-bound coactivator or corepressor proteins.

identical to those that exert nuclear actions. Indeed, it is now established that
ERs localize in most of the subcellular compartments, including the cytoplasm
and the cell membrane.[3] The study of some cell membrane-initiated effects of
estrogens has indeed provided a pioneering evidence that nonclassical effects of
estrogens may exist. Between these seminal studies are the identification of the
regulation of cell membrane ion channels,[4] of G-protein-coupled receptors,[5] of
tyrosine kinases and mitogen-activated protein kinases (MAPK),[6] the activation of adenylate cyclase production,[7] and of phospholipase C activation[8] and
more recently the activation of phosphatidylinositol 3-OH kinase[9,10] (FIG. 2).

Recent research has actually expanded a lot of our understanding of the biological meaning of these actions, showing that the rapid effects of ERs are not
independent from the traditional signaling events leading to regulation of gene
expression. Rather, there is a tight interconnection between the nongenomic
signaling pathways recruited by estrogens and changes in gene expression. For
example, the activation of PI3K by ER-α is required to achieve the activation
of the expression of a wide set of estrogen target genes in endothelial cells[11]
(FIG. 3).

Nongenomic signaling of estrogens seems to be particularly important in
so-called estrogen "nontarget" tissues. These sites are those that, because

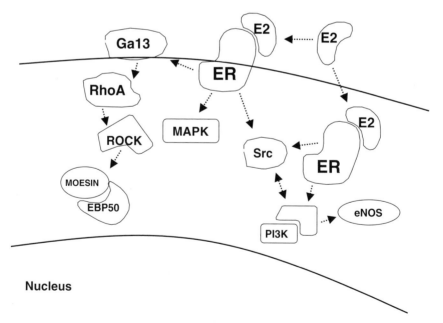

FIGURE 2. Extranuclear signaling actions of ERs. ERs can also act at the cell membrane or in the cytoplasm by interacting and activating different signaling intermediates.
Between these, well-recognized targets of ERs outside the nucleus are MAPK, and PI3K as
well as G proteins such as G-α13.

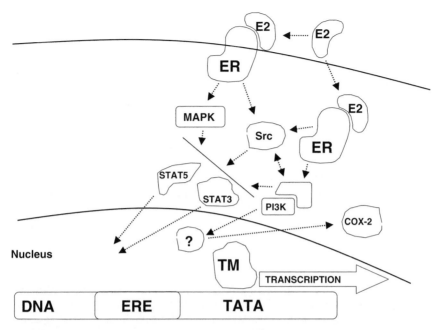

FIGURE 3. Integration of extranuclear and nuclear actions of ERs. Via the activation of extranuclear signaling mechanisms, ERs impact gene expression via signaling cascades that result into the modification of the activity of transcription factors.

of the relatively lower concentration of steroid hormones receptors, have been in the past neglected as possible steroid-regulated sites. Between these sites are the cardiovascular system and the central nervous system. Instead, while growing evidence indicates that there is roughly no cell where steroid hormones unable to exert regulatory actions, nongenomic mechanisms are found to play a prominent role in the modulation of these tissues by steroids.

ESTROGENS AND THE CARDIOVASCULAR SYSTEM

Among the nonreproductive targets of sex steroids, the cardiovascular system provides a paramount example of a system where the rapid actions of estrogens play a critical role in the determination of the functional effects of these hormones.[2]

In fact, estrogens mediate several relevant effects on vascular cells, inducing rapid vasodilatation,[2,9,10,12–17] exerting anti-inflammatory activity,[18–21] as well as stimulating endothelial growth and migration.[22] The final outcome of these actions is possibly a protective action on the vessels from atherosclerotic degeneration.[23,24]

Between many different mechanisms, estrogens regulate vasodilatation, inducing nitric oxide (NO) synthesis and release in endothelial cells.[2] NO is a central controller of vascular function, a potent vasodilator as well as an anti-inflammatory molecule.

The principal player in this set of actions enrolled by ER is the NO synthase, endothelial nitric oxide synthase (eNOS). This enzyme is finely controlled through a variety of mechanisms by estrogens, including gene expression regulation and rapid modifications of enzyme activity.[25] These latter actions are independent of gene expression and depend in part on the activation of MAPK or tyrosine kinase–dependent pathways.[25] However, the major part of the rapid activation of eNOS in human endothelial cells is mediated by a signaling cascade that involves the interaction of ER-α with the regulatory subunit of the phosphatidylinositol 3-OH kinase.[9,10] This interaction leads to PI3K activation, followed by the recruitment of the Ser-/Thr- kinase, Akt. This kinase phosphorylates eNOS, therefore triggering its activation.

While a short estrogen treatment induces a rapid activation of eNOS with an increased synthesis and release of NO that occurs within minutes, a longer exposure to estrogen promotes eNOS gene expression, leading to a further increase of NO synthesis.[25] To this extent, recent evidence indicates that the activation of PI3K is required in order to achieve the induction of the expression of a large set of endothelial genes, including eNOS,[26] suggesting a strong interrelation between extranuclear and nuclear signaling cascades.

The activation of the ER-α/PI3K signaling pathway by estrogen has important pathophysiological implications *in vivo*, as estrogen induces a dramatic reduction in leukocyte adhesion to endothelial cells in vessels after ischemia/reperfusion, which is completely reversed by treatment with PI3K and eNOS inhibitors.[9] In addition, corticosteroids have been shown to reduce the ischemic area in mouse hearts exposed to an experimental coronary artery occlusion model through the activation of PI3K and eNOS.[27]

In addition to these previously described rapid actions of sex steroids, we have recently described a novel and intriguing action of estrogen in endothelial cells. Through the activation of a cell-membrane-initiated signaling pathway involving a G-protein, ER-α dynamically regulates the assembly of the actin cytoskeleton and therefore cell interaction with the extracellular matrix and migration.[22] This signaling cascade is recruited by the interaction of the C-terminal portion of cell membrane ER-α with the G-protein G-α13, which leads to the activation of the small GTPase RhoA and thus of the Rho-associated kinase, ROCK-2.[22] This chain of events leads to the rapid activation of the actin-regulatory protein moesin. This cascade of events ensues within minutes of estradiol administration, resulting in changes of cell morphology and in the development of specialized cell membrane structures such as ruffles and pseudopodia that are necessary for cell movement.[22] More recent data from our laboratory indicates that this mechanism is common also to other cell types, including cancer cells, such as breast cancer cells. In these cells, the activation of this signaling pathway is related to the ability of cancer cells to move in the surrounding environment and to invade three-dimensional matrices (T. Simoncini, unpublished data).

CONCLUSIONS

Although the work of the past recent years has highlighted with growing detail the molecular basis of some of the rapid actions of ERs, there is still a large number of extranuclear effects of sex steroid hormones that have yet to be characterized. For instance, it is still not completely established whether there are physiological or pathophysiological conditions where nongenomic signaling by steroid hormone receptors may be particularly important *in vivo*.

ER nontranscriptional signaling mechanisms are particularly important at the vascular level, through which estrogens induce fundamental actions resulting in the control of the vascular tone, the remodeling of the vessel wall, and in antiatherogenic effects. Understanding the molecular mechanisms through which these actions are exerted represents an important key to engineering newer pharmacological tools for the prevention of cardiovascular disease in postmenopausal women.

REFERENCES

1. TRUSS, M. & M. BEATO. 1993. Steroid hormone receptors: interaction with deoxyribonucleic acid and transcription factors. Endocr. Rev. **14:** 459–479.
2. SIMONCINI, T. & A. R. GENAZZANI. 2003. Non-genomic actions of sex steroid hormones. Eur. J. Endocrinol. **148:** 281–292.
3. PEDRAM, A., M. RAZANDI & E. R. LEVIN. 2006. Nature of functional estrogen receptors at the plasma membrane. Mol. Endocrinol. **20:** 1996–2009.
4. NAKAJIMA, T. *et al.* 1995. 17beta-estradiol inhibits the voltage-dependent L-type Ca2+ currents in aortic smooth muscle cells. Eur. J. Pharmacol. **294:** 625–635.
5. KELLY, M. J. *et al.* 1999. Rapid effects of estrogen to modulate G protein-coupled receptors via activation of protein kinase A and protein kinase C pathways. Steroids **64:** 64–75.
6. MIGLIACCIO, A. *et al.* 1996. Tyrosine kinase/p21ras/MAP-kinase pathway activation by estradiol-receptor complex in MCF-7 cells. EMBO J. **15:** 1292–1300.
7. ARONICA, S.M., W.L. KRAUS & B. S. KATZENELLENBOGEN.1994. Estrogen action via the cAMP signaling pathway: stimulation of adenylate cyclase and cAMP-regulated gene transcription. Proc. Natl. Acad. Sci. USA **91:** 8517–8521.
8. LE MELLAY, V., B. GROSSE & M. LIEBERHERR. 1997. Phospholipase C beta and membrane action of calcitriol and estradiol. J. Biol. Chem. **272:** 11902–11907.
9. SIMONCINI, T. *et al.* 2000. Interaction of oestrogen receptor with the regulatory subunit of phosphatidylinositol-3-OH kinase. Nature **407:** 538–541.

10. SIMONCINI, T., E. RABKIN & J. K. LIAO. 2003. Molecular basis of cell membrane estrogen receptor interaction with phosphatidylinositol 3-kinase in endothelial cells. Arterioscler. Thromb. Vasc. Biol. **23:** 198–203.
11. LEVIN, E.R. 2005. Integration of the extranuclear and nuclear actions of estrogen. Mol. Endocrinol. **19:** 1951–1959.
12. SIMONCINI, T. & A. R. GENAZZANI. 2000. Raloxifene acutely stimulates nitric oxide release from human endothelial cells via an activation of endothelial nitric oxide synthase. J Clin. Endocrinol. Metab. **85:** 2966–2969.
13. SIMONCINI, T. *et al.* 2002. Genomic and nongenomic mechanisms of nitric oxide synthesis induction in human endothelial cells by a fourth-generation selective estrogen receptor modulator. Endocrinology **143:** 2052–2061.
14. SIMONCINI, T., A.R. GENAZZANI & J. K. LIAO. 2002. Nongenomic mechanisms of endothelial nitric oxide synthase activation by the selective estrogen receptor modulator raloxifene. Circulation **105:** 1368–1373.
15. SIMONCINI, T. *et al.* 2004. Tibolone activates nitric oxide synthesis in human endothelial cells. J. Clin. Endocrinol. Metab. **89:** 4594–4600.
16. SIMONCINI, T. *et al.* 2005. Differential estrogen signaling in endothelial cells upon pulsed or continuous administration. Maturitas **50:** 247–258.
17. SIMONCINI, T. *et al.* 2005. Activation of nitric oxide synthesis in human endothelial cells by red clover extracts. Menopause **12:** 69–77.
18. SIMONCINI, T., R. De Caterina & A. R. GENAZZANI. 1999. Selective estrogen receptor modulators: different actions on vascular cell adhesion molecule-1 (VCAM-1) expression in human endothelial cells. J. Clin. Endocrinol. Metab. **84:** 815–818.
19. SIMONCINI, T. *et al.* 2000. Estrogens and glucocorticoids inhibit endothelial vascular cell adhesion molecule-1 expression by different transcriptional mechanisms. Circ. Res. **87:** 19–25.
20. SIMONCINI, T. & A. R. GENAZZANI. 2000. Direct vascular effects of estrogens and selective estrogen receptor modulators. Curr. Opin. Obstet. Gynecol. **12:** 181–187.
21. SIMONCINI, T. & A. R. GENAZZANI. 2000. Tibolone inhibits leukocyte adhesion molecule expression in human endothelial cells. Mol. Cell. Endocrinol. **162:** 87–94.
22. SIMONCINI, T. *et al.* 2006. Estrogen receptor {alpha} interacts with G{alpha}13 to drive actin remodeling and endothelial cell migration via the RhoA/Rho Kinase/Moesin pathway. Mol. Endocrinol. **20:** 1756–1771.
23. MENDELSOHN, M.E. & R. H. KARAS. 1999. The protective effects of estrogen on the cardiovascular system. N. Engl. J. Med. **340:** 1801–1811.
24. MENDELSOHN, M.E. & R. H. KARAS. 2005. Molecular and cellular basis of cardiovascular gender differences. Science **308:** 1583–1587.
25. CHAMBLISS, K.L. & P. W. SHAUL. 2002. Estrogen modulation of endothelial nitric oxide synthase. Endocr. Rev. **23:** 665–686.
26. PEDRAM, A. *et al.* 2002. Integration of the non-genomic and genomic actions of estrogen. Membrane-initiated signaling by steroid to transcription and cell biology. J. Biol. Chem. **277:** 50768–50775.
27. Hafezi-Moghadam, A. *et al.* 2002. Acute cardiovascular protective effects of corticosteroids are mediated by non-transcriptional activation of endothelial nitric oxide synthase. Nat. Med. **8:** 473–479.

Estrogens in Human Vascular Diseases

MARIAM KLOUCHE

Bremen Centre for Laboratory Medicine, 28205 Bremen, Germany

ABSTRACT: Estrogens are correlated with a lower incidence of atherosclerotic vascular disease, but also provide a protective effect on neovascular disorders, such as Kaposi's sarcoma (KS). Estrogens mediate indirect antiatherosclerotic vascular effects by reducing low-density lipoprotein (LDL) levels and by influencing fibrinolysis, and they exert direct actions on vascular cells including vascular relaxation and vasodilatation, thus reducing progression of the lesion. It is increasingly appreciated that the estrogenic effects are mediated not only by the classic genomic action via the specific nuclear hormone receptors ERα and ERβ, but also by distinct rapid, nongenomic actions. Vascular cells have the capacity to express different types of estrogen receptors, and we provide evidence for selective expression of estrogen receptor subtypes on different human vascular cell types. Moreover, we give an overview on the vascular effects of estrogens, selective estrogen receptor modulators (SERMs), and androgens on normal and malignant vascular cells, with particular focus on the protective estrogenic potential on the vasculature.

KEYWORDS: estrogen; androgen; ERβ; vascular; smooth muscle; IL-6; VEGF

INTRODUCTION

Cardiovascular diseases continue to constitute the leading cause of death in both men and women. However, the prevalence of cardiovascular morbidity and mortality is significantly lower in premenopausal woman compared to men, but steadily increases after menopause.[1–3] This apparent disparity has been attributed to the protective effects of estrogens, while the potential promoting role of androgens has received comparably little attention.[4,5] Although premenopausal women enjoy relative cardiovascular protection, estrogen replacement therapy has not shown cardiovascular benefits in postmenopausal women,[6,7] suggesting that the effects of estrogens on the cardiovascular system are much more complex than previously thought. The discovery of a second estrogen receptor subtype, the ERβ, and the recognition of the selective distribution of the ERs, in addition to the disclosure of at least two novel types

Address for correspondence: Prof. Dr. Mariam Klouche, Bremer Zentrum für Laboratoriumsmedizin, Friedrich-Karl-Str. 22, 28205 Bremen, Germany. Voice: +49-421- 4307-233; fax: +49-421-4307-534.
e-mail: mariam.klouche@laborzentrum-bremen.de

Ann. N.Y. Acad. Sci. 1089: 431–443 (2006). © 2006 New York Academy of Sciences.
doi: 10.1196/annals.1386.032

of nongenomic estrogen action, have recently broadened the understanding of the spectrum of estrogen action mechanisms.

The apparent protection for females and the predilection for males is not a unique feature of cardiovascular diseases, but is even more prominent in neovascular disorders, particularly Kaposi's sarcoma (KS).[8] This multifocal vascular neoplasm occurs almost exclusively in males.

PROTECTIVE EFFECTS OF ESTROGENS ON CARDIOVASCULAR DISEASES

The incidence of cardiovascular disease is lower in premenopausal woman compared to men, and the steady increase after the onset of menopause is assumed to result from declining endogenous estrogen levels and loss of the cardioprotective effects.[1-3] While the cardiovascular protective effect of estrogen before menopause is undebated, the effect of postmenopausal estrogen therapy on the risk of cardiovascular disease remains controversial. After hormone replacement in postmenopausal woman, only a selective reduction of the vascular atherosclerotic risk was shown for coronary heart disease, but not for stroke.[9] Moreover, in woman with preexisting cardiovascular diseases after the onset of menopause, two recent trials—the Heart and Estrogen/Progestin Replacement Study (HERS)[6] and the Estrogen Replacement and Atherosclerosis trial (ERA)[7]—which used angiographically verified endpoints, have failed to confirm the capacity of hormone replacement therapy to mediate cardioprotective effects. Thus, estrogens appear to induce beneficial preventive effects primarily at a very early stage of atherosclerotic vascular disease, which does not apply to the secondary prevention in woman with advanced atherosclerotic vascular disease.

GENDER EFFECTS ON NEOVASCULAR DISEASES

The apparent protective effect of estrogen is not limited to developing atherosclerotic vascular diseases, but is also obvious in other proliferative neovascular disorders with inflammatory components, such as Kaposi's sarcoma KS occurs primarily in males, with a rate from 1:5 to 1:20 compared to that in woman.[8] The multifocal neovascular neoplasm contains inflammatory elements and constitutes one of the most common neoplasms complicating AIDS.[10] The predominant cell type are spindle cells, which share features of endothelial cells and of smooth muscle cells,[11,12] suggesting that KS cells constitute primitive mesenchymal cells that can form vascular channels. KS is a human herpes virus type 8 (HHV8)-associated disease. Notably, the prevalence of the causal herpes virus is equivalent in men and woman.[13] Thus, the protection of woman from this neovascular disorder is even more prominent compared to atherosclerotic vascular disease. Clinically, the vascular neoplasm is responsive to treatment with biological response modifiers, which act on expression of viral genes.[14] While we are able to show an ameliorating effect of estrogens of KS cell proliferation and proinflammatory signaling, androgens were not only metabolized but also induced mitogenic effects on KS cells (Klouche and Carruba, submitted for publication).

ESTROGEN-REGULATED GENES IN VASCULAR CELLS

Principally, all cellular components of the vascular wall may respond to estrogens, including the different vascular endothelial cell types, vascular smooth muscle cells, cardiac myocytes and fibroblasts, which together play important roles in cardiovascular health and disease (TABLE 1). Estrogen participates in the regulation of several genes which are crucially involved in the pathogenesis of inflammatory and proliferative vascular diseases, including atherosclerosis.[15] Directly influenced genes include molecules active in cell–cell communication, such as adhesion molecules, hormone receptors, and particularly genes

TABLE 1. Estrogen-regulated genes in vascular cells

Regulated vascular function	Genes involved	Vascular cell type involved
Cell adhesion	↑ E-selectin/ CD62 E	EC
	↑ VCAM/ CD106	EC, VSMC
	↓ of cytokine-induced ICAM-1, VCAM-1 and E-selectin expression	EC
	↓ of nicotine-induced VCAM-1 and E-selectin expression	EC
Inflammation	↑ Cylooxygnenase-1 (COX-1)	EC
	↑ Prostacyclin synthase (PGI2)	EC, VSMC
	↓ MCP-1 expression	EC, VSMC
Vascular remodeling	↑ Matrix metalloproteinase	EC, VSMC
	↑ Endothelin-1	EC
	↑ Collagen	VSMC
	↑ Elastin	VSMC
	↑ c-fos	EC, VSMC
Angiogenesis and vascular cell proliferation	Direct growth inhibition	VSMC
	Inhibition of angiotensin II-induced proliferation	VSMC
	↓ Neointima formation	VSMC
	Cell proliferation	EC
Vascular relaxation	↑ Endothelial nitric oxide synthase (eNOS)	EC
	↑ Inducible nitric oxide synthase	EC
	↑ cGMP	
Signaling molecules	↑ Phosphoinositol-3 (PI3)	EC
	↑ MAP-kinase	EC
Hormone response	↑ Progesterone receptor	EC

involved in inflammation, vascular remodeling, angiogenesis, and vascular tone; an overview is given in TABLE 1.

EXPRESSION AND DISTRIBUTION OF ESTROGEN
RECEPTORS ON VASCULAR CELLS

To date two estrogen receptors, the classic estrogen receptor alpha (ER-α), and a second receptor, the ERβ, have been identified.[16,17] Despite considerable homology, both receptors are structurally and functionally distinct. Both ER subtypes differ in their tissue distribution,[18] C-terminal ligand-binding domains,[18,19] the N-terminal transactivation DNA-binding domain,[18,20] and the selective activation of estrogen-responsive promoters, suggesting different regulatory functions. The estrogen and androgen receptors form part of the nuclear hormone receptor family of steroid-activated transcription factors. Of note, the estrogen receptor is the only known member of the steroidal family of nuclear hormone receptors, which occurs in two different subtypes.

Several studies have demonstrated the presence of functional estrogen receptors in human and animal vascular cells, including different endothelial cells and vascular smooth muscle cells (VSMCs).[21,22] Depending on the cell type, the localization, and the distribution, the relative expression levels of the ERα and the ERβ may vary considerably, and each subtype may be predominantly expressed under distinct conditions on the same cell type.[18] In humans, both estrogen receptors have been described to be present in vascular endothelial cells. The relative extent of ER expression and the role of these receptor subtypes, particularly in other vascular cell types, is not conclusively known.[17] We and others have shown unique expression of the ERβ on human VSMCs.[23-26] On vascular cells, the ER-β is functionally active.[27] The vasculoprotective effect of the ERβ was confirmed in an *in vivo* model using the selective ERβ agonist biochanin A.[28] Of note, in dilated and thickened varicose veins, vascular remodeling was correlated with ERβ expression.[29] The pathophysiologic relevance of these findings was underlined by a recent study, showing that genetic variants of the estrogen receptor correlate with the risk of myocardial infarction.[30] Moreover, recent data suggest that, besides the ER, expression of the AR also correlates inversely with more extensive vascular disease development, particularly when present during the early stages.[4]

In addition to normal vascular smooth muscle cells, we have shown selective expression of the ERβ and the androgen receptor (AR) in human neovascular KS cells. We have shown previously the induction of local acute-phase protein pentraxin-3 (PTX-3) expression in KS spindle cells by the viral homologue of human IL-6 (vIL-6).[31] Virokine expression allows direct activation of the interleukin-6 receptor[32,33] and is likely to promote tumor progression. In the presence of proinflammatory cytokines of the

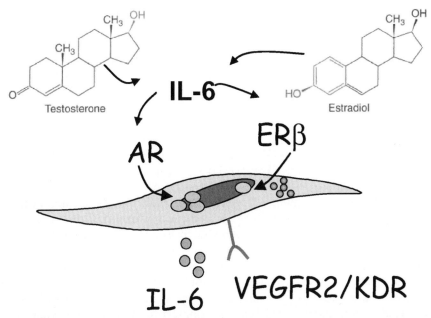

FIGURE 1. Interaction between proinflammatory cytokines and steroid hormone receptor expression on KS cells. IL-6 and other members of the IL-6 family of proinflammatory cytokines induced an upregulation of the ERβ and the androgen receptor on human KS cells, thereby increasing responsiveness to the natural hormones. Depending on the relative balance of the natural estrogens and androgens, this coactivation may eventually lead to vascular tumor promotion or suppression.

IL-6 family or of vIL-6, which can be produced by spindle cells, expression of both steroid hormone receptors was upregulated, indicating a close interaction between the inflammatory and proliferative vascular alterations (FIG. 1).

MOLECULAR MECHANISMS OF ESTROGEN ACTION ON VASCULAR CELLS

Classically, steroid hormone action involves activation of steroid hormone receptors, which are ligand-activated transcription factors that interact with the promoter regions of various genes and regulate gene expression.[34] Once bound to the specific receptors, estrogen induces dimerization and activation, thereby stabilizing the ligated receptor complex. After translocation in the nucleus, specific palindromic gene regions within estrogen-responsive elements are bound that regulate gene expression. This genomic activation pathway requires hours and may persist up to days until gene expression is induced. Moreover, ERα and ERβ may form homo- as well as heterodimers, which add a further degree of complexity to the cellular activation profile.[35] Thus not only the relative expression level of ERα and ERβ in vascular tissues, but also the differences in DNA-binding activity between ERα/ERβ homo- or heterodimers contribute to the varying functional activity of the ERs in target cells. In addition to this complexity, the estrogen receptors may even be activated by different growth factors in the absence of the specific ligand estrogen.[36]

RAPID NONGENOMIC EFFECTS OF ESTROGENS IN VASCULAR CELLS

While the steroid hormone estrogen is traditionally thought to control transcriptional activation through the classical nuclear estrogen receptor pathway, evidence for rapid alternative nongenomic signaling events, which occur within minutes, is accumulating (TABLE 2). The nongenomic pathway of estrogen action possibly involves targeting of a membrane ER to functional signaling modules in membrane caveolae, such as G-proteins or receptor-tyrosine kinases, enabling the rapid activation of mitogen-activated protein kinase (MAPK) and of phosphatidylinositol 3-Akt (PI3k/Akt) kinase pathways, and endothelial NO synthase (eNOS).[37] Besides the classic nuclear receptors, functionally distinct membrane surface-bound isoforms of the ERα and ERβ have been described which arise from the same transcript as the nuclear receptors.[38,39] This type of estrogen-mediated cellular activation profile involves putative estrogen-binding elements, which are located in specialized domains in the plasma membrane and act as molecular scaffolds required for rapid, nongenomic estrogen-mediated activation of downstream signaling pathways. In 2004, the novel caveolin-binding protein striatin was identified as the molecular anchor that localizes ERα to the membrane and organizes the ERα-eNOS membrane signaling complex in vascular endothelial cells.[40]

Recently, a new additional transmembrane G-protein-coupled receptor for estrogens was found which is uniquely localized to the endoplasmic reticulum.[41] This activation was independent of the estrogen receptors and may

TABLE 2. Rapid nongenomic vascular effects of estrogens

Rapid vasodilatation
eNOS-derived NO
Rapid vascular relaxation
eNOS- and iNOS-derived NO
cGMP
Endothelial rounding
↓ Cell adhesion (leukocytes)

NOS = nitric oxide synthase.

mark the detection of a second pathway of nongenomic estrogen signaling. Several studies have demonstrated independent regulation of nongenomic and genomic ER-dependent signaling, providing conceptual support for the potential development of "pathway-specific" selective ER modulators.

MODULATION OF VASCULAR FUNCTIONS BY ESTROGENS

Until recently, the protective vascular and cardiovascular effects of estrogens were mainly attributed to indirect systemic effects on lipoprotein metabolism, as well as to their influence on hemostasis and fibrinolysis[1–3] and on platelets[42] (TABLE 3). This concept is mainly based on the fact that atherogenic lipoproteins are central promotors of the atherosclerotic lesion progression. We have shown previously that atherogenic lipoproteins have the capacity to interact with lesional complement[43] and to induce the expression of chemokines,[44] of local acute-phase proteins,[45] of matrix metalloproteinases,[46] as well as of proinflammatory cytokines.[47,48] Thus, estrogen-mediated lowering of low-density lipoprotein (LDL) levels may indirectly attenuate lesion progression by reducing availability of atherogenic lipoproteins. By influencing the hemostatic and fibrinolytic system, estrogens may further counteract deleterious effects on fibrinolytic systems induced by atherogenic lipoproteins,[46] together constituting an important cause of cardiovascular complications. The attenuation of cytokine-mediated[49] or endothelial toxic[50] effects by estrogens represents a further important regulatory mechanism for the maintenance of vascular homeostasis. Thus, estrogens ameliorate the local vascular reactivity to proinflammatory cytokines.

TABLE 3. Vascular protective effects of estrogens

Indirect estrogen-mediated effects
Lipoprotein metabolism
↓ LDL
↓ Lipoprotein-(a)
↑ HDL
Fibrinolysis
↓ Plasminogen-activator-inhibitor-1 (PAI-1)
↓ Tissue-type plasminogen activator (tPA)
Coagulation
↓ Prothombotic proteins
Anti-inflammation
↓ of induced platelet-leukocyte-aggregates
Direct estrogen-mediated effects
Vasodilatation
Vessel relaxation
↓ Lesion progression
↑ Re-endothelialization

DIRECT ACTIONS OF ESTROGENS ON VASCULAR CELLS

Now, the contribution of the direct effects of estrogens on different vascular cell types to cardiovascular protection is increasingly recognized (TABLE 3). Direct actions of estrogens on vascular cells include rapid nongenomic effects on vasodilatation and relaxation as well as the classic genomic effects, requiring the presence of the specific nuclear receptors. Collectively, these data show that the vasculature forms part of the important estrogen target tissues, like the reproductive and hepatic tissues, and bone.

Physiologically, estrogens regulate the vascular tone, and play a protective role during the vascular response to injury.[1,2] Estrogens increase vascular relaxation and mediate acute vasodilatation in men and women via both rapid nongenomic pathways and classic delayed gene expression mechanisms. The rapid estrogen effects on vascular tone are primarily mediated by calcium-dependent signaling mechanisms, which converge on the activation of the endothelial (eNOS) or inducible nitric oxide synthase (iNOS), resulting in a local net increase of nitric oxide (NO). Nongenomic NOS activation has also been demonstrated for selective estrogen receptor modulators (SERMs), and may therefore provide a physiologically relevant target for selection of SERMs with vascular protective activity.

Besides the participation in the physiologic regulation of the vascular tone, estrogens mediate protective cardiovascular effects after injury. In the course of vascular stress, estrogens limit vascular smooth muscle cell proliferation and pathologic increases in vascular medial area, which was confirmed in a model using ERα/β knockout mice model treated with 17β-estradiol.[1,2] Moreover, physiologic replacement with 17β-estradiol allowed the reduction in infarct size and restricted cardiomyocyte apoptosis after myocardial infarction.[51] Particularly during the early stages of atherogenesis, estrogens inhibit the initiation and early progression of fatty streaks. By contrast, in established and advanced lesions, the presence of estrogen does not apparently alter the pathologic process.[52]

EFFECT OF ESTROGEN ON ANGIOGENESIS

Physiologic estrogen-regulated angiogenesis is a fundamental process for reproduction, and includes processes from cyclic endometrial angiogenesis to uterine changes during pregnancy.[53] In endometrial cells, 17β-estradiol has been shown to induce expression and secretion of members of the vascular endothelial growth factor (VEGF) family,[54] which constitutes one of the central regulators of developmental and adult angiogenesis and homeostasis.[55] In vivo, members of the VEGF family induce a potent angiogenic response, increase vascular permeability, and act as survival factor for endothelial cells.

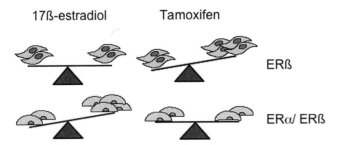

FIGURE 2. Estrogen receptor subtype distribution determines functional response to estrogens or SERMs. In human endothelial cells, which coexpress the ERα and the ERβ, estrogen mediated notable cell proliferation, while in arterial vascular smooth muscle cells, which express uniquely the ERβ in the absence of the ERα, estrogens produced no mitogenic effect. By contrast, tamoxifen induced only VSMC proliferation and lacked any effect on EC mitogenesis. This indicates that ER subtype distribution determines functional reactivity of the cells to natural hormones or receptor agonists/antagonists.

The angiogenic effects of VEGF are mediated by two types of receptors, both members of the receptor tyrosine kinase (RTK) family—the VEGFR-1/Flt-1 and the VEGFR-2/KDR—which can be regulated by the antiangiogenic soluble form sFlt-1.[56] Estrogen-mediated induction of VEGFR-1/KDR expression has been shown in endometrial capillaries.[57] This mechanism involves an indirect paracrine induction of the RTK via 17β-estradiol-stimulated VEGF expression.

In human vascular endothelial and smooth muscle cells, we show that 17β-estradiol induced expression of all three types of VEGF receptors. While in endothelial cells, E2 predominantly induced the active receptors, allowing pronounced EC proliferation, in VSMC, a comparable induction of the proangiogenic and antiangiogenic soluble receptors was observed, which did not permit induction of proliferation (FIG. 2). In contrast, tamoxifen, as one older member of the SERM family, produced no net effect on endothelial cells, but induced VEGF receptors in vascular smooth muscle cells. Of note, androgens induced a more than 200-fold expression of the VEGF receptors in vascular cells, mediating pronounced susceptibility to the mitogenic action of members of the VEGF family. In conclusion, in cells like VSMC and KS, which exclusively expressed the ERβ, the selective estrogen receptor agonist/antagonist tamoxifen induced expression of VEGF receptors. In contrast, in EC, which coexpressed the ERα and the ERβ, expression of the tyrosine kinase receptors was not altered in the presence of tamoxifen. We conclude that different distribution of ERs and the different relative stimulation capacity of natural 17β-estradiol and SERMs may be exploited for the use in directed vascular cell manipulation, for example, in promotion versus suppression of angiogenesis.

SUMMARY

Estrogens play a dichotomous role in normal vascular development and vascular diseases by promoting physiologic angiogenesis, but protecting from neovascular and inflammatory vascular diseases. The disclosure of the additional ERβ with a different functional activation profile, and the recent description of different nongenomic activation pathways, add to understanding the complexity of the estrogen effects in vascular diseases. We provide evidence for a different activation potential of estrogen in vascular and neovascular cells uniquely expressing the ERβ. Finally, the distinctive activation profiles of SERMs with respect to the distinct distribution of ER subtypes on vascular cells, and particularly the contribution of androgens, constitute promising targets for the directed manipulation of vascular homeostasis.

ACKNOWLEDGMENTS

Part of the experiments regarding VEGF-R expression after activation with 17β-estradiol is nonpublished data from the medical thesis of Claudia Winker de Pena.

REFERENCES

1. MENDELSOHN, M.E. & R.H. KARAS. 1999. The protective effects of estrogen on the cardiovascular system. N. Engl. J. Med. **340:** 1801–1811.
2. MENDELSOHN, M.E. 2002. Protective effects of estrogen on the cardiovascular system. Am. J. Cardiol. **89:** 12E–17E.
3. MENDELSOHN, M.E. & R.H. KARAS. 2005. Molecular and cellular basis of cardiovascular gender differences. Science **308:** 1583–1587.
4. LIU, P.Y., R.C. CHRISTIAN, M. RUAN, *et al.* 2005. Correlating androgen and estrogen steroid receptor expression with coronary calcification and atherosclerosis in men without known coronary artery disease. J. Clin. Endocrinol. Metab. **90:** 1041–1046.
5. KHALIL, R.A. 2005. Sex hormones as potential modulators of vascular function in hypertension. Hypertension **46:** 249–254.
6. VITTINGHOFF, E., M.G. SHLIPAK, P.D. VAROSY, *et al.* 2003. Heart and Estrogen/Progestin Replacement Study Research Group. Risk factors and secondary prevention in women with heart disease: the Heart and Estrogen/Progestin Replacement Study. Ann. Intern. Med. **138:** 81–89.
7. HERRINGTON, D.M., D.M. REBOUSSIN, K.P. KLEIN, *et al.* 2000. The Estrogen Replacement and Atherosclerosis (ERA) study: study design and baseline characteristics of the cohort. Control Clin. Trials **21:** 257–285.
8. GOEDERT, J.J., F. VITALE, C. LAURIA, *et al.* 2002. Classical Kaposi's Sarcoma Working Group. Risk factors for classical Kaposi's sarcoma. J. Natl. Cancer Inst. **94:** 1712–1718.

9. STAMPFER, M.J., G.A. COLDITZ, W.C. WILLETT, *et al*. 1991. Postmenopausal estrogen therapy and cardiovascular disease. Ten-year follow-up from the nurses' health study. N. Engl. J. Med. **325:** 756–762.

10. FRIEDMAN-KIEN, A.E. & B.R. SALTZMAN. 1990. Clinical manifestations of classical, endemic African, and epidemic AIDS-associated Kaposi's sarcoma. J. Am. Acad. Dermatol **22:** 1237–1250.

11. BOSHOFF, C., Y. ENDO, P.D. COLLINS, *et al*. 1997. Angiogenic and HIV-inhibitory functions of KSHV-encoded chemokines. Science **278:** 290–294.

12. ENSOLI, B. & M.C. SIRIANNI. 1998. Kaposi's sarcoma pathogenesis: a link between immunology and tumor biology. Crit. Rev. Oncog. **9:** 107–124.

13. CALABRO, M.L., J. SHELDON, A. FAVERO, *et al*. 1998. Seroprevalence of Kaposi's sarcoma-associated herpesvirus/human herpesvirus 8 in several regions of Italy. J. Hum. Virol **1:** 207–213.

14. KREUTER, A., H. RASOKAT, M. KLOUCHE, *et al*. 2005. Liposomal pegylated doxorubicin versus low-dose recombinant interferon-alfa-2a in the treatment of advanced classic Kaposi's sarcoma; retrospective analysis of three German centers. Cancer Investigation **23:** 653–659.

15. LING, S., P. KOMESAROFF & K. SUDHIR. 2006. Cellular mechanisms underlying the cardiovascular actions of oestrogens. Clin. Sci. (Lond) **111:** 107–118.

16. KUIPER, G.G., E. ENMARK, M. PELTO-HUIKKO, *et al*. 1996. Cloning of a novel receptor expressed in rat prostate and ovary. Proc. Natl. Acad. Sci. USA **93:** 5925–5930.

17. MOSSELMAN, S., J. POLMAN & R. DIJKEMA. 1996. ERbeta: identification and characterization of a novel human estrogen receptor. FEBS Lett. **392:** 49–53.

18. KUIPER, G.G., B. CARLSSON, K. GRANDIEN, *et al*. 1997. Comparison of the ligand binding specificity and transcript tissue distribution of estrogen receptors alpha and beta. Endocrinology **138:** 863–870.

19. PAECH, K., P. WEBB, G.G. KUIPER, *et al*. 1997. Differential ligand activation of estrogen receptors ERalpha and ERbeta at AP1 sites. Science **277:** 1508–1510.

20. WADE, C.B., S. ROBINSON, R.A. SHAPIRO & D.M. DORSA. 2001. Estrogen receptor (ER)alpha and ERbeta exhibit unique pharmacologic properties when coupled to activation of the mitogen-activated protein kinase pathway. Endocrinology **142:** 2336–2342.

21. RUBANYI, G.M., K. KAUSER & A. JOHNS. 2002. Role of estrogen receptors in the vascular system. Vascul. Pharmacol. **38:** 81–88.

22. DEROO, B.J. & K.S. KORACH. 2006. Estrogen receptors and human disease. J. Clin. Invest. **116:** 561–570.

23. CHRISTIAN, R.C., P.Y. LIU, S. HARRINGTON, *et al*. 2006. Intimal estrogen receptor (ER)beta, but not ERalpha expression, is correlated with coronary calcification and atherosclerosis in pre- and postmenopausal women. J. Clin. Endocrinol. Metab. **91:** 2713–2720.

24. BRENNER, R.M. & O.D. SLAYDEN. 2004. Steroid receptors in blood vessels of the rhesus macaque endometrium: a review. Arch. Histol. Cytol. **67:** 411–416.

25. HODGES, Y.K., L. TUNG, X.D. YAN, *et al*. 2000. Estrogen receptors alpha and beta: prevalence of estrogen receptor beta mRNA in human vascular smooth muscle and transcriptional effects. Circulation **101:** 1792–1798.

26. CRITCHLEY, H.O., R.M. BRENNER, T.A. HENDERSON, *et al*. 2001. Estrogen receptor beta, but not estrogen receptor alpha, is present in the vascular endothelium of

the human and nonhuman primate endometrium. J. Clin. Endocrinol Metab. **86:** 1370–1378.

27. LIANG, M., E. EKBLAD, J.A. GUSTAFSSON & B.O. NILSSON. 2001. Stimulation of vascular protein synthesis by activation of oestrogen receptor beta. J. Endocrinol **171:** 417–423.

28. SCHREPFER, S., T. DEUSE, T. MUNZEL, *et al.* 2006. The selective estrogen receptor-beta agonist biochanin A shows vasculoprotective effects without uterotrophic activity. Menopause **13:** 489–499.

29. KNAAPEN, M.W., P. SOMERS, H. BORTIER, *et al.* 2005. Smooth muscle cell hypertrophy in varicose veins is associated with expression of estrogen receptor-beta. J. Vasc. Res. **42:** 8–12.

30. SHEARMAN, A.M., J.A. COOPER, P.J. KOTWINSKI, *et al.* 2006. Estrogen receptor alpha gene variation is associated with risk of myocardial infarction in more than seven thousand men from five cohorts. Circ. Res. **98:** 590–592.

31. KLOUCHE, M., N. BROCKMEYER, C. KNABBE & S. ROSE-JOHN. 2002. Human herpesvirus 8-derived viral IL-6 induces PTX3 expression in Kaposi's sarcoma cells. AIDS **16:** F9–F18.

32. MÜLLBERG, J., T. GEIB, T. JOSTOCK, *et al.* 2000. IL-6 receptor independent stimulation of human gp130 by viral IL-6. J. Immunol. **164:** 4672–4677.

33. KLOUCHE, M., G. CARRUBA, L. CASTAGNETTA & S. ROSE-JOHN. 2004. Virokines in the pathogenesis of cancer—focus on human herpesvirus 8. Ann. N.Y. Acad. Sci. **1028:** 329–339.

34. MANGELSDORF, D.J., C. THUMMEL, M. BEATO, *et al.* 1995. The nuclear receptor superfamily: the second decade. Cell **83:** 835–839.

35. COWLEY, S.M., S. HOARE, S. MOSSELMAN & M.G. PARKER. 1997. Estrogen receptors alpha and beta form heterodimers on DNA. J. Biol. Chem. **272:** 19858–19862.

36. SMITH, C.L. 1998. Cross-talk between peptide growth factor and estrogen receptor signaling pathways. Biol. Reprod. **58:** 627–632.

37. MENDELSOHN, M.E. 2002. Genomic and nongenomic effects of estrogen in the vasculature. Am. J. Cardiol. **90:** 3F–6F.

38. COLLINS, P. & C. WEBB. 1999. Estrogen hits the surface. Nat. Med. **5:** 1130–1131.

39. CHAMBLISS, K.L., I.S. YUHANNA, R.G. ANDERSON, *et al.* 2002. ERbeta has nongenomic action in caveolae. Mol. Endocrinol. **16:** 938–946.

40. LU, Q., D.C. PALLAS, H.K. SURKS, *et al.* 2004. Striatin assembles a membrane signaling complex necessary for rapid, nongenomic activation of endothelial NO synthase by estrogen receptor alpha. Proc. Natl. Acad. Sci. USA **101:** 17126–17131.

41. REVANKAR, C.M., D.F. CIMINO, L.A. SKLAR, *et al.* 2005. A transmembrane intracellular estrogen receptor mediates rapid cell signaling. Science **307:** 1625–1630.

42. ROSIN, C., M. BRUNNER, S. LEHR, *et al.* 2006. The formation of platelet-leukocyte aggregates varies during the menstrual cycle. Platelets **17:** 61–66.

43. BHAKDI S., M. TORZEWSKI, M. KLOUCHE & M. HEMMES. 1999. Complement and atherogenesis: binding of CRP to degraded, non-oxidized LDL enhances complement activation. Arterioscler. Thromb. Vasc. Biol. **19:** 2348–2354.

44. KLOUCHE, M., S. GOTTSCHLING, V. GERL, *et al.* 1998. Atherogenic properties of enzymatically degraded LDL: selective induction of MCP-1 and cytotoxic effects on human macrophages. Arterioscler. Thromb. Vasc. Biol. **18:** 1376–1385.

45. KLOUCHE, M., G. PERI & C. KNABBE. 2004. Cholesterol-loading induces expression of pentraxin-3 by human vascular smooth muscle cells. Atherosclerosis **175:** 221–228.

46. MAY, A.E., R. SCHMIDT, Bö BÜLBÜL, *et al.* 2005. Plasminogen and matrix metallo-proteinase activation by enzymatically modified LDL in monocytes and smooth muscle cells. Thrombosis Haemostasis **93:** 710–715.

47. KLOUCHE, M., S. BHAKDI, S. HEMMES & S. ROSE-JOHN. 1999. Novel path to the activation of vascular smooth muscle cells: upregulation of gp130 creates an autocrine activation loop by IL-6 and its soluble receptor. J. Immunol. **163:** 4583–4589.

48. KLOUCHE, M., S. ROSE-JOHN, W. SCHMIEDT & S. BHAKDI. 2000. Enzymatically degraded, nonoxidized LDL induces human vascular smooth muscle cell activation, foam cell transformation, and proliferation. Circulation **101:** 1799–1805.

49. LING, S., L. ZHOU, H. LI, *et al.* 2006. Effects of 17beta-estradiol on growth and apoptosis in human vascular endothelial cells: influence of mechanical strain and tumor necrosis factor-alpha. Steroids **71:** 799–808.

50. WANG, Y., Z. WANG, L. WANG, *et al.* 2006. Estrogen down-regulates nicotine-induced adhesion molecule expression via nongenomic signal pathway in endothelial cells. Int. Immunopharmacol. **6:** 892–902.

51. PATTEN, R.D. & R.H. KARAS. 2006. Estrogen replacement and cardiomyocyte protection. Trends Cardiovasc. Med. **16:** 69–75.

52. ROSENFELD, M.E., K. KAUSER, B. MARTIN-MCNULTY, *et al.* 2002. Estrogen inhibits the initiation of fatty streaks throughout the vasculature but does not inhibit intraplaque hemorrhage and the progression of established lesions in apolipoprotein E deficient mice. Atherosclerosis **164:** 251–259.

53. PERROT-APPLANAT, M., M. ANCELIN, H. BUTEAU-LOZANO, *et al.* 2000. Ovarian steroids in endometrial angiogenesis. Steroids **65:** 599–603.

54. BAUSERO, P., M. BEN-MAHDI, J. MAZUCATELLI, *et al.* 2000. Vascular endothelial growth factor is modulated in vascular muscle cells by estradiol, tamoxifen, and hypoxia. Am. J. Physiol. Heart Circ. Physiol **279:** H2033–H2042.

55. CEBE-SUAREZ, S., A. ZEHNDER-FJALLMAN & K. BALLMER-HOFER. 2006. The role of VEGF receptors in angiogenesis; complex partnerships. Cell Mol. Life Sci. **63:** 601–615.

56. FERRARA, N., H.P. GERBER & J. LECOUTER. 2003. The biology of VEGF and its receptors. Nat. Med. **9:** 669–676.

57. HERVE, M.A., G. MEDURI, F.G. PETIT, *et al.* 2006. Regulation of the vascular endothelial growth factor (VEGF) receptor Flk-1/KDR by estradiol through VEGF in uterus. J. Endocrinol. **188:** 91–99.

Implications of Recent Clinical Trials of Postmenopausal Hormone Therapy for Management of Cardiovascular Disease

JACQUES E. ROSSOUW

Women's Health Initiative, National Heart, Lung, and Blood Institute, Rockville, Bethesda, Maryland 20892, USA

ABSTRACT: Estrogen therapy, originally used for the treatment of menopausal vasomotor symptoms, had by 1990 become a mainstay for the prevention of coronary heart disease (CHD) in postmenopausal women. The recommendations for use of estrogen in CHD were based on epidemiologic, animal, and laboratory data. However, a series of clinical trials published from 1998 onward have failed uniformly to confirm a CHD benefit. When the disappointing results of the secondary prevention trials were announced, there was widespread anticipation of more promising results from the primary prevention trials of the Women's Health Initiative (WHI). The WHI trials in generally healthy women also did not provide evidence of benefit, and the use of HT for disease prevention is now discouraged. In response, some commentators have incorrectly stated that the WHI was not a true primary prevention trial. A more appropriate way to frame the question is whether the effects of HT on cardiovascular disease (CVD) differ by age or years since menopause. Some preliminary data suggest that more recently menopausal women starting HT could be at lower risk of CHD (but not stroke) than women more distant from the menopause. However, even if ongoing studies provide evidence that HT can slow the initiation of early atherosclerosis in younger women, this is unlikely to translate into a reconsideration of the use of HT for the prevention of disease, because the long-term effects on cardiovascular events are unknown and unknowable, HT has other adverse effects, and there are more effective and safer ways of preventing cardiovascular disease.

KEYWORDS: estrogen; progestin; postmenopausal hormone therapy; cardiovascular disease; women

Address for correspondence: Jacques E. Rossouw, M.D., Women's Health Initiative, National Heart, Lung, and Blood Institute, Rockledge 2, Room 8106, 6701 Rockledge Drive, Bethesda, MD 20892, USA. Voice: 301-435-6669; fax: 301-480-5158.
e-mail: rossouwj@nih.gov

Ann. N.Y. Acad. Sci. 1089: 444–453 (2006). © 2006 New York Academy of Sciences.
doi: 10.1196/annals.1386.046

INTRODUCTION

Conjugated equine estrogens (CEEs) were first approved in the United States for menopausal symptoms and hormone replacement therapy in 1942, but only came into widespread use in the 1960s and early 1970s after publications and speaking tours by gynecologist Dr. Robert Wilson. He espoused the notion that menopause is a state of hormone deficiency akin to castration, and that the estrogen needed to be "replaced" to ensure health and happiness.[1] The "feminine forever" fountain-of-youth premise of his book is captured in the title, and in passages such as "In the entire realm of medicine, there are few forms of therapy with a more consistent record of beneficence." His ideas were widely promoted in the popular press. The increasing use of hormone "replacement" therapy occurred despite warning signals from the Coronary Drug Project in men, a set of lipid-lowering trials in which the high-dose CEE arms were stopped early because of increased risk of thrombosis and cardiovascular disease.[2] In addition, there was emerging knowledge from observational studies in young women that use of the oral contraceptive pill was associated with increased risk of thrombosis, stroke, and coronary heart disease (CHD).[3] In 1975 a set of papers in the *New England Journal of Medicine* showed a strong association between unopposed estrogen use and risk of endometrial cancer, after which prescriptions plummeted, only to resume during the late 1970s when it was demonstrated that the addition of a progestin would protect against endometrial cancer.[4,5] The return to large-scale use during the 1980s and 1990s was increasingly for indications other than menopausal symptoms: prevention of osteoporosis and cardiovascular disease. Evidence for the hypothesis that estrogen could prevent osteoporosis was strong and based on observational data, mechanistic studies, and small clinical trials of bone mineral density. Evidence for prevention of cardiovascular disease also appeared to be reasonably strong, including observational data, small trials of lipids and other intermediate outcomes, and animal studies.[6,7] The Food and Drug Administration had approved prevention of osteoporosis as an indication, but not that for CHD. The heavily promoted hypothesis that estrogen could prevent chronic disease had another effect: prescriptions were more often written for older women well beyond the menopause, and for longer periods of time.

THE INFLUENCE OF OBSERVATIONAL STUDIES SHOWING AN ASSOCIATION OF HORMONE THERAPY WITH REDUCED RISK OF CHD

During the 1990s it was the conventional wisdom that estrogen would prevent CHD. Several authoritative bodies recommended this off-label use, especially for women at high risk, that is, women who already had had a heart attack.[8–11] This thinking was based on observational studies suggesting that risk reduction in hormone users was at least as great, and possibly even greater, in women with prior heart disease as in healthy women.[6,11] There was less evidence for estrogen in combination with a progestin, and some uncertainty as to whether the risk reduction would be of a similar magnitude.[12] The upshot was that by the early 1990s, the great majority of internists, family doctors, cardiologists, and gynecologists in the United States were prescribing estrogen for prevention of heart disease. Though it was recognized that estrogen could also increase the risk of breast cancer, the twin benefits of potential reduction in heart disease and fractures were thought to outweigh the risk of breast cancer.[12]

The most persuasive data in support of the putative benefit for coronary disease was that from several dozen observational studies; however, such studies are subject to a variety of systematic biases that could lead them to overestimate benefit, if any.[13,14] In general, women who elect to take hormone therapy, or for whom therapy is prescribed, tend to be better educated and healthier to start with. Those that remain on therapy in the longer term are a highly selected group of compliant women who have not suffered any adverse effects. Because the practice guidelines and the prescription patterns of physicians were well ahead of the evidence, there was a clear need for randomized controlled clinical trials to test whether or not hormone therapy might indeed be of benefit to women with and without existing cardiovascular disease.

THE IMPACT OF CLINICAL TRIALS OF HORMONE THERAPY TO PREVENT CHD

Because benefit was deemed to be most likely in women with existing heart disease, and because their higher background rates allowed for a smaller sample size, most of the planned trials were in women with clinical or angiographic evidence of coronary disease. The Heart and Estrogen/Progestin Replacement Study (HERS) was the first of the large-scale trials to report its results, and they were disappointing.[15] Overall, combined CEE and medroxy-progesterone (MPA) did not affect the incidence of CHD events; furthermore, during the first year there was a significant increase in CHD risk. With longer follow-up the risk decreased and reversed toward the end of the original study. This pattern can be seen as one of no overall effect, but a redistribution of events within the trial period. The questions are whether the initial increase was due to some triggering of acute thrombotic events in an existing complicated lesion, and whether the later decrease in risk was due to a longer-term effect of lipid lowering, or whether it was simply a survivor effect in the less susceptible women. During the posttrial follow-up (during which almost half of the participants continued their active medication) there was no suggestion of a continued benefit and the overall result remained neutral, supporting a conclusion that HT has no overall effect on CHD beyond the triggering of early events in susceptible women.[16] The possibility that several years of HT might reduce existing atherosclerosis was dealt a further blow when a series of angiographic trials showed no benefit in reducing the progression of atherosclerosis.[17–19]

After the publication of HERS, the conventional wisdom was revised to a view that HT is not effective for secondary prevention, and there was a general expectation that the results of the Women's Health Initiative (WHI) trials of HT would yield different results. The WHI trials studied generally healthy women, though a small proportion of women with existing cardiovascular disease were included. On average, the risk profile of the cohort was better than in the general U.S. population, as evidenced by their low CHD rates (about half of that in the general population). Two parallel trials were conducted: the trial of CEE plus MPA (CEE + MPA) in women with an intact uterus enrolled 16,608 women aged 50–79 years, and the trial of CEE alone in women who had had a hysterectomy enrolled 10,739 women. The trials were planned to have a follow-up of 8.4 years, but both ended before that. The trial of CEE + MPA was terminated after an average follow-up of 5.6 years because of increased risks of breast cancer, CHD, stroke, and pulmonary embolism, which were not offset by decreased risks of hip fracture and colorectal cancer.[20] The trial of CEE was terminated after 7.1 years average follow-up because of increased risk of stroke, no effect on the primary outcome of CHD, no overall benefit, and little probability that the results would change with additional follow-up.[21] A substudy of participants in both trials aged 65–79 years showed increased risks of dementia and minimal cognitive impairment.[22] Other risks included those of gallbladder disease and urinary incontinence.[23,24] Though vasomotor symptoms improved in the 12–17% of women who had moderate/severe symptoms at baseline, the overall health-related quality of life was not improved.[25,26] There were some differences between the two trials: in the CEE + MPA, but not in the CEE trial, the CHD and breast cancer risks were increased. Colorectal cancer risk appeared to be decreased in the CEE + MPA trial only. The effects were similar for stroke, dementia, and venous thrombosis (increased risk) and for hip fracture (decreased risk).

The publication of the WHI CEE + MPA trial results in July 2002 was attended by a considerable amount of attention from the media, the public, and the medical profession. By July 2003, the U.S. prescriptions for the particular CEE + MPA formulation (Prempro) had dropped by 66% and overall HT prescriptions dropped by 38%.[27] The findings led to a revision of the package inserts for all HT formulations, including statements that HT should not be used for the prevention of CVD, and if used for approved indications it should be used at the lowest dose and shortest duration needed to obtain the therapeutic effect. In addition, HT was relegated to second-line status for the prevention of osteoporosis. The practice guidelines of many professional organizations were revised to include statements similar to those in the Food and Drug

Administration guidance; however, some individuals remained convinced that HT does have a cardioprotective effect if initiated early enough, and disputed that WHI truly was a primary prevention trial.[28,29]

CAN THE OBSERVATIONAL STUDIES AND THE CLINICAL TRIALS BE RECONCILED?

The current conventional wisdom is that menopausal estrogen therapy (with or without a progestin) should not be initiated or continued for the purpose of preventing cardiovascular disease. This is diametrically opposed to the conventional wisdom prevalent at the time of planning the WHI program. However, there is an emergent wisdom that hormone therapy may offer cardiovascular protection (or at least do no harm) if started early in the menopause.[30] Those who subscribe to this view cite differences in study populations between observational studies and the clinical trials that may have modified the effect of HT on CHD. An examination of the Nurses' Health Study (NHS) and WHI cohorts indicates some differences in risk factors: NHS women had slightly higher rates of ever smoking (60% vs. 50%), but lower rates of hypertension (18% vs. 28%), being overweight (38% vs. 70%), having diabetes mellitus (3% vs. 4%), or a history of coronary disease (0% vs. 4%).[31] However, with the exception of the small proportion of women with existing disease admitted to the trials, the existence of risk factors does not imply that the trials were not primary prevention. Primary prevention is defined as an intervention in persons without diagnosed clinical disease. Preclinical disease may exist, but such persons are included in the concept of primary prevention. On the other hand, primordial prevention intervenes on risk factors at an earlier stage before preclinical disease. Because hormone treatment was typically started in adulthood, neither observational studies of HT use nor clinical trials can qualify as being primordial prevention, but both can represent primary prevention. Nonetheless, primary prevention encompasses such a wide spectrum of health status that it remains possible that there were substantive differences between the primary prevention observational studies and the primary prevention clinical trials. This is not true for the secondary prevention observational studies and the clinical trials, where by definition established disease is present at baseline.

Possibly the most informative differences in respect of primary prevention are that the age range in NHS was lower (30–63 years compared to 50–79 years in WHI) and most of the women started HT at menopause and (presumably) had vasomotor symptoms, while most women in WHI commenced study HT many years subsequent to the menopause and did not have vasomotor symptoms. However, it should be noted that with 8,832 women aged 50–59 years the WHI trials constitute the largest randomized trial experience of HT in younger women, that 26% of women in the CEE + MPA trial and 48% in the CEE trial had used HT in the past or were using them at baseline, and 12% and

17%, respectively, reported having moderate/severe vasomotor symptoms at baseline.[20,21] The existence of subgroups that overlap with those in the NHS and other observational studies provides an opportunity to try to reconcile the divergent findings between clinical trials and observational studies, by examining whether characteristics such as age, years since menopause, prior use of hormone therapy, or presence of vasomotor symptoms modify the effects of HT. Baseline CHD risk factors are unlikely to explain the more adverse findings for CHD in WHI, because subgroup analyses did not suggest that women with these factors (including prior CVD) had a greater increase in risk of CHD on hormone therapy than women without the factors. However, other subgroup analyses have suggested a possible role for years since menopause (in the CEE + MPA trial) or age (in the CEE trial).[32,33] Prior use of HT did not appear to influence the results. Further, more detailed analyses of the possible interactions of age, years since menopause, and presence of vasomotor symptoms on HT effect on CHD are under way.

The theoretical model for a role of age (or years since menopause) in modifying the effect of HT can be conceptualized as three different effects of estrogen depending on the underlying state of the arteries: retardation of the initiation of the earliest stages of atherosclerosis (impaired endothelial function, fatty streaks) in young adults, no effect on progression of existing raised lesions in middle age, and triggering of clinical events in complicated lesions (erosion or rupture of unstable plaque, with subsequent thrombosis and occlusion).[31] Mechanistic studies in animals and in the laboratory support estrogen effects in the first, angiographic trials in the second, and large clinical outcome trials plus limited mechanistic studies in the third stage. Unfortunately, by the time most women reach the age of menopause, they are likely to have raised lesions and a small proportion will also have complicated lesions. Hence, it is not at all clear whether there is a potential for clinical benefit in preventing CHD at middle age, though there may be for women who start HT at a younger age (e.g., women who undergo premature surgical menopause). At best, it may turn out that women undergoing a natural menopause at the average age of 50–59 years are not at any substantially increased risk from HT for several years, in part because they are at very low absolute risk whether or not they take HT. What is very clear is that initiation of HT does not protect against CHD in women older than 60 years, and that HT increases the risk in the first year or two after therapy is begun. Even if there is a "window of opportunity" at middle age where there is no harm, one cannot assume that the lack of harm will continue with prolonged therapy as women and their arteries age. A further caveat against thinking that the age of initiation explains the different results of observational studies and clinical trials is that the observational studies predicted equal or even greater benefit in women with existing heart disease or atherosclerosis. We know that this cannot be true, given the results of the angiographic trials and the clinical outcome trials. Hence, at a minimum, the observational studies overestimate any potential benefit.

Unlike CHD, the risk of stroke on HT does not appear to be modified by age or years since menopause.[34,35] This is consistent with the observational studies which suggest an increased risk of stroke in the same populations, with the same drugs, and the same dosages at which the studies suggested benefit for CHD. It is unclear why stroke and CHD should react differently to HT, but one possibility is that stroke is less dependent on the favorable lipid changes on HT, and is affected more adversely by the prothrombotic effects of HT.

RESEARCH QUESTIONS

Some of the research questions that remain are whether lower doses of estrogen, or different routes of administration, different types and regimens of progestin, or selective estrogen receptor modulators (SERMs) may have different effects on CHD risk. Trials of SERMs have thus far yielded results similar to those of HT: increased risk of stroke and no effect on CHD risk.[36] If the gender difference in CHD by age is informative at all in relation to estrogen and progestin, then nonoral estradiol and progesterone starting at a younger age would be the most likely candidates for offering protection against CHD. Transdermal estradiol avoids the first-pass hepatic circulation, and thus has much less effect on coagulation factors and on CRP. Use of transdermal estradiol appears to be associated with less risk of venous thromboembolism than do oral estrogens, but whether this has any clinical implication for CHD or stroke has not been adequately tested.[37] Similarly, the effects of lower doses of estrogen and of progesterone (either orally or intravaginally) have not been adequately tested. Surrogate outcome trials using carotid intima-media thickness or coronary artery calcification as indicators of effect on atherosclerosis are testing lower doses of oral CEE, transdermal estadiol, and oral or vaginal progesterone in younger women.[38,39] Favorable results from these surrogate trials will be somewhat reassuring for younger women considering the use of HT in the shorter term for the relief of symptoms, or even for women with osteoporosis as an initial therapy before switching to bisphosphonates, raloxifene, or other therapies at an older age.

While it is possible that these trials will demonstrate a slowing of the onset of early lesions, such findings would be unlikely to change the current paradigm that HT should not be used for the prevention of CHD. HT has other effects beyond any effect on atherosclerosis, and in particular the prothrombotic and proinflammatory effects may be important for the triggering of clinical events. The short-term trials cannot answer the question of whether continued estrogen use over many decades will overcome the inevitable age-related degeneration of arterial health. In addition, long-term HT is associated with increasing risk of breast cancer. Given the availability of other well-proven, effective, and safe strategies for preventing CHD, there will be no need to rely on HT for this indication. Favorable results from the surrogate outcome trials are also unlikely to lead to a definitive trial with clinical outcomes, given the very large number or younger women that would need to be enrolled, and the very long-term follow-up that would be needed. Such large and long-duration trials are at this point the sole strategy that might change the current paradigm. The history of estrogen and heart disease has been permeated with "magical thinking" ever since the days of Robert Wilson. A recent commentary points out that the observational epidemiology that provided respectability to the idea of cardio-protection ignored some hard realities; the contradiction with the trials in men and the adverse effects of oral contraceptives in women; that mechanism does not prove causality; and that it is not possible to adjust for all confounders.[40] Without proof that initiating estrogen at an earlier age, or that transdermal estrogen or newer SERMs have a different effect, any assumption that they do could well be another exercise in "magical thinking" that ignores contrary evidence. There are no other examples of cardio-protective drugs that work in women but not in men, and there are no examples of drugs that work in primary (or primordial) prevention, but not in secondary prevention.[40]

CLINICAL IMPLICATIONS

The implications of what we have learned thus far from the clinical trials vary by specialty. Cardiologists, who have a vast armamentarium of strategies to choose from, no longer see any role for HT in prevention of CHD. Endocrinologists and internists focusing on prevention of osteoporosis face a more limited role for HT at lower dose and for shorter periods than used in the past. Other effective and safe drugs are preferred as first line for the prevention of osteoporosis. Gynecologists who are looking to treat menopausal vasomotor symptoms have been advised to reconsider the need for women with less severe symptoms, and to exhaust other options first. If HT is used, it should be used at the lowest dose and the shortest duration needed, with periodic evaluation of whether there is a continuing need.

CONCLUSIONS

Postmenopausal HT has come full circle. It started as a therapy to treat vasomotor symptoms and vaginal dryness, and it has returned to that status. It is no longer recommended for the prevention of chronic disease, and even its use for osteoporosis prevention is now more limited. Increasing attention is being paid to the issue of whether the short-term use of HT in more recently menopausal women for the relief of symptoms has been discouraged to a greater extent than needs be, given the very low absolute risks of major disease and the possibility that HT may retard atherosclerosis if initiated early. However, the return of HT for the prevention of CHD appears unlikely (even if initiated early), because of the trial findings and unresolvable uncertainties surrounding long-term use.

REFERENCES

1. WILSON, R.A. 1966. Feminine Forever. Evans. New York, NY.
2. ANON. 1970. The Coronary Drug Project. Initial findings leading to modifications of its research protocol. JAMA **214:** 1303–1313.
3. ORY, H.W. 1977. Association between oral contraceptives and myocardial infarction. JAMA **237:** 2619–2622.
4. SMITH, D.C., R. PRENTICE, D.J. THOMPSON, et al. 1975. Association of exogenous estrogen and endometrial carcinoma. N. Engl. J. Med. **293:** 1164–1167.
5. ZIEL, H.K. & W.D. FINKLE. 1975. Increased risk of endometrial carcinoma among users of conjugated estrogens. N. Engl. J. Med. **293:** 1167–1170.
6. STAMPFER, M.J. & G.A. COLDITZ. 1990. Estrogen replacement therapy and coronary heart disease: a quantitative assessment of the epidemiologic evidence. Prev. Med. **20:** 47–63.
7. LOBO, R.A. 1990. Estrogen and cardiovascular disease. Ann. N. Y. Acad. Sci. **592:** 286–294.
8. ANON. 1992. Hormone replacement therapy. ACOG Technical Bulletin Number 166–April 1992 (replaces No. 93, June 1986). Int. J. Gynaecol. Obstet. **41:** 194–202.
9. ANON. 1992. Guidelines for counseling postmenopausal women about preventive hormone therapy. American College of Physicians. Ann. Intern. Med. **117:** 1038–1041.
10. ANON. 1993. Summary of the second report of the National Cholesterol Education Program (NCEP) Expert Panel on Detection, Evaluation, and Treatment of High Blood Cholesterol in Adults (Adult Treatment Panel II). JAMA **269:** 3015–3023.
11. MOSCA, L., J.E. MANSON S.E. SUTHERLAND, et al. 1997. Cardiovascular disease in women. A statement for healthcare professionals from the American Heart Association. Circulation **96:** 2468–2482.
12. GRADY, D., S.M. RUBIN, D.B. PETITTI, et al. 1992. Hormone therapy to prevent disease and prolong life in postmenopausal women. Ann. Intern. Med. **117:** 1016–1037.
13. ROSSOUW, J.E. 1996. Estrogens for prevention of coronary heart disease. Putting the brakes on the bandwagon. Circulation. **94:** 2982–2985.
14. SOTELO, M.M. & S.R. JOHNSON. 1997. The effects of hormone replacement therapy on coronary heart disease. Endocrinol. Metab. Clin. North Am. **26:** 313–328.
15. HULLEY, S., D. GRADY, T. BUSH, et al. 1998. Randomized trial of estrogen plus progestin for secondary prevention of coronary heart disease in postmenopausal women. JAMA **280:** 605–613.
16. GRADY, D., D. HERRINGTON, V. BITTNER, et al. 2002. Cardiovascular disease outcomes during 6.8 years of hormone therapy: Heart and Estrogen/Progestin Replacement Study follow-up (HERS II). JAMA **288:** 49–57.
17. HERRINGTON, D.M., D.M. REBOUSSIN, K.B. BROSNIHAN, et al. 2000. Effects of estrogen replacement on the progression of coronary-artery atherosclerosis. N. Engl. J. Med. **343:** 522–529.
18. WATERS, D.D., E.L. ALDERMAN, J. HSIA, et al. 2002. Effects of hormone replacement therapy and antioxidant vitamin supplements on coronary atherosclerosis in postmenopausal women: a randomized controlled trial. JAMA **288:** 2432–2440.
19. HODIS, H.N., W.J. MACK, S.P. AZEN, et al. 2003. Hormone therapy and the progression of coronary-artery atherosclerosis in postmenopausal women. N. Engl. J. Med. **349:** 535–545.

20. WRITING GROUP FOR THE WOMEN'S HEALTH INITIATIVE INVESTIGATORS. 2002. Risks and benefits of estrogen plus progestin in healthy postmenopausal women. JAMA **288:** 321–333.
21. WOMEN'S HEALTH INITIATIVE STEERING COMMITTEE. 2004. Effects of conjugated equine estrogen in postmenopausal women with hysterectomy: the Women's Health Initiative Randomized Controlled Trial. JAMA **291:** 1701–1712.
22. SHUMAKER, S., C. LEGAULT, L. KULLER, *et al.* 2004. Conjugated equine estrogens and incidence of probable dementia and mild cognitive impairment in post-menopausal women. JAMA **291:** 2947–2958.
23. CIRILLO, D., R. WALLACE, R. RODABOUGH, *et al.* 2005. Effect of estrogen therapy on gallbladder disease. JAMA **293:** 330–339.
24. HENDRIX, S.L., B.B. COCHRANE, I.E. NYGAARD, *et al.* 2005. Effects of estrogen with and without progestin on urinary incontinence. JAMA **293:** 935–948.
25. HAYS, J., J. OCKENE, R. BRUNNER, *et al.* 2003. Effects of estrogen plus progestin on health-related quality of life. N. Engl. J. Med. **348:** 1839–1854.
26. BRUNNER, R.L., M. GASS, A. ARAGAKI, *et al.* 2005. Effects of conjugated equine estrogen on health-related quality of life in postmenopausal women with hysterectomy: results from the Women's Health Initiative Randomized Clinical Trial. Arch. Intern. Med. **165:** 1976–1986.
27. HERSH, A.L., M.L. STEFANICK & R.S. STAFFORD. 2004. National use of post-menopausal hormone therapy. JAMA **291:** 47–53.
28. SPEROFF, L. 2005. Clinical appraisal of the Women's Health Initiative. J. Obstet. Gynaecol. Res. **31:** 80–93.
29. NAFTOLIN, F., H.S. TAYLOR,, R. KARAS,, *et al.* 2004. The Women's Health Initiative could not have detected cardioprotective effects of starting hormone therapy during the menopausal transition. Fertil. Steril. **81:** 1498–1501.
30. MANSON, J.E., S. BASSUK & S. HARMAN. 2006. Postmenopausal hormone therapy: new questions and the case for new clinical trials. Menopause **13:** 139–147.
31. ROSSOUW, J.E. 2005. Coronary heart disease in menopausal women: implications of primary and secondary prevention trials of hormones. Maturitas **51:** 51–63.
32. MANSON, J.E., J. HSIA, K.C. JOHNSON, *et al.* 2003. Estrogen plus progestin and the risk of coronary heart disease. N. Engl. J. Med. **349:** 523–534.
33. HSIA, J., R.D. LANGER, J.E. MANSON, *et al.* 2006. Conjugated equine estrogens and coronary heart disease: the Women's Health Initiative. Arch. Intern. Med. **166:** 357–365. Erratum in Arch. Intern. Med. **166:** 759.
34. HENDRIX, S.L., S. WASSERTHEIL-SMOLLER, K.C. JOHNSON, *et al.* 2006. Effects of conjugated equine estrogen on stroke in the Women's Health Initiative. Circulation **113:** 2425–2434.
35. WASSERTHEIL-SMOLLER, S., S.L. HENDRIX, M. LIMACHER, *et al.* 2003. Effect of estrogen plus progestin on stroke in postmenopausal women: the Women's Health Initiative: a randomized trial. JAMA **289:** 2673–2684.
36. STEFANICK, M.L. 2006. Risk-benefit profiles of raloxifene for women. N. Engl. J. Med. **355:** 190–192.
37. LOWE, G.D.O. 2004. Hormone replacement therapy and cardiovascular disease: increased risks of venous thromboembolism and stroke, and no protection from coronary heart disease. J. Intern. Med. **256:** 361–374.
38. HARMAN, S.M., E.A. BRINTON, M. CEDARS, *et al.* 2005. KEEPS: The Kronos Early Estrogen Prevention Study. Climacteric **8:** 3–12.
39. NCT00114517 available at www.clinicaltrials.gov (accessed August 14, 2006)
40. PETITTI, D. 2004. Commentary: hormone replacement therapy and coronary heart disease: four lessons. Int. J. Epidemiol. **33:** 461–463.

Association between the Polymorphism of CCR5 and Alzheimer's Disease

Results of a Study Performed on Male and Female Patients from Northern Italy

CARMELA RITA BALISTRERI,[a] MARIA PAOLA GRIMALDI,[a]
SONYA VASTO,[a] FLORINDA LISTI,[a] MARTINA CHIAPPELLI,[a,b]
FEDERICO LICASTRO,[b] DOMENICO LIO,[a] CALOGERO CARUSO,[a]
AND GIUSEPPINA CANDORE[a]

[a]Gruppo di Studio sull' Immunosenescenza, Dipartimento di Biopatologia e Metodologie Biomediche, Università di Palermo, Palermo, Italy

[b]Dipartimento di Patologia Sperimentale, Università di Bologna, Bologna, Italy

ABSTRACT: Alzheimer's disease (AD) is the most common cause of dementia in Western society. The prevalence of AD is greater in women than in men, largely due to longevity and survival differences favoring women. However, some studies suggest that incidence rates may really be increased in women. One possible factor influencing AD incidence in women is the loss of ovarian estrogens production after menopause, which might be involved in AD pathogenesis. Estrogens seem to influence some neuronal functions. Many of these actions appear beneficial (i.e., neuroprotective action against a variety of insults, as oxidative stress, and reduction of β-amyloid plaques formation). Furthermore, several studies have shown that proinflammatory genotypes seem to significantly contribute to AD risk. In the present study, we evaluated whether the anti-inflammatory allele of chemokine receptor CCR5 is a component of the genetic protective background versus AD neuronal degeneration. We genotyped for $\Delta 32$ (a 32-bp deletion of the CCR5 gene that causes a frameshift at amino acid 185) in 191 AD patients (133 women and 58 men; age range: 53–98 years; mean age: 74.88 ± 8.44) and 182 controls (98 women and 84 men; age range: 65–93; mean age 73.21 ± 8.24) from northern Italy. No different distribution of the CCR$\Delta 32$ deletion in the two cohorts was clearly evident. Statistical analysis by gender stratification, demonstrated no differences in genotype distribution and allelic frequency both in women and in men. Further, studies should focus on identification of proinflammatory genetic variants involved in AD pathogenesis in women.

Address for correspondence: Giuseppina Candore, Ph.D., Gruppo di Studio sull'Immunosenescenza, Dipartimento di Biopatologia e Metodologie Biomediche, Corso Tukory 211, 90134 Palermo, Italy. Voice: +39-09-1655-5932; fax: +39-09-1655-5933.
e-mail: gcandore@unipa.it

Ann. N.Y. Acad. Sci. 1089: 454–461 (2006). © 2006 New York Academy of Sciences.
doi: 10.1196/annals.1386.012

KEYWORDS: Alzheimer's disease; CCR5; immunogenetics; inflammation; women

INTRODUCTION

Alzheimer's disease (AD) is a neurological disorder that presently affects 20–30 million individuals around the world.[1] It is the most common neurodegenerative disease associated with aging.[2] It can also be classified as a complex multifactorial disease, such as cardiovascular diseases, because there are both genetic and environmental factors that result in the phenotypic expression of what is clinically called AD.[3] Because of the demographic shifts and remarkable medical advances of the last century, aging populations are now the fastest growing portions of the population, and women constitute a majority of this population because of their increased life expectancy relative to that of males.[1] Thus, women would appear to be at special risk for AD, possibly because of the loss of ovarian estrogens production after menopause, which might be involved in AD pathophysiology.[4] Indeed, estrogens seem to influence several neuronal functions.[5] Many of these actions appear to be neuroprotective against a variety of insults, as oxidative stress, excitatory neurotoxicity, and ischemia.[6] A further putatively beneficial action of estrogens in the brain is the reduction in β-amyloid (Aβ) formation.[7]

On the other hand, inflammation plays a key role in AD pathogenesis. Indeed, as shown by the amyloid cascade/neuroinflammation hypothesis,[8–10] the key component of the AD neurodegeneration is an upregulation of inflammatory cytokines, acute-phase proteins, and other proinflammatory mediators causing the neurodegenerative changes. In particular, there is growing evidence that chemokines and their receptors are upregulated in reactive microglial cells in the AD brain,[11, 12] and they may play a role in the recruitment and accumulation of microglial cells at Aβ sites in senile plaques.[13] Indeed, some immunohistochemical studies demonstrated that the activated microglial cells in both control and AD brain present an increased expression of chemokine receptor CCR5, suggesting that CCR5 receptor might play a role in the regulation of brain immune response in AD.[14]

Besides, CCR5 protein (chemokine-CC motif-receptor 5 provided by HUGO Gene Nomenclature Committee) is a cell-surface receptor that binds the β-chemokines involved in migration toward an increasing concentration of chemokines, monocytes, NK cells, and some T cells. So, this chemiotatic response results in recruitment of leukocytes to the inflammatory site.[15–17] This molecule is also involved in the binding and entry of human immunodeficiency virus (HIV) into target cells. In particular, in the CCR5 gene a 32-base pair deletion (Δ32) resulting in a nonfunctional receptor, which could be responsible for the relative or absolute resistance to HIV-1 infection,[18] has been found. Furthermore, recently it has been suggested that CCR5 Δ32 polymorphism has a protective effect towards some inflammatory diseases.[17]

In this study, we aimed to see whether the anti-inflammatory allele CCR5Δ32 is a component of the genetic protective background protective versus AD neurodegeneration. To this end, we studied AD patients and age-matched controls from northern Italy and, to assess the role of gender, the data were separately analyzed in men and women.

MATERIALS AND METHODS

The study included 191 AD patients (133 women and 58 men; age range: 53–98 years; mean age: 74.88 ± 8.44), from northern Italy. All AD subjects were diagnosed as having probable AD according to NINCDS–ADRDA and DSM-III-R criteria.[19,20] Cognitive performances and alterations were measured according to the Mini Mental State Evaluation (MMSE) and the Global Deterioration Scale (GDS). All AD cases were defined as sporadic because the family history did not mention any first-degree relative with dementia. Besides, 80% of AD patients showed clinical onset of the disease after 65 years of age (late-onset AD, LOAD) and 20% before this age (early-onset AD, EOAD). Furthermore, a large number of the patients ($n = 187$) were followed up for 2 years and cognitive performances recorded. Longitudinal cognitive decline was assessed by MMSE scores according to the published method[21] and patients were divided into three groups with different degree of deterioration rate (fast = decrement of more than five points/year; intermediate = 2–4.9 points/year; slow = less that 2 points/year). Controls were 182 unrelated individuals (98 women and 84 men; age range: 65–93; mean age 73.21 ± 8.24) randomly selected from a nursing home. These subjects had complete neurological and medical examinations that showed that they were free of significant illness. The controls were collected from the same population of the patients' cohort. Patients and controls were assessed to have parents and grandparents born in northern Italy to ensure ethnicity. Consequently, possible confounding effects, such as the inclusion in the study of members of different ethnic groups, have been minimized. Informed consent was obtained from all patients and controls according to Italian law.

Blood specimens were collected in tripotassium EDTA sterile tubes and DNA extracted was genotyped for two single nucleotide polymorphisms (SNPs): CCR5Δ32 and ApoE-ε4. The procedure for detecting the CCR5Δ32 SNP was based on polymerase chain reaction (PCR) amplification, according to published methods.[22] Briefly, we mixed one couple of 3' and 5' allele-specific primer in a 25 μL total volume that contained DNA template, 1.50 mM magnesium chloride, 9.8 mM ammonium sulfate, 39.6 mM Tris, 200 μM dNTPs, and 0.2U Taq-Gold polymerase (Applera Italia, Monza, Italy). Cycling was performed at 95°C for 10 min, followed by 35 cycles at 94°C for 30 sec, 59°C for 30 sec, and 72°C for 30 sec. The patterns of the two alleles (+Δ32 and

TABLE 1. Genotype distribution of Δ32CCR5 deletion in 191 AD patients and 182 age-matched controls from northern Italy

Subjects	Genotypes			Alleles	
	Δ32−/Δ32−	Δ32−/Δ32+	Δ32+/Δ32+	Δ32−	Δ32+
AD patients	173	18	0	364 (95.3%)	18 (4.7%)
Age-matched Controls	165	17	0	347 (95.4%)	17 (4.6%)

All the genotypes were in HWE. No different distribution of CCR5(Δ32 genotypes was obtained in two cohorts. No different distribution of CCR5(Δ32 alleles was obtained between two cohorts.

−Δ32) were detected by electrophoresis on 2% agarose. Furthermore, the allelic APOE-ε4 polymorphism was assessed by a PCR-based method.[23]

Allele and genotypic frequencies of two analyzed SNPs were evaluated by gene count. Significant differences in frequency, among the groups, were calculated by χ^2 test (3×2, 2×2 tables, where appropriate). Furthermore, odds ratio (OR) with confidence interval (CI) and its significance were calculated. The data were tested for the goodness-of-fit between the observed and expected genotype frequencies according to the Hardy–Weinberg equilibrium (HWE) by χ^2 test. Besides, we evaluated the synergistic effects between CCR5 and APOE polymorphisms by logistic regression analysis. We also analyzed the allelic frequencies of CCR5Δ32 deletion according to gender in AD patients and controls by χ^2 test. In addition, the genotype distribution of CCR5Δ32 SNP was analyzed by χ^2 test in three groups of AD patients with different degrees of cognitive decline (fast, intermediate, slow).[21]

RESULTS

We found no significant differences in the genetic distribution and allelic frequency of CCR5 polymorphism between the two studied groups (TABLE 1). Furthermore, we analyzed the allelic frequencies of CCR5Δ32 deletion according to gender in AD patients and controls. No statistical difference was observed among the allele frequency of CCR5Δ32 deletion by stratification according to gender in AD patients and controls (TABLE 2).

Besides, when compared to wild-type/wild-type genotypes, the OR for CCR5Δ32 allele-carrying genotypes was 0.9 (95% CI = 0.4–1.9, $P = 0.078$). In addition, we studied the synergistic effects between CCR5 and APOE polymorphisms by logistic regression analysis. There was no interaction between carriage of CCR5Δ32 allele and the APOE ε4 allele: in the presence of the APOE ε4 allele, the risk of CCR5Δ32 allele carriers (OR = 5.64, 95% CI = 3.56–10.8) was double that of CCR5Δ32 allele noncarriers (OR = 2.82, 95% CI = 3.78–11.2), but the interaction was not significant.

TABLE 2. Allele frequencies of CCR5(Δ32 deletion analyzed according to gender in AD (133 female and 58 male) patients and controls (98 female and 84 male), from northern Italy

	Female		Male	
	AD Patients ($n = 133$)	Controls ($n = 98$)	AD Patients ($n = 58$)	Controls ($n = 84$)
Alleles				
CCR5Δ32−	252 (94.7%)	188 (96%)	112 (96.5%)	159 (94.6%)
CCR5Δ32+	14 (5.3%)	8 (4%)	4 (3.5%)	9 (5.4%)

No statistically significant differences in the allele frequency of CCR5Δ32 deletion were observed, stratifying according to gender AD patients and controls.

Finally, analyzing the genotype distribution of CCR5Δ32 deletion in groups of AD patients with different degrees of cognitive decline (fast, intermediate, slow), no significant difference was observed.

DISCUSSION

There is growing evidence that AD Aβ deposition is associated with a local inflammatory response, which is initiated by the activation and migration of microglia in inflammatory sites.[10,24–26] Besides, it has been recently demonstrated that the recruitment of microglial cells in senile plaques is induced by chemokines and their receptors upregulated in AD brain.[11,12,27] In particular, it has been observed that CCR5 receptor is overexpressed on microglial cells of AD brain, and many of these reactive microglia were found associated with amyloid deposits.[14] So, this receptor seems to be involved in AD pathogenesis and its expression seems to be induced by aggregated Aβ peptides.[14] Indeed, aggregated Aβ peptides have been shown to stimulate the expression of a range of proinflammatory genes, and a recent study demonstrated that the most highly induced genes in human postmortem brain microglia stimulated with Aβ belonged to the chemokine family.[28] On the other hand, it has been recently suggested that CCR5 is involved in the plaque atherosclerotic development. This receptor is expressed on macrophages, Th1 and Th2 lymphocytes, aortic smooth muscle cells, and coronary endothelial cells, and CCR5 ligands have been detected in plaques.[29–35] Furthermore, recent preliminary genetic studies showed that the CCR5Δ32 variant of gene CCR5 protects individuals from early acute myocardial infarction (AMI) and severe CHD. Thus, the allelic variant CCR5Δ32 may have a protective role against AMI as consequence of an attenuated inflammatory response, which would determine a slower progression of atherosclerotic lesion among CCR5Δ32 carriers.[36–38]

Taking into account that the CCR5 deletion seem to represent a factor protective for AMI disease, the aim of this study was to evaluate whether CCR5 genotype is also a component of the genetic protective background against AD. Analyzing our data, we found no significant differences in the genetic distribution and allelic frequency of CCR5 polymorphism between the two studied groups. Furthermore, no statistical difference was observed among the allele frequency of CCR5Δ32 deletion by stratification according to gender in AD patients and controls. In addition, we studied the synergistic effects between CCR5 and APOE polymorphisms by logistic regression analysis. There was no interaction between carriage of CCR5Δ32 allele and the APOE ε4 allele. So, this study indicated that CCR5 is not a protective factor against AD. Besides, our data are in agreement with three recent reports.[39-41] Statistical analysis by gender stratification demonstrated no differences in genotype distribution and allelic frequency both in women and men. Further, studies should focus on identification of proinflammatory genetic variants involved in AD pathogenesis in women.

Finally, the different results of studying the association between CCR5 deletion and inflammatory age-related diseases seem to suggest a different mechanism of recruitment of monocyte lineage cells in the two types (senile and atheroclerotic) of plaques.

ACKNOWLEDGMENTS

This work was supported by grants from the Italian Ministry of Education, University and Research to C.C. and G.C. C.R.B., M.P.G and, S.V., M.C. are Ph.D. students at Pathobiology Ph.D. course (directed by C.C.) of Palermo University and this work is in partial fulfillment of the requirement for the Ph.D. The collaboration of Dr. Massimo Franceschi (Department of Neurology, Santa Maria Hospital, Castellanza [VA], Italy) in the selection of patients and controls is warmly acknowledged.

REFERENCES

1. SELKOE, D.J. 2005. Defining molecular targets to prevent Alzheimer disease. Arch. Neurol. **62:** 192–195.
2. LICASTRO, F. *et al.* 2005. Innate immunity and inflammation in ageing: a key for understanding age-related diseases. Immun. Ageing **2:**8.
3. CARUSO, C. *et al.* 2003. Genetics of neurodegenerative disorders. N. Engl. J. Med. **349:** 193–194.
4. HENDERSON, V.W. 2006. Estrogen-containing hormone therapy and Alzheimer's disease risk: understanding discrepant inferences from observational and experimental research. Neuroscience **138:** 1031–1039.
5. HENDERSON, V.W. *et al.* 2000. Estrogen for Alzheimer's disease in women: randomized, double-blind, placebo-controlled trial. Neurology **54:** 295–301.
6. ALKAYED, N.J. *et al.* 2000. Neuroprotective effects of female gonadal steroids in reproductively senescent female rats. Stroke **31:** 161–168.

7. PETANCESKA, S.S. *et al.* 2000. Ovariectomy and 17beta-estradiol modulate the levels of Alzheimer's amyloid beta peptides in brain. Exp. Gerontol. **35:** 1317–1325.
8. EIKELENBOOM, P. *et al.* 2002. Neuroinflammation in Alzheimer's disease and prion disease. Glia **40:** 232–239.
9. ROGERS, J. *et al.* 2002. Microglia and inflammatory mechanisms in the clearance of amyloid beta peptide. Glia **40:** 260–269.
10. STREIT, W.J. 2004. Microglia and Alzheimer's disease pathogenesis. J. Neurosci. Res. **77:** 1–8.
11. AKIYAMA, S. *et al.* 2000. Inflammation and Alzheimer's disease. Neurobiol. Aging **21:** 383–421.
12. BAJETTO, A. *et al.* 2002. Characterization of chemokines and their receptors in the central nervous system: physiopathological implications. J. Neurochem. **82:** 1311–1329.
13. STREIT, W.J. 2001. Chemokines and Alzheimer's disease. Neurobiol. Aging **22:** 909–913.
14. XIA, M.Q. *et al.* 1998. Immunohistochemical study of the beta-chemokine receptors CCR3 and CCR5 and their ligands in normal and Alzheimer's disease brains. Am. J. Pathol. **153:** 31–37.
15. PREMACK, B.A. & T.J. SCHALL. 1996. Chemokine receptors: gateways to inflammation and infection. Nat. Med. **11:** 1174–1178.
16. SAMSON, M. *et al.* 1996. Molecular cloning and functional expression of a new human CC-chemokine receptor gene. Biochemistry **11:** 3362–3367.
17. LOCATI, M. *et al.* 2005. Chemokines and their receptors: roles in specific clinical conditions and measurement in the clinical laboratory. Am. J. Clin. Pathol. **123:** S82–S95.
18. SAMSON, M. *et al.* 1996. Resistance to HIV-1 infection in Caucasian individuals bearing mutant alleles of the CCR-5 chemokine receptor gene. Nature **382:** 722–725.
19. AMERICAN PSYCHIATRIC ASSOCIATION. 1987. Diagnostic and statistical manual of mental disorders: DSM-III-R. Third revised edition.American Psychiatric Association. Washington DC.
20. MCKHANN, G. *et al.* 1984. Clinical diagnosis of Alzheimer's disease: report of the NINCDS-ADRDA Work Group under the auspices of Department of Health and Human Service Task Force on Alzheimer's Disease. Neurology **34:** 939–944.
21. DOODY, R.S. *et al.* 2001. A method for estimating progression rates in Alzheimer's disease. Arch. Neurol. **58:** 449–454.
22. GLAS, J. *et al.* 2003. The Delta 32 mutation of the chemokine-receptor 5 gene neither is correlated with chronic hepatitis C nor does it predict response to therapy with interferon-alpha and ribavirin. Clin. Immunol. **108:** 46–50.
23. LICASTRO, F. *et al.* 2000. Gene polymorphism affecting alpha-1-antichymotrypsin and interleukin-1 plasma levels increases Alzheimer's disease risk. Ann. Neurol. **48:** 388–391.
24. WEINER, H.L. & D. Frenkel. 2006. Immunology and immunotherapy of Alzheimer's disease. Nat. Rev. Immunol. **6:** 404–416.
25. SASTRE, M. *et al.* 2006. Contribution of inflammatory processes to Alzheimer's disease: molecular mechanisms. Int. J. Dev. Neurosci. **24:** 167–176.
26. LUCAS, S.M. *et al.* 2006. The role of inflammation in CNS injury and disease. Br. J. Pharmacol. **147:** S232–S240.

27. RANSOHOFF, R.M. 2002. The chemokine system in neuroinflammation: an update. J. Infect. Dis. **186:** S152–S156.
28. WALKER, D.G. *et al.* 2001. Gene expression profiling of amyloid beta peptide-stimulated human post-mortem brain microglia. Neurobiol. Aging **22:** 957–966.
29. ROTTMAN, J.B. *et al.* 1997. Cellular localization of the chemokine receptor CCR5. Am. J. Pathol. **151:** 1341–1351.
30. BERGER, O. *et al.* 1999. CXC and CC chemokine receptors on coronary and brain endothelia. Mol. Med. **5:** 795–805.
31. SCHECTER, A.D. *et al.* 2000. Human vascular smooth muscle cells possess functional CCR5. J. Biol. Chem. **275:** 5466–5471.
32. MACH, F. 2001. The role of chemokines in atherosclerosis. Curr. Atheroscler. Rep. **3:** 243–251.
33. MACK, M. *et al.* 2001. Expression and characterization of the chemokine receptors CCR2 and CCR5 in mice. J. Immunol. **166:** 4697–4704.
34. HANSSON, G.K. 2005. Inflammation, atherosclerosis, and coronary artery disease. N. Engl. J. Med. **352:** 1685–1695.
35. VEILLARD, N.R. *et al.* 2005. Simvastatin modulates chemokine and chemokine receptor expression by geranylgeranyl isoprenoid pathway in human endothelial cells and macrophages. Atherosclerosis. Epub ahead of print.
36. GONZALEZ, P. *et al.* 2001. Genetic variation at the chemokine receptors CCR5/CCR2 in myocardial infarction. Genes Immunity **2:** 191–195.
37. SZALAI, C. *et al.* 2001. Involvement of polymorphisms in the chemokine system in the susceptibility for coronary artery disease (CAD). Atherosclerosis **158:** 233–239.
38. CANDORE, G. *et al.* 2006. Opposite role of proinflammatory alleles in acute myocardial infarction and longevity. Ann. N.Y. Acad. Sci. **1067:** 270–275.
39. COMBARROS, O. *et al.* 2004. The chemokine receptor CCR5-Delta32 gene mutation is not protective against Alzheimer's disease. Neurosci. Lett. **366:** 312–314.
40. HUERTA, C. *et al.* 2004. Chemokines (RANTES and MCP-1) and chemokine-receptors (CCR2 and CCR5) gene polymorphisms in Alzheimer's and Parkinson's disease. Neurosci. Lett. **370:** 151–154.
41. GALIMBERTI, D. *et al.* 2004. CCR2-64I polymorphism and CCR5Delta32 deletion in patients with Alzheimer's disease. J. Neurol. Sci. **225:** 79–83.

7-Nitroindazole Protects Striatal Dopaminergic Neurons against MPP$^+$-Induced Degeneration

An *in Vivo* Microdialysis Study

VINCENZO DI MATTEO,[a] ARCANGELO BENIGNO,[b]
MASSIMO PIERUCCI,[a] DAVIDE ANTONIO GIULIANO,[b]
GIUSEPPE CRESCIMANNO,[b] ENNIO ESPOSITO,[a]
AND GIUSEPPE DI GIOVANNI[b]

[a]*Istituto di Ricerche Farmacologiche "Mario Negri," Consorzio Mario Negri Sud, 66030 Santa Maria Imbaro (CH), Italy*

[b]*Dipartimento di Medicina Sperimentale, Sezione di Fisiologia Umana, "G. Pagano," Università degli Studi di Palermo, 90134 Palermo, Italy*

ABSTRACT: The neuropathological hallmark of Parkinson's disease (PD) is the selective degeneration of dopaminergic (DAergic) neurons in the substantia nigra pars compacta (SNc). In this study, using a microdialysis technique, we investigated whether an inhibitor of neuronal nitric oxide synthase (nNOS), 7-nitrindazole (7-NI), could protect against DAergic neuronal damage induced by *in vivo* infusion of 1-methyl-4-phenylpiridinium iodide (MPP$^+$) in freely moving rats. Experiments were performed over 2 days in three groups of rats: (*a*) nonlesioned, (*b*) MPP$^+$-lesioned, and (*c*) 7-NI pretreated MPP$^+$-lesioned rats. On day 1, control rats were perfused with an artificial CSF, while 1 mM MPP$^+$ was infused into the striatum for 10 min in the other two groups. The infusion of the MPP$^+$ produced a neurotoxic damage of the SNc DA neurons and increased striatal DA levels. On day 2, 1 mM MPP$^+$ was reperfused for 10 min into the striata of each rat group and DA levels were measured as an index of neuronal cell integrity. The limited rise of DA following MPP$^+$ reperfusion in the MPP$^+$-lesioned rats was due to toxin-induced neuronal loss and was reversed by pretreatment with 7-NI (50 mg/kg, intraperitoneally) on day 1, indicating a neuroprotective effect by inhibiting NO formation. These results indicate that neuronally derived NO partially mediates MPP$^+$-induced neurotoxicity. The similarity between the MPP$^+$ model and PD suggests that NO may play a significant role in its etiology.

Address for correspondence: Dr. Giuseppe Di Giovanni, Dipartimento di Medicina Sperimentale, Sezione di Fisiologia Umana, "G. Pagano," Università degli Studi di Palermo, 90134 Palermo, Italy. Voice: +39-0916555821; fax: +39-0916555823.
e-mail: g.digiovanni@unipa.it

Ann. N.Y. Acad. Sci. 1089: 462–471 (2006). © 2006 New York Academy of Sciences.
doi: 10.1196/annals.1386.015

KEYWORDS: Parkinson's disease; *in vivo* microdialysis; corpus striatum; nitric oxide; MPP$^+$

INTRODUCTION

Parkinson's disease (PD) is a neurological disorder that affects movement, balance, and fine motor control. These impairments are related to the progressive degeneration of dopaminergic (DAergic) neurons in the substantia nigra pars compacta (SNc), with a concomitant reduction of striatal DA levels.[1,2] The pathogenesis of PD is a complex of multifactorial, genetic, and environmental events. Important factors include formation of free radicals, impaired mitochondrial activity, increased sensitivity to apoptosis, excitotoxicity, and inflammation.[3,4] Although the mechanisms involved in nigral degeneration in PD are unknown, evidence from postmortem studies suggests the involvement of reactive oxygen species (ROS) and oxidative stress,[5–7] partly arising from an increased DA metabolism, which causes the production of free radical species.[5,8]

Several *in vitro* and *in vivo* studies indicate that nitric oxide (NO) transmission is involved in DAergic neuronal damage induced by toxins, such as 1-methyl-4-phenyl-1,2,3,6-tetrahydropyridine (MPTP) or its pyridinium ion (MPP$^+$)[9–12] but its mechanism is still unknown and some data are controversial.[13] On the basis of the above considerations, the aim of this study was to investigate the potential protective effect of 7-nitroindazole (7-NI), a relatively specific neuronal inhibitor of nitric oxide synthase (nNOS), against degeneration of the nigrostriatal system induced by MPP$^+$. To this purpose, MPP$^+$ was perfused by *in vivo* reverse microdialysis, into the striata of conscious, freely moving rats, and DA extracellular output was measured in the perfusion fluid at 20-min intervals. Twenty-four hours later, 1 mM MPP$^+$ was perfused again to challenge intact DAergic neurons. The amount of DA released after a second perfusion (challenge) of MPP$^+$ was considered an index of intact DAergic neurons.[14–16]

MATERIALS AND METHODS

Male Sprague–Dawley rats (Charles River, Calco, Italy) weighing 340 g to 380 g were used. The animals were kept at constant room temperature (21 $\pm$ 1°C) and relative humidity (60 $\pm$ 5%) under a regular light–dark schedule (light 8.00–20.00 h). Food and water were freely available. Procedures involving animals and their care were conducted in conformity with the institutional guidelines that are in compliance with national (D.L. n. 116, G.U., suppl. 40, 18 Febbraio 1992) and international laws and policies (*EEC Council Directive 86/609, OJ L 358,1, Dec. 12, 1987; NIH Guide for the Care and Use of Laboratory Animals*, NIH Publication N. 85-23, 1985 and Guidelines for the Use of Animals in Biomedical Research.*)

*Thromb. Haemost. **58**: 1078–1084.

Rats were anesthetized with chloral hydrate (400 mg/kg, i.p.) and placed on a stereotaxic instrument (David Kopf Instruments, Tujunga, USA). A microdialysis guide cannula for CMA/12 probe was implanted over the left corpus striatum (AP = 0.8, L = 3.0, V = −3.0 from the dura surface and respect to the bregma), according to the atlas of Paxinos and Watson (1986), and permanently fixed to the skull with stainless steel screws and methylacrylic cement. A microdialysis probe (CMA/12, 3-mm length, 500-μm outer diameter, Carnegie Medicine, Stockholm, Sweden), connected to a two-channel liquid swivel (Carnegie Medicine, Stockholm, Sweden), was lowered through the guide cannula to reach a depth of 6 mm below the dura surface. The rats were placed in a CMA/120 system for freely moving animals (Carnegie Medicine, Stockholm, Sweden). The probe was perfused overnight at a constant rate of 0.30 μL/min by means of a microperfusion pump (Harvard Apparatus syringe infusion pump 22, USA) with an artificial cerebrospinal fluid (aCSF) composed of 147 mM Na$^+$, 2.7 mM K$^+$, 1 mM Mg^{2+}, 1.2 mM Ca^{2+}, 154.1 mM Cl$^-$, adjusted to pH 7.4 with 2 mM sodium-phosphate buffer. The experiments were performed 24 h (day 1) and 48 h (day 2) after probe implantation in awake, freely moving animals. The corpus striatum was perfused at a flow rate of 1 μL/min, and every 20 minutes samples of perfusate were collected and immediately assayed by high-performance liquid chromatography (HPLC) with electrochemical detection.

After establishing a steady baseline level in three consecutive samples (control value), MPP$^+$ iodide, dissolved in aCSF solution, was administered for 10 min and sampling was continued for 2 h. On day 1, MPP$^+$ (1 mM) was perfused through the microdialysis probe to induce neurodegeneration. On day 2, MPP$^+$ (1 mM) was reperfused (challenge) for 10 min in each rat perfused on day 1.

Dialysate samples were analyzed by reverse-phase HPLC coupled with electrochemical detection. The mobile phase was composed of 70 mM NaH$_2$PO$_4$, 0.1 mM Na$_2$EDTA, 0.7 mM triethylamine, 0.1 mM octylsulfonic acid, and 10% methanol, adjusted to pH 4.8 with orthophosphoric acid. This mobile phase was delivered at 1 mL/min flow rate (Pump 420, Kontron Instruments, Milano, Italy) through a Hypersil column (C18, 4.6 × 150 mm, 5 μm, Sigma Aldrich Chemicals, USA). Samples were injected manually into the HPLC and detection of DA was carried out with a coulometric detector (Coulochem II, ESA, Bedford, MA, USA) coupled to a dual-electrode analytic cell (model 5014). The potential of the first electrode was set at −175 mV and the second at +175 mV. Under these conditions, the sensitivity for DA was 0.35 pg/20 μL with a signal-to-noise ratio of 3:1.

All pharmacological treatments were performed following the stabilization of DA levels in the perfusate. A stable baseline, defined as three consecutive samples in which DA content varied by less than 10%, was generally obtained 150–180 min after the beginning of the perfusion (stabilization period). 7-NI was freshly diluted in a solution of DMSO (10% in peanut oil). 7-NI was given intraperitoneally (i.p.) in a volume of 2 mL/kg body weight. The dose of 7-NI (50 mg/kg, i.p.) was chosen on the basis of previous data.[17] 7-NI was given 1 h before neurotoxin.

Dopamine content in each sample was expressed as the absolute dialysate levels in nmol/L (without considering probe recovery). Data correspond to mean ± SEM values of absolute DA levels obtained in each experimental group. Data were analyzed by one-way analysis of variance (ANOVA) with repeated measures, followed by the Fisher's protected least significance difference *post hoc* test (Fisher's PLSD) to allow multiple comparisons between groups. All statistical analyses were performed with StatView^{TM} version 5.0.1 (SAS Institute Inc., Cary, NC, USA).

MPP$^+$ and 7-NI were purchased from Sigma-Aldrich, Milano, Italy.

RESULTS

Day 1

Perfusion of the 1 mM MPP$^+$ for 10 min, at day 1, produced a strong increase in the extracellular output of DA peaking at 40 min after the perfusion of the neurotoxin. The administration of 7-NI (50 mg/kg, i.p.), 1 h before infusion of MPP$^+$, did not modify the extracellular DA release induced by the neurotoxin, which appears to indicate that it does not affect the DA-uptake mechanism (FIG. 1A). The total amount of DA, measured as the sum of DA released in five consecutive samples (100 min) after MPP$^+$ perfusion, was similar in the two groups (7-NI+MPP$^+$ vs. MPP$^+$) (see FIG. 1B).

Day 2

To check the integrity of the DA-system, 1 mM MPP$^+$ was perfused for 10 min one day after (day 2) the first infusion of MPP$^+$. The challenge with MPP$^+$ produced a maximal DA extracellular output 40 min after its infusion in all rats. MPP$^+$ perfusion produced a maximal DA increase of 905 ± 111 nmol in the nonlesioned rats (aCSF/MPP$^+$, $n = 5$), 320 ± 33 in the MPP$^+$-lesioned rats (MPP$^+$/MPP$^+$, $n = 7$) and 679 ± 148 nmol in the lesioned rats pretreated with 7-NI (7-NI+MPP$^+$/MPP$^+$, $n = 6$) (FIG. 2A). The limited rise of DA following the MPP$^+$ reperfusion was due to toxin-induced neuronal loss and was reversed by pretreatment with 7-NI. The total amounts of DA, released in 100 min, were reduced in MPP$^+$-lesioned rats, challenged with MPP$^+$ on day 2 as compared to controls ($P < 0.01$ vs. aCSF/MPP$^+$ at Fisher's PLSD test). 7-NI restored the total amount of released DA ($P < 0.05$ and $P < 0.01$ vs. MPP$^+$(MPP$^+$ group at Fisher's PLSD test; FIG. 2B). The limited rise of DA following the second MPP$^+$ perfusion was due to previous toxin-induced neuronal loss and was reversed by pretreatment with 7-NI.

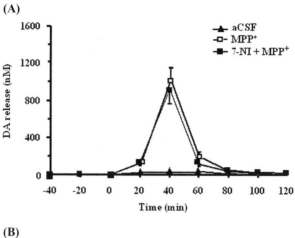

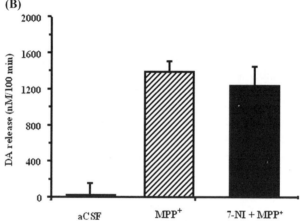

FIGURE 1. (A) Effect of 7-NI on MPP$^+$-induced increase in DA extracellular lev-els in the corpus striatum on day 1. A first group of rats was infused only with aCSF (▲, aCSF, $n = 5$). A second group was treated with 1 mM MPP$^+$ infused at time 0 for 10 min (□, MPP$^+$, $n = 7$). The third group received 7-NI (50 mg/kg, i.p.) 1 h before 1 mM MPP$^+$ (■, 7-NI+MPP$^+$, $n = 6$). Each data point represents mean ± SEM of absolute levels of DA, without considering probe recovery. Statistical analysis (one-way ANOVA) did not reveal differences between MPP$^+$ and 7-NI+ MPP$^+$ groups. **(B)** Effect of 7-NI on DA total output, measured as the sum of five (100 min) consecutive samples after perfusion of MPP$^+$ in the corpus striatum on day 1. The aCSF group did not receive any toxin ($n = 5$). The second group (MPP$^+$) was perfused with 1 mM MPP$^+$ for 10 min ($n = 7$). The third group (7-NI+MPP$^+$) received 7-NI (50 mg/kg, i.p.) 1 h before 1 mM MPP$^+$ ($n = 6$). Each column shows mean ± SEM of absolute levels of DA, without considering probe recovery. Statistical analysis (one-way ANOVA) revealed no differences between MPP$^+$ and 7-NI+ MPP$^+$ groups.

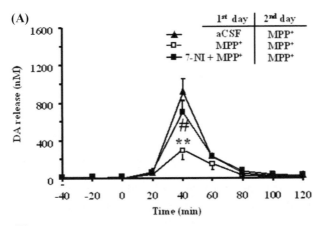

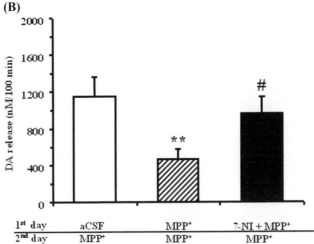

FIGURE 2. (A) Effect of 7-NI on MPP⁺-induced DA depletion in the corpus striatum of MPP⁺-lesioned rats on day 2. Each data point represents mean ± SEM of absolute levels of DA, without considering probe recovery. Statistical analysis shows that 1 mM MPP⁺ perfused on day 2 in aCSF rats (▲, aCSF/MPP⁺, $n = 5$) induced a significant increase of DA release. 7-NI (50 mg/kg i.p.) given 1 h before 1 mM MPP⁺ on day 1 (■, 7-NI+MPP⁺/MPP⁺, $n = 6$) prevented MPP⁺-induced decrease in DA release (□, MPP⁺/MPP⁺, $n = 7$) (one-way ANOVA, followed by Fisher's PLSD *post hoc* test: ** $P < 0.01$ MPP⁺/MPP⁺ vs. aCSF/MPP⁺, #$P < 0.05$ 7-NI+MPP⁺/MPP⁺ vs. MPP⁺/MPP⁺). **(B)** Effect of 7-NI on total DA output measured as the sum of five (100 min) consecutive samples after perfusion of MPP⁺ 24 h after MPP⁺ lesion in the corpus striatum. 7-NI (50 mg/kg i.p.) given 1 h before 1 mM MPP⁺ on day 1 ($n = 6$) prevented MPP⁺-induced decrease of DA release (one-way ANOVA, followed by Fisher's PLSD *post hoc* test: **$P < 0.01$ MPP⁺/MPP⁺ vs. aCSF/MPP⁺, #$P < 0.05$ 7-NI+MPP⁺/ MPP⁺ vs. MPP⁺/MPP⁺).

DISCUSSION

Our results have shown that the inhibition of the NO system by pretreatment with 7-NI can have a protective effect against neuronal damage induced by intrastriatal infusion of MPP^+ by a microdialysis approach in conscious rats. MPP^+ used in this study was found to induce degeneration of nigrostriatal DA-containing neurons; the toxin perfused into the striatum is accumulated by DAergic terminals and then retrogradely transported in the cell bodies of DAergic neurons, causing cell degeneration and loss.[18–20] MPP^+ apparently causes a defect of complex I of the mitochondrial respiratory chain. The interruption of ATP supply increases ROS production and consequently causes nigral cell death in a way similar to that found in PD.[20–22]

Under our experimental conditions, short perfusion of MPP^+ induced a comparable impairment of DAergic striatal nerve terminals, associated with a massive increase in DA efflux 40 min after toxin injection, on day 1. A second challenge with MPP^+, 24 h later, caused a limited output of extracellular DA in MPP^+-lesioned rats, and this was considered an index of the damage produced by the neurotoxins.[14–16] 7-NI, a potent nNOS inhibitor, given 1 h before perfusion with the neurotoxins, on day 1, partially restored the cell's ability to release DA after the second MPP^+ challenge, showing a protective effect against MPP^+ toxic effects on DAergic neurons.

Although the etiology of PD is complex, a significant body of data from clinical and experimental models suggests a role for oxidative stress as a causative agent inducing DA neurodegeneration.[1,6,23] Dopamine catabolism by monoamine oxidase (MAO) induces the formation of hydrogen peroxide, thus rendering DA-containing neurons particularly liable to oxidative stress.[5,8,24] Furthermore, oxidation of DA by enzymatic and nonenzymatic mechanisms produces neuromelanin, which potentiates hydroxyl radical formation when combined with iron.[5] Increased nigral DA metabolism is associated with the production of hydrogen peroxide, which, together with iron, may be converted into ·OH, reacting very rapidly with almost every molecule found in living cells, including DNA, membrane lipids, and amino acids.[6,20,25] The increased DA turnover could itself enhance basal production of hydrogen peroxide and cause a depletion of reduced glutathione (GSH) stores, leading to further overproduction of toxic hydroxyl radicals, as a consequence of impaired GSH scavenging activity. Thus, PD etiology could be explained by a genetic susceptibility to environmental or endogenous agents, leading to oxidative damage in a neuronal population that is naturally under oxidative stress.[20]

The role of oxidative stress in the pathogenesis of MPTP/MPP^+-induced DAergic degeneration, has been suggested.[26–32] Numerous studies have proposed that nNOS inhibitors, including 7-NI, may reduce DAergic neuronal degeneration, both *in vitro* and *in vivo* through antioxidative mechanisms.[9–13] Our study showed that 7-NI almost completely counteracted the neurotoxicity induced by MPP^+ perfusion in the rat striatum, as indicated by electrochemical measurements of DA. Our data suggest that the neuroprotective effect of 7-NI against MPP^+-induced DA striatal depletion is probably due to a block in the rise of the toxic peroxynitrite ($ONOO^-$) produced by the combination of NO and $\cdot OH$ induced by MPP^+, as has been shown by previous studies.[12,33] Peroxynitrite is a highly reactive molecule, a potent oxidizing agent known to initiate lipid peroxidation in biological membranes, hydroxylation, and nitration of aromatic amino acid residues, and sulfhydryl oxidation of proteins.[34-36]

Nevertheless, 7-NI in our study did not modify extracellular DA output after the first perfusions with MPP^+, suggesting that it did not affect DA uptake or metabolism, a piece of evidence in contrast with findings in other studies.[37,38] Furthermore, it has been shown that 7-NI could act as a competitive inhibitor of MAO type B as well, an effect that contributes to the 7-NI protection against MPTP toxicity.[39] Indeed, MAO-B catalyzes the metabolic activation of MPTP to MPP^+ that is ultimately responsible for neurotoxicity.[40,41] Under our conditions this effect might be totally ruled out, having used the MPP^+ ion directly.

In conclusion, this study shows a protective effect of 7-NI on MPP^+-induced neurodegeneration, following *in vivo* microdialytic perfusion in conscious rats. These results therefore provide further evidence that the inhibition of the NO system may be useful for the treatment of neurodegenerative diseases such as PD.

ACKNOWLEDGMENTS

We want to thank Ms. Samantha Austen for the English revision of the manuscript.

REFERENCES

1. JELLINGER, K. 1989. Pathology of Parkinson's Disease. *In* Handbook of Experimental Pharmacology. D.B. Calne, Ed.: Vol. 8: 47–112. Springer, Berlin.
2. SCHERMAN, D. *et al.* 1989. Striatal dopamine deficiency in Parkinson's disease: role of aging. Ann. Neurol. **26:** 551–557.
3. DI GIOVANNI, G. *et al.* 2007. Biochemical and therapeutic effects of antioxidants in the treatment of Parkinson's disease. *In* The Basal Ganglia Pathophysiology: Recent Advances. G. Di Giovanni, Ed.: Research Signpost, India. In press.
4. VON BOHLEN UND HALBACH, O., A. SCHOBER & K. KRIEGLSTEIN. 2004. Genes, proteins, and neurotoxins involved in Parkinson's disease. Prog. Neurobiol. **73:** 151–177.
5. JENNER, P. *et al.* 1992. Oxidative stress as a cause of nigral cell death in Parkinson's disease and incidental Lewy body disease. The Royal Kings and Queens Parkinson's Disease Research Group. Ann. Neurol. **32:** S82–S87.
6. SIMONIAN, N.A. & J.T. COYLE. 1996. Oxidative stress in neurodegenerative diseases. Annu. Rev. Pharmacol. Toxicol. **36:** 83–106.
7. MARK, R.J. *et al.* 1997. A role for 4-hydroxynonenal, an aldehydic product of lipid peroxidation, in disruption of ion homeostasis and neuronal death induced by amyloid beta-peptide. J. Neurochem. **68:** 255–264.

8. DEXTER, D.T. *et al.* 1991. Alterations in the levels of iron, ferritin and other trace metals in Parkinson's disease and other neurodegenerative diseases affecting the basal ganglia. Brain **114:** 1953–1975.

9. WATANABE, H. *et al.* 2004. Protective effects of neuronal nitric oxide synthase inhibitor in mouse brain against MPTP neurotoxicity: an immunohistological study. Eur. Neuropsychopharmacol. **14:** 93–104.

10. KUROSAKI, R. *et al.* 2002. Role of nitric oxide synthase against MPTP neurotoxicity in mice. Neurol. Res. **24:** 655–662.

11. PRZEDBORSKI, S. *et al.* 1996. Role of neuronal nitric oxide in 1-methyl-4-phenyl-1,2,3,6-tetrahydropyridine (MPTP)-induced dopaminergic neurotoxicity. Proc. Natl. Acad. Sci. **93:** 4565–4571.

12. SCHULZ, J.B. *et al.* 1995. Inhibition of neuronal nitric oxide synthase by 7-nitroindazole protects against MPTP-induced neurotoxicity in mice. J. Neurochem. **64:** 936–939.

13. BARC, S. *et al.* 2001. Impairment of the neuronal dopamine transporter activity in MPP(+)-treated rat was not prevented by treatments with nitric oxide synthase or poly(ADP-ribose) polymerase inhibitors. Neurosci. Lett. **314:** 82–86.

14. ROLLEMA, H. *et al.* 1986. Brain dialysis in conscious rats reveals an instantaneous massive release of striatal dopamine in response to MPP$^+$. Eur. J. Pharmacol. **126:** 345–346.

15. SANTIAGO, M., A. MACHADO & J. CANO. 2001. Validity of a quantitative technique to study striatal dopaminergic neurodegeneration by *in vivo* microdialysis. J. Neurosci. Methods **108:** 181–187.

16. DI MATTEO, V. *et al.* 2006. Aspirin protects striatal dopaminergic neurons from neurotoxin-induced degeneration: an *in vivo* microdialysis study. Brain Res. **1095:** 167–177.

17. DI GIOVANNI, G. *et al.* 2003. Nitric oxide modulates striatal neuronal activity via soluble guanylyl cyclase: an *in vivo* microiontophoretic study in rats. Synapse **48:** 100–107.

18. GLINKA, Y., M. GASSEN & M.B.H. YOUDIM. 1997. Mechanism of 6-hydroxydopamine neurotoxicity. J. Neural. Transm. **50:** 55–66.

19. LOTHARIUS, J., L.L. DUGAN & K.L. O'MALLEY. 1999. Distinct mechanisms underlie neurotoxin-mediated cell death in cultured dopaminergic neurons. J. Neurosci. **19:** 1284–1293.

20. BLUM, D. *et al.* 2001. Molecular pathways involved in the neurotoxicity of 6-OHDA, dopamine and MPTP: contribution to the apoptotic theory in Parkinson's disease. Prog. Neurobiol. **65:** 135–172.

21. NICKLAS, W.J., I. VYAS & R.E. HEIKKILA. 1985. Inhibition of NADH-linked oxidation in brain mitochondria by 1-methyl-4-phenyl-pyridine, a metabolite of the neurotoxin, 1-methyl-4-phenyl-1,2,5,6-tetrahydropyridine. Life Sci. **36:** 2503–2508.

22. PRZEDBORSKI, S. & M. VILA. 2001. MPTP: a review of its mechanisms of neurotoxicity. Clin. Neurosci. Res. **1:** 407–418.

23. HORNYKIEWICZ, O. 1989. Ageing and neurotoxins as causative factors in idiopathic Parkinson's disease—a critical analysis of the neurochemical evidence. Prog. Neuropsychopharmacol. Biol. Psychiatry **13:** 319–328.

24. ZIGMOND, M.J., T.G. HASTINGS & R.G. PEREZ. 2002. Increased dopamine turnover after partial loss of dopaminergic neurons: compensation or toxicity? Parkinsonism Relat. Disorders **8:** 389–393.

25. LANG, A.E. & A.M. LOZANO. 1998. Parkinson's disease: first of two parts. New Engl. J. Med. **339:** 1044–1053.

26. AUBIN, N. *et al.* 1998. Aspirin and salicylate protect against MPTP-induced dopamine depletion in mice. J. Neurochem. **71:** 1635–1642.
27. OBATA, T. 1999. Reserpine prevents hydroxyl radical formation by MPP+ in rat striatum. Brain Res. **828:** 68–73.
28. MOHANAKUMAR, K.P., D. MURALIKRISHNAN & B. THOMAS. 2000. Neuroprotection by sodium salicylate against 1-methyl-4-phenyl-1,2,3,6-tetrahydropyridine-induced neurotoxicity. Brain Res. **864:** 281–290.
29. OBATA, T. & S. KUBOTA. 2001. Protective effect of tamoxifen on 1-methyl-4-phenylpyridine-induced hydroxyl radical generation in the rat striatum. Neurosci. Lett. **308:** 87–90.
30. TEISMANN, P. & B. FERGER. 2001. Inhibition of the cyclooxygenase isoenzymes COX-1 and COX-2 provide neuroprotection in the MPTP-mouse model of Parkinson's disease. Synapse **39:** 167–174.
31. SAIRAM, K. *et al.* 2003. Non-steroidal anti-inflammatory drug sodium salicylate, but not diclofenac or celecoxib, protects against 1-methyl-4-phenyl pyridinium-induced dopaminergic neurotoxicity in rats. Brain Res. **966:** 245–252.
32. MAHARAJ, D.S. *et al.* 2004. Acetaminophen and aspirin inhibit superoxide anion generation and lipid peroxidation, and protect against 1-methyl-4-phenyl pyridinium-induced dopaminergic neurotoxicity in rats. Neurochem. Int. **44:** 355–360.
33. MATTHEWS, R.T., L. YANG & M.F. BEAL. 1997. S-methylthiocitrulline, a neuronal nitric oxide synthase inhibitor, protects against malonate and MPTP neurotoxicity. Exp. Neurol. **143:** 282–286.
34. BECKMAN, J.S. 1991. The double-edged role of nitric oxide in brain function and superoxide-mediated injury. J. Dev. Physiol. **15:** 53–59.
35. BECKMAN, J.S. *et al.* 1992. Kinetics of superoxide dismutase- and iron-catalyzed nitration of phenolics by peroxynitrite. Arch. Biochem. Biophys. **198:** 438–445.
36. SZABO, C. & V.L. DAWSON. 1998. Role of poly(ADP-ribose) synthetase in inflammation and ischaemia-reperfusion. Trends Pharmacol. Sci. **19:** 287–298.
37. KISS, J.P., G. ZSILLA & E.S. VIZI. 2004. Inhibitory effect of nitric oxide on dopamine transporters: interneuronal communication without receptors. Neurochem. Int. **45:** 485–489.
38. VOLZ, T.J. & J.O. SCHENK. 2004. L-arginine increases dopamine transporter activity in rat striatum via a nitric oxide synthase-dependent mechanism. Synapse **54:** 173–182.
39. CASTAGNOLI, K. *et al.* 1997. The neuronal nitric oxide synthase inhibitor 7-nitroindazole also inhibits the monoamine oxidase-B-catalyzed oxidation of 1-methyl-4-phenyl-1,2,3,6-tetrahydropyridine. Chem. Res. Toxicol. **10:** 364–368.
40. CHIBA, K., A. TREVOR & N. CASTAGNOLI JR. 1984. Metabolism of the neurotoxic tertiary amine, MPTP, by brain monoamine oxidase. Biochem. Biophys. Res. Commun. **120:** 574–578.
41. MARKEY, S.P. *et al.* 1984. Intraneuronal generation of a pyridinium metabolite may cause drug-induced parkinsonism. Nature **311:** 464–467.

Age-Related Inflammatory Diseases

Role of Genetics and Gender in the Pathophysiology of Alzheimer's Disease

GIUSEPPINA CANDORE,[a] CARMELA R. BALISTRERI,[a]
MARIA P. GRIMALDI,[a] SONYA VASTO,[a] FLORINDA LISTÌ,[a]
MARTINA CHIAPPELLI,[a,b] FEDERICO LICASTRO,[b] DOMENICO LIO,[a]
AND CALOGERO CARUSO[a]

[a]*Gruppo di Studio sull' Immunosenescenza, Dipartimento di Biopatologia e
Metodologie Biomediche, Università di Palermo, Palermo 90134, Italy*

[b]*Dipartimento di Patologia Sperimentale, Università di Bologna, Italy*

ABSTRACT: Alzheimer's disease (AD) is a heterogeneous and progressive
neurodegenerative disease which in Western societies mainly accounts
for clinical dementia. A high proportion of women are affected by this
disease, especially at a very advanced age, which might to a large extent be associated with the fact that women live longer. However, some
studies suggest that incidence rates may be really increased in women.
For this reason the influence of estrogens on the brain and the decrease
of it during menopause are of special interest. After menopause, circulating levels of estrogens markedly decline, influencing several brain
processes predicted to influence AD risk. The control of estrogens on
oxidative stress, inflammation, and the cerebral vasculature might also
be expected to increase AD risk. During the Women's Health Initiative
Memory Study—a randomized, placebo-controlled trial of women 65–
79 years of age—oral estrogen plus progestin was seen to double the rate
of developing dementia, with risk appearing soon after the treatment
was initiated. On the basis of current evidence, hormone therapy (HT)
is thus not indicated for the prevention of AD. Inflammation clearly occurs in pathologically vulnerable regions of the AD brain and the search
for genetic factors influencing the pathogenesis of AD has led to the
identification of numerous gene polymorphisms that act as susceptibility modifiers. Accordingly, several reports have indicated that the risk of
AD is substantially influenced by several genetic polymorphisms in the
promoter region, or other untranslated regions, of genes encoding inflammatory mediators. Here we review several data suggesting that inflammatory genetic variation may contribute to higher AD susceptibility in
women too. All together this information may represent the basis both for

Address for correspondence: Giuseppina Candore, Ph.D., Gruppo di Studio sull'Immunosenescenza,
Dipartimento di Biopatologia e Metodologie Biomediche, Corso Tukory 211, 90134 Palermo, Italy.
Voice: +39-09-1655-5932; fax: +39-09-1655-5933.
  e-mail: gcandore@unipa.it

Ann. N.Y. Acad. Sci. 1089: 472–486 (2006). © 2006 New York Academy of Sciences.
doi: 10.1196/annals.1386.008

future recognition of individuals at risk as well as for a pharmacogenomic approach in achieving drug responsiveness.

KEYWORDS: Alzheimer's disease; genetics; inflammation; estrogens; CD14; toll-like receptors; cyclooxygenases; lipoxygenases

INTRODUCTION

Alzheimer's disease (AD) is a progressive neurodegenerative disease, which in Western societies accounts for the majority of cases of clinical senile dementia.[1,2] AD is characterized by global cognitive dysfunction, especially memory loss, behavior or personality changes, and impairments in the performance of activities of daily living. Neuropathological hallmarks of AD are neuritic plaques and neurofibrillary tangles.[3,4] Neuritic plaques are extracellular deposits of the beta-amyloid peptide (Aβ); these plaques are usually in a milieu of reactive astrocytes, activated microglia, degenerating axons, and dendrites.[5] Neurofibrillary tangles are intracellular depositions of hyperphosphorylated degenerate filaments, which result from aggregations of the microtubular protein tau, frequently conjugated with ubiquitin.[3,5] As these cellular changes progress, brain atrophy and neuronal loss in the hippocampus, temporal cortex, and limbic area are observed.[6] β-amyloid peptides are derived from proteolytic activity of proteinases, namely β- and γ-secretases, on amyloid precursor protein (APP).[7] The APP is a trans-membrane glycoprotein ubiquitously expressed (it is also present on platelets), produced by the endoplasmatic reticulum and mainly involved in neuronal and dendritic growth and synapse formation. Actually, the enzyme α-secretase, cutting the N-terminal of Aβ, protects it from amyloidogenic changes, whereas the enzyme β-secretase, by cutting the N-terminal of Aβ, induces conformational changes in the peptide. The latter is the substrate of γ-secretase, which influences the appearance of $A\beta_{42}$ amyloid protein. There is evidence that presenilins (PS1 and PS2) function as γ-secretase enzymes, which are responsible for the final proteolytic cleavage of APP, resulting in the production of β-amyloid peptides.[8] The wild-type presenilins predominantly produce short peptides ($A\beta_{1-40}$). The peptide $A\beta_{40}$, which constitutes more the 90% of the secreted Aβ protein, is more soluble and less amyloidogenic compared to the $A\beta_{42}$ isoform. Presenilin mutations, on the other hand, cause an increased production of longer peptides ($A\beta_{1-42}$). The great part of amyloid tissue is constituted by $A\beta_{42}$ isoform, which is highly amyloidogenic. This peptide is highly neurotoxic especially on account of the self-aggregation and its capacity to form insoluble plaques either *in vitro* or *in vivo*.[9,10]

In fewer than 1% of all cases of AD, there are causative single gene mutations in one of the three major genes for APP, PS1, or PS2, or in still unknown genes. Mutations in these genes are linked to autosomal dominant early-onset familial AD. Late-onset AD (that is, >95% of all cases of AD) manifests above the age of 65 years with an aging-dependent exponentially growing incidence.[4,7–10] In Europe, AD accounts for 54% of the overall forms of dementia, although the prevalence among people above 65 years of age seems higher with a score of 4.4%. The prevalence of this disease is age-dependent and shows higher incidence in women. The values range from 1.1% among women from 65 to 69 years of age to 36% for women above 95 years of age, while the incidence in males of these ages ranges from 2.2% to 31.6%.[11]

Age is the first and foremost risk factor in AD. The prevalence of AD is approximately 1% between 65 and 69 years and is higher than 60% in individuals over 80–85 years of age.[12] Although the mean age of AD onset is around 80 years, early-onset disease, defined arbitrarily as the illness occurring before the age of 60 years, can occur, although is rare. Thus, early-onset cases make up about 6–7% of all cases of AD. A good number of early-onset cases are familial, with an autosomal dominant pattern of inheritance and high penetrance. AD may not be an inevitable accompaniment of the aging process, but a disease with significant genetic roots; genetics is important not only in predicting susceptibility, but also age of onset in the elderly.[4,5,10]

Another risk factor is female gender; in fact, as discussed above, AD is more common among women than men by a ratio of 1.2 to 1.5, in large part due to longevity and survival differences favoring women, but some studies suggest that incidence rates may be indeed increased for women.[13–15] A possible factor influencing AD incidence in women is the loss of ovarian estrogen production after menopause, because estrogens might be involved in AD pathophysiology (see next paragraph).

ROLE OF ESTROGENS

In recent years, accumulated evidence shows that estrogens also play very important roles in various nonreproductive organs throughout the body, including the central nervous system (CNS).[16] Cumulative evidence from basic science and clinical research suggests that estrogens play a significant neuromodulatory and neuroprotective role in the brain, which underlies their ability to ameliorate symptoms associated with Parkinson's disease and tardive dyskinesia[17–19] and decrease the incidence and delay the onset of AD.[20–22] Subsets of neurons possess intraneuronal receptors for estrogen.[23] The complex of estrogens and its receptor translocates into the cell nucleus, where it regulates transcription of target genes. Through interactions with membrane receptor, estrogens also influence neuronal functions in ways that do not require genomic interactions.[24] A number of estrogen actions have the potential to affect AD incidence or AD symptoms.[25] Estrogens, for example, are neuroprotective against a variety of experimental insults, including oxidative stress, excitatory neurotoxicity, and ischemia;[26,27] they can promote the growth of nerve processes and modulate synaptic plasticity.[28,29] Other putatively benefical actions include increase of cerebral blood flow, enhancing glucose transport into the brain and reductions in β-amyloid formation.[30–32] The cessation of ovarian estrogen production in postmenopausal women might facilitate Aβ deposition by increasing the local concentrations of Aβ in brain. In addition, 17 beta-estradiol treatment is associated with diminution of brain Aβ levels, suggesting that modulation of Aβ metabolism may be one of the ways by which estrogen replacement therapy might prevent or delay the onset of AD or both in postmenopausal women.[32] However, some estrogen actions might be harmful. Proinflammatory effects could be deleterious[33] and prothrombotic properties of some estrogens could adversely affect the cerebral vasculature.[34]

With the loss of ovarian estrogen production after menopause, estrogen-containing hormone therapy (HT) might be expected to influence the risk of AD.[15] The relation between HT and AD risk has been the focus of a number of observational studies. Although observational findings generally support the hypothesis that HT reduces AD risk, these results are seemingly in contrast with conclusions from Women's Health Initiative Memory Study (WHIMS), a large experimental study in the United States designed to assess cognitive consequences of HT.[35–38] In that study, in the Estrogen + Progestin trial, the hazard ratio (a measure of relative risk) for dementia was doubled for women assigned to active treatment compared with controls. In the estrogen-alone trial, the hazard ratio was also higher for women allocated to the estrogen group, although the increase was not statistically significant. There are several possibilities for the divergent findings and discrepant conclusions between results of the WHIMS trial and those of observational studies. Bias and unrecognized confounding in observational research are the leading candidates for the discrepant results; studies are also distinguished by differences in outcome measures, HT formulations, prevalence of menopausal symptoms among study participants, and participant age; finally, there is the timing of HT initiation in relation to menopause: "the critical window hypothesis." Better human studies are essential before this important issue can be settled for the group of younger perimenopausal and postmenopausal women most likely to consider HT in the future.[15]

On the other hand, it is known that there is a sexual dimorphism in the immune response. Males of many species are more susceptible than females to infections caused by parasites, fungi, bacteria, and viruses. One proximate cause of sex differences in infection is differences in endocrine–immune interactions. Specifically, males may be more susceptible to infection than females because sex steroids, specifically androgens in males and estrogens in females, modulate several aspects of host immunity.[33,39,40] So the increased prevalence of AD in women might be also linked to the long-life premenopausal effect of estrogens on immune-inflammatory responses involved in AD. The process of the disease requires, in fact, a long time to develop, as demonstrated by the increased incidence of AD in subjects exposed to head trauma 40 years before the disease's occurrence.[41]

ROLE OF INFLAMMATION

The first hint that inflammation plays a part in AD emerged when researchers noted that patients with rheumatoid arthritis had an unusually low incidence of the neurodegenerative disease.[42] Further studies suggested that nonsteroidal anti-inflammatory drugs, used in arthritis patients, were the key of the protective effect. There are a lot of published epidemiological studies demonstrating that people who are known to be taking anti-inflammatory drugs considerably reduce their odds of developing AD, and population studies have confirmed this negative association.[43–45] Note that anti-inflammatory drugs do not only inhibit ciclo-oxygenase, but also activate the receptor PPARγ (peroxisome proliferator–activated receptor γ), which is a transcription factor that works by shutting down the expression of proinflammatory genes in mononucleate phagocyte.[46] The long-term prospective association between dementia and the well-known inflammation marker high-sensitivity C-reactive protein (CRP) was evaluated in a cohort of Japanese American men who were seen in the second examination of the Honolulu Heart Program (1968–1970) and who were subsequently re-examined 25 years later for dementia in the Honolulu-Asia Aging Study (1991–1996). In a random subsample of 1,050 Honolulu-Asia Aging Study cases and noncases, high-sensitivity CRP concentrations were measured from serum taken at the second examination; dementia was assessed in a clinical examination that included neuroimaging and neuropsychological testing and was evaluated using international criteria. Compared with men in the lowest quartile (<0.34 mg/L) of high-sensitivity CRP, men in the upper three quartiles had a threefold significantly increased risk for all dementias combined, AD, and vascular dementia.[47] These data are in agreement with the hypothesis that long-life pathogen burden is involved in the pathophysiology of age-related diseases (see next paragraph).[48] On the whole, these data clearly demonstrate the importance of proinflammatory phenotype in the occurrence of AD. Scientists do not refer to the acute inflammation, that is, increased blood flow and entry of white blood cells into tissue in response to injury or infection, resulting in swelling, redness, and pain, but to chronic inflammation. Reduced to its simplest term, inflammation is a teleonomic response to eliminate the initial cause of cell injury as well as the necrotic cells and tissues resulting from the original insult. If tissue health is not restored or in response to stable low-grade irritation (as in AD in response to Aβ deposition), inflammation becomes a chronic condition that continuously erodes the surrounding tissues. In fact, in chronic inflammatory immune responses, tissue injury and healing proceed simultaneously. The lateral damage caused by this type of inflammation usually accumulates slowly, sometimes asymptomatically for years, and can lead to severe tissue deterioration. A characteristic feature of chronic inflamed tissues is the presence of an increased number of monocytes, as well as monocyte-derived tissue macrophages, that is, microglial cells in the brain.[49]

Immunohistochemical studies have shown that the plaques and tangles of AD are heavily infiltrated with activated glial cells and inflammatory factors, such as cytokines, chemokines, complement components, and acute-phase proteins, colocalize as secondary components in senile plaques or are overproduced in AD brains.[50] Activated glial cells surround the depositions of amyloid attempting to phagocytose and degrade amyloid component.[42,51] Microglial cells also recruit astrocytes, which become activated. Following activation, both cell types produce acute-phase proteins, complement components, prostaglandins (PGs), and cytokines.[52,53] Actually, the microglial cell is a high producer of free radicals and the generation of reactive oxygen species contributes to damage neurons. Because Aβ represents pathogenetic molecules, the innate immune system is clearly making an initial attempt to protect the brain by clearing these potentially toxic products.[42] The hypothesis is that the intractable nature of the plaques and tangles stimulates a chronic inflammatory reaction to clear this debris. However, chronic inflammation can be injurious to host tissue, as is clearly illustrated in rheumatoid arthritis (see also above). Besides, the brain might be particularly vulnerable because neurons are postmitotic and cannot be replaced if lost. Chronically activated microglia and astrocytes can kill adjacent neurons by the release of highly toxic products such as reactive oxygen intermediates, nitric oxide, proteolytic enzymes, complement factors, or excitatory amino acids. Proinflammatory cytokines seem to be involved in APP metabolism and in the Aβ peptide production. In addition, they enhance Aβ production and inhibit APP production on the whole and the soluble fraction of APP with neuronal protective effect. Acute-phase proteins also play a role during chronic inflammation of the brain in AD because they bind amyloid and promote fibrillar formation and deposition.[50,54–56]

ROLE OF GENETICS OF INFLAMMATION

A body of evidence has accumulated showing that gene variants in inflammatory genes may modulate the development and the clinical history of chronic inflammatory disease. Indeed, the search for genetic factors influencing the pathogenesis of AD has lead to the identification of numerous gene polymorphisms that act as susceptibility modifiers.[56–58] As such, they appear to modify the risk of developing AD, but they are neither necessary nor sufficient to cause the disease. Accordingly, several reports have appeared indicating that the risk of AD is substantially influenced by several polymorphisms in the promoter region, and other untranslated regions, of genes encoding inflammatory mediators.[54,59–62] Alleles that favor increased expression of the inflammatory mediators or decreased expression of anti-inflammatory mediators are more frequent in patients with AD than in controls.[54,59,63] The polymorphisms are fairly common in the general population, so there is a strong likelihood that any given individual will inherit one or more of the high-risk alleles.[56–58,63,64]

In particular, proinflammatory cytokines are believed to play a pathogenetic role in age-related diseases, and genetic variations located within their promoter regions (mostly single nucleotide polymorphisms [SNPs]) have been shown to influence the susceptibility to age-related diseases by increasing gene transcription and therefore cytokine production.[48,63] Recently, we performed a series of meta-analysis on some cytokine polymorphisms and AD (our unpublished observations). We examined the role of the following functional single nucleotide polymorphisms IL-1β –511, IL-1β +3953, IL-6 –174, IL-10 –1082. Concerning IL-1β –511 SNP, the genotype TT is associated with early-onset AD; the same result is obtained with the genotype TT of an IL-1β +3953 SNP, whereas meta-analysis on IL-6 –174 SNP demonstrated no significant association with AD risk. Finally, meta-analysis on IL-10 gene (anti-inflammatory) showed that the –1082GG genotype, associated with an increased production of IL-10, is a protective factor for AD. So, cytokine genes play a relevant role in AD pathophysiology (FIG. 1).

Concerning other genes of innate immunity, a key role should be played by the toll-like receptor (TLR)-4, CD14, cyclooxygenase (COX) and lipoxygenase (LOX) genes (FIG. 1). As reported by some recent studies, the microglial cell

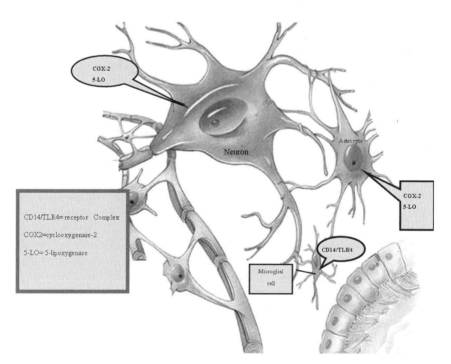

FIGURE 1. Involvement of inflammatory molecules in pathophysiology of AD.

activation has a fundamental role in the inflammatory pathogenesis of AD,[65] as stated by the amyloid cascade/neuroinflammation hypothesis.[65–68] The former is responsible for the production of the neurotoxic substances, such as reactive oxygen and nitrogen species, proinflammatory cytokines, complement proteins, and other inflammatory mediators that bring important neurodegenerative changes.[66,67,69–71] Some studies have suggested that activation of microglial cells may be induced throughout the binding of Aβ peptides. Several membrane proteins expressed on microglial cells seem to be implicated in Aβ peptide binding. In particular, Fassenbender *et al.*[72] have demonstrated that the CD14/TLR4 receptor complex binds highly hydrophobic Aβ peptide aggregates, suggesting the production of neurotoxic substances.[68,71–75] A further, not mutually, alternative explanation on the key role of microglial activation may be related to the role of CD14/TLR4 as LPS receptor. In fact, some studies have linked infections to other relevant age-related inflammatory diseases such as atherosclerosis because the total burden of infections at various sites may affect the progression of atherosclerosis and elicit clinical symptoms. This can be due to remote signaling by inflammatory mediators that activate immune cells in the atherosclerotic plaques through CD14 TLR4 activation.[66,74,75] So it should to be biologically possible that functional variation in the TLR4 and CD14 genes might influence the susceptibility to sporadic AD. This might be the case for the allelic variants of CD14 and TLR4 genes. In particular, a common adenine-to-guanine substitution in TLR4 gene, 896 nucleotides downstream of the transcription start site (+896), causes the replacement of an aspartic acid residue by a glycine at amino acid 299 (Asp299Gly). This missense polymorphism has recently generated great interest as it leads to an attenuated efficacy of LPS signaling and a reduced capacity to elicit inflammation.[76] The carriage of at least one minor 299Gly allele is associated with a diminished risk of vascular events,[75,77] as well as successful aging in humans.[78,79] As regards the CD14 gene, a common biallelic (C/T) polymorphism at position −260 has been described, and several recent reports indicate that CD14 T/T genotype is a risk factor for some clinical complications of atherosclerosis.[80,81]

As previously stated, there are a lot of published epidemiological studies demonstrating that people who are known to be taking anti-inflammatory drugs considerably reduce their odds of developing AD and population studies have confirmed this negative association.[43–45] The anti-inflammatory drugs inhibit the cyclooxygenases, which are the key enzymes in the conversion of arachidonic acid to different bioactive lipid moieties, collectively called PGs. In the early 1990s, it was shown that there are at least two isoforms of this enzyme, COX-1 and COX-2, and that the latter is responsible for the formation of PGs at the site of inflammation.[82] COXs play a key role in the pathophysiological process of inflammatory diseases. The COX2 enzyme has been detected in different cell types of the CNS, but its expression seems to be primarily neuronal.[83–85] Reports about astrocytes are conflicting. Moreover in the brain of the patient with AD its expression correlates with amyloid plaque density and neurofibrillary tangles. In fact, a study has demonstrated that an increase in neuronal expression of COX-2 is implied in the progression of ischemic brain damage.[86] The gene for COX-2 has been mapped to 1q25, which is located between 1q23 and 1q31, two regions to which genetic linkage to AD has been reported.[84–86] Recently a number of polymorphisms have been described in the promoter region of the COX-2 gene that likely regulate its transcription; but only one polymorphism, located at position −765, has been shown to be functional.[87,88] It has shown that the polymorphism −765C/G is associated with a low promoter activity and decreased inflammatory molecules.[89]

As regards lipoxygenases, they are a family of lipid-peroxidizing enzymes that insert molecular oxygen into free as well as esterified polyunsaturated fatty acids.[90] The cysteinyl-leukotrienes (cys-LTs) are lipid mediators, generated by the 5-lipoxygenase (5-LO) pathway. This enzyme has been described in neurons and also in some glial cells throughout the cerebrum, basal ganglia, and hippocampus. Compared with controls, a significant increase of LTs was observed in cerebrospinal fluid from AD and mild cognitive impairment, which correlated with lipid peroxidation and tau protein levels. So the activation of this enzyme occurs early in the course of AD, before the onset of overt dementia, thereby implicating LOX-mediated lipid peroxidation in the pathogenesis of AD.[91] Accordingly, recent studies have shown that LOX polymorphisms involved in a decreased expression of LOX-5 are less represented in AD patients and in patients affected by more severe atherosclerosis.[92–95] It has been proposed that an overexpressed 5-LOX gene could significantly increase the brain's vulnerability to neurodegeneration.[96] The expression of this gene is diminished in individuals with a mutation in the core promoter of the gene 5-LOX (on chromosome 10q11.2). Hence, it has been hypothesized[97] that 5-LOX promoter polymorphism could affect the onset of AD and/or influence the response of Alzheimer's patients to treatment with anti-inflammatory 5-LOX inhibitors.

Our preliminary results obtained in patients and controls from northern Italy demonstrate that polymorphisms of these inflammatory molecules are associated with AD (TABLE 1). As shown in the table, in some studies these associations are observed only in male's or only in females.

TABLE 1. Studies on the association of the proinflammatory gene polymorphisms in male and female AD patients and age-related controls from northern Italy

Gene polymorphisms	Significance		
	Men + Women	Men	Women
CD14 −C260T	Yes	No	No
TLR4 +A896G	Yes	No	Yes
5LOX −G1761A	Yes	No	No
COX-2 −G765C	Yes	Yes	No

NOTE: Unpublished observations.

CONCLUSIONS

AD is a multifactorial disease—that is, one cause is not sufficient for the disease to develop—and therefore AD might be the result of a cumulative effect which contributes with different timing to achieve a threshold where the chance for developing the disease is very high. Difference in inflammatory status can contribute to draw a risk phenotype. Therefore, these studies are meant to detect and utilize a risk profile that allows early identification of individuals susceptible to disease as well as pharmacogenomic design of the right dose for a desired effect in age-related diseases such as AD. It is intriguing that in some studies, independently of the sample size, the significance of some polymorphisms was found to be different in men and women. Further studies are necessary to demonstrate that this is not due to chance, but rather to an interaction between polymorphisms and gender (see above the sexual dimorphism in immune response).

The study of novel drugs that selectively interfere with the sequence of events triggered by the genetic mechanism(s) underlying the inflammatory related disease may be a good example of how genotyping is incorporated into clinical drug therapy in order to bridge the gap between pharmacogenetic research and clinical application. Taking into account the immune-inflammatory genes we have reviewed in the present paper, we can formulate the following working hypothesis for the therapeutic treatment of subjects with severe risk factors for AD before the clinical appearance of the disease. In particular: (*a*) The occurrence of a high-risk genetic profile linked to the presence of high-responder alleles of proinflammatory cytokines or of low-responder alleles of anti-inflammatory cytokines might suggest the treatment with biologics as monoclonal antibodies directed versus the proinflammatory cytokines. (*b*) Subjects, carriers of high-responder TLR4 and CD14 polymorphisms, might be selected for a clinical trial of antibiotic prophylaxis for the prevention of AD because the long-life pathogen burden is thought to be involved in the pathophysiology of this disease. (*c*) Finally, concerning the COX and LOX genes, the presence of high-responder alleles suggests the possibility of preventive treatment with specific inhibitors of eicosanoids or their enzymes.

ACKNOWLEDGMENTS

This work was supported by grants from the Italian Ministry of Education, University and Research to G.C. and C.C. C.R.B., M.P.G., S.V., and M.C. are Ph.D. students in the pathobiology Ph.D. program (directed by Calogero Caruso) of Palermo University and this work is in partial fulfillment of the requirement for the Ph.D. The collaboration of Dr. Massimo Franceschi (Department of Neurology, Santa Maria Hospital, Castellanza [VA], Italy) in the selection of patients and controls is warmly acknowledged.

REFERENCES

1. HELMER, C. *et al.* 2001. Mortality with dementia: results from a French prospective community-based cohort. Am. J. Epidemiol. **154:** 642–648.

2. ARONSON, M.K. *et al.* 1991. Dementia. Age-dependent incidence, prevalence, and mortality in the old old. Arch. Intern. Med. **151:** 989–992.

3. TROJANOWSKI, J.Q. *et al.* 1997. Strategies for improving the postmortem neuropathological diagnosis of Alzheimer's disease. Neurobiol. Aging **18:** S75–S79.

4. SELKOE, D.J. 2001. Alzheimer's disease: genes, proteins, and therapy. Physiol. Rev. **81:** 741–766.

5. MAIMONE, D. *et al.* 2001. Pharmacogenomics of neurodegenerative diseases. Eur. J. Pharmacol. **413:** 11–29.

6. MCKHANN, G. *et al.* 1984. Clinical diagnosis of Alzheimer's disease: report of the NINCDS-ADRDA Work Group under the auspices of Department of Health And Human Services Task Force on Alzheimer's Disease. Neurology **34:** 939–944.

7. MATHISEN, P.M. 2003. Gene discovery and validation for neurodegenerative diseases. Drug Discov. Today **8:** 39–46.

8. WOLFE, M.S. 2001. Gamma-secretase inhibitors as molecular probes of presenilin function. J. Mol. Neurosci. **17:** 199–204.

9. ESLER, W.P. *et al.* 2001. A portrait of Alzheimer secretases–new features and familiar faces. Science **293:** 1449–1454.

10. HUTTON, M. *et al.* 1998. Genetics of Alzheimer's disease. Essays Biochem. **33:** 117–131.

11. Available at http://ec.europa.eu/health/ph_information/dissemination/diseases Accessed Oct. 23, 2006.

12. HY, L.X. *et al.* 2000. Prevalence of AD among whites: a summary by levels of severity. Neurology **55:** 198–204.

13. GAO, S. *et al.* 1998. The relationships between age, sex, and the incidence of dementia and Alzheimer disease: a meta-analysis. Arch. Gen. Psychiatry **55:** 809–815.

14. LAUNER, L.J. *et al.* 1999. Rates and risk factors for dementia and Alzheimer's disease: results from EURODEM pooled analyses. EURODEM Incidence Research Group and Work Groups. European Studies of Dementia. Neurology **52:** 78–84.

15. HENDERSON, V.W. 2006. Estrogen-containing hormone therapy and Alzheimer's disease risk: understanding discrepant inferences from observational and experimental research. Neuroscience **138:** 1031–1039.

16. AMANTEA, D. *et al.* 2005. From clinical evidence to molecular mechanisms underlying neuroprotection afforded by estrogens. Pharmacol. Res. **52:** 119–132.

17. BEDARD, P.J. *et al.* 1977. Estrogens and the extrapyramidal system. Lancet **2:** 1367–1368.

18. CYR, M. *et al.* 2002. Estrogenic modulation of brain activity: implications for schizophrenia and Parkinson's disease. J. Psychiatry Neurosci. **27:** 12–27.

19. CURRIE, L.J. *et al.* 2004. Postmenopausal estrogen use affects risk for Parkinson disease. Arch. Neurol. **61:** 886–888.

20. PAGANINI-HILL, A. *et al.* 1996. Estrogen replacement therapy and risk of Alzheimer disease. Arch. Intern. Med. **156:** 2213–2217.

21. HENDERSON, V.W. 1997. Estrogen replacement therapy for the prevention and treatment of Alzheimer's disease. CNS Drugs **8:** 343–351.

22. BRINTON, R.D. 2004. Impact of estrogen therapy on Alzheimer's: a fork in the road? CNS Drugs **18:** 405–422.

23. SHUGHRUE, P.J. *et al.* 1997. Comparative distribution of estrogen receptor-alpha and -beta mRNA in the rat central nervous system. J. Comp. Neurol. **388:** 507–525.
24. TORAN-ALLERAND, C.D. 2004. Minireview: a plethora of estrogen receptors in the brain: where will it end? Endocrinology **145:** 1069–1074.
25. HENDERSON, V.W. 2000. Hormone Therapy and the Brain: A Clinical Perspective on the Role of Estrogen. Parthenon Publishing. New York, NY.
26. ALKAYED, N.J. *et al.* 2000. Neuroprotective effects of female gonadal steroids in reproductively senescent female rats. Stroke **31:** 161–168.
27. GOODMAN, Y. *et al.* 1996. Estrogens attenuate and corticosterone exacerbates excitotoxicity, oxidative injury, and amyloid beta-peptide toxicity in hippocampal neurons. J. Neurochem. **66:** 1836–1844.
28. BRINTON, R.D. *et al.* 1997. 17 beta-estradiol enhances the outgrowth and survival of neocortical neurons in culture. Neurochem. Res. **22:** 1339–1351.
29. FOY, M.R. *et al.* 2000. Estrogen and neural plasticity. Curr. Direct. Psychol. Sci. **9:** 148–152.
30. OHKURA, T. *et al.* 1995. Estrogen increases cerebral and cerebellar blood flows in postmenopausal women. Menopause **2:** 13–18.
31. BISHOP, J. *et al.* Estradiol enhances brain glucose uptake in ovariectomized rats. Brain Res. Bull. **36:** 315–320.
32. PETANCESKA, S.S. *et al.* 2000. Ovariectomy and 17 beta-estradiol modulate the levels of Alzheimer's amyloid beta peptides in brain. Neurology **54:** 2212–2217.
33. CUSHMAN, M. *et al.* 1999. Effect of postmenopausal hormones on inflammation-sensitive proteins: the Postmenopausal Estrogen/Progestin Interventions (PEPI) Study. Circulation **100:** 717–722.
34. ROSENDAAL, F.R. *et al.* 2002. Female hormones and thrombosis. Arterioscler. Thromb. Vasc. Biol. **22:** 201–210.
35. HOGERVORST, E. *et al.* 2000. The nature of the effect of female gonadal hormone replacement therapy on cognitive function in post-menopausal women: a meta-analysis. Neuroscience **101:** 485–512.
36. YAFFE, K. *et al.* 1998. Estrogen therapy in postmenopausal women: effects on cognitive function and dementia. JAMA **279:** 688–695.
37. SHUMAKER, S.A. *et al.* 2003. Estrogen plus progestin and the incidence of dementia and mild cognitive impairment in postmenopausal women: the Women's Health Initiative Memory Study: a randomized controlled trial. JAMA **289:** 2651–2662.
38. SHUMAKER, S.A. *et al.* 2004. Women's Health Initiative Memory Study. Conjugated equine estrogens and incidence of probable dementia and mild cognitive impairment in postmenopausal women: Women's Health Initiative Memory Study. JAMA **291:** 2947–2958.
39. KLEIN, S.L. 2000. The effects of hormones on sex differences in infection: from genes to behavior. Neurosci. Biobehav. Rev. **24:** 627–638.
40. ROBERTS, C.W. *et al.* 2001. Sex-associated hormones and immunity to protozoan parasites. Clin. Microbiol. Rev. **14:** 476–488.
41. JELLINGER, K. 2004. Head injury and dementia. Curr. Opin. Neurol. **17:** 719–723.
42. McGEER, E.G. *et al.* 1998. The importance of inflammatory mechanisms in Alzheimer disease. Exp. Gerontol. **33:** 371–378.
43. BREITNER, J.C. *et al.* 1994. Inverse association of anti-inflammatory treatments and Alzheimer's disease: initial results of a co-twin control study. Neurology **44:** 227–232.
44. BREITNER, J.C. *et al.* 2001. Do nonsteroidal antiinflammatory drugs reduce the risk of Alzheimer's disease? N. Engl. J. Med. **345:** 1567–1568.

45. IN T'VELD, B.A. *et al.* 2001. Nonsteroidal antiinflammatory drugs and the risk of Alzheimer's disease. N. Engl. J. Med. **345:** 1515–1521.
46. BERNARDO, A. *et al.* 2005. Nuclear receptor peroxisome proliferator-activated receptor-gamma is activated in rat microglial cells by the anti-inflammatory drug HCT1026, a derivative of flurbiprofen. J. Neurochem. **92:** 895–903.
47. SCHMIDT, R. *et al.* 2002. Early inflammation and dementia: a 25-year follow-up of the Honolulu-Asia Aging Study. Ann. Neurol. **52:** 168–174.
48. CANDORE, G. *et al.* 2006. Biology of longevity: role of the innate immune system. Rejuvenation Res. **9:** 143–148.
49. MITCHELL, R.N. & R.S. COTRAN. 2003. Acute and chronic inflammation. *In* Robbins Basic Pathology. V. Kumar *et al.*, Eds.: 33–60. Saunders. Philadelphia, PA.
50. LICASTRO, F. *et al.* 2000. Increased plasma levels of interleukin-1, interleukin-6 and alpha-1-antichymotrypsin in patients with Alzheimer's disease: peripheral inflammation or signals from the brain? J. Neuroimmunol. **103:** 97–102.
51. MCGEER, P.L. *et al.* 1994. Neuroimmune mechanisms in Alzheimer disease pathogenesis. Alzheimer Dis. Assoc. Disord. **8:** 149–158.
52. MRAK, R.E. *et al.* 1995. Glial cytokines in Alzheimer's disease: review and pathogenic implications. Hum. Pathol. **26:** 816–823.
53. GRIFFIN, W.S. *et al.* 1998. Glial-neuronal interactions in Alzheimer's disease: the potential role of a "cytokine cycle" in disease progression. Brain Pathol. **8:** 65–72.
54. LICASTRO, F. *et al.* 2000. Gene polymorphism affecting alpha1-antichymotrypsin and interleukin-1 plasma levels increases Alzheimer's disease risk. Ann. Neurol. **48:** 388–391.
55. DE LUIGI, A. *et al.* 2001. Inflammatory markers in Alzheimer's disease and multi-infarct dementia. Mech. Ageing Dev. **122:** 1985–1995.
56. LICASTRO, F. *et al.* 2003. Brain immune responses cognitive decline and dementia: relationship with phenotype expression and genetic background. Mech. Ageing Dev. **124:** 539–548.
57. CARUSO, C. *et al.* 2003. Genetics of neurodegenerative disorders. N. Engl. J. Med. **349:** 193–194.
58. KAMBOH, M.I. 2004. Molecular genetics of late-onset Alzheimer's disease. Ann. Hum. Genet. **68:** 381–404.
59. LICASTRO, F. *et al.* 2005. A new promoter polymorphism in the alpha-1-antichymotrypsin gene is a disease modifier of Alzheimer's disease. Neurobiol. Aging **26:** 449–453.
60. LIO, D. *et al.* 2006. Tumor necrosis factor-alpha-308A/G polymorphism is associated with age at onset of Alzheimer's disease. Mech. Ageing Dev. **127:** 567–571.
61. RAINERO, I. *et al.* 2004. Association between the interleukin-1alpha gene and Alzheimer's disease: a meta-analysis. Neurobiol. Aging **25:** 1293–1298.
62. SERIPA, D. *et al.* 2005. Genotypes and haplotypes in the IL-1 gene cluster: analysis of two genetically and diagnostically distinct groups of Alzheimer patients. Neurobiol. Aging **26:** 455–464.
63. LIO, D. *et al.* 2003. Interleukin-10 promoter polymorphism in sporadic Alzheimer's disease. Genes Immun. **4:** 234–238.
64. LICASTRO, F. *et al.* 2005. Innate immunity and inflammation in ageing: a key for understanding age-related diseases. Immun. Ageing **2:** 8.
65. LUCAS, S.M. *et al.* 2006. The role of inflammation in CNS injury and disease. Br. J. Pharmacol. **147:** S232–S240.

66. EIKELENBOOM, P. *et al.* 2002. Neuroinflammation in Alzheimer's disease and prion disease. Glia **40:** 232–239.
67. ROGERS, J. *et al.* 2002. Microglia and inflammatory mechanisms in the clearance of amyloid beta peptide. Glia **40:** 260–269.
68. STREIT, W.J. 2004. Microglia and Alzheimer's disease pathogenesis. J. Neurosi. Res. **77:** 1–8.
69. AKIYAMA, S. *et al.* 2000. Inflammation and Alzheimer's disease. Neurobiol. Aging **21:** 383–421.
70. MCGEER, E.G. *et al.* 2001. Innate immunity in Alzheimer's disease: a model for local inflammatory reactions. Mol. Interv. **1:** 22–29.
71. BSIBSI, M. *et al.* 2002. Broad expression of Toll-like receptors in the human central nervous system. J. Neuropathol. Exp. Neurol. **61:** 1013–1021.
72. FASSBENDER, K. *et al.* 2004. The LPS receptor (CD14) links innate immunity with Alzheimer's disease. FASEB J. **18:** 203–205.
73. LOTZ, M. *et al.* 2005. Amyloid beta peptide 1–40 enhances the action of Toll-like receptor-2 and -4 agonists but antagonizes Toll-like receptor-9-induced inflammation in primary mouse microglial cell cultures. J. Neurochem. **94:** 289–298.
74. ARROYO-ESPLIGUERO, R. *et al.* 2004. CD14 and toll-like receptor 4: a link between infection and acute coronary events? Heart **90:** 983–988.
75. KIECHL, S. *et al.* 2002. Toll-like receptor 4 polymorphisms and atherogenesis. N. Engl. J. Med. **347:** 185–192.
76. ARBOUR, N.C. *et al.* 2000. TLR4 mutations are associated with endotoxin hyporesponsiveness in humans. Nat. Genet. **25:** 187–191.
77. AMEZIANE, N. *et al.* 2003. Association of the Toll-like receptor 4 gene Asp299Gly polymorphism with acute coronary events. Arterioscler Thromb. Vasc. Biol. **23:** e61–e64.
78. BALISTRERI, C.R. *et al.* 2005. Role of TLR4 receptor polymorphisms in boutonneuse fever. Int. J. Immunopathol. Pharmacol. **18:** 655–660.
79. BALISTRERI, C.R. *et al.* 2004. Role of Toll-like receptor 4 in acute myocardial infarction and longevity. JAMA **292:** 2339–2340.
80. HUBACEK, J.A. *et al.* 1999. C(-260)–>T polymorphism in the promoter of the CD14 monocyte receptor gene as a risk factor for myocardial infarction. Circulation **99:** 3218–3220.
81. ITO, D. *et al.* 2000. Polymorphism in the promoter of lipopolysaccharide receptor CD14 and ischemic cerebrovascular disease. Stroke **31:** 2661–2664.
82. SMITH, W.L. *et al.* 2000. Cyclooxygenases: structural, cellular, and molecular biology. Annu. Rev. Biochem. **69:** 145–182.
83. HO, L. *et al.* 1999. Regional distribution of cyclooxygenase-2 in the hippocampal formation in Alzheimer's disease. J. Neurosci. Res. **57:** 295–303.
84. HOOZEMANS, J.J. *et al.* 2001. Cyclooxygenase expression in microglia and neurons in Alzheimer's disease and control brain. Acta Neuropathol. (Berl.) **101:** 2–8.
85. OKA, A. *et al.* 1997. Induction of cyclo-oxygenase 2 in brains of patients with Down's syndrome and dementia of Alzheimer type: specific localization in affected neurones and axons. Neuroreport **8:** 1161–1164.
86. NOGAWA, S. *et al.* 1997. Cyclo-oxygenase-2 gene expression in neurons contributes to ischemic brain. Neuroscience **17:** 2746–2755.
87. LEVY-LAHAD, E. *et al.* 1995. A familial Alzheimer's disease locus on chromosome 1. Science **269:** 970–973.

88. TAY, A. *et al.* 1994. Assignment of the human prostaglandin-endoperoxide synthase 2 (PTGS2) gene to 1q25 by fluorescence in situ hybridization. Genomics **23:** 718–719.

89. PAPAFILI, A. *et al.* 2002. Common promoter variant in cyclooxygenase-2 represses gene expression: evidence of role in acute-phase inflammatory response. Arterioscler. Thromb. Vasc. Biol. **22:** 1631–1636.

90. BRASH, A.R. 1999. Lipoxygenases: occurrence, functions, catalysis, and acquisition of substrate. J. Biol. Chem. **274:** 23679–23682.

91. YAO, Y. *et al.* 2005. Elevation of 12/15 lipoxygenase products in AD and mild cognitive impairment. Ann. Neurol. **58:** 623–626.

92. JALA, V.R. *et al.* 2004. Leukotrienes and atherosclerosis: new roles for old mediators. Trends Immunol. **25:** 315–322.

93. QU, T. *et al.* 2001. 5-Lipoxygenase (5-LOX) promoter polymorphism in patients with early-onset and late-onset Alzheimer's disease. J. Neuropsychiatry Clin. Neurosci. **13:** 304–305.

94. LUSIS, A.J. *et al.* 2004. Genetic basis of atherosclerosis, part I, new genes and pathways. Circulation **110:** 1868–1873.

95. DWYER, J.H. *et al.* 2004. Arachidonate 5-lipoxygenase promoter genotype, dietary arachidonic acid, and atherosclerosis. N. Engl. J. Med. **350:** 29–37.

96. MANEV, H. *et al.* 2000. Putative role of neuronal 5-lipoxygenase in an aging brain. FASEB J. **14:** 1464–1469.

97. MANEV, H. *et al.* 2006. 5-Lipoxygenase (ALOX5) and FLAP (ALOX5AP) gene polymorphisms as factors in vascular pathology and Alzheimer's disease. Med. Hypotheses. **66:** 501–503.

A Study of Serum Immunoglobulin Levels in Elderly Persons That Provides New Insights into B Cell Immunosenescence

FLORINDA LISTÌ,[a] GIUSEPPINA CANDORE,[a]
MARIA ASSUNTA MODICA,[a] MARIANGELA RUSSO,[a]
GABRIELE DI LORENZO,[b] MARIA ESPOSITO-PELLITTERI,[b]
GIUSEPPINA COLONNA-ROMANO,[a] ALESSANDRA AQUINO,[a]
MATTEO BULATI,[a] DOMENICO LIO,[a] CLAUDIO FRANCESCHI,[c]
AND CALOGERO CARUSO[a]

[a]Gruppo di Studio sull'Immunosenescenza, Dipartimento di Biopatologia e Metodologie Biomediche, Università di Palermo, Palermo, Italy

[b]Dipartimento di Medicina Clinica e delle Patologie Emergenti, Università di Palermo, Palermo, Italy

[c]Dipartimento di Patologia Sperimentale and Centro Interdipartimentale "L. Galvani," Università di Bologna, Bologna, Italy, and Istituto Nazionale di Riposo e Cura per Anziani, Ancona, Italy

ABSTRACT: The literature on immunosenescence has focused mainly on T cell impairment. With the aim of gaining insight into B cell immunosenescence, we investigated the serum immunoglobulin levels in a cohort of 166 subjects (20–106 years). Serum IgG (and IgG subclasses) were quantified by the nephelometric technique, IgE by CAP system fluorescence enzyme immunoassay, and IgD by radial immunodiffusion (RID). There was an age-related increase of IgG and IgA; the IgG age-related increase was significant only in men, but IgG1 levels showed an age-related increase both in men and women, whereas IgG3 showed an age-related increase only in men. IgE levels remain unchanged, whereas IgD and IgM serum levels decreased with age; the IgM age-related decrease was significant only in women, likely due to the relatively small sample of aged men. Thus, in the elderly the B cell repertoire available to respond to new antigenic challenge is decreased. A lot of memory IgD− B cells are filling immunological space and the amount of naïve IgD+ B cells is dramatically decreased. This shift away from a population of predominantly naïve B cells obviously reflects the influences of cumulative exposure to foreign pathogens over time. These age-dependent B cell changes indicate

Address for correspondence: Giuseppina Candore, Ph.D., Gruppo di Studio sull'Immunosenescenza, Dipartimento di Biopatologia e Metodologie Biomediche, Corso Tukory 211, 90134 Palermo, Italy. Voice: +39-09-1655-5932; fax: +39-09-1655-5933.
e-mail: gcandore@unipa.it

Ann. N.Y. Acad. Sci. 1089: 487–495 (2006). © 2006 New York Academy of Sciences.
doi: 10.1196/annals.1386.013

that advanced age is a condition characterized by lack of clonotypic immune response to new extracellular pathogens. In any event, the increase of memory B cells and the loss of naïve B cells, as measured by serum IgD levels, could represent hallmarks of immunosenescence and could provide useful biomarkers possibly related to the life span of humans.

KEYWORDS: B cell; centenarians; elderly; immunosenescence; immunoglobulins

INTRODUCTION

The modifications of the immune system in the elderly are generally seen as deterioration of the immune system, that is, immunosenescence. On the other hand, immunosenescence is a complex process involving multiple reorganizational and developmentally regulated changes, rather than a simple unidirectional decline of whole functions. However, immunosenescence is largely responsible for the diminished ability of older individuals to overcome infection.[1-4]

Immunosenescence is claimed to be principally a result of the declining effectiveness of T cells. Lifelong and chronic antigenic load is the major driving force of immunosenescence, which has an impact on human life span by reducing the number of virgin antigen-nonexperienced T cells, and, simultaneously, filling the immunological space with expanded clones of memory and effector, antigen-experienced T cells. Gradually, the T cell population shifts to a lower ratio of naïve to memory cells, the thymus pumps out fewer naïve T cells with age and those T cells remaining, especially the CD8+ subset, also show increased oligoclonality with age. So, the repertoire of cells available to respond to antigenic challenge from previously unencountered pathogens is shrinking.[4-8]

In contrast to T cells, no evidence for a loss of B cell function has been seemingly found as neither the total number of B cells or immunoglobulin (Ig) secreting cells have been shown to be profoundly decreased with age.[9] However, the B cell repertoire is influenced by aging during an actual immune response, where the spectrum of expressed Ig genes, as well as the frequency of somatic mutations, affects the quality, though not necessarily the quantity, of the antibody response. What appears as an intrinsic defect in somatic mutations seems to be caused by suppressive influences exerted *in vivo* by aged CD4+ T cells,[3,9-11] possibly reflecting both the age-associated shift from type 1 to type 2 cytokine patterns[4,12] and the age-related impairment of the CD40–CD40L system.[11,13] Finally, one of the most dramatic examples of age-associated repertoire change is the appearance of oligoclonal expansions of CD5 B cells producing antibodies against self-antigens, albeit with no known pathophysiological consequences.[3,9,11]

In a recent paper, we have focused on B cells in the aged by studying the expression of some surface markers. In particular, in the elderly and in centenarians there was an increase of CD27+ B cells with a decrease of CD27− B lymphocytes.[14] These data seem of some importance. In fact, CD27 is considered a marker of primed memory cells and its engagement promotes the differentiation of memory B cells into plasma cells.[15] The decrement of virgin CD27− B lymphocytes cells and the concurrent increase of memory CD27+ B lymphocytes can be one of the events that might have an impact on the antibody repertoire of the elderly.[14] In fact, chronic antigenic load might fill immunological space with expanding clones of memory, antigen-experienced B cells, which affect the clonotypic immune response to new extracellular pathogens.

In this study, with the aim of gaining insight into B cell immunosenescence, we investigated the serum Ig levels in young and old persons and in centenarians.

MATERIALS AND METHODS

Sera were collected from Sicilian people: 46 healthy young adults (age <66 years, 30 women, and 16 men), 85 healthy aged persons (66–96 years, 63 women and 22 men), and 35 centenarians (≥ 99 years, 24 women and 11 men). None of the selected subjects was affected by neoplastic, infectious, or autoimmune disease, nor had they received any drug influencing immune functions at the time of the study. The study was approved by the University Hospital Ethics Committee and all the subjects gave written informed consent. Blood venous samples were withdrawn from the subjects under basal condition at 9:00 AM and allowed to clot; after centrifugation, serum was stored in aliquots at −70°C until analysis.

The concentrations of IgM, IgA, IgG, and IgG subclasses were determined by a nephelometric technique (Array System 360, Beckman Coulter, Cassina De' Pecchi, Provincia di Milano, Italy). The nephelometric quantification is based upon the reaction of a monospecific anti-immunoglobulin-specific antiserum with the human Ig to be determined. The generated immune complexes are quantified by measuring the side-scattered light. The nephelometer is calibrated by measurement of a series of turbidity standards. The monospecific antisera were purchased from Beckman Coulter. The concentrations in the test samples are calculated relative to the calibration curves, obtained with the nephelometric standard sera. The amount of IgD in each serum sample was determined by the use of radial immunodiffusion (Medic, Pavone Canavese, Provincia di Torino, Italy). Serum samples (20 μL) were deposited in the gel with monoclonal antibodies anti-IgD and incubated at room temperature (≅ 20°C) in a damp chamber for 48 h. The IgD concentration was determined

TABLE 1. Age- related serum concentrations of immunoglobulins (mean and 95% CI)

	21–43 years ($n = 46$)	66–96 years ($n = 85$)	99–108 years ($n = 35$)
IgG mg/L	9,780 (8,711–10,861)	10,688 (9,911–10,865)	13,045 (12,047–14,042)
IgA mg/L	1,898 (1,650–2,146)	3,211 (2,834–3,588)	4,739 (4,049–4,218)
IgM mg/L	1,407 (1,203–1,611)	1,079 (927–1,232)	1,011 (893–1,128)
IgD IU/mL	23.7 (14.2–33.2)	7.3 (2.4–12.3)	3.2 (2.5–3.8)
IgE kU/L	119.2 (66.5–171.9)	189.5 (57.5–321.5)	172.1 (71.1–273.2)

Spearman's rank significant correlation between age and serum immunoglobulins concentrations: IgG = 0.0004; IgA < 0.0001; IgM = 0.002; IgD < 0.0001.

by evaluating the diameters of immunoprecipitates and converting them with a table conversion. Total serum IgE levels were quantified by CAP-system fluorescence enzyme immunoassay (FEIA) (Pharmacia, Uppsala, Sweden), using UNICAP 100, according to the manufacturer's instruction. Serum concentrations of IgD are presented as IU/mL. Total serum IgE values are expressed in kU/L. All the other Ig serum concentrations are presented as mg/L.

The results were expressed as mean (95% CI) and differences between genders were analyzed by the Mann–Whitney U-test. The rank correlations between concentration of serum Igs and age were calculated by Spearman's rank coefficient.

RESULTS

TABLE 1 shows the summary of age-related Ig serum concentrations (mean and 95% CI). There was a significant positive correlation with age for IgG and IgA values (respectively $= 0.0004$ and < 0.0001 by Spearman's rank coefficient), whereas there was a significant negative correlation with age for IgM and IgD values (respectively $= 0.002$ and < 0.0001). No significant age-related changes in IgE values were observed. By analyzing data according to the gender (TABLE 2), significant age-related correlation was maintained in women for IgA (< 0.0001), IgM ($= 0.001$), IgD (< 0.0001) and in men for IgG ($= 0.0001$), IgA (< 0.0001), and IgD ($= 0.01$). Serum IgM concentrations were reduced in young men when compared with young women ($P < 0.05$). No other differences were found between women and men.

TABLE 3 shows the summary of age-related serum concentrations of IgG subclasses (mean and 95% CI). There was a significant positive correlation with age for IgG_1 and IgG_3 values (respectively $= 0.0009$ and $= 0.009$). No significant age-related changes in IgG_2 and IgG_4 values were observed. By analyzing data according to gender (TABLE 4), significant age-related correlation was maintained in women for IgG_1 ($= 0.01$) and in men for IgG_1 ($= 0.01$) and IgG_3 ($= 0.02$). No differences were found between women and men.

TABLE 2. Age- and gender-related serum concentration of immunoglobulins (mean and 95% CI)

	Women (*n* = 117)		
	21–43 years (*n* = 30)	66–96 years (*n* = 63)	99–108 years (*n* = 24)
IgG mg/L	10,284 (9,056–11,512)	10,350 (9,546–1,158)	12,820 (11,515–14,125)
IgA mg/L	1,857 (1,600–2,113)	3,060 (2,652–3,468)	5,292 (3,849–6,734)
IgM mg/L	1,584 (1,312–1,857)	1,166 (973–1,356)	1,055 (885–1,224)
IgD IU/mL	28.5 (15.6–41.5)	4.6 (2.4– 6.8)	3.2 (2.3–3.9)
IgE kU/L	68.2 (26.8–109.6)	103.2 (49.5–156.9)	131.9 (22.7–241.0)
	Men (*n* = 49)		
	21–43 years (*n* = 16)	66–96 years (*n* = 22)	99–108 years (*n* = 11)
IgG mg/L	8,858 (6,653 –11,063)	11,652 (9,648–1,365.)	13,535 (11,848–15,222)
IgA mg/L	1,974 (1,398–255)	3,643 (2,736–4,550)	5,292 (3,849–6,734)
IgM mg/L	1,075 (835–1,316)	831 (646–1,016)	915 (838–992)
IgD IU/mL	14.5 (1.5–27.6)	15.1 (3.7–34.0)	3.3 (2.0–4.6)
IgE kU/L	214.9 (89.2–340.6)	436.5 (64.4–937.6)	259.9 (19.3–500.6)

Serum IgM concentrations were reduced in young men compared with young women ($P < 0.05$). No other differences were found between women and men in the same groups.

Spearman's rank significant correlation between age and serum immunoglobulins concentrations in women: IgA < 0.0001; IgM $= 0.001$; IgD < 0.0001.

Spearman's rank significant correlation between age and serum immunoglobulins concentrations in men: IgG $= 0.0001$; IgA < 0.0001; IgD $= 0.01$.

Concerning the difference that we observed between women and men, our data are in agreement with previous results showing that IgA, IgM, and IgE serum levels are influenced by sex, although we cannot exclude the existence of regulator genes of immunoglobulin synthesis on heterochromosome since B cell diseases and immunoglobulin deficiencies are linked genetically to the X chromosome.[16]

DISCUSSION

It is well known that immune function declines with aging. It is assumed that this decline concerns cell-mediated immunity more than humoral responses.

TABLE 3. Age-related serum concentrations of IgG subclasses of (mean and 95% CI)

	21–43 years (*n* = 46)	66–96 years (*n* = 85)	99–108 years (*n* = 35)
IgG_1 mg/L	7,239 (6,603–7,874)	8,802 (7,478– 10,126)	9,542 (8,631–9,176)
IgG_2 mg/L	5,849 (404–4,643)	4,657 (404–5,270)	4,758 (4,308–5,208)
IgG_3 mg/L	1,127 (633–1,621)	920 (814–1,026)	1,090 (876–914)
IgG_4 mg/L	676 (450–902)	752 (606–898)	709 (572–847)

Spearman's rank significant correlation between age and serum subclasses of IgG concentrations. $IgG_1 = 0.0009$; $IgG_3 = 0.009$.

TABLE 4. Age- and gender-related serum concentration of IgG subclasses (mean and 95%CI)

	Women ($n = 117$)		
	21–43 years ($n = 30$)	66–96 years ($n = 63$)	99–108 years ($n = 24$)
IgG_1 mg/L	6,890 (6,159–7,621)	8,605 (7,132–10,077)	9,412 (8,102–10,722)
IgG_2 mg/L	5,158 (4,360–5,956)	4,633 (3,897–5,370)	4,925 (4,352–5,498)
IgG_3 mg/L	1,358 (613–2,123)	905 (782–1,027)	1,057 (834–1,280)
IgG_4 mg/L	592 (453–731)	722 (556–888)	707 (515–899)

	Men ($n = 49$)		
	21–43 years ($n = 16$)	66–96 years ($n = 22$)	99–108 years ($n = 11$)
IgG_1 mg/L	7,891 (6,626–7,576)	9,367 (6,255–12,478)	9,825 (8,970–10,668)
IgG_2 mg/L	7,120 (1,707–12,533)	4,725 (3,543–5,907)	4,394 (3,604–5,184)
IgG_3 mg/L	675 (538–812)	965 (740–1,190)	1,164 (613–1,714)
IgG_4 mg/L	834 (198–551)	839 (512–1,165)	715 (538–891)

No differences were found between females and males in the same groups.
Spearman's rank significant correlation between age and serum subclasses of IgG concentrations in women: $IgG_1 = 0.01$.
Spearman's rank correlation between age and serum immunoglobulins concentrations in men: $IgG_1 = 0.01$; $IgG_3 = 0.02$.

However, the B cell system is also affected, as suggested by the increased incidence of autoantibodies, monoclonal gammopathies, and chronic lymphocytic leukemia in the elderly.[3–11] In particular, immunoglobulin levels may show age-related changes. Several reports in the past have regarded the study of serum immunoglobulin levels in the elderly, with the aim of both determining the normal values for clinical laboratory and of exploring the age-related pathophysiology of the humoral responses.[17] The number of subjects under study and their age was different in the various studies; nevertheless, three decades ago, hyperimmunoglobulinemia was claimed to be a characteristic of the elderly.[18] On the whole, the results demonstrated that IgG and IgA serum levels increase with age, whereas IgM levels remain unchanged and IgE and IgD decrease with age. Besides, among IgG subclasses, IgG1, 2, and 3 showed a significant increase, whereas IgG4 did not.[17,19,20]

To the best of our knowledge no papers before ours have been published on the relationship between age and all immunoglobulin class serum levels in the same sample under study; besides, our paper includes the largest number of centenarians studied so far. So, taking into account our results and the above discussed findings, we can conclude that there is an age-related increase of IgG and IgA; the IgG age-related increase was significant only in men, but IgG1 levels showed an age-related increase both in men and women, whereas IgG3 showed an age-related increase only in men. On the other hand, IgE levels remain unchanged, as already shown by us,[21] whereas IgD and IgM serum levels decreased with age; the IgM age-related decrease was significant only in women, likely due to the relatively small sample of aged men. Present and previous data on unchanged levels of IgE make questionable the statement that the incidence of allergic diseases decreases with age.[21] Most important are the data on the other immunoglobulins. In fact, the age-related increase of IgG and IgA and, conversely, the age-related decrease of IgM and particularly of IgD seem to be of some importance in order to gain insight into B cell immunosenescence.

Secreted IgD is present in small amounts in the human serum. Regulation of the synthesis still remains uncertain, but it has been argued that an independent mechanism, possibly genetically determined, is important in the basal production, although its levels seemingly depend on the amount of IgD+ B cells.[22–24] Within the germinal centers activated naïve IgD+ B cells undergo vigorous proliferation, somatic hypermutation of Ig V region genes, isotype switching, interaction with antigens, antigen-driven selection, and differentiation into memory B cells, which proliferate rapidly in response to antigens and produce large amounts of antibodies.[15,25] The classical criterion of memory B cells is the lack of expression of membrane IgD and CD38 or the expression of switched IgG, IgA, and IgE; however, CD27 antigen represents a key marker for memory B cells and the definitive marker of all memory B cells is the presence of somatically mutated high-affinity antigen receptors.[25,26] So, adult-circulating B cells may be separated into three subpopulations: IgD+CD27− naïve B cells, nonswitched memory B cells IgD+CD27+, and IgDCD27+ switched memory B cells.[27,28] In fact, CD27+ B cells carry somatic mutated V-region genes, indicating that they are memory cells, representing unclass-switched memory B cells.[26] Thus, IgD+CD27+ B cells are an independent subpopulation of memory B cells and may play a crucial role in secondary immune response by their prompt synthesis of high-affinity IgM. The percentages of IgD+CD27+ memory B cells increase during childhood and adulthood, peak at about 40 years of age, and then decline in the aged, determining a poor secondary humoral immunity by IgM.[28]

The present results, showing that the levels of IgM and IgD are negatively age-related whereas IgG and IgA are positively related, demonstrate, then, that in the elderly a B cell repertoire available to respond to new antigenic challenge is decreased. We can presume that a lot of memory IgD− B cells are filling immunological space and the amount of naïve IgD+ B cells is dramatically decreased. This shift away from a population of predominantly naïve B cells obviously reflects the influences of cumulative exposure to foreign pathogens over time. These age-dependent B cell changes documented by present and previous studies[14,28] indicate that advanced age, *per se*, is a condition characterized by lack of clonotypic immune response to new extracellular pathogens. In any event, our results are suggesting that the increase of memory B cells and the loss of naïve B cells, as measured by serum IgD levels, could represent hallmarks of immunosenescence and could provide useful biomarkers possibly related to the life span of humans. Since information on the senescence of

B cells is of obvious interest, further studies are necessary to confirm these results by extending the number of markers used to characterize the cells.

ACKNOWLEDGMENTS

This work was supported by grants from the Italian Ministry of Education, University and Research (ex 605) to G.C., G.D.L., G.C.R., D.L., and C.C. Funds from the Italian Ministry of Health (Determinanti Immunogenetici di Salute nell'anziano: un confronto interregionale) to C.C. are also acknowledged. The "Immunosenesence Research Group" coordinated by Prof. C. Caruso in association with INRCA was enlarged through a joint contract (Longevity and Elderly Disability Biological Markers). F.L. and M.E.P. are Ph.D. students at Pathobiology Ph.D. course (directed by C.C.) of Palermo University and this work is submitted in partial fulfillment of the requirement for the Ph.D.

REFERENCES

1. FRANCESCHI, C. *et al.* 1995. The immunology of exceptional individuals: the lesson of centenarians. Immunol. Today **16:** 12–16.
2. COSSARIZZA, A. *et al.* 1997. Cytometric analysis of immunosenescence. Cytometry **27:** 297–313.
3. GLOBERSON, A. & R.B. EFFROS. 2000. Ageing of lymphocytes and lymphocytes in the aged. Immunol. Today **21:** 515–521.
4. PAWELEC, G. *et al.* 2002. T cells and aging. Front. Biosci. **7:** d1056–1183.
5. FRANCESCHI, C. *et al.* 2000. Human immunosenescence: the prevailing of innate immunity, the failing of clonotypic immunity, and the filling of immunological space. Vaccine **18:** 1717–1720.
6. FAGNONI, F.F. *et al.* 2000. Shortage of circulating naive CD8(+) T cells provides new insights on immunodeficiency in aging. Blood **95:** 2860–2868.
7. PAWELEC, G. *et al.* 2004. Is immunosenescence infectious? Contribution of persistent herpes viruses to immunosenescence and influence on human longevity. Trends Immunol. **25:** 406–410.
8. PAWELEC, G. *et al.* 2005. Human immunosenescence: is it infectious? Immunol. Rev. **205:** 257–268.
9. WEKSLER, M.E. 2000. Changes in the B-cell repertoire with age. Vaccine **18:** 1624–1628.
10. MILLER, R.A. 1996. The aging immune system: primer and prospectus. Science **273:** 70–74.
11. WEKSLER, M.E. & P. SZABO. 2000. The effect of age on the B-cell repertoire. J. Clin. Immunol. **20:** 240–249.
12. CARUSO, C. *et al.* 1996. Cytokine production pathway in the elderly. Immunol. Res. **15:** 84–90.
13. LIO, D. *et al.* 1998. Interleukin-12 release by mitogen-stimulated mononuclear cells in the elderly. Mech. Ageing Dev. **102:** 211–219.
14. COLONNA-ROMANO, G. *et al.* 2003. B cells in the aged: CD27, CD5, and CD40 expression. Mech Ageing Dev. **124:** 389–393.

15. AGEMATSU, K. *et al.* 2000. CD27: a memory B-cell marker. Immunol. Today **21:** 204–206.

16. MODICA, M.A. *et al.* 1989. Blood IgA, IgM and IgE levels are influenced by sex and HLA phenotype. Exp. Clin. Immunogenet. **6:** 251–257.

17. PAGANELLI, R. *et al.* 1994. Humoral immunity in aging. Aging Clin. Exp. Res. **6:** 143–150.

18. RADL, J. *et al.* 1975. Immunoglobulin patterns in humans over 95 years of age. Clin. Exp. Immunol. **22:** 84–90.

19. TIETZ, N.W. *et al.* 1992. Laboratory values in fit aging individuals—sexagenarians through centenarians. Clin. Chem. **38:** 1167–1185.

20. HARALDSSON, A. *et al.* 2000. Serum immunoglobulin D in infants and children. Scand. J. Immunol. **51:** 415–418.

21. DI LORENZO, G. *et al.* 2003. A study of age-related IgE pathophysiological changes. Mech. Ageing Dev. **124:** 445–448.

22. LIO, D. *et al.* 1992. IgD serum levels are influenced by HLA-DR phenotype. Dis. Markers **10:** 105–108.

23. LITZMAN, J. *et al.* 1997. Serum IgD levels in children under investigation for and with defined immunodeficiency. Int. Arch. Allergy Immunol. **114:** 54–58.

24. PREUD'HOMME, J.L. *et al.* 2000. Structural and functional properties of membrane and secreted IgD. Mol. Immunol. **37:** 871–887.

25. KLEIN, U. *et al.* 1998. Somatic hypermutation in normal and transformed human B cells. Immunol. Rev. **162:** 261–280.

26. BANCHEREAU, J. & F. ROUSSET. 1992. Human B lymphocytes: phenotype, proliferation, and differentiation. Adv. Immunol. **52:** 125–262.

27. GROTH, C. *et al.* 2002. Impaired up-regulation of CD70 and CD86 in naive (CD27-) B cells from patients with common variable immunodeficiency (CVID). Clin. Exp. Immunol. **129:** 133–139.

28. SHI, Y. *et al.* 2003. Functional analysis of human memory B-cell subpopulations: IgD+CD27+ B cells are crucial in secondary immune response by producing high affinity IgM. Clin. Immunol. **108:** 128–137.

Role of Proinflammatory Alleles in Longevity and Atherosclerosis

Results of Studies Performed on −1562C/T MMP-9 in Centenarians and Myocardial Infarction Patients from Sicily

DOMENICO NUZZO,[a] SONYA VASTO,[a] CARMELA R. BALISTRERI,[a] DANIELE DI-CARLO,[a] FLORINDA LISTÌ,[a] GREGORIO CAIMI,[b] MARCO CARUSO,[b] ENRICO HOFFMANN,[b] EGLE INCALCATERRA,[b] DOMENICO LIO,[a] CALOGERO CARUSO,[a] AND GIUSEPPINA CANDORE[a]

[a]Gruppo di Studio sull' Immunosenescenza, Dipartimento di Biopatologia e Metodologie Biomediche, Università di Palermo, Palermo, Italy

[b]Dipartimento di Medicina Interna, Malattie Cardiovascolari e Nefrourologiche, Università di Palermo, Palermo, Italy

ABSTRACT: Centenarians are characterized by marked delay or escape from age-associated diseases that cause mortality at earlier ages. Jointly, atherosclerosis and its complications, such as myocardial infarction (AMI), significantly contribute to mortality in the elderly. Inflammation is a key component of atherosclerosis and inflammatory genes are good candidates for the risk of the development of atherosclerosis. Genetic traits contribute to the risk of AMI and allelic variations in inflammatory genes should boost the risk of disease. If proinflammatory genotypes significantly contribute to the risk of AMI, alleles associated with disease susceptibility should not be included in the genetic background favoring longevity. Hence, genotypes of natural immunity should play an opposite role in atherosclerosis and longevity. Metalloproteinase (MMPs) are involved in tissue remodeling and therefore play a remarkable role in inflammation-based disease. MMPs are a family of Zn^{2+}-dependent enzymes with proteolytic activity against connective tissue proteins such as collagens, proteoglycans, and elastin, which appear to play important roles in the development and progression of the atherosclerotic lesion. There is evidence indicating a role played by the MMPs in the weakening of atherosclerotic plaque which predisposes to lesion disruption. In this study we performed a genetic study on −1562C/T MMP-9 sin-

Address for correspondence: Giuseppina Candore, Ph.D., Gruppo di Studio sull'Immunosenescenza, Dipartimento di Biopatologia e Metodologie Biomediche, Corso Tukory, 211, 90134 Palermo, Italy. Voice: +39-091-655-5932; fax: +39-091-655-5933.

e-mail: gcandore@unipa.it

Ann. N.Y. Acad. Sci. 1089: 496–501 (2006). © 2006 New York Academy of Sciences.
doi: 10.1196/annals.1386.048

gle nucleotide polymorphism (SNP) in order to discern a possible role in AMI. We analyzed the distribution of this SNP in 115 AMI patients, 123 controls, and 34 centenarians from Sicily. We found no significant differences in the genetic distribution and allelic frequency of −1562C/T MMP-9 SNP between the studied groups. The present results are not in agreement with our previous findings, strengthening our hypothesis that genetic background protection against cardiovascular disease is a relevant component of the longevity trait, at least in the generation of Italian male centenarians under study. However, present results do not exclude that differential expression of MMP-9 playing an opposite role in AMI and longevity because other kinds of regulation might be more relevant than those linked to the SNP under study.

KEYWORDS: inflammation; infarction; longevity; metalloproteases; polymorphism

INTRODUCTION

In atherosclerosis, deposition of oxidized low-density lipoproteins (ox-LDL) represents the initial event. This is followed by infiltration of circulating monocytes, which convert to macrophages and take up ox-LDL to become foam cells. Activated lymphocytes also occur in atherosclerotic plaques at all stages of its progression, and other inflammatory cells are also present. Formation of a distinct fibrous cap over a large lipid core occurs only as a late consequence of atherosclerosis. The lipid core arises because macrophages die by apoptosis and spill their lipid contents. The plaque cap is formed by migration of vascular smooth muscle cells. Catastrophic rupture or surface erosion of the fibrous cap underlies fatal coronary thrombosis and myocardial infarction (AMI), which is the leading cause of premature death in developed countries. Plaque rupture, which accounts for more than 80% of fatal cases of AMI, occurs in regions of high tangential stress and where collagen is depleted. The implication is that matrix destruction weakens the plaque to the point where it can no longer resist the cyclical strain caused by the cardiac cycle.[1–5]

Metalloproteases (MMPs) are a family of Zn^{2+}-dependent enzymes with proteolytic activity against connective tissue proteins such as collagens, proteoglycans, and elastin, which appear to play important roles in the development and progression of the atherosclerotic lesion. The role of MMPs has been shown to be involved in vascular smooth muscle cell migration and proliferation, in which the matrix-degrading activity of these enzymes confer the ability to break down the surrounding connective tissue barriers. Moreover, there is also evidence indicating a role played by the MMPs in the weakening of atherosclerotic plaque that predisposes to lesion disruption. The most common locations where disruption occurs are the lateral regions of the plaque, where macrophage accumulation is accompanied by a local loss of connective tissue. The polymorphisms that have been identified thus far often affect the promoter region of the MMP gene and thereby influence critical steps in the binding of transcription factors or the overall efficiency of transcription. These polymorphisms have been shown to influence MMP gene expression and be associated with susceptibility of coronary atherosclerosis and subsequent acute coronary syndromes. Among all the different metalloproteases particular importance has been given to MMP-9.[6-9]

We hypothesized that functional $-1562C/T$ MMP-9 single nucleotide polymorphism (SNP)[9] of MMP-9 can actively control gene expression and play a role in the cap rupture in atherosclerosis, contributing to the onset of AMI. To test our hypothesis we set up a study including patients affected by acute AMI, controls and centenarians belonging to our homogeneous Sicilian population. We have analyzed the distribution of the SNP in centenarians, because our previous studies have demonstrated that alleles associated with AMI susceptibility are not included in the genetic background favoring longevity.[10,11] Individuals with exceptional longevity indeed possess genetic factors that modulate ageing processes and, in particular, are protective against cardiovascular diseases.[12] So, pro/anti-inflammatory alleles have a role in determining susceptibility or resistance to immune-inflammatory diseases, including atherosclerosis, and reciprocally in determining or not the possibility to reach the extreme limit of life. Besides, centenarian genetic background studies may contribute to clarify the role of key genetic components influencing age-associated diseases which are characterized by a multifactorial etiology, as AMI.[10,11]

MATERIALS AND METHODS

We analyzed the distribution of the polymorphism in 115 AMI patients, 123 controls and 34 centenarians. We enrolled young patients admitted at the Cardiac Unit of Palermo University Hospital (Italy), as they were affected by AMI (109 men, 6 women). To improve the power of our analysis, we selected cases genetically loaded for early-onset AMI (<46 years).[13] The diagnosis of AMI was based on typical electrocardiographic and enzymatic criteria and confirmed by echocardiography and coronary angiography. The healthy, age-matched control group (100 men, 23 women) was recruited among students or staff personnel who were checked and judged to be in good health on the basis of their clinical history and on blood tests (complete blood cell count, erythrocyte sedimentation rate, glucose, urea nitrogen, creatinine, electrolytes, C-reactive protein, liver function tests, iron, proteins, cholesterol, triglycerides). A second control group consisted of 34 Sicilian centenarians (12 women, 22 men). Centenarian age was verified by researching archival records in the City Hall and/or church registries, paying attention to the concordance between reported age and personal chronologies (age of marriage and of military service for men, age of first and last pregnancy for women, age of children, among others). These subjects did not have any cardiac risk factors or major age-related diseases (e.g., CAD, severe cognitive impairment, severe physical impairment, clinically evident cancer, or renal insufficiency), although some had decreased auditory and visual acuity. The Sicilian ethnicity of all subjects was confirmed by having all four grandparents born in Sicily; immigration and intermarriage has historically been rare. The study was approved by the Hospital Ethics Committee and informed consent was obtained from all subjects. DNA was genotyped for −1562C/T MMP-9 SNP according to published methods.[9] Allele and genotypic frequencies of the analyzed polymorphism were evaluated by gene count. Significant differences in frequency among the groups were calculated by χ^2 test (3 × 3, 3 × 2 tables, where appropriate). The data were tested for the goodness of fit between the observed and expected genotype frequencies according to Hardy-Weinberg equilibrium (HWE) by χ^2 test. We also analyzed the allelic frequencies of polymorphism according to gender in patients and controls by χ^2 test.

RESULTS AND DISCUSSION

We found no significant differences in the genetic distribution and allelic frequency of −1562C/T MMP-9 SNP between the studied groups (TABLE 1). Furthermore, we analyzed the allelic frequencies the of the MMP-9 polymorphism according to gender in patients, controls and centenarians. No statistically significant difference was observed among the allele frequencies by stratification according to gender (data not shown).

Present results are not in agreement with our previous results, strengthening our hypothesis that genetic background protecting against cardiovascular disease is a relevant component of the longevity trait, at least in the generation of Italian male centenarians under study.[14] In fact, the proinflammatory alleles of these inflammatory genes—pyrin (i.e., the gene responsible for familial Mediterranean fever; 2080G); the coreceptor for lipopolysaccharide (TLR4 A896); the chemokine receptor (CCR5 Δ 32); the Gap junction channel protein regulating leukocyte recruitment (Cx37 + 1019T); the enzymes involved in ecosanoid production (−765G COX-2 and −1708A LOX); the anti-inflammatory IL-10 cytokine (–A108); and the proinflammatory TNF-α

TABLE 1. Frequency of genotypes and alleles for −1562C/T MMP-9 SNP in 115 young AMI patients, in 123 healthy age-related controls, and 34 centenarians from Sicily

	CC	CT	TT	−1562C	−1562T
AMI patients	73 (63.5%)	39 (33.9%)	3 (2.6%)	185 (80.4%)	45 (19.6%)
Young controls	86 (69.9%)	36 (29.3%)	1 (0.8%)	208 (84.6%)	38 (15.4%)
Centenarians	22 (64.7%)	12 (35.3%)	0 (0%)	56 (82.4%)	12 (17.6%)

NOTE: The distribution of genotypes was in HWE. Genotype and allele frequencies were not significantly different between the groups.

cytokine (–G308A)—were significantly over-represented in AMI patients and under-represented in the oldest old and centenarians, whereas age-related controls displayed intermediate values[10,11,14,15] (unpublished observations). What we have said is applicable for the male gender; further studies are necessary to validate this hypothesis in women.[15]

The activity of MMPs is tightly regulated at the level of gene transcription and is also regulated by their secretion in an inactive zymogen form that requires extracellular activation and co-secretion of the tissue inhibitors of MMPs (TIMPs). Thus, increased gene transcription, enhanced activation, and reduced activity of TIMPs can individually or together create a milieu for increased matrix proteolysis. MMPs can be activated by other proteases and increased MMP production can be induced by ox-LDL and other inflammatory stimuli as well as hemodynamic stress. In particular, production of MMP-9 by macrophages is mediated by a prostaglandin (PG) E2/cAMP-dependent pathway.[8,16–18]

The present results do not exclude that differential expression of MMP-9 playing an opposite role in AMI and longevity. In fact, the other kinds of regulation briefly previously discussed might be more relevant than those linked to the SNP under study.

ACKNOWLEDGMENTS

This work was supported by grants from the Ministry of Education, University and Research, ex60% to Calogero Caruso and Giuseppina Candore and the Ministry of Health (Markers genetici di sindrome coronarica acuta e valutazione della L-arginina nella prevenzione di eventi ischemici). Domenico Nuzzo, Sonya Vasto, and Carmela R. Balistreri are Ph.D. students in the pathobiology Ph.D. course directed by Calogero Caruso of Palermo University, and this work is in partial fulfillment of the requirement for the Ph.D.

REFERENCES

1. ROSS, R. 1999. Mechanisms of disease. Atherosclerosis: an inflammatory disease. N. Engl. J. Med. **340**: 115–126.
2. HANSSON, G.K. *et al.* 2002. Innate and adaptive immunity in the pathogenesis of atherosclerosis. Circ. Res. **91**: 281–291.
3. STARY, H.C. 1990. The sequence of cell and matrix changes in atherosclerotic lesions of coronary arteries in the first forty years of life. Eur. Heart J. **11**(Suppl. E): 3–19.
4. LIBBY, P. & M. AIKAWA. 2002. Stabilization of atherosclerotic plaques: new mechanisms and clinical targets. Nat. Med. **8**: 1257–1262.
5. DAVIES, M.J. 2000. Coronary disease: the pathophysiology of acute coronary syndromes. Heart **83**: 361–366.

6. LUTTUN, A. *et al.* 2000. The role of proteinases in angiogenesis, heart development, restenosis, atherosclerosis, myocardial ischemia, and stroke: insights from genetic studies. Curr. Atheroscler. Rep. **2:** 407–416.

7. ZHANG, B. *et al.* 1999. Functional polymorphism in the regulatory region of gelatinase B gene in relation to severity of coronary atherosclerosis. Circulation **99:** 1788–1794.

8. CIPOLLONE, F. & M.L. FAZIA. 2006. Cox-2 and atherosclerosis. J. Cardiovasc. Pharmacol. **47S1:** S26–S36.

9. GORACY, J. *et al.* 2003. The C(-1562)T polymorphism in the promoter of the matrix metalloproteinase-9 (MMP-9) gene and coronary atherosclerosis. Pol. Arch. Med. Wewn. **110:** 1275–1281.

10. CANDORE, G. *et al.* 2006. Biology of longevity: role of the innate immune system. Rejuvenation Res. **9:** 143–148.

11. CANDORE, G. *et al.* 2006. Opposite role of pro-inflammatory alleles in acute myocardial infarction and longevity: results of studies performed in a Sicilian population. Ann. N. Y. Acad. Sci. **1067:** 270–275.

12. TERRY, D.F. *et al.* 2003. Cardiovascular advantages among the offspring of centenarians. J. Gerontol. A. Biol. Sci. Med. Sci. **58:** M425–M431.

13. MARENBERG, M.E. *et al.* 1994. Genetic susceptibility to death from coronary heart disease in a study of twins. N. Engl. J. Med. **330:** 1041–1046.

14. CARUSO, C. *et al.* 2005. Inflammation and life-span. Science **307:** 208 [letter].

15. CANDORE, G. *et al.* 2006. Immunogenetics, gender and longevity. Ann. N. Y. Acad. Sci. This volume.

16. BREW, K. *et al.* 2000. Tissue inhibitors of metalloproteinases: evolution, structure and function. Biochim. Biophys. Acta **1477:** 267–283.

17. GALIS, Z.S. *et al.* 1994. Increased expression of matrix metalloproteinases and matrix degrading activity in vulnerable regions of human atherosclerotic plaques. J. Clin. Invest. **94:** 2493–2503.

18. CIPOLLONE, F. *et al.* 2001. Overexpression of functionally coupled cyclooxygenase-2 and prostaglandin E synthase in symptomatic atherosclerotic plaques as a basis of prostaglandin E (2)-dependent plaque instability. Circulation **104:** 921–927.

Association between Platelet Glycoprotein Ib-α and Myocardial Infarction

Results of a Pilot Study Performed in Male and Female Patients from Sicily

GIUSEPPINA CANDORE,[a] GIUSEPPINA PIAZZA,[a]
ANTONINO CRIVELLO,[a] MARIA PAOLA GRIMALDI,[a]
VALENTINA ORLANDO,[a] MARCO CARUSO,[b] GREGORIO CAIMI,[b]
ENRICO HOFFMANN,[b] EGLE INCALCATERRA,[b] DOMENICO LIO,[a]
AND CALOGERO CARUSO[a]

[a]Gruppo di Studio sull'Immunosenescenza, Dipartimento di Biopatologia e Metodologie Biomediche , Università di Palermo, Palermo, Italy

[b]Dipartimento di Medicina Interna, Malattie Cardiovascolari e Nefrourologiche, Università di Palermo, Palermo, Italy

ABSTRACT: Myocardial infarction (AMI) is a complex multifactorial disorder. Platelet adhesion and thrombosis are pivotal events in the development of atherosclerotic lesions. Occlusive thrombus is almost exclusively initiated by plaque rupture and adhesion of platelets to subendothelial von Willebrand factor (vWf) by its specific platelet receptor, the α-chain of glycoprotein (GP) Ib-IX-V complex of the human platelet-specific antigens (HPA). Two polymorphisms have been reported in the sequence of GPIb-α. The first, a C/T transition at nucleotide 1018 results in an amino acid dimorphism (Thr/Met) at residue 145 of GPIb-α, which is located within the vWF-binding domain of the receptor. The second is a T/C polymorphism in the Kozak sequence at position −5 from the initiator ATG. This affects the receptor density on the platelet surface. We assessed 1018 C/T and −5 T/C Kozak polymorphisms to see whether they are associated with AMI in homogeneous populations of Sicilian patients with AMI. To this end, we have analyzed the distribution of 1018 C/T and −5 T/C Kozak polymorphisms in 105 young Sicilian patients (<46 years) and 110 healthy age-related controls, by PCR–SSP and PCR–RFLP. Our results demonstrate no significant differences in the frequency of 1018 C/T and −5 T/C Kozak polymorphism between patients with AMI and controls. Stratifying by gender, there is no

Address for correspondence: Giuseppina Candore, Ph.D., Gruppo di Studio sull'Immunosenescenza, Dipartimento di Biopatologia e Metodologie Biomediche, Corso Tukory 211, 90134 Palermo, Italy. Voice: +39-09-1655-5932; fax: +39-09-1655-5933.
e-mail: gcandore@unipa.it

Ann. N.Y. Acad. Sci. 1089: 502–508 (2006). © 2006 New York Academy of Sciences.
doi: 10.1196/annals.1386.011

difference between male and female patients and control data. Thus, our results indicate that the HPA-2 polymorphisms are not associated with an increased risk for AMI at early onset (< 46 years) both in men and in women.

KEYWORDS: coagulation; myocardial infarction; platelet glycoprotein Ib-α; polymorphisms

INTRODUCTION

Platelets play a key role in acute coronary syndromes and acute myocardial infarction (AMI), as demonstrated by histopathologic findings and clinical observations showing the efficacy of antiplatelet therapies for these disorders. The glycocalyx layer on the external membrane contains a series of complex glycoprotein molecules (GPs), which are classified from GP-I to GP-X. The platelet membrane GPs act as receptors for many adhesive proteins, such as collagen, von-Willebrand factor (vWF), fibronectin, ADP, thrombin, and so on, which bring about platelet adhesion, activation, and aggregation. These prominent features in thrombus formation are pivotal events in the complications of atherosclerotic lesions.[1,2]

The GP Ib/IX/V complex, in particular, is the major platelet surface receptor for vWF. It is composed of four subunits—GP Ib-α, GP Ib-β, GP IX, and GP V— that are synthesized from different genes. GP Ib-α and GP Ib-β are linked by a disulfide bridge, while GP IX and GP V join the complex noncovalently. The vWF binding site is localized on the N-terminal domain of GP Ib-α.[3] When the arterial vessel wall has been injured under high shear stress and arterial subendothelial structures have been exposed, platelets adhere to the subendothelial extracellular matrix. Under conditions of high shear stress, this first adhesion is mediated by the contact between immobilized subendothelial von Willebrand factor and the GP Ib/IX/V receptor complex.[4] This adhesion is initially reversible and allows platelets to tether and to roll over the thrombogenic surface and it causes intraplatelet signaling, resulting in the activation of other platelet receptors, like GP Ia/IIa or GP VI.[5] The binding of these complexes to subendothelial collagen mediates the stationary and stable adhesion of platelets and subsequent platelet activation. The last step is platelet aggregation and the formation of a platelet-rich plug that is mediated by the binding of the divalent or multivalent ligands, fibrinogen, or vWF, to GP IIb/IIIa.[6]

The GP complex expresses several polymorphic antigenic determinants on their surface, which are called human platelet-specific antigens (HPAs). HPAs have conventionally been defined as antigens exclusively present on platelets and on megakaryocytes. It is now clear, however, that most of these antigens have a broader tissue distribution and are expressed on receptor molecules involved in cell–matrix interactions.[7]

Two polymorphisms have been reported in the sequence of GPIb-α. The first, a C/T transition at nucleotide 1018 results in an amino acid dimorphism

(Thr/Met) at residue 145 of GPIb-α, which is located within the vWF-binding domain of the receptor.[8] The second is a T/C polymorphism in the Kozak sequence at position −5 from the initiator AUG.[9] From previous studies of the translation initiation site, the nucleotides preceding the AUG initiator Codon are thought to be important in translation efficiency in eukaryotic cells.[10] The original consensus Kozak sequence contains nucleotide C at position −5, and therefore the switch to T at the −5 position of GPIb-α may theoretically decrease translation efficiency of the receptor. Afshar-Khargan *et al.*[9] reported an association between the C allele of the Kozak dimorphism and increased platelet GPIb-IX-V receptor levels both *in vitro* and *in vivo*.[9] In this study, we tried to determine whether 1018 C/T and −5 T/C Kozak polymorphisms are associated with AMI in homogeneous populations of Sicilian patients.

MATERIALS AND METHODS

We analyzed the distribution of polymorphisms in 105 AMI patients and 110 controls. We enrolled young patients admitted at the Cardiac Unit of Palermo University Hospital (Italy) for AMI (95 men, 10 women, <46 years of age). The diagnosis of AMI was based on typical electrocardiographic and enzymatic criteria and confirmed by echocardiography and coronary angiography. The healthy, age-matched control group (100 men, 15 women) was recruited among students or staff personnel who were checked and judged to be in good health on the basis of their clinical history and on blood tests (complete blood cell count, erythrocyte sedimentation rate, glucose, urea nitrogen, creatinine, electrolytes, C-reactive protein, liver function tests, iron, proteins, cholesterol, triglycerides). The Sicilian ethnicity of the participants at the study was established by confirming that all four grandparents were born in Sicily; immigration and intermarriage have historically been rare.

Blood specimens were collected in tripotassium EDTA sterile tubes, and DNA was extracted and processed for genotyping. For detection of the Kozak polymorphism, the sequence of the upstream primer was 5′-GAGAGAAGGACGGAGTCGAG-3′ and that of the downstream primer was 5′-GGTTGTGTCTTTCGGCAGG-3′. We used the RFLP-PCR technique. Samples were restriction-digested using 2U PPu MI at 37°C for several hours. Digestion of the amplified product from T/T produced 3 bands (125 base pair, 157 bp, 175 bp), from C/C 2 bands (125 bp and 332 bp), and from heterozygotes C/T 4 bands (125bp, 157 bp, 175 bp, and 332 bp).[11] The HPA-2 polymorphism, Tre145Met was detected by allele-specific hybridization, using the common upstream primer 5′-GATGGGACGCTGCCAGTGCTG-3′ with either the downstream primer for Thr 5′-CTTCTCCAGCTTGGGTGTGGGCG-3′, or the downstream primer for Met 5′- CTTCTCCAGCTTGGGTGTGGGCA-3′.

TABLE 1. Genotype distribution and allele frequency for Kozak -5T/C polymorphism in 105 young patients (< 46 years) and 110 age-related controls from Sicily

	Genotypes			Alleles	
	CC	CT	TT	C	T
Patients	1 (1%)	22 (21%)	82 (78%)	24 (11%)	186 (89%)
Controls	3 (3%)	18 (16%)	89 (81%)	24 (11%)	196 (89%)

The distribution of genotypes was in HWE. Genotype and allele frequencies were not significantly different between the two groups.

The PCR amplification was performed in a final volume of 20 μL, containing 50–100 ng of DNA template, 0.2U of Taq DNA polymerase, 0.2mM of dNTPs mix, PCR Buffer10 × (10 mM Tris-HCl pH 8.3; 50 mM KCl), 1.5 mM of $MgCl_2$ and 1 pmol/L of each primer. The final mix was amplified with a PCR thermal sequencer and the procedure was carried out as follows. The reaction was heated to 95°C for 5 min for denaturation, followed by 33 cycles with denaturation at 95°C for 40 sec, annealing at 63°C for 40 sec, and extension at 72°C for 3 min. The amplified products were separated by electrophoresis on a 2% agarose gel. Ethidium bromide staining of the agarose gel was used to detect the amplified fragments.

Allele and genotypic frequencies of two analyzed polymorphisms were evaluated by gene count. Significant differences in frequency, among the groups, were calculated by χ^2 test (3 × 2, 2 × 2 tables, where appropriate). The data were tested for the goodness-of-fit between the observed and expected genotype frequencies according to Hardy–Weinberg equilibrium (HWE) by χ^2 test. We also analyzed the allelic frequencies of HPA polymorphisms according to gender in patients and controls by χ^2 test.

RESULTS AND DISCUSSION

We found no significant differences in the genetic distribution and allelic frequency of both HPA polymorphisms between the two studied groups

TABLE 2. Genotype distribution and allele frequency for 145 Met/Thr polymorphism in 105 young patients (< 46 years) and 110 age-related controls from Sicily

	Genotypes			Alleles	
	Met/Met145	Met/Thr 145	Thr/Thr145	145Met	145Thr
Patients	2 (2%)	25 (24%)	78 (74%)	29 (14%)	181 (86%)
Controls	2 (2%)	22 (20%)	86 (78%)	26 (12%)	194 (88%)

The distribution of genotypes was in HWE. Genotype and allele frequencies were not significantly different between the two groups.

(TABLES 1 and 2). Furthermore, we analyzed the allelic frequencies of HPA polymorphisms according to gender in patients and controls. No statistical difference was observed among the allele frequencies by stratification according to gender in patients and controls (data not shown).

Coronary atherosclerosis with plaque disruption resulting in superimposed thrombosis is the main pathological mechanism of acute coronary syndromes, with the amount and extent of associated thrombus formation affecting the final clinical outcome.[12] The composition of thrombi found in arterial thrombosis is predominantly that of a platelet-rich core attached to an underlying atheromatous plaque in an epicardial coronary artery.[13] Blood passing through arteries that have been narrowed by atheroma will be subjected to higher local shear forces, resulting in an increased risk of thrombotic occlusion through the shear-dependent vWF and GPIb/IX/V interaction. It therefore appears that platelet adhesion to vascular subendothelium and subsequent platelet aggregation are critical elements in the mechanism of coronary thrombosis.[14]

The roles of vWF–GPIb/IX/V interaction in the development of complications of atherosclerosis have been implicated in several reports.[15] Agents that block either vWF or GPIb/IX/V inhibited and delayed coronary occlusion in animal models.[16] Elevated plasma levels of vWF are a poor prognostic factor of coronary heart disease as well as an independent risk factor for subsequent acute coronary events in patients with angina pectoris. Participation of vWF–GPIb/IX/V in cardiovascular diseases (CVD), however, is not well understood, although shear-induced platelet aggregation was enhanced in ischemic CVD.[17]

To date, there is no direct evidence showing a relation between the GPIb-α genotype and the functional difference of platelet. It is possible that replacement of threonine by methionine at residue 145, which is located within the vWF and thrombin-binding domain of this receptor, might affect the structure and function of this receptor. It is also possible that the effect of 145T/M genotype is merely a reflection of the functional differences caused by the other polymorphism on the coding sequence, the "repeat polymorphism," located in the macroglycopeptide portion, which is in linkage disequilibrium with 145T/M. In reported results the genotype with Met-allele (T/M and M/M genotypes) was associated with CVD in the Korean population.[18] These results agree with those obtained by Gonzalez–Conejero et al. but contradict the results reported by Carlsson et al.[19,20] These findings are compatible with a published study on the association of GPIb-α genotype with coronary artery disease.[21] The nucleotide −5C Kozak sequence variant of GPIb-α was recently associated with increased translational efficiency and increased platelet surface density of the GPIb-IX-V receptor on platelets as well as transfected cells expressing the complex. These findings support the possibility of the Kozak sequence C allele as a candidate genetic susceptibility marker for atherothrombotic disease.[22]

However, no statistically significant differences were observed in our work, likely because of the younger age of our patients with respect to the previous studies. Thus, it is possible that these polymorphisms are risk factors for AMI in aged but not in younger people, where the genetics of inflammation plays a more relevant role.[23-28]

ACKNOWLEDGMENTS

This work was supported by grants from the Ministry of Education, University and Research, ex 60% to C.C. and G.C. and the Ministry of Health (Markers genetici di sindrome coronarica acuta e valutazione della L-arginina nella prevenzione di eventi ischemici). A.C. and M.P.G. are Ph.D. students at Pathobiology Ph.D. course (directed by C.C.) of Palermo University and this work is in partial fulfillment of the requirement for the Ph.D.

REFERENCES

1. DEL ZOPPO, G.J. 1998. The role of platelets in ischemic stroke. Neurology **51**:S9–S14.
2. HARKER, L.A. 1998. Therapeutic inhibition of platelet function in stroke. Cerebrovasc. Dis. **8**: S8–S18.
3. WARE, J. 1998. Molecular analyses of the platelet glycoprotein Ib-IX-V receptor. Thromb. Haemost. **79**: 466–478.
4. FREDRICKSON, B.J. *et al.* 1998. Shear-dependent rolling on von Willebrand factor of mammalian cells expressing the platelet glycoprotein Ib-IX-V complex. Blood **92**: 3684–3693.
5. FURIHATA, K. *et al.* 2002. Influence of platelet collagen receptor polymorphisms on risk for arterial thrombosis. Arch. Pathol. Lab. Med. **126**: 305–309.
6. SHATTIL, S.J. *et al.* 1998. Integrin signaling: the platelet paradigm. Blood **91**: 2645–2657.
7. NEWMAN, P.J. *et al.* 1995. Human platelet alloantigens: recent findings, new perspectives. Thromb. Hemost. **74**: 234–239.
8. KUIJPERS, R. *et al.* 1992. NH2-terminal globular domain of human platelet glycoprotein Ib alpha has a methionine 145/threonine145 amino acid polymorphism, which is associated with the HPA-2 (Ko) alloantigens. J. Clin. Invest. **89**: 381–384.
9. AFSHAR-KHARGHAN, V. *et al.* 1999. Kozak sequence polymorphism of the glycoprotein (GP) Ibalpha gene is a major determinant of the plasma membrane levels of the platelet GP Ib-IX-V complex. Blood **94**: 186–191.
10. KOZAK, M. 1987. An analysis of 5′-noncoding sequences from 699 vertebrate messenger RNAs. Nucleic Acids Res. **15**: 8125–8148.
11. BAKER, R.I. *et al.* 2001. Platelet glycoprotein Iba Kozak polymorphism is associated with an increased risk of ischemic stroke. Blood **98**: 36–40.
12. FUSTER, V. *et al.* 1992. The pathogenesis of coronary artery disease and the acute coronary syndromes. N. Engl. J. Med. **326**:310–318.
13. DAVIES, M.J. *et al.* 1989. Factors influencing the presence or absence of acute coronary thrombi in sudden ischemic death. Eur. Heart J. **10**: 203–208.

14. FUSTER, V. *et al.* 1990. Atherosclerotic plaque thrombosis: evolving concepts. Circulation **82**: II47–II59.
15. NICHOLS, T.C. *et al.* 1991. Role of von Willebrand factor in arterial thrombosis. Studies in normal and von Willebrand disease pigs. Circulation **83**: IV56–IV64.
16. YAO, S.K. *et al.* 1994. Blockade of platelet membrane glycoprotein Ib receptors delays intracoronary thrombogenesis, enhances thrombolysis, and delays coronary artery reocclusion in dogs. Circulation **89**: 2822–2828.
17. JANSSON, J.H. *et al.* 1991. von Willebrand factor in plasma: a novel risk factor for recurrent myocardial infarction and death. Br. Heart J. **66**: 351–355.
18. PARK, S. *et al.* 2004. Association of gene polymorphisms of platelet glycoprotein Ia and IIb/IIIa and myocardial infarction and extent of coronary artery disease in Korean population. Yonsei Med. J. **45**: 428–434.
19. GONZALEZ-CONEJERO, R. *et al.* 1998. Polymorphisms of platelet membrane glycoprotein Ib associated with arterial thrombotic disease. Blood **92**: 2771–2776.
20. CARLSSON, L.E. *et al.* 1997. Polymorphisms of the human platelet antigens HPA-1, HPA-2, HPA-3, and HPA-5 on the platelet receptors for fibrinogen (GPIIb/IIIa), von Willebrand factor (GPIb/IX), and collagen (GPIa/IIa) are not correlated with an increased risk for stroke. Stroke **28**: 1392–1395.
21. MURATA, M. *et al.* 1997. Coronary artery disease and polymorphisms in a receptor mediating shear stress-dependent platelet activation. Circulation **96**: 3281–3286.
22. DOUGLAS, H. *et al.* 2002. Platelet membrane glycoprotein Ibalpha gene −5T/C Kozak sequence polymorphism as an independent risk factor for the occurrence of coronary thrombosis. Heart **87**: 70–74.
23. BALISTRERI, C.R. *et al.* 2004. Role of toll-like receptor 4 in acute myocardial infarction and longevity. JAMA **292**: 2339–2340.
24. BALISTRERI, C.R. *et al.* 2006. Association between +1059G/C CRP polymorphism and acute myocardial infarction in a cohort of patients from Sicily: a pilot study. Ann. N. Y. Acad. Sci. **1067**: 276–281.
25. CANDORE, G. *et al.* 2006. Opposite role of pro-inflammatory alleles in acute myocardial infarction and longevity: results of studies performed in the Sicilian population. Ann. N. Y. Acad. Sci. **1067**: 270–275
26. CANDORE, G. *et al.* 2006. Biology of longevity: role of the innate immune system. Rejuvenation Res. **9**: 143–148.
27. GRIMALDI, M.P. *et al.* 2006. Role of the pyrinM694V (A2080G) allele in acute myocardial infarction and longevity: a study in the Sicilian population. J. Leukoc. Biol. **79**: 611–615.
28. LIO, D *et al.* 2004. Opposite effects of IL-10 common gene polymorphisms in cardiovascular diseases and in successful ageing: genetic background of male centenarians is protective against coronary heart disease. J. Med. Genet. **41**: 790–794.

Genetic Control of Immune Response in Carriers of Ancestral Haplotype 8.1

The Study of Chemotaxis

GIUSEPPINA CANDORE, CARMELA R. BALISTRERI,
ANNA MARIA CAMPAGNA, ALFREDO COLOMBO, IRENE CUPPARI,
DANIELE DI-CARLO, MARIA P. GRIMALDI, VALENTINA ORLANDO,
GIUSEPPINA PIAZZA, SONYA VASTO, DOMENICO LIO,
AND CALOGERO CARUSO

*Gruppo di Studio sull'Immunosenescenza, Dipartimento di Biopatologia e
Metodologie Biomediche, Università di Palermo, Palermo, Italy*

ABSTRACT: In all caucasian populations the association of an impressive
number of autoimmune diseases with genes from the HLA-B8, DR3 haplotype that is part of the ancestral haplotype (AH) 8.1 HLA-A1, Cw7,
B8, TNFAB*a2b3, TNFN*S, C2*C, Bf*s, C4A*Q0, C4B*1, DRB1*0301,
DRB3*0101, DQA1*0501, DQB1*0201 has been reported by different
research groups. This haplotype, which is more common in northern Europe, is also associated with a number of immune system dysfunctions in
healthy subjects. Analyzing the data according to gender, some dysfunctions are observed in women but not in men, in agreement with the role
of X-linked genes and/or estrogens in the development and progression
of autoimmune diseases. It has been proposed that a small number of
genes within the 8.1 AH modify immune responsiveness and hence affect
multiple immunopathological diseases. In this article, we demonstrate
that neutrophil chemotaxis is significantly decreased in carriers of this
AH, suggesting that this impairment may also be related to the increased
occurrence of autoimmune diseases in these individuals.

KEYWORDS: ancestral haplotype; autoimmune diseases; chemotaxis;
HLA; immune response

INTRODUCTION

The ancestral haplotype (AH) 8.1 (HLA-A1, Cw7, B8, TNFAB*a2b3,
TNFN*S, C2*C, Bf*s, C4A*Q0, C4B*1, DRB1*0301, DRB3*0101,

Address for correspondence: Giuseppina Candore, Ph.D., Gruppo di Studio sull'Immunosenescenza,
Dipartimento di Biopatologia e Metodologie Biomediche, Corso Tukory 211, 90134 Palermo, Italy.
Voice: +39-09-1655-5932; fax: +39-09-1655-5933.
e-mail: gcandore@unipa.it

Ann. N.Y. Acad. Sci. 1089: 509–515 (2006). © 2006 New York Academy of Sciences.
doi: 10.1196/annals.1386.003

DQA1*0501, DQB1*0201) is a caucasoid haplotype which is more common in northern Europe. Subjects with this haplotype have a higher risk of developing specific autoimmune diseases than do those without these alleles. In particular, this association has been reported with genes from the HLA-B8, DR3 haplotype, which is a part of this AH. In healthy subjects, the 8.1 AH is also associated with several dysfunctions of the immune system by altering the balance of cytokines produced. Analyzing the data according to gender, some dysfunctions are observed in women but not in men, in agreement with the role of X-linked genes and/or estrogens in the development and progression of autoimmune diseases. The most significant change concerns the type 1 responses, which are decreased in contrast with the type 2 humoral responses, which are increased. The type 2 profile plays an important role in the increased incidence of autoimmune disease in 8.1 carriers by an increased blood lymphocyte spontaneous apoptosis and an increased production of some autoantibodies (TABLE 1).[1–12] An excess of apoptotic cells, involved in the increased production of autoantigens, seems to be provided by a high concentration, genetically determined, of tumor necrosis factor (TNF)-α.[4, 11] In addition, 8.1 AH is characterized by a null allele of C4A gene.[4, 12] This allele does not code for a functional C4A protein, which likely plays an anti-inflammatory role, being specialized in the opsonization and immunoclearance processes. So, this genetic defect seems to be associated with an increased production of autoantibodies directed against cells that have undergone apoptosis and are not efficiently disposed of on account of a reduced antigenic clearance. The decrement of the type 1 responses should cause, moreover, a decrease of macrophages, neutrophils, and natural killer functions as well as defects of T cell activation.[4, 8, 10, 12–14]

To verify this seeming paradox of a decreased type 1 inflammatory responses in healthy subjects carrying 8.1 AH, we studied neutrophil function in these subjects and in healthy controls negative for this AH. As a model of neutrophil functionality we studied *in vitro* Boyden chemotaxis, the easiest method to use and standardize chemotaxis.[15]

MATERIALS AND METHODS

We studied 30 subjects (age range 30–50 years old, 15 women and 15 men) in good health. The subjects did not show any clinical symptoms of infection or fever and the subjects did not undergo any pharmacological therapy that could modify the immune responses.

Polymorphonuclear leukocytes (PMNs) were separated by centrifugation on Lympholyte-poly (Cedarlane Laboratories, Hornby, Canada), which is a mixture of sodium metrizoate and dextran 500. This mixture is ideally suited for isolation of PMN from human whole blood. The mononuclear cells and PMNs are separated into two distinct bands free from red blood cells. The PMNs were suspended to a final concentration of 1×10^6 cells/mL in

TABLE 1. Immune response parameters observed in healthy carriers of the 8.1 AH

Immunological alterations observed	Effects of the 8.1 AH
Autoantibodies	Increased
Blood activated T cells	Increased
Blood immune complexes	Increased
Blood lymphocytes	Reduced
In vitro T cell activation	Reduced
Lymphocyte apoptosis	Increased
Macrophage function	Reduced
Natural killer activity	Reduced
Neutrophil chemotaxis	Reduced
Antibody response to EBV, HBV, and influenza virus	Reduced
T cell response to mitogens	Reduced
Type 1 cytokine production	Reduced
Type 2 cytokine production	Increased

Values obtained from 8.1 donors were compared with those obtained from "negative" individuals and were found significantly increased or reduced. Note that when these data have been analyzed, taking into account the gender, some dysfunctions have been observed in women but not in men, according to the data, conferring an important role of X-linked genes and/or estrogens in the development and progression of autoimmune diseases (for references see text).

Hanks' solution supplemented with 1% of bovine serum albumin. A 0.2 mL volume of each cell suspension was incubated in the upper compartment of a Boyden chamber (Chem-Fmlp microfilter, FAR Italia, Italy) separated from the lower compartment by a 3-μM pore membrane filter (13-mm diameter, 150-μm thickness). Each sample was incubated in two different chambers in the presence (sample C) or not (sample R) of chemotactic factor N-formyl-methionyl-leucyl-phenylalanine (FMLP) at 37°C for 1 h. At the end of the incubation, the chambers were emptied and the filters removed, fixed in ethanol, washed in distilled water, and stained with Harris' hematoxylin. PMN migrating through the filters were counted in at least 10 fields ($\times$400). Results were expressed as chemotaxis index (CI) that is, C/R $\times$ 100. Reference values were between 175 and 145 μM ($C = 40$ and $R = 65$ μm).[15–17]

For HLA typing, blood specimens were collected in tripotassium EDTA sterile tubes; DNA was extracted from 30 healthy subjects (age range between 30 and 50 years) and processed for genotyping. DNA samples were amplified for HLA-B8, DR3 alleles by the polymerase chain reaction sequence-specific

TABLE 2. Chemotactic index (mean $\pm$ SD) of 6 healthy subjects carrying (AH) 8.1 and 24 subjects not carrying the haplotype

Haplotype	Chemotactic index	Significance by Student's *t*-test
A.H . 8.1 +	148.50 $\pm$ 7.33	$P < 0.0075$
A.H. 8.1 −	161.95 $\pm$ 4.11	

primer (PCR-SSP) multiplex. PCR products were obtained after amplification in a 12.5 μL volume containing 20 ng of genomic DNA template, 0.5 U of Taq DNA polymerase, 200 μM dNTP, $1\times$ buffer containing (10 mmol/L Tris-HCl pH 8.3, 50 mmol/L KCl), 2 mmol/L $MgCl_2$, and 0.2 pmol/L of each of the primers HLA allele specific. The HLA-DR3 allele was amplified through two different primers: DR17-1F 5'gTTTCTTggAgTACTCTACgTC; DR17-1R 5'gTCCACCCggCCCCgCT; DR17-2F 5'gACggAgCgggTgCggTA; DR17-2R CTgCACTgTgAAgCTCTCCA, and the HLA-B8 allele was drawn as follows: forward B8 5' gAC Cgg AAC ACA CAg ATC TT; reverse B8-1 5' CCT CCA ggT Agg CTC TgT C; reverse B8-2 5' CCg CgC gCT CCA gCg Tg. Cycling was performed as follows: 5 cycles of 95°C for 1 min (denaturating), 65°C for 1 min (annealing), 72°C for 2 min (extension), followed by 25 cycles in which the annealing temperature was lowered to 55°C. Ten microliters of each PCR reaction was run on a 2% agarose gel. The HLA-B8,DR3 alleles were defined by the presence or absence of PCR products of 112 bp.

Value given as mean $\pm$ SD was compared between 8.1 AH positive- and -negative subjects using Student's t-test. Difference was considered significant when it attained a P value < 0.05.

RESULTS AND DISCUSSION

The chemotactic indexes of 6 subjects carrying AH 8.1 and 24 subjects negative for the haplotype are reported in TABLE 2. Data show that neutrophil chemotaxis is significantly decreased in carriers of this haplotype. Because of the small number of subjects under study it was not possible to analyze data according to gender. However, this haplotype is also characterized by an impairment in neutrophil chemotaxis.

Concerning the mechanisms of this type 1 response defect, it has to be remembered that carriers of this haplotype show an impairment of type 1 cytokine production. Neutrophils are phagocytic cells recruited from the circulation via chemoattractant signals and a complex network of adhesion molecules. They participate in acute inflammatory reactions as the first line of defence against pathogens, but are also implicated in the pathogenesis of inflammatory diseases. In inflammation, neutrophils roll along the endothelial wall of postcapillary venules and sample inflammatory signals. The ability of cells to sense external chemical cues and respond by directionally migrating towards them is a fundamental process called chemotaxis. This phenomenon is essential for many biological responses in the human body, including the invasion of neutrophils to sites of inflammation. Chemotaxis is a fundamental biological process in which a cell migrates following the direction of a spatial cue. Chemotaxis is composed of two independent, but interrelated processes—motility and directionality—both of which are regulated by extracellular stimuli, chemoattractants and cytokines. These chemoattractants act as immediate mediators of inflammatory responses by regulating leukocyte recruitment, infiltration, homing, and trafficking as well as of their development and function. In particular the type 1 cytokine IL-12 binds specifically to human neutrophils and this binding leads to the activation of human neutrophils, so this cytokine plays a relevant role in chemotaxis.[18–22] Thus, the decreased production of type 1 cytokine IL-12 observed in the haplotype carriers (TABLE 1 and our unpublished observations) might be responsible for the decreased chemotaxis observed in these subjects.

Genetic studies have shown that individuals with certain HLA alleles have a higher risk of specific autoimmune disease than those without these alleles. Particularly, the association in all caucasian populations of an impressive number of autoimmune diseases with genes from the HLA-B8,DR3 haplotype that is part of the AH 8.1 HLA-A1, Cw7, B8, TNFAB*a2b3, TNFN*S, C2*C, Bf*s, C4A*Q0, C4B*1, DRB1*0301, DRB3*0101, DQA1*0501, DQB1*0201 has been reported by different research groups. This haplotype is also associated in healthy subjects with a number of immune system dysfunctions. We have proposed that a small number of genes within the 8.1 AH modify immune responsiveness and hence affect multiple immunopathologic diseases. This AH carries a single segment characterized by no C4A gene. This null allele does not code for a functional C4A protein that likely plays an anti-inflammatory role, being specialized in the opsonization and immunoclearance processes. So, this genetic defect has been claimed to allow an increased production of autoantibodies directed against cells that have undergone apoptosis and are not efficiently disposed of because of a reduced antigenic clearance. In fact, in the AH carriers the simultaneous high setting of TNF-α may supply the autoantigens by providing an excess of apoptotic cells, which drives the autoimmune response.[1–14] On the other hand, the impairment of chemotaxis might also be relevant to the occurrence of autoimmunity in these subjects. In fact, the relative inabi-lity linked to chemotactic impairment of AH 8.1ositive subjects to remove some kinds of an-tigenic stimuli from the body determines the persistence of an-tigen that may be responsible for the autoimmune responses. For instance, in HLA-B8,DR3ositive mothers whose platelet group is HPA-1-negative, the inability to remove fetal platelets leads to neonatal al-loimmune trombocytopenia when the fetus is HPA-1-positive.[23] Accordingly, we have demonstrated that HLA-B8,DR3ositive indi-viduals may present an increased number of circulating T lympho-cytes displaying the surface markers characteristic of T cell activation.[24] This increased number of activated blood T cells may reflect a cellular activation caused by persistent an-tigenic stimulation. A clinically relevant autoimmune response will develop only in the presence of other immunologic abnormalities.

ACKNOWLEDGMENTS

This work was supported by grants from the Ministry of Education, University and Research, ex 60% to C.C. and G.C. C.R.B., M.P.G., and S.V. are

Ph.D students in the Pathobiology Ph.D curriculum (directed by C. Caruso) of Palermo University. This work is in partial fulfillment of the requirement for the Ph.D.

REFERENCES

1. KLEIN, J. & A. SATO. 2000. The HLA system. N. Engl. J. Med. **343:** 782–786, 702–709.
2. GRUEN, J.R. & S.M. WEISSMAN. 1997. Evolving views of the major histocompatibility complex. Blood **90:** 4252–4265.
3. DAWKINS, R. *et al*. 1999. Genomics of the major histocompatibility complex: haplotypes, duplication, retroviruses and disease. Immunol. Rev. **167:** 275–304.
4. PRICE, P. *et al*. 1999. The genetic basis for the association of the 8.1 ancestral haplotype (A1, B8, DR3) with multiple immunopathological diseases. Immunol. Rev. **167:** 257–274.
5. DAVIDSON, A. & B. DIAMOND. 2001. Autoimmune diseases. N. Engl. J. Med. **345:** 340–350.
6. CARUSO, C. *et al*. 2000. HLA, aging and longevity: a critical reappraisal. Hum. Immunol. **61:** 942–949.
7. MODICA, M.A. *et al*. 1993. The HLA-B8,DR3 haplotype and immune response in healthy subjects. Immunol. Infect. Dis. **3:** 119–127.
8. LIO, D. *et al*. 1997. Modification of cytokine patterns in subjects bearing the HLAB8, DR3 phenotype: implications for autoimmunity. Cytokines Cell. Mol. Ther. **3:** 217–224.
9. CARUSO, C. *et al*. 1996. Major histocompatibility complex regulation of cytokine production. J. Interferon Cytokine Res. **16:** 983–988.
10. CANDORE, G. *et al*. 1998. Biological basis of the HLA-B8,DR3 associated progression of acquired immune deficiency virus syndrome. Pathobiology **66:** 33–37.
11. LIO, D. *et al*. 2001. A genetically determined high setting of TNF-α influences immunological parameters of HLA-B8,DR3 positive subjects: implications for autoimmunity. Human. Immunol. **62:** 705–713.
12. CANDORE, G. *et al*. 2003. Pathogenesis of autoimmune diseases associated with 8.1 ancestral haplotype: a genetically determined defect of C4 influences immunological parameters of healthy carriers of the haplotype. Biomed. Pharmacother. **57:** 274–277.
13. WALPORT, M.J. 2001. Complement. N. Engl. J. Med. **344:** 1140–1144, 1058–1066.
14. CANDORE, G. *et al*. 2002. Pathogenesis of autoimmune diseases associated with 8.1 ancestral haplotype: effect of multiple gene interactions. Autoimmun. Rev. **1:** 29–35.
15. DI LORENZO, G. *et al*. 1999. Granulocyte and natural killer activity in the elderly. Mech. Ageing Dev. **108:** 25–38.
16. FERRANTE, A. & T.H. THONG. 1980. Optimal conditions for simultaneous purification of mononuclear and polymorphonuclear leucocytes from human blood by the Hypaque-Ficoll method. J. Immunol. Methods **36:** 109–117.
17. PATRONE, F. *et al*. 1980. *In vitro* effects of synthetic chemotactic peptides on neutrophil function. Int. Arch. Allergy Appl. Immunol. **62:** 316–323.
18. LEY, K. 2002. Integration of inflammatory signals by rolling neutrophils. Immunol. Rev. **186:** 8–18.

19. COLLISON, K. *et al.* 1998. Evidence for IL-12-activated Ca2+ and tyrosine signaling pathways in human neutrophils. J. Immunol. **161:** 3737–3745.
20. GREGORY, S.H. & E.J. WING. 2002. Neutrophil-Kupffer cell interaction: a critical component of host defenses to systemic bacterial infections. J. Leukoc. **72:** 239–248.
21. BAGORDA, A. *et al.* 2006. Chemotaxis: moving forward and holding on to the past. Thromb. Haemost. **95:** 12–21.
22. GOUWY, M. *et al.* 2005. Synergy in cytokine and chemokine networks amplifies the inflammatory response. Cytokine Growth Factor Rev. **16:** 561–580.
23. WILLIAMSON, L.M. *et al.* 1998. The natural history of fetomaternal alloimmunization to the platelet-specific antigen HPA-1a (PlA1, Zwa) as determined by antenatal screening. Blood **92:** 2280–2287.
24. MODICA, M.A. *et al.* 1990. Markers of T lymphocyte activation in HLA-B8, DR3 positive individuals. Immunobiology **181:** 257–266.

Immunogenetics, Gender, and Longevity

GIUSEPPINA CANDORE,[a] CARMELA R. BALISTRERI,[a]
FLORINDA LISTÌ,[a] MARIA P. GRIMALDI,[a] SONYA VASTO,[a]
GIUSEPPINA COLONNA-ROMANO,[a] CLAUDIO FRANCESCHI,[b,c]
DOMENICO LIO,[a] GRAZIELLA CASELLI,[d] AND CALOGERO CARUSO[a]

[a]*Gruppo di Studio sull' Immunosenescenza, Dipartimento di Biopatologia e
Metodologie Biomediche, Università di Palermo, Palermo, Italy*

[b]*Dipartimento di Patologia Sperimentale e Centro Interdipartimentale Luigi
Galvani, Università di Bologna, Bologna, Italy*

[c]*I.N.R.C.A., Dipartimento di Scienze Gerontologiche, Ancona, Italy*

[d]*Dipartimento di Scienze Demografiche, Università di Roma "La Sapienza,"
Rome, Italy*

ABSTRACT: In this article we discuss relevant data on aging, longevity,
and gender with particular focus on inflammation gene polymorphisms
which could affect an individual's chance to reach the extreme limit
of human life. The present review is not an extensive revision of the
literature, but rather an expert opinion based on selected data from
the authors' laboratories. In 2000–2005 in the more developed regions,
the life expectancy at birth is 71.9 years for men (78.3 in Japan) and
79.3 years for women (86.3 in Japan). Indeed, gender accounts for important differences in the prevalence of a variety of age-related diseases.
Considering people of far-advanced age, demographic data document
a clear-cut prevalence of females compared to males, suggesting that
sex-specific mortality rates follow different trajectories during aging. In
Italy this female/male ratio is relatively lower (about 5/1; F/M ratios are
usually 5–6:1 in other developed countries), but significant differences
have been observed between Italian regions in the distribution of centenarians by gender—from two women per man in the South to more
than eight in certain regions in the North. Thus, a complex interaction of
environmental, historical, and genetic factors, differently characterizing
the various parts of Italy, likely plays an important role in determining
the gender-specific probability of achieving longevity. This can be due
to gender-specific cultural and anthropological characteristics of Italian
society in the last 100 years. Age-related immunoinflammatory factors
increase during proinflammatory status, and the frequency of pro/anti-
inflammatory gene variants also show gender differences. There is some
suggestion that people genetically predisposed to weak inflammatory

Address for correspondence: Prof. Calogero Caruso, Gruppo di Studio sull'Immunosenescenza,
Dipartimento di Biopatologia e Metodologie Biomediche, Corso Tukory 211, 90134 Palermo, Italy.
Voice: +39-09-1655-5911; fax: +39-09-1655-5933.
 e-mail: marcoc@unipa.it

Ann. N.Y. Acad. Sci. 1089: 516–537 (2006). © 2006 New York Academy of Sciences.
doi: 10.1196/annals.1386.051

activity may be at reduced chance of developing coronary heart disease (CHD) and, therefore, may achieve longer lifespan if they avoid serious life-threatening infectious disease thoroughout life. Thus, the pathogen burden, by interacting with host genotype, could determine the type and intensity of the immune-inflammatory response responsible for both proinflammatory status and CHD. These findings point to a strong relationship between the genetics of inflammation, successful aging, and the control of cardiovascular disease, but seem to suggest that the evidence for men is much stronger. The importance of these studies lies in the fact that half of the population (males) lives approximately 10% shorter lives than the other half (females). Understanding the different strategies that men and women seem to follow to achieve longevity may help us to comprehend better the basic phenomenon of aging and allow us to search for safe ways to increase male lifespan.

KEYWORDS: aging; immune response; inflammation; longevity

AGEING

Aging is a postmaturational process that, because of a diminished homeostasis and increased organism vulnerability, causes a reduction of the response to environmental stimuli. The progressive decrease in physiological capacity and the reduced ability to respond to stresses lead to increased susceptibility and vulnerability to disease. Thus, mortality due to all causes increases exponentially with aging. Aging involves all the cells, tissues, organs, and organisms and is modulated by external factors. In diverse tissues various markers of aging have been described: the increase of lipofuscin (age pigment) and the increased cross-linking in extracellular matrix molecules such as collagen are well known in the elderly. Cross-sectional and longitudinal studies show several modifications of such physiological functions as glomerular filtration and the heart rate. These modifications are not always present in all the individuals and in all the organs in the body. So, the speed of aging is different between the individuals of the same species, but in the same individual it could also be different in different organs: frequently there is a cognitive insufficiency whereas the locomotor system is fully efficient or vice versa. More interestingly, studies of gene expression have demonstrated that in the aged several genes show an increase or a decrease in expression. Usually the genes overexpressed are active in stress conditions, such as inflammation.[1–5]

According to evolutionary theories, all animals represent an optimal compromise aimed at securing gene propagation, and so evolutionary pressures select for the ability to procreate and to take care of offspring. Thus, old age has not planned in evolution, as further demonstrated by the lack of old animals in the wilderness. As matter of the fact, we can find them only in the zoos and in domesticated species such as dogs and cats. Exceptions are elephants and turtles, which live for a very long time on account of physical reasons that make them not easily plundered.[3,6] Because aging has a negligible impact on organisms in their natural environment we can conclude that: (i) aging is not genetically programmed to limit the population size, and (ii) selection does not directly work on the aging process. However, the existence of genes that, interacting with the environment, can influence aging and longevity has been clearly demonstrated, as discussed below.

In aging studies, two parameters are usually taken in consideration: life expectancy and the maximum lifespan potential (MLSP). The life expectancy at birth, also known as the average lifespan, represents the mean number of years lived. The other parameter represents instead the age of the longest-lived member(s) of the population or species. Improvements in hygiene and preventive and curative medicine as well as socioeconomic developments have led to an increase of the human mean life expectancy, which allows ever larger proportions of the population to reach an age that is far beyond that of the reproductive phase, but the MLSP has remained constant between 100 and the 122 years (as the French women Jeanne Calment died in Arles at the age of 122 and a half years).[7] Undeniably, the improvement in public health has reduced the principal causes of mortality in the elderly, allowing an increasing number of individuals to reach the maximum lifespan age. If, in the future, the greater causes of death such as cardiovascular disease were to be drastically reduced, life expectancy would yet increase, while the MLSP should be marginally affected.[2,8]

In Western countries the mortality rate increases 25 times more in individuals over 60 years old when compared to people 25–44 years of age.[2] The mortality rate slows down, reaching a plateau as far as the extreme limit of life is drawing near. Most likely mortality decelerates because frailer individuals drop out of the population, leaving behind a more robust cohort that continues to survive. So, the distribution of certain genotypes and other survival-related attributes in a cohort changes with older and older age. This process is termed demographic selection. Because persons drop out of the population because of death from cardiovascular disease, for example, the distribution of certain genotypes in a cohort changes with increasing age.[9,10] This effect is exemplified by the drop-out of the apolipoproteinE ε-4 allele among the extreme old. One of its counterparts, the ε-2 allele, increases in frequency with advanced age among caucasians. Presumably the drop-out of the ε-4 allele is a result of its association with premature mortality secondary to heart disease.[11]

THEORIES OF AGING

To adequately explain the "aging phenotype," different theories have been postulated. However, the proposed theories to explain the senescence process can be gathered in two groups: the stochastic theories and the genetic-evolutionary ones. In any case, the theories have to take into account that humans and animals are structurally designed as a compromise to guarantee optimal survival until the time of reproduction based on natural selection that is effective until that age.[3]

The stochastic theories consider chance as the decisive factor. Aging should be caused by random damage to molecules that retain critical functions along the metabolite pathway. One theory implies that the accumulation of somatic mutations might be caused by background radiation; moreover, the DNA repair ability should also be an important factor because is correlated with the life expectancy of different species.[12,13] Other theories take into account posttranslational processes (oxidation and glycosylation) that increase during life and cause protein alteration and subsequently organ dysfunction. A good example is the role of the low-density lipoproteins (LDLs) oxidized in atherosclerosis.[14,15] Ultimately, to the stochastic theories belongs the free radicals theory, suggesting that free radicals are accumulated in the organisms over time. Oxidants are mainly produced as byproducts of normal aerobic metabolism, but also by phagocytic cells and during lipid peroxidation: this process is harmful for almost all the constituents of the body and overall for DNA and mitochondria. In physiological conditions there is equilibrium between the endogenous production of free radical and their neutralization. An excess of free radical production is called oxidative stress. Numerous experimental studies have shown an inverse correlation between free radical production and duration of life.[16] Many inflammatory diseases typical of the elderly, such as atherosclerosis and Alzheimer's disease, are also related to a prevalence of oxidant versus antioxidant reactions.[17] The enthusiastic acceptance of the role of free radicals in the process of aging has suggested the employment of some kind of food—for instance, vegetables, fruit, red wine—and the use of vitamins (C and E) known to be excellent antioxidants.

The developmental-genetic theories are based on the concept of senescence as a fundamental part of the life development. This consideration originates from the observation that the maximum duration of the life is species-specific and from the human data on the hereditary component of longevity (see below). Both in the nematode *Caenorhabditis elegans*, and in *Drosophila melanogaster*, mutants have been identified accountable for life longer extension. Mutations reducing the activity of a gene called *daf-2*, which among other effects seem to slow metabolism, could double the lifespan of *Caenorhabditis elegans*. Since then, studies in animal models have identified dozens of other genes that influence longevity.[7,18,19]

In human beings, longevity runs in families, whether these genes are longevity genes or genes involved in the control of age-related diseases. In any case, evolutionary theory and empirical evidence suggest that aging is a process of gradual accumulation of damage in cells and tissues of the body. Thus, genes implicated in aging and longevity are implicated in the network of cell maintenance systems, including immune system genes. In fact, the increase in causes of death in people over 65 years when compared with those of individuals between 25 and 44 years old are heart disease, 92-fold; cancer, 43-fold; stroke, greater than 100-fold; chronic lung disease, greater than 100-fold; and pneumonia and influenza, 89-fold.[2] These data suggest a key role for both clonotypic and natural immunity in the control of the survival of the elderly because the susceptibility to these diseases depends in part on a good and functional immune system.[20-22] Therefore, longevity may be correlated with optimal functioning of the immune system, while the aging of immune system, immunosenescence, is the consequence of the continuous attrition caused by chronic antigenic overload. Concomitantly, the antigenic load results in the progressive generation of inflammatory responses involved in age-related diseases. Most of the parameters affected by immunosenescence appear to be under genetic control, and research is addressing this point. Thus immunosenescence fits with basic assumptions of evolutionary theories of aging, such as antagonistic pleiotropy. In fact, the immune system, by neutralizing infectious agents, plays a beneficial role until the time of reproduction and parental care, but, by determining a chronic inflammation, can play a detrimental one late in life, in a period largely not foreseen by evolution.[4,21]

LONGEVITY

Aging and longevity depend on historical, environmental, stochastic, and genetic factors. Trends in Russia, where male life expectancy tumbled during the hardships that followed the fall of Communism, provide a stark reminder of the link between longevity and economic prosperity.[7] Exceptional longevity tends to run in families, although whether this is primarily a result of shared genes or shared environment is unclear (see below). Around the 1970s, in all industrialized countries, the progressive decline of mortality (1–2% per year) in individuals over 80 years old has increased about 20 times the number of oldest old people, that is, centenarians. Centenarians represent a cohort of select survivors who have, at least, markedly delayed diseases that often cause mortality in the general population at significantly younger ages.[23,24] So, centenarians may be a human model of disease-free or at the least, disease-delayed aging. A number of studies have been performed to search for factors that could play a role in such a survival advantage; hence these individuals can provide very useful information for biologic and genetic knowledge of aging. Thus far, no particular environmental trait, such as diet, economic status, or level of education has been found to significantly correlate with the ability to survive to extreme old age.[9,25-28]

The continuation of the decline in mortality at older age means that an increasing number of individuals are becoming centenarians. Women are more likely to cross this threshold, and to such an extent that in low-mortality Western countries there are 5–7 women per man beyond this age. In fact, if one wants to live a long life, it helps to be born female or at least not to indulge in typically reckless male behavior. One extra year is biologically inborn, and 5 or 6 years can be ascribed to differences in social behavior between the sexes, because men take more risks, In fact, the difference in mortality between men and women is not only a question of biologic sex; but it is also a question of "socially constructed sex," a question of gender. Behavioral and environmental factors clearly play a role in determining excess male mortality. Beyond a slight biologic advantage for females, excess male mortality results from the emergency of typically male "man-made diseases." Work-related risk in industrial activity, alcoholism, smoking, and car accidents are the main factors contributing to excess male mortality. An aspect to be highlighted is that the attitude women generally have concerning their body, their health, and their lifestyle is very different from that of men.[7]

In the more developed regions, the life expectancy at birth in 2000–2005 is 71.9 years for men and 79.3 years for women. The highest values are in Japan and are, respectively, 79.3 and 86.3 years for men and women.[29] Females also live longer than males in many other species; for instance, in the laboratory, female Wistar rats live on average 14% longer than males. The fact that this phenomenon also occurs in animals other than humans indicates that it cannot be only attributed to sociological factors, but might reflect specific biological characteristics of both genders. A role for the sex hormones, testosterone in males and estrogen in females, in the gender differences in lifespan seen in mammals is widely claimed.[30]

The role of testosterone in decreasing males' lifespan has also been attributed to the link between this hormone and the male characteristics of aggression and competitiveness, as well as libido. Estrogens, on the other hand, have beneficial effects on the cardiovascular system, because they reduce LDL cholesterol and increase concentrations of high-density lipoprotein (HDL) cholesterol, whereas testosterone also increases blood concentrations of LDL and decreases concentrations of HDL cholesterol, so that men are more prone than women to cardiovascular diseases and stroke.[30–32]

Estrogens also exhibit antioxidant properties *in vivo* by upregulating the expression of the genes encoding antioxidant enzymes. In experimental animals estrogens are responsible for the lower mitochondrial free-radical production observed in females as compared with males. Estrogens should elicit this effect by upregulating expression of the genes encoding mitochondrial antioxidant enzymes.[30]

Besides, there is known sexual dimorphism in the immune response. There is overwhelming evidence that sex-associated hormones can also modulate immune responses and consequently directly influence the outcome of infection, so affecting survival and longevity.[33,34]

FEMININITY RATIO (FR) IN LONGEVITY

Gender accounts for important differences in the incidence and prevalence of a variety of age-related diseases. Considering people of far-advanced age, demographic data document a clear-cut prevalence of females compared to males, suggesting that sex-specific mortality rates follow different trajectories during aging. Gender differences in the health status of centenarians are also reported, because male centenarians are less heterogeneous and more healthy than female centenarians.[35] The importance of these studies lies in the fact that half of the population (males) live approximately 10% shorter lives than the other half (females). An understanding of the reasons for this difference in longevity may help us to better understand the basic phenomenon of aging and allow us to search for safe ways to increase male lifespan.

In the present review, we discuss data from two separate studies performed on Italian and Sardinian centenarians.[36,37] In Italy this ratio is relatively lower (about 5/1) (F/M ratios are usually 5–6:1 in other developed countries),[38] but significant differentials have been observed between Italian regions in the distribution of centenarians by gender, from two women per man in the South to over eight in certain regions in the North.[39] In fact, at the age of 99 years the national FR in Italy is 3.86 women per man for the 1900/1901 cohort, but it is 5.07 in Lombardy, 6.89 in the Veneto, 2.31 in Calabria, and 2.13 in Sicily. These regional disparities have triggered a number of enquiries about the possible role of specific genetic characteristics.[36,39]

In order to explain these differentials, characterized by a North/South axis, Robine et al.[36] have studied the evolution of the femininity ratio (FR), using a longitudinal approach to follow the aging process in two cohorts born in 1900/1901. Taking into account that there are very great differences in death rates in Italy from one region to another, especially after the age of 60 years, and that these differences vary widely from one gender to the other and among regions, their hypothesis was that regional differences in mortality beyond the age of 60 years explained the FRs observed today among centenarians. To make this approach feasible, the effects of migration need to be taken account of, because migration concerns men rather women. It is by comparing the number of centenarians not with the number of births but with the number of survivors of these cohorts at age 60 years (centenarian rate) that one can eliminate the influence of the migration process, because its effect becomes negligible after the age of 60 years.[36] The assessment of the total number of centenarians in Italy per 10,000 births and, respectively, per 10,000 individuals aged 60 years, will clarify this point. For the cohorts under study, the total number is 17.2 for men and 70.0 for women and, respectively, 41.0 for men and 141.0 for women. These centenarian rates differ widely from one region to another. It is especially low for men in northern Italy and for women in southern Italy, but show a different distribution taking into account the number of centenarians per 10,000 individuals aged 60 years. Although always low for men in northern

Italy, the number is particularly high in southern Italy (63.1 in Sicily). On the other hand, differences in the population of women are much smaller, ranging from 139.5 in the Veneto to 121.5 in Lombardy. Hence the birth ratio points to a deficit in centenarian women in the two southern regions, whereas, in contrast, the centenarian rate shows a deficit of centenarian men in the two northern regions and a strong excess in the two southern regions. Only migration can explain the contrasting deficits observed by comparing the centenarian rates with the numbers of births.[36]

As expected, the FR at birth does not vary significantly from the North to the South of Italy, remaining in the range of 0.94–0.95 females per male at birth. At the age of 59 years, the higher mortality of men results in an FR of 1.12 women per man in Italy as a whole, with a little regional variation. The relatively high level of emigration of men compared with that of women in southern Italy could have been expected to lead to a greater FR among those aged 59 years in these regions: only a mortality differential favorable to men can have offset to this extent the effect of migration on the FR. At the age of 60 years, when the migration effect has become negligible, there is still no significant difference in the FR between any of the regions for the 1900/1901 cohort. Beyond this age, differences in FR between the regions are therefore due to mortality differentials alone. This explains the considerable difference in FR at the age of 99 years observed between the North and South of Italy previously quoted. These data highlight how the differences in mortality between the sexes and the regions after the age of 60 years produce the FRs observed among centenarians in the Italian regions.[36]

This study highlights the significant differences in FRs and mortalities observed at the age of 100 years between regions in Italy in 2001. Most of these differences can be explained by mortality differentials after the age of 60 years and in particular between the ages of 60 and 85 years. The high mortality of men in the North and their low mortality in the South explain most of the results: an increased FR in the North and a reduced ratio in the South. The mortality differentials among women play only a minor role, except in Sicily, where high mortality after the age of 75 years, for the most recent cohort, reduces the FR further still. The high mortality of Italian men in the North compared with the South has been the subject of a number of studies, which have highlighted the role of cancer, especially lung cancer, and ischemic diseases in excess mortality. In women, excess mortality from cerebrovascular causes and diabetes in the South, notably in Sicily (see below), compensates for excess mortality from cancer and ischemic diseases in the North, thus explaining why the total mortality varies little from one region to another.[36]

Concerning Sardinian centenarians, the area more or less coinciding with the province of Nuoro has a higher number of centenarians than elsewhere, in particularly for men. In fact, the FR among centenarians in Sardinia is 2.7:1 in comparison to about 5:1 for Italy. There is widespread consensus that the presence of a greater or lesser number of centenarians is largely due to mortality differentials at age 80–100 years.[40] A recent study has been performed to cast light on knowledge of elderly mortality differentials, total and by cause of death, in Sardinia, and attempts to verify the hypothesis that the number of centenarians largely depends on mortality features between 80 and 100 years.[37] To do so, an analysis was conducted of age and sex mortality trends over time at province and municipality level. Results fully confirmed the underlying hypothesis. A 2001 analysis on Sardinians born between 1880 and 1900 as part of the AKEA project[41e] showed that the area with the highest number of centenarians groups together inland adjacent municipalities in the province of Nuoro. Here, for 1990–1994, male life expectancy at age 80 is 8.7 years compared with a regional average of 7.5 years, while that for women is 11.1 and 8.3 years compared with a regional average of 12 years.[37] This zone is part of a wider area where the number of centenarians continues to outstrip the regional average and where life expectancy at age 80 years for the same period is 8.2 for men and 8.7 years for women, once again topping the regional average.[37] Aside from some exceptions it can largely be said that analogies between low mortality at ages 80 years and over and the presence of centenarians is confirmed. A further goal of the AKEA project is to ascertain the causes of death responsible for geographic differences in mortality. Sardinians are at an advantage compared to Italians and they enjoy lower cardiovascular mortality. In zones with the lowest mortality in Sardinia, deaths from these diseases are lower than elsewhere. Besides offering an explanation for such differences, these findings indicate the existence of a specific genetic or environmental factor(s) that protect(s) Sardinian men. This research shows that besides having "good" genes, a favorable environment is also essential for longevity. Equally crucial is the ability to preserve one's health from external "assaults" that can curtail an individual's potential lifespan.[37]

Thus, a complex interaction of environmental, historical, and genetic factors, differently characterizing the various parts of Italy, likely plays an important role in determining the gender-specific probability of achieving longevity.[35–37] 1

GENETICS OF LONGEVITY

The idea that the longevity is based on genetic background is supported by many scientific studies. Nevertheless the lifestyle, habits, type of employment, and level of education also play a relevant role.[42] Data obtained in a study of Scandinavian twins suggest that lifespan is influenced by genetics for 25%.[43] But these studies have not been carried out on nonagenarians and centenarians, so they do not have information about the maximum lifespan. However,

---

[e]The AKEA project directed by Luca Deiana of Sassari University, is the first of a serces of project studying Sardinian centenarians. The name AKEA is derived from an expression in the Sardinian dialect that means "may you live 100 years!"

centenarian siblings have an increased probability of a prolonged existence and the age at death of the centenarian parents is higher than the expectancy of their birth cohort. It is perhaps unsurprising that parents and siblings of centenarians are themselves relatively long-lived. Given the rarity of life-long mortality differences between social groups defined in other ways, these findings suggest a substantial familial component in differentiating exceptionally long-lived individuals from the rest of the population. Obviously, as previously stated, a familiar trait could be environmental, behavioral, or genetic. On the other hand, in general, environmental characteristics of siblings such as socioeconomic status, lifestyles, and region of residence are likely to diverge as they grow older. Thus if the survival advantage of the siblings of centenarians is mainly due to environmental factors, the advantage should decline with age. Because the relative risk of becoming centenarians remains stable over a wide age range, the advantage should be attributable more to genetic than to environmental factors. Moreover, families in which longevity is presented as a main factor belong to different ethnic groups, with a different degree of education, a different partner-economic level, and a different style of life, and hence the importance of the genetic factors.[9,25–28] In the present review we focus on the role of the genes that control immune-inflammatory responses.

GENETICS OF LONGEVITY: ROLE OF HLA

The major histocompatibility complex (MHC) is traditionally divided into the class I, class II, and class III regions (FIG. 1). Class I and class II molecules are highly polymorphic heterodimeric glycoproteins, which take up antigenic peptides intracellularly and emerge on the cell surface, where they present processed peptide fragments to the T lymphocyte receptor. Thus they can restrict and regulate T cell responses against specific antigens. These are the bases for the antigen-specific control of the immune response. The response depends on the ability of histocompatibility molecules to bind some peptides and not others. Thus, survival and longevity might be associated with a positive or negative selection of alleles that respectively confer resistance or susceptibility to infectious disease(s). Besides, genetic studies have shown that persons who have certain HLA (the human MHC) alleles have a higher risk of specific immune-mediated diseases than do persons without these alleles. The associations vary in strength, and in all the diseases studied, several other genes in addition to those of the HLA region are likely to be involved. An intriguing feature of the MHC is the occurrence of particular combinations of alleles, at loci across this 4-Mb region, more frequently than would be expected based on the frequencies of individual alleles. This nonrandom association of alleles gives rise to highly conserved haplotypes that appear to be derived from a common remote ancestor, so-called ancestral haplotypes (AHs). This term underlines the fact that conserved, population-specific haplotypes are continuous sequences de-

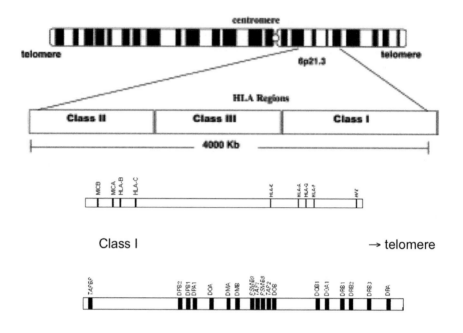

FIGURE 1.   The HLA region encompasses over 4 Mb of DNA (~0.1% of the genome) on the chromosome band 6p21.3 and its extensive characterization has recently culminated in the determination of the nucleotide sequence of the entire region, confirming the presence of ~220 genes. The MHC is traditionally divided into the class I, class II, and class III regions. There are some 20 class I genes in the HLA region; three of these, HLA-A, B, and C, the so-called classic, or class Ia genes, are the main actors in the immunologic theatre. Besides, there are nonclassical HLA class Ib molecules characterized by a limited polymorphism and a restricted expression pattern. HFE is the most telomeric HLA class Ib gene. The class II genes code for the α and β polypeptide chains of the class II molecules. The designation of their loci on chromosome 6 consists of three letters: the first (D) indicates the class, the second (M, O, P, Q, or R) the family, and the third (A or B) the chain (α or β, respectively). The class III region, which has been redefined as the ~730 kb of DNA extending from NOTCH4 to BAT1, is now known to contain at least 62 genes.

rived with little, if any, change from an ancestor of all those now carrying all or part of the haplotype. These AHs determine a nonrandom assortment of alleles at neighboring loci, referred to as "linkage disequilibrium."[44–48]

The studies studying the association between longevity and HLA are generally difficult to interpret on account of major methodological problems. However, as reported by Caruso et al.,[44,45] some of them, well designed and performed, suggest an HLA effect on longevity. In studies performed in caucasoids, an increase in HLA-DR11 (that is a HLA-DR5 split) in Dutch women over 85 years was observed. The same laboratory performed a further study and, by using a "birth-place-restricted comparison" in which the origin of all the subjects was ascertained, the authors were able to confirm that aging in women was positively associated with HLA-DR5.[49,50] Two French studies confirmed the relevance of HLA-DR11 to longevity in aged populations.[51,52] This increase is consistent with the protective effects of this allele in viral diseases, as HLA-DR5, or its subtype HLA-DR11, frequencies have been shown to be decreased in some viral diseases.[44,45] Finally, an association between longevity and the AH 8.1 (or part of this haplotype, i.e., HLA-B8,DR3) apparently emerges. The 8.1 AH is a common Caucasoid haplotype, unique in its association with a wide range of immunopathological diseases and in healthy subjects with a large array of immune dysfunctions.[46,47] An excess of this AH in oldest old men has been reported in French and in Northern Irish populations. This association appears to be gender-specific. In fact, a Greek study showed a significant decrease of 8.1 AH in aged women.[53–55] So, the immune changes typical of the 8.1 AH should contribute to early morbidity and mortality in elderly women, who are more susceptible to autoimmune diseases than men, and to longevity in elderly men. Thus, these studies seem to suggest that HLA-DR11 in women and HLA-B8,DR3 in men may be considered markers of successful aging.[49–55] However, in a longitudinal study, in which a total of 919 subjects aged 85 years and older, were HLA-typed and followed up for at least 5 years, no HLA-association with mortality was found.[56] Besides, in Sardinian centenarians we did not observe the associations demonstrated in the other well-planned and designed studies discussed above.[57] Moreover, a study set out to specifically confirm the previously reported increase in the frequency of the 8.1 AH in aged men of the Northern Irish population did not reveal any statistically significant haplotype frequency differences between the aged cohort of individuals in comparison to the younger controls. However, a striking decrease was observed when the aged women (13.1%) were compared to the control women (17.8%).[58]

The HLA HFE gene codes for a class I α chain, which seemingly no longer participates in immunity, because it has lost its ability to bind peptides due to a definitive closure of the antigen binding cleft that prevents peptide binding and presentation. The HFE protein, expressed in crypt enterocytes of the duodenum, regulates the iron uptake by intestinal cells because it has acquired the ability to form a complex with the receptor for iron-binding transferrin. The C282Y mutation (a cysteine-to-tyrosine mutation at amino acid 282) in this gene has been identified as the main genetic basis of hereditary hemochromatosis. It destroys its ability to make up a heterodimer with β2-microglobulin. The defective protein fails to associate to the transferrin receptor and the complex cannot be transported to the surface of the duodenal crypt cells. As a consequence, in homozygous people two to three times the normal amount of iron is absorbed from food by the intestine. It has been suggested that an estimated 60–70 generations ago, C282Y mutation occurred in the HFE gene of a Celtic individual who is the ancestor of the more than 5% of caucasoids now carrying the allele. It has been claimed that the great expansion of Celtic people could be in part explained by the widespread presence of this HFE gene mutation. This gave to heterozygous carriers selective advantages on the basis of improved survival during infancy, childhood, and pregnancy, by leading to increased iron absorption and accumulation of larger body iron stores because ancient diet consisted mainly in iron-poor grains and cereals, whereas meat was highly uncommon.[48,59] This evolutionary significance of these mutations suggests their possible role in survival and longevity. We have recently reported that C282Y mutation may confer a selective advantage in term of longevity to Sicilian women. Our data seem to suggest that possession of C282Y allele, known to be associated with an increase of iron uptake, significantly increases only in women the possibility to reach longevity. In this respect, it has to be remembered that for the generation of elderly people under study, lifestyle, including diet, was quite different for men and women. Considering the historical and social contest in which the generation of women under study lived, we have suggested that that possession of iron-sparing alleles significantly increases the possibility to reach longevity in women. For instance, in Sicily, a lot of pregnancies and an iron-poor diet, consisting mainly in grains, vegetables, and fruits, were yet the rule for the women born at the beginning of last century; in fact meat was highly uncommon and in any case it was put aside for men and children.[60] These considerations can also contribute to explaining, at least in part, the previous data on female mortality in southern Italy.

On the whole these findings clearly show that HLA/longevity associations are population-specific, being heavily affected by the population-specific genetic and environmental history (selection by different kinds of infectious diseases or lifestyle for HFE). These associations are gender-related, so gene variants representing a genetic advantage for one gender are not automatically relevant for the other gender in terms of successful aging, for the reasons previously outlined.

GENETICS OF LONGEVITY: ROLE OF GENETICS OF INFLAMMATION

Theoretically, a proinflammatory profile should be associated with longevity, but this is not the case. The process of life for the individual is the struggle to preserve its integrity. However, the preservation of the integrity of the organism comes with a price—systemic inflammation.[61] Why the innate immune system activates is not clear, but increased exposure to infectious agents or cumulative damage to tissues could spark the change.[4,5] The inflammation is not *per se* a negative phenomenon: it is the response of the immune system to the aggression of viruses or bacteria. The problem is that the human organism, in the course of evolution, has been set to live 40 or 50 years.

Nowadays the immune system must be active for more decades than in past centuries. This very long activity leads to a chronic inflammation that slowly but inexorably damages all the organs: this is a typical phenomenon linked to aging and, as discussed by Licastro *et al.*,[22] it is considered the major risk factor for all the chronic age-related diseases. Other well-known factors, as cholesterol levels in coronary heart disease (CHD), maintain their importance; differences in the inflammatory state can explain why high cholesterol levels do not always determine the cardiovascular disease.[10] So, it is emergent evidence that polymorphic alleles of inflammatory cytokines, involved in high cytokine production, are related to unsuccessful aging as atherosclerosis and Alzheimer's disease; reciprocally, controlling inflammatory status may allow to us better attain successful aging.[21]

Some of our recent evidence has, in fact, linked cytokine polymorphisms with longevity and differential longevity between males and females in the Italian population (TABLE 1).[62] A study performed on Italian centenarians reported that those individuals who are genetically predisposed to produce high levels of IL-6 during aging, that is, C-negative men at IL-6 –174 C/G single nucleotide polymorphism (SNP) have a reduced capacity to reach the extreme limits of human lifespan.[63] Moreover, more recent data indicate that –1082G IL-10 SNP, associated with a high production of the cytokine, is increased among Italian male centenarians.[10,64,65] These findings allow hypothesizing that different alleles at different cytokine gene coding for pro- (IL-6) or anti-inflammatory (IL-10) cytokines may affect the individual lifespan expectancy by influencing the type and intensity of the immune-inflammatory responses against environmental stressors. In aged women inflammation is important too, but the differences in lifespan seem to be not directly related to it. These results have not been fully confirmed in other populations; again, they are population-specific, being heavily affected by the population-specific genetic and environmental history.[62]

TABLE 1. Studies on cytokine gene polymorphisms in young, elderly, and centenarians from Italy

Gene polymorphism	Centenarians	Elderly (age)	Young (age)	Results
IL-6 –174 C/G	68♂	150♂(60–99)		↓ GG
IL-6 –174 C/G	255♀	227♀(60–99)		No change
IL-10 –1082A/G	31♂		161♂ (18–60)	↑ GG
IL-10 –1082A/G	159♀		99♀ (18–60)	No change
IL-10 –1082A/G	72♂		115♂ (22–60)	↑ GG
IL-10 –1082A/G	102♀		112♀ (22–60)	No change
IL-10 –1082A/G	54♂		110♂ (18–60)	↑ GG
TNF-α -308G/A	72♂		115♂ (18–60)	No change
TNF-α -308G/A	102♀		112♀ (18–60)	No change

NOTE: ↑ and ↓ refer to significant ($P < 0.05$) increase or respectively decrease of alleles or genotypes with respect to control population. For references see text.

Male centenarians are people who seem genetically equipped for defeating major age-related diseases because they present SNP in the immune system genome which, regulating the immune-inflammatory responses, seems to be associated with longevity. Moreover, centenarians are characterized by marked delay or escape from age-associated diseases that, on average, cause mortality at earlier ages.[23,24] In addition, centenarian offspring have an increased likelihood of surviving to 100 years and showed a reduced prevalence of age-associated diseases, such as cardiovascular disease, and lower prevalence of cardiovascular risk factors.[66] Thus, genes involved in CHD may play an opposite role in human longevity.[67,68]

Atherosclerosis and its complications contribute significantly to increased morbidity and mortality rate in older people. Inflammation is a key component of atherosclerosis and inflammatory genes are, therefore, good candidates for the risk of developing atherosclerosis. Differences in the genetic regulation of immune-inflammatory processes might partially explain why some people, but not others, develop the disease and why some develop a greater inflammatory response than others. Accordingly, common gene polymorphisms regulating high inflammatory molecule production have been associated with atherosclerosis. Conversely, those associated with a positive control of inflammation might play a protective role against atherosclerosis.[67]

If proinflammatory genotypes significantly contribute to the risk of CHD, alleles associated with disease susceptibility should not be included in the genetic background favoring longevity. Hence, we hypothesized that genotypes of natural immunity might play an opposite role in atherosclerosis and longevity. Trying to confirm our hypothesis, we are studying the role of proinflammatory alleles in acute myocardial infarction (AMI) and in longevous subjects in our homogeneous Sicilian population. To improve the power of our study, we select cases genetically loaded for having early AMI onset (<46 years).[67,68]

The proinflammatory alleles of the following inflammatory genes—pyrin (i.e., the gene responsible for familial Mediterranean fever) (2080G), the coreceptor for lipopolysaccharide (TLR4 A896), the chemokyne receptor (CCR5 Δ 32), the Gap junction channel protein regulating leukocyte recruitment (Cx37 + 1019T), the enzymes involved in ecosanoid production (−765G COX-2 and −1708A LOX), the anti-inflammatory IL-10 cytokine (−A108) and proinflammatory TNF-α cytokine (-G308A)—were significantly over-represented in AMI patients and under-represented in oldest old and centenarians, whereas age-related controls displayed intermediate values (Refs. 21, 68, and 72, and unpublished observations). These results strengthen the hypothesis that genetic background protecting against cardiovascular disease is a relevant component of the longevity trait, at least in the generation of Italian male centenarians under study.[68–70] The results obtained in the Italian patients and centenarians might also depend on the differential importance of classical risk factors for atherosclerosis and AMI in the Italian population because the traditional Mediterranean diet may affect the incidence and prevalence of AMI.

So, it is possible that these polymorphisms are not relevant for longevity (and atherosclerosis) in north European populations, where a rich meat diet is the major risk factor for cardiovascular diseases.[62,67,73,74]

CONCLUSIONS

In this article we discuss relevant data on aging, longevity, and gender with particular focus on inflammation gene polymorphisms which could affect the individual's chance to reach the extreme limit of human life. The present review is not an extensive revision of the literature, but rather an expert opinion based on selected data from authors' laboratories.

Centenarians have lived most of their life in an environment quite different from that we experience today. In the last years enormous demographic and epidemiological changes have occurred that have changed our lifestyle. In other words, to study centenarians means to perform a sort of archeological research that has to consider the historical and anthropological characteristics of the population of men and women under study. Type of occupation, migration, mortality related to labor, diseases and nutritional status, wars, and childbearing can impinge differently on later survival and FR in longevity. Accordingly, studies performed in different parts of Italy have disclosed differences related to geography and sex. As discussed in this review, a strict biological and reductionist approach is insufficient to account for the observed differences; a new integrated approach, including demography and anthropology, appears to be necessary to unravel the complex interaction between the environmental/cultural and biological/genetic components responsible for gender difference in longevity.[35]

The immunogenetics of aging and longevity is both complex and intriguing. Indeed, the longevity phenotype is strongly affected by lifestyle and stochastic and environmental factors and by complex epistatic and pleiotropic gene effects. The genetics of aging and longevity is highly unusual and most probably represents a post-reproduction genetic scenario, where the force of selection progressively fades in the later decades of life.[75,76] Species are not programmed to get older, but to survive. Senescence and disease age-related are the price for a high fitness-reproduction, so aging seems to be the only available way to live a long life. In a human heterogeneous population, the ability to maintain a good response to "stressors" should have a Gaussian distribution. Centenarians could represent the extreme tail of this plot: they represent the best kind of adaptability to environmental conditions. Centenarian offspring have a marked increased probability of longevity and show a reduced prevalence of age-associated diseases, particularly those related to cardiovascular disease and cardiovascular risk factors.[66] For the generation of male centenarians under study that means to be equipped with a genetic background and lifestyle that delivers resistance to CHD. This also means that common genetic risk factors, as identified on the basis of specific diseases, are not the key of longevity and

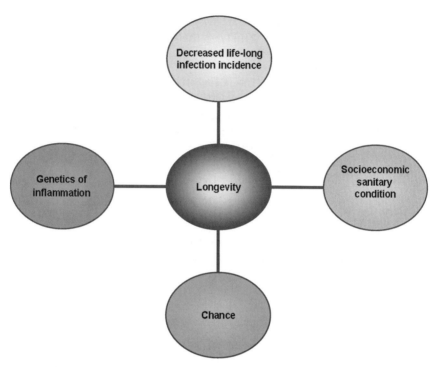

FIGURE 2. The factors influencing longevity in the generation of male centenarians under study.

the effect that these genes have on the mortality rate of the global population seems to be not relevant.[45,56] Accordingly, the genes that control the natural immunity (inflammation) seem more significant than the genes of the HLA system that control the specific immunity against the single pathogens.

Finally, our data prompt considerations on the role that antagonistic pleiotropy[6] plays in diseases and in longevity. The aging of the immune system, immunosenescence, is the consequence of the continuous attrition caused by chronic antigenic overload. The antigenic load results in the progressive generation of inflammatory responses involved in age-related diseases.[20–22] So, immunosenescence fits with the basic assumptions of evolutionary theories of aging, such as antagonistic pleiotropy. In fact, the immune system, by neutralizing infectious agents, plays a beneficial role until the time of the reproduction and parental care. Subsequently, by determining a chronic inflammation, these factors play a detrimental role late in life, in a period largely unforeseen by evolution. Genetic backgrounds promoting proinflammatory responses may play opposite roles in CHD and in longevity, such that CHD are a late consequence of an evolutionary proinflammatory response highly charged and programmed to resist infections in earlier life. Genetic polymorphisms responsible for a low inflammatory response might result in an increased chance of long lifespan in an environment with a reduced antigen (i.e., pathogens) load, such as a modern-day health environment, and may also permit a lower-grade survivable inflammatory response to atherogenesis and atherosclerosis-related disease. These findings point to a strong relationship between the genetics of inflammation, successful aging, and the control of cardiovascular disease; however, they do seem to suggest that the evidence for men is much stronger, whereas in females the situation seems to be quite different, indicating that males and females may follow different trajectories toward extreme longevity.[35]

In conclusion in the present review we have tried to clarify the different environmental and immunogenetics factors involved in the differential longevity of men and women (FIG. 2). We did not discuss the relevance of the stochastic events in longevity. The relevance of chance in our life is less a matter of study of science, but rather of philosophy or, even better, of poetry.

ACKNOWLEDGMENTS

This work was supported by grants from the Ministry of Education, University and Research, ex60% to Calogero Caruso and G.C. and the Ministry of Health (Markers genetici di sindrome coronarica acuta e valutazione della L-arginina nella prevenzione di eventi ischemici). Carmela R. Balistreri, Maria P. Grimaldi, and Sonya Vasto are Ph.D. students in the Pathobiology Ph.D. curriculum (directed by C. Caruso) of Palermo University and this work is in partial fulfillment of the requirement for the Ph.D. The "Immunosenesence Research Group" coordinated by Prof. C. Caruso in association with INRCA was enlarged through a joint contract (Longevity and elderly disability biological markers).

REFERENCES

1. WEINDRUCH, R. *et al.* 2002. Gene expression profiling of aging using DNA microarrays. Mech. Ageing. Dev. **123:** 177–193.
2. TROEN, B.R. 2003. The biology of aging. Mt. Sinai J. Med. **70:** 3–22.
3. WICK, G. *et al.* 2003. A Darwinian-evolutionary concept of age-related diseases. Exp. Gerontol. **38:** 13–25.
4. FRANCESCHI, C. *et al.* 2000. Inflamm-aging. An evolutionary perspective on immunosenescence. Ann. N.Y. Acad. Sci. **908:** 208–218.
5. FRANCESCHI, C. *et al.* 2000. The network and the remodeling theories of aging: historical background and new perspectives. Exp. Gerontol. **35:** 879–896.
6. NESSE, R.M. & G.C. WILLIAMS. 1995. Evolution and Healing. The New Science of Darwinian Medicine. Weidenfeld and Nicolson. United Kingdom.
7. ABBOTT, A. 2004. Ageing: growing old gracefully. Nature **428:** 116–118.
8. ROUSH, W. 1996. Live long and prosper? Science **273:** 42–46.

9. PERLS, T. *et al.* 2002. The genetics of aging. Curr. Opin. Genet. Dev. **12:** 362–369.
10. LIO, D. *et al.* 2004. Opposite effects of IL-10 common gene polymorphisms in cardiovascular diseases and in successful ageing: genetic background of male centenarians is protective against coronary heart disease. J. Med. Genet. **41:** 790–794.
11. PANZA, F. *et al.* 2004. Vascular genetic factors and human longevity. Mech. Ageing Dev. **125:** 169–178.
12. HART, R.W. & R.B. SETLOW. 1974. Correlation between deoxyribonucleic acid excision-repair and life-span in a number of mammalian species. Proc. Natl. Acad. Sci. USA **71:** 2169–2173.
13. DORIA, G. & D. FRASCA. 2000. Genetic factors in immunity and aging. Vaccine **18:** 1591–1595.
14. CERAMI, A. *et al.* 1987. Glucose and aging. Sci. Am. **256:** 90–96.
15. STADTMAN, E.R. 2001. Protein oxidation in aging and age-related diseases. Ann. N.Y. Acad. Sci. **928:** 22–38.
16. SALVIOLI, S. *et al.* 2006. Genes, Ageing and Longevity in Humans: Problems, Advantages and Perspectives. Free Radic. Res. In press.
17. FINKEL, T. & N.J. HOLBROOK. 2000. Oxidants, oxidative stress and the biology of ageing. Nature **408:** 239–247.
18. HONDA, Y. & S. HONDA. 2002. Oxidative stress and life span determination in the nematode *Caenorhabditis elegans*. Ann. N.Y. Acad. Sci. **959:** 466–474.
19. KAPAHI, P. *et al.* 2004. Regulation of lifespan in *Drosophila* by modulation of genes in the TOR signaling pathway. Curr. Biol. **14:** 885–890.
20. FRANCESCHI, C. *et al.* 2000. Human immunosenescence: the prevailing of innate immunity, the failing of clonotypic immunity, and the filling of immunological space. Vaccine **18:** 1717–1720.
21. CANDORE, G. *et al.* 2006. Biology of longevity: role of the innate immune system. Rejuvenation Res. **9:** 143–148.
22. LICASTRO, F. *et al.* 2005. Innate immunity and inflammation in ageing: a key for understanding age-related diseases. Immun. Ageing **2:** 8.
23. FRANCESCHI, C. *et al.* 1995. The immunology of exceptional individuals: the lesson of centenarians. Immunol. Today **16:** 12–16.
24. FRANCESCHI, C. & M. BONAFE. 2003. Centenarians as a model for healthy aging. Biochem. Soc. Trans. **31:** 457–461.
25. PERLS, T. 2002. Life-long sustained mortality advantage of siblings of centenarians. Proc. Natl. Acad. Sci. USA **99:** 8442–8447.
26. PERLS, T. *et al.* 2002. What does it take to live to 100? Mech. Ageing Dev. **123:** 231–242.
27. PERLS, T. & D. TERRY. 2003. Understanding the determinants of exceptional longevity. Ann. Intern. Med. **139:** 445–449.
28. PERLS, T. & D. TERRY. 2003. Genetics of exceptional longevity. Exp. Gerontol. **38:** 725–730.
29. World Population Prospects: The 2004 Revision. Available at www. unpopulation.org.
30. VINA, J. 2005. Why females live longer than males: control of longevity by sex hormones. Sci. Aging Knowledge Environ. **8:** pe17.
31. MENDELSOHN, M.H. & R.H. KARAS. 1999. The protective effects of estrogen on the cardiovascular system. N. Engl. J. Med. **340:** 1801–1811.
32. WEIDEMANN, W. & H. HANKE. 2002. Cardiovascular effects of androgens. Cardiovasc. Drug Rev. **20:** 175–198.

33. KLEIN, S.L. *et al.* 2000. The effects of hormones on sex differences in infection: from genes to behaviour. Neurosci. Biobehav. Rev. **24:** 627–638.
34. ROBERTS, C.W. *et al.* 2001. Sex-associated hormones and immunity to protozoan parasites. Clin. Microbiol. Rev. **14:** 476–488.
35. FRANCESCHI, C. *et al.* 2000. Do men and women follow different trajectories to reach extreme longevity? Italian Multicenter Study on Centenarians. Aging Clin. Exp. Res. **12:** 77–84.
36. ROBINE, J.M. *et al.* 2006. Differentials in the femininity ratio among centenarians: variations between northern and southern Italy from 1870. Popul. Stud. **60:** 99–113.
37. CASELLI, G. & R.M. LIPSI. 2006. Survival differences among the oldest old in Sardinia: who, what, where, and why? Demogr. Res. **14:** 267–294.
38. ROBINE, J.M. & G. CASELLI. 2005. An unprecedented increase in the number of centenarians. Genus **61:** 57–82.
39. PASSARINO, G. *et al.* 2002. Male/female ratio in centenarians: a possible role played by population genetic structure. Exp. Gerontol. **37:** 1283–1289.
40. JEUNE, B. & J.W. VAUPEL. 1995. Exceptional Longevity: From Prehistory to the Present. Odense University Press. Odense.
41. POULAIN, M. *et al.* 2004. Identification of a geographic area characterized by extreme longevity in the Sardinia island: the AKEA study. Exp. Gerontol. **39:** 1423–1429.
42. COURNIL, A. & T.B. KIRKWOOD. 2001. If you would live long, choose your parents well. Trends Genet. **17:** 233–235.
43. LJUNGQUIST, B. *et al.* 1998. The effect of genetic factors for longevity: a comparison of identical and fraternal twins in the Swedish Twin Registry. J. Gerontol. A Biol. Sci. Med. Sci. **53:** M441–M446.
44. CARUSO, C. *et al.* 2000. HLA, aging, and longevity: a critical reappraisal. Hum. Immunol. **61:** 942–949.
45. CARUSO, C. *et al.* 2001. Immunogenetics of longevity. Is major histocompatibility complex polymorphis relevant to the control of human longevity? A review of literature data. Mech. Ageing. Dev. **122:** 445–462.
46. CANDORE, G. *et al.* 2002. Pathogenesis of autoimmune diseases associated with 8.1 ancestral haplotype: effect of multiple gene interactions. Autoimmun. Rev. **1:** 29–35.
47. CANDORE, G. *et al.* 2003. Pathogenesis of autoimmune diseases associated with 8.1 ancestral haplotype: a genetically determined defect of C4 influences immuno-logical parameters of healthy carriers of the haplotype. Biomed. Pharmacother. **57:** 274–277.
48. KLEIN, J. & A. SATO. 2000. The HLA system. N. Engl. J. Med **343:** 702–709; 782–786.
49. LAGAAY, A.M. *et al.* 1991. Longevity and heredity in humans. Association with the human leukocyte antigen phenotype. Ann. N.Y. Acad. Sci. **621:** 78–89.
50. IZAKS, G.J. *et al.* 2000. The effect of geographic origin on the frequency of HLA antigens and their association with ageing. Eur. J. Immunogenet. **27:** 87–92.
51. IVANOVA, R. *et al.* 1998. HLA-DR alleles display sex-dependent effects on survival and discriminate between individual and familial longevity. Hum. Mol. Genet. **7:** 187–194.
52. HENON, N. *et al.* 1999. Familial versus sporadic longevity and MHC markers. J. Biol. Regulat. Homeost. Agent **13:** 27–30.

53. PROUST, J. *et al.* 1982. HLA and longevity. Tissue Antigens **19:** 168–173.
54. REA, I.M. & D. MIDDLETON. 1994. Is the phenotypic combination A1B8Cw7DR3 a marker for male longevity? J. Am. Geriatr. Soc. **42:** 978–983.
55. PAPASTERIADES, C. *et al.* 1997. HLA phenotypes in healthy aged subjects. Gerontology **43:** 176–181.
56. IZAKS, G.J. *et al.* 1997. The association between human leucocyte antigens (HLA) and mortality in community residents aged 85 and older. J. Am. Geriatr. Soc. **45:** 56–60.
57. LIO, D. *et al.* 2003. Association between the HLA-DR alleles and longevity: a study in Sardinian population. Exp. Gerontol. **38:** 313–318.
58. ROSS, O.A. *et al.* 2003. HLA haplotypes and TNF polymorphism do not associate with longevity in the Irish. Mech. Ageing Dev. **124:** 563–567.
59. CANDORE, G. *et al.* 2002. Frequency of the HFE Gene Mutations in Five Italian Populations. Blood Cells Mol. Dis. **29:** 267–273.
60. LIO, D. *et al.* 2002. Association between the MHC class I gene HFE polymorphisms and longevity: a study in Sicilian population. Genes Immun. **3:** 20–24.
61. BROD, S.A. 2000. Unregulated inflammation shortens human functional longevity. Inflamm. Res. **49:** 561–570.
62. REA, I.M. *et al.* Cytokine gene polymorphisms and longevity. *In* Cytokine Gene Polymorphisms in Multifactorial Conditions. Koen Vandenbroeck, Ed. CRC Press. Boca Raton, FL.
63. BONAFE, M. *et al.* 2001. A gender-dependent genetic predisposition to produce high levels of IL-6 is detrimental for longevity. Eur. J. Immunol. **31:** 2357–2361.
64. LIO, D. *et al.* 2002. Gender specific association between –1082 IL-10 promoter polymorphism and longevity. Genes Immun. **3:** 30–33.
65. LIO, D. *et al.* 2003. Inflammation, genetics, and longevity: further studies on the protective effects in men of IL-10 -1082 promoter SNP and its interaction with TNF-alpha -308 promoter SNP. J. Med. Genet. **40:** 296–299.
66. TERRY, D.F. *et al.* 2003. Cardiovascular advantages among the offspring of centenarians. J. Gerontol. A Biol. Sci. Med. Sci. **58:** M425–M431.
67. CANDORE, G. *et al.* Cytokine gene polymorphisms and atherosclerosis. *In* Cytokine Gene Polymorphisms in Multifactorial Conditions. Koen Vandenbroeck, Ed. CRC Press. Boca Raton, FL.
68. CANDORE, G. *et al.* 2006. Opposite role of pro-inflammatory alleles in acute myocardial infarction and longevity: results of studies performed in a Sicilian population. Ann. N.Y. Acad. Sci. **1067:** 270–275.
69. CARUSO, C. *et al.* 2005. Inflammation and life-span. Science **307:** 208 [letter].
70. CANDORE, G. *et al.* 2006. Inflammation, longevity, and cardiovascular diseases: role of polymorphisms of TLR4. Ann. N.Y. Acad Sci. **1067:** 282–287.
71. GRIMALDI, M.P. *et al.* 2006. Role of the pyrin M694V (A2080G) allele in acute myocardial infarction and longevity: a study in the Sicilian population. J. Leukoc. Biol. **79:** 611–615.
72. BALISTRERI, C.R. *et al.* 2004. Role of toll-like receptor 4 in acute myocardial infarction and longevity. JAMA **292:** 2339–2340.
73. MASSARO, M. *et al.* 1999. Direct vascular antiatherogenic effects of oleic acid: a clue to the cardioprotective effects of the Mediterranean diet. Cardiologia **44:** 507–513.
74. BARZI, F. *et al.* GISSI-PREVENZIONE INVESTIGATORS. 2003. Mediterranean diet and all-causes mortality after myocardial infarction: results from the GISSI-Prevenzione trial. Eur. J. Clin. Nutr. **57:** 604–611.

75. FRANCESCHI, C. *et al.* 2005. Genes involved in immune response/inflammation, IGF1/insulin pathway and response to oxidative stress play a major role in the genetics of human longevity: the lesson of centenarians. Mech. Ageing Dev. **126:** 351–361.
76. CAPRI, M. *et al.* 2006. The genetics of human longevity. Ann. N.Y. Acad. Sci. **1067:** 252–263.

Estrogens and Autoimmune Diseases

MAURIZIO CUTOLO,[a] SILVIA CAPELLINO,[a] ALBERTO SULLI,[a]
BRUNO SERIOLI,[a] MARIA ELENA SECCHI,[a] BARBARA VILLAGGIO,[a]
AND RAINER H. STRAUB[b]

[a]Research Laboratory and Division of Rheumatology, Department of Internal
Medicine, University of Genova, Viale Benedetto XV, 6, 16132 Genova, Italy

[b]Laboratory of Neuroendocrineimmunology, Department of Internal Medicine,
University Hospital, Regensburg, Germany

ABSTRACT: Sex hormones are implicated in the immune response, with
estrogens as enhancers at least of the humoral immunity and androgens
and progesterone (and glucocorticoids) as natural immune-suppressors.
Several physiological, pathological, and therapeutic conditions may
change the serum estrogen milieu and/or peripheral conversion rate, including the menstrual cycle, pregnancy, postpartum period, menopause,
being elderly, chronic stress, altered circadian rhythms, inflammatory
cytokines, and use of corticosteroids, oral contraceptives, and steroid
hormonal replacements, inducing altered androgen/estrogen ratios and
related effects. In particular, cortisol and melatonin circadian rhythms
are altered, at least in rheumatoid arthritis (RA), and partially involve
sex hormone circadian synthesis and levels as well. Abnormal regulation of aromatase activity (i.e., increased activity) by inflammatory cytokine production (i.e., TNF-alpha, IL-1, and IL-6) may partially explain
the abnormalities of peripheral estrogen synthesis in RA (i.e., increased
availability of 17-beta estradiol and possible metabolites in synovial fluids) and in systemic lupus erythematosus, as well as the altered serum
sex-hormone levels and ratio (i.e., decreased androgens and DHEAS).
In the synovial fluids of RA patients, the increased estrogen concentration is observed in both sexes and is more specifically characterized by
the hydroxylated forms, in particular 16alpha-hydroxyestrone, which is
a mitogenic and cell proliferative endogenous hormone. Local effects of
sex hormones in autoimmune rheumatic diseases seems to consist mainly
in modulation of cell proliferation and cytokine production (i.e., TNF-
alpha, Il-1, IL-12). In this respect, it is interesting that male patients with
RA seem to profit more from anti-TNFalpha strategies than do female
patients.

KEYWORDS: sex hormones; autoimmune diseases; rheumatoid arthritis;
systemic lupus erythematosus; estrogens; androgens; circadian rhythms

Address for correspondence: Maurizio Cutolo, M.D., Research Laboratory and Division of Rheumatology, Department of Internal Medicine, University of Genova, Viale Benedetto XV, 6, 16132 Genova,
Italy. Voice: +39-(0)10-353-7994; fax: +39-(0)10-353-8885.
e-mail: mcutolo@unige.it

Ann. N.Y. Acad. Sci. 1089: 538–547 (2006). © 2006 New York Academy of Sciences.
doi: 10.1196/annals.1386.043

SEX HORMONES AND AUTOIMMUNE DISEASES

Epidemiological evidence indicates that during the fertile period women are more often affected by rheumatic diseases than men, particularly autoimmune diseases.[1] As a matter of fact, rheumatic disorders with autoimmune involvement such as rheumatoid arthritis (RA) or systemic lupus erythematosus (SLE) result from the combination of several predisposing factors, which include the relationships between epitopes of the trigger agent (i.e., virus) and histocompatibility epitopes (i.e., human leukocyte antigen [HLA]), latitude effects, the status of the stress response system including the hypothalamic-pituitary-adrenocortical axis (HPA) and the sympathetic nervous system (SNS), and mainly the effects of the gonadal hormones (hypothalamic-pituitary-gonadal axis—HPG).[2,3]

The pre- or postmenopausal serum sex hormonal status is a further factor influencing the rate of rheumatic diseases. It is therefore important, whenever possible, to evaluate epidemiologic data broken down into age (e.g., 10-year age band) and sex-specific group before making inferences.[4] Obviously, sex hormones seem to play an important role as modulators of both disease onset and perpetuation and they show circadian rhythms together with cortisol.[5]

Sex hormones are implicated in the immune response, with estrogens as enhancers at least of humoral immunity and androgens and progesterone (and glucocorticoids) as natural immune-suppressors[4,5] (see FIG. 1A). Low concentrations of gonadal and adrenal androgen [testosterone (T)/dihydrotestosterone (DHT), dehydroepiandrosterone (DHEA) and its sulfate (DHEAS), respectively] levels, as well as reduced androgen/estrogen ratio, have been detected in serum and body fluids (i.e., blood, synovial fluid [SF], smears, saliva) of male and female RA patients, as well as in SLE, supporting the possible pathogenic role for the decreased levels of the immune-suppressive androgens.[6] However, with respect to serum levels of estrogens, interestingly they are not significantly changed, which is in complete contrast to androgen levels in RA patients (reduced).[4]

Several physiological, pathological, and therapeutic conditions may change the serum estrogen milieu and/or peripheral conversion rate, including the menstrual cycle, pregnancy, postpartum period, menopause, being elderly, chronic stress, altered circadian rhythms (i.e., cortisol/melatonin), inflammatory cytokines, and use of corticosteroids, oral contraceptives, and steroid hormonal replacements, inducing altered androgen/estrogen ratios and related effects.[5–7] Recently, it was shown that at physiological concentrations, 17-beta estradiol and a combination of downstream estrogens stabilized or increased immune stimuli–induced tumor necrosis factor (TNF) secretion.[8] These effects are dependent on the presence of physiological concentrations of cortisol and are therefore related to its circadian rhythms.[8]

As a matter of fact, sex hormones can also exert local actions (paracrine) in the tissues in which they are formed or enter the circulation and both T

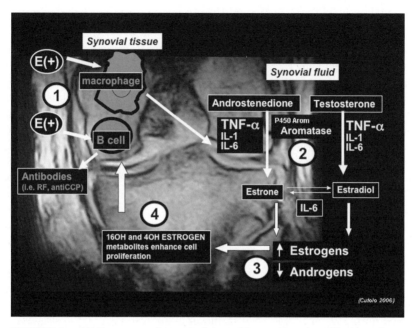

FIGURE 1. (**A**) Estrogens enhance the humoral immunity and proliferation of monocytes/macrophages. (**B**) The proinflammatory cytokines (e.g., tumor necrosis factor alpha, IL-1β, IL-6) have been found to accelerate the metabolic conversion of estrogens from androgens by inducing the synovial tissue aromatases. (**C**) Therefore, increased concentrations of estrogens (and low androgens) are observed at the level of the synovial fluid of RA patients of both sexes. (**D**) Estrogen hydroxylated metabolites, in particular 16alpha-hydroxyestrone, exert mitogenic and cell proliferative effects.

and 17-beta estradiol seem to exert dose- and time-dependent effects on cell growth and apoptosis.[2,4] These effects, as well as important influences on gene promoter of Th1/Th2 cytokines and the recently discovered increased SF estrogen concentrations might suggest new interesting roles for estrogens, at least in RA.[8–11]

PERIPHERAL SEX HORMONE METABOLISM IN AUTOIMMUNE DISEASES

Several findings suggest an accelerated metabolic conversion of upstream androgen precursors to 17-beta estradiol in RA and SLE patients. The 17-beta estradiol, as the aromatic product of the gonadal steroid metabolic pathway and the result of peripheral conversion from the adrenal androgen DHEA, recognizes as upstream precursors different hormones such as DHEA, testosterone and progesterone.

As a matter of fact, a very large number of studies and reviews have shown in the last 20 years reduced serum concentrations of DHEAS, testosterone, and progesterone in both male and female RA/SLE patients.[12,13] These data strongly support an accelerated peripheral metabolic conversion of upstream androgen precursors to 17-beta estradiol.

High estrogen concentrations have been found particularly in synovial fluids of RA patients of both sexes. The appropriate explanation might originate from recent studies showing that the inflammatory cytokines (i.e., TNFα, IL-6, IL-1), particularly increased in RA synovitis, are able to markedly stimulate the aromatase activity in peripheral tissues[14,15] (see FIG. 1B).

As a matter of fact, the aromatase enzyme complex is involved in the peripheral conversion of androgens (testosterone and androstenedione) to estrogens (estrone and estradiol, respectively). In tissues rich in macrophages a significant correlation was found between the aromatase activity and the IL-6 production, and aromatase has been also found in synoviocytes.[16] Therefore, the increased aromatase activity induced by locally produced inflammatory cytokines (i.e., TNFα, IL-1, IL-6) might explain the altered balance resulting in lower androgens and higher estrogens in the synovial RA fluids, as well as their effects on synovial cells, first described in our research[17] (see FIG. 1C).

The role of local sex hormone concentrations at the level of inflammatory foci is of great value in order to explain the modulatory effects exerted by these hormones on the immune-inflammatory reaction.

Men with RA have a higher than normal frequency of low testosterone levels. Interestingly, in a recent study, DHEAS and estrone concentrations have been found lower and estradiol was found higher in male RA patients compared with healthy controls.[18]

In this study, estrone did not correlate with any disease variable, whereas estradiol correlated strongly and positively with all measured indices of inflammation. Men with RA had aberrations in all sex hormones analyzed, although only estradiol consistently correlated with inflammation.[18] The low levels of estrone and DHEAS may depend on a shift in the adrenal steroidogenesis towards the glucocorticoid pathway, whereas increased conversion of estrone to estradiol seemed to be the cause for the high estradiol levels (effect of the 17beta-hydroxysteroid dehydrogenase).

In SLE patients the aromatase activity evaluated in skin and subcutaneous tissue, showed a tendency toward an increase when compared to control subjects.[19] Among SLE patients, the aromatase activity varied inversely with disease activity and the patients had decreased androgen and increased estrogen serum levels.[19] Therefore, tissue aromatase activity showed significant direct correlation with estrogen levels in SLE patients.

These data suggest that abnormal regulation of aromatase activity (i.e., increased activity) may partially explain the abnormalities of peripheral estrogen synthesis (i.e., increased availability of 17-beta estradiol and possible metabolites) in SLE, as well as the altered serum sex-hormone levels and ratio (i.e., decreased androgens and DHEAS) (see FIG. 1C).

Similarly, a recent study by Straub proposed that the urinary excretion of hydroxyestrogens (namely, 16α-hydroxyestrone and 2-hydroxyestrogens) reflects the production in the tissues, because no respective hydroxylase activity is expected in the urine.[20,21]

On the other hand, as recently reviewed, peripheral estrogen hydroxylation was found increased in both men and women with SLE and the estrogenic metabolites have been reported to increase B cell differentiation and to activate T cells.[22]

THE ROLE OF THE ESTROGEN METABOLITES

Therefore, the elevated serum levels of 16α-hydroxyestrone, already described in SLE patients, indicate that disease in men differs from diseases in women to the extent that only 16 alpha-hydroxyestrone was elevated in men, whereas women had elevations of both 16 alpha-hydroxyestrone and estriol.[23] These data suggest abnormal patterns of 17-beta estradiol metabolism which may lead to increased estrogenic activity in SLE patients.

A similar phenomenon is described in the synovial fluids of RA patients where the increased estrogen concentration observed in both sexes are more specifically characterized by the hydroxylated forms, in particular 16alpha-hydroxyestrone, which is a mitogenic and cell proliferative endogenous hormone[17,20] (see FIG. 1D). In these studies, the molar ratio of free estrogens/free androgens was found significantly higher in RA synovial fluids.

Two important aspects must be considered. Total serum levels of 17-beta estradiol are not typically outside of physiologic ranges in RA, as well as in SLE patients of both sexes, and the reported alterations in estrogen metabolism are again observed in both male and female patients, as recently reviewed.[24,25]

Therefore, it is intriguing that gender may not influence the entire phenomenon and that the gonadal production of the sex hormones is not responsible for the observed metabolic results, because most of the measured metabolites are converted in the periphery, which is largely independent of gender. The phenomenon seems only dependent on the inflammatory state of the tissues, and the common mechanisms in both RA and SLE patients might indicate that is also a disease-unspecific phenomenon.

Furthermore, 17-beta estradiol is thought to play a dual pro- and anti-inflammatory role in chronic inflammatory diseases that was found related to low and high concentrations, respectively. In the light of these data, it is possible that the phenomenon might just depend on different dose-related rate of peripheral 17-beta estradiol conversion to pro- or anti-inflammatory metabolites, such as 16α-hydroxyestrone or naturally occurring antagonists (i.e., 2-hydroxyestrogens), respectively.[26]

POSSIBLE MECHANISMS OF IMMUNOMODULATION BY SEX HORMONES: THE CLINICAL EVIDENCE

Macrophages release cytokines such as tumor necrosis factor alpha (TNF alpha), interleukin-1 (IL-1), and IL-6, which, for example, modulate the symptoms at least of RA. Macrophage release of these cytokines can be modulated by estrogen by different ways. Fc gamma receptor type IIIA (CD16a) is a receptor expressed on macrophages that selectively binds IgG molecules, an important rheumatoid factor in RA. Binding of CD16 by anti-CD16 monoclonal antibodies stimulates macrophage cytokine release. In a recent study, estrogen can modulate proinflammatory cytokine release from activated monocytes and/or macrophages, in particular through modulation of CD16 expression.[27]

On the other hands, recent studies have shown that 16α-hydroxyestrone was far more potent than 17-beta estradiol in exerting cell proliferative activities (Fig. 1). More recently we tested in cultured human myeloid monocytic cells (THP-1), differentiated into activated macrophages (M), the effects of 17-beta estradiol and testosterone in order to evaluate their influence on cell proliferation and apoptosis.[28] The effects were evaluated on the NF-κB activity, as a complex of molecules modulating cellular activation. Testosterone was found to exert proapoptotic effects and to reduce M proliferation, whereas 17-beta estradiol induced opposite effects by interfering with NF-κB activities.[28] Therefore, these results seem to support the hypothesis of a sex hormone modulation of cell growth and apoptosis.

In another study, 17-beta estradiol was found to increase IgG and IgM production by peripheral blood mononuclear cells (PBMCs) from SLE patients, which leads to elevated levels of polyclonal IgG, including IgG anti-dsDNA by enhancing B cell activity via interleukin 10 (IL-10).[19] These latter results should also be replicated in the presence of 16α-hydroxyestrone as well as with the naturally occurring 2-hydroxylated antiestrogen. In fact, in a recent study it has been shown that disease activity in SLE patients was negatively correlated to urinary concentrations of 2-hydroxylated estrogens.[21]

Estrogens are confirmed as one of the risk factors in autoimmunity. Interesting changes of serum estrogens have been found during pregnancy in SLE patients and have been found correlated with cytokine variations.[29,30] The major hormonal alteration observed during pregnancy in SLE patients was an unexpected lack of estrogen serum level increase, and, to a lesser extent, progesterone serum level increase, during the second and even more in the third trimester of gestation.[29] This lack of increase probably was due to placental compromise. In addition, a lower than expected increase of IL-6 in the third trimester of gestation and persistently high levels of IL-10 during pregnancy seem to be the major alterations of the cytokine milieu in the peripheral circulation of pregnant patients with SLE.[30]

Therefore, these steroid hormone and cytokine variations may result in a lower humoral immune response activation, probably related to a change in the estrogen/androgen balance, which in turn could account for a more immunosuppressive effect exerted by cytokines on disease activity as observed during the third trimester in pregnant SLE patients.[29]

Because cyclophosphamide-induced ovarian failure has been reported to be protective against flare-ups of SLE, a recent study evaluated whether patients with SLE experience a decrease in disease activity after natural menopause.[31] Differences in disease activity scores (mean and maximum) and the number of visits to a rheumatologist's office were only significant when the fourth year before menopause was compared with the fourth year after menopause. Disease activity was found to be mild during the premenopausal and postmenopausal periods in women with SLE. A modest decrease, especially in the maximum disease activity, was seen after natural menopause.[31] A role might also be played by the effects of behavioral conditions at different latitudes, such as was observed by comparing cortisol, melatonin, and inflammatory cytokines between northern (Estonia) and southern (Italy) Europe.[2,5,6]

CONCLUSIONS

Sex hormones can exert local (paracrine) actions in the tissues in which they are formed and an accelerated peripheral metabolic conversion of upstream androgen precursors to 17-beta estradiol and even conversion to more estrogenic metabolites is observed at least in RA/SLE patients. Cortisol and melatonin circadian rhythms are altered, at least in RA, and partially involve also sex hormone circadian synthesis and levels.[32]

Local effects of sex hormones in autoimmune rheumatic diseases seems to consist mainly in modulation of cell proliferation and cytokine production. In this respect, it is interesting that male patients with RA seem to profit more from anti-TNFalpha strategies than do female patients.[33]

Because male patients have elevated levels of circulating androgens in comparison with female patients, this probably leads to a relatively higher local aromatase-mediated production of proinflammatory estrogens in men with RA compared with women with the disease. Therefore, blockade of TNF-induced upregulation of aromatase would particularly increase the level of androgens in male as compared with female patients with RA, and this can lead to a better clinical outcome, already reported in male patients.[34]

All these data further suggest caution in exogenous estrogen administration in patients with autoimmune diseases (i.e., oral contraceptive pills, estrogen replacements, induction of ovulation), and offer the prospect of novel and improved applications of hormonal or/and antihormonal immunotherapy (i.e., antiestrogens, receptor modulators, antagonist metabolites, and androgenic compounds).

ACKNOWLEDGMENTS

Neuroendocrine studies in RA were partially supported by the EULAR Study Group on Neuroendocrine Immunity in Rheumatic Diseases (NEIRD) and the First Executive Programme of the cultural, educational, scientific, and technological co-operation between Italy and Estonia (2005–2008, program 5) and were supported by the Ministery for Foreign Affairs of Italy and the Ministeries of Culture, Education and Research of Estonia.

REFERENCES

1. BIJLSMA, J.W., A. MASI, R.H. STRAUB, *et al.* 2006. Neuroendocrine immune system involvement in rheumatology. Ann. N. Y. Acad. Sci. **1069:** xviii–xxiv.
2. CUTOLO, M., G.J. MAESTRONI, K. OTSA, *et al.* 2005. Circadian melatonin and cortisol levels in rheumatoid arthritis patients in winter time: a north and south Europe comparison. Ann. Rheum. Dis. **64:** 212–216.
3. STRAUB, R.H. & M. CUTOLO. 2006. Does stress influence the course of rheumatic diseases? Clin. Exp. Rheumatol. **24:** 225–228.
4. CUTOLO, M. 2003. Gender and the rheumatic diseases: epidemiological evidence and possible biologic mechanisms. Ann. Rheum. Dis. **62:** 3.
5. CUTOLO, M., B. VILLAGGIO, K. OTSA, *et al.* 2005. Altered circadian rhythms in rheumatoid arthritis patients play a role in the disease's symptoms. Autoimmun. Rev. **4:** 497–502.
6. CUTOLO, M., K. OTSA, O. AAKRE, *et al.* 2005. Nocturnal hormones and clinical rhythms in rheumatoid arthritis. Ann. N. Y. Acad. Sci. **1051:** 372–378.
7. STRAUB, R.H., F. BUTTGEREIT & M. CUTOLO. 2005. Benefit of pregnancy in inflammatory arthritis. Ann. Rheum. Dis. **64:** 801–803.
8. JANELE, D., T. LANG, S. CAPELLINO, *et al.* 2006. Effects of testosterone, 17-beta estradiol, and downstream estrogens on cytokine secretion from human leukocytes in the presence and absence of cortisol. Ann. N. Y. Acad. Sci. **1069:** 168–182.
9. KAWASAKI, T., T. USHIYAMA, K. INOUE, *et al.* 2000. Effects of estrogen on interleukin-6 production in rheumatoid fibroblast-like synoviocytes. Clin. Exp. Rheumatol. **18:** 743–745.
10. LI, Z.G., V.A. DANIS & P.M. BROOKS. 1993. Effect of gonadal steroids on the production of IL-1 and IL-6 by blood mononuclear cells *in vitro*. Clin. Exp. Rheumatol. **11:** 157–162.
11. CUTOLO, M., B. VILLAGGIO, P. MONTAGNA, *et al.* 2004. Synovial fluid estrogens in rheumatoid arthritis. Autoimmun. Rev. **3:** 193–198.
12. BIJLSMA, J.W.J., R.H. STRAUB, A.T. MASI, *et al.* 2002. Neuroendocrine immune mechanisms in rheumatic diseases. Trends Immunol. **23:** 59–76.
13. LAHITA, R.G., H.L. BRADLOW, E. GINZLER, *et al.* 1987. Low plasma androgens in women with sustemic lupus erythematosus. Arthritis Rheum. **30:** 241–248.
14. MACDIARMID, F., D. WANG & L.G. DUNCAN. 1994. Stimulation of aromatase activity in breast fibroblasts by tumor necrosis factor α. Mol. Cell. Endocrinol. **106:** 17–21.

15. PUROHIT, A., M.W. GHILCHIC & L. DUNCAN. 1995. Aromatase activity and interleukin-6 production by normal and malignant breast tissues. J. Clin. Endocrinol. Metab. **80:** 3052–3058.
16. LE BAIL, J., B. LIAGRE, P. VERGNE, et al. 2001. Aromatase in synovial cells from postmenopausal women. Steroids **66:** 749–757.
17. CASTAGNETTA, L., M. CUTOLO, O. GRANATA, et al. 1999. Endocrine end-points in rheumatoid arthritis. Ann. N. Y. Acad. Sci. **876:** 180–192.
18. TENGSTRAND, B., K. CARLSTRON, L. FELLANDER-TSAI, et al. 2003. Abnormal levels of serum dehydroepiandrosterone, estrone, and estradiol in men with rheumatoid arthritis: high correlation between serum estradiol and current degree of inflammation. J. Rheumatol. **30:** 2338–2343.
19. FOLOMEEV, M., M. DOUGADOS, J. BEAUNE, et al. 1992. Plasma sex hormones and aromatase activity in tissues of patients with systemic lupus erythematosus. Lupus **1:** 191–195.
20. CASTAGNETTA, L.A., G. CARRUBA, M. CUTOLO, et al. 2003. Increased estrogen formation and estrogen to androgen ratio in the synovial fluid of patients with rheumatoid arthritis. J. Rheumatol. **30:** 2597–2605.
21. WEIDLER, C., P. HARLE, J. SCHEDEL, et al. 2004. Patients with rheumatoid arthritis and systemic lupus erythematosus have increased renal excretion of mitogenic estrogens in relation to endogenous antiestrogens. J. Rheumatol. **31:** 489–494.
22. KANDA, N., T. TSUCHIDA & K. TAMAKI. 1999. Estrogen enhancement of anti-double-stranded DNA antibody and immunoglobulin G production in peripheral blood mononuclear cells from patients with systemic lupus erythematosus. Arthritis Rheum. **42:** 328–337.
23. LAHITA, R.G., H.L. BRADLOW, H.G. KUNKEL, et al. 1979. Alterations of estrogen metabolism in systemic lupus erythematosus. Arthritis Rheum. **22:** 1195–1198.
24. CUTOLO, M., A. SULLI , B. SERIOLO, et al. 2003. New roles for estrogens in rheumatoid arthritis. Clin. Exp. Rheumatol. **21:** 687–690.
25. MCMURRAY, R.W. & W. MAY. 2003. Sex hormones and systemic lupus erythematosus: review and meta-analysis. Arthritis Rheum. **48:** 2100–2110.
26. CUTOLO, M. 2004. Estrogen metabolites: increasing evidence for their role in rheumatoid arthritis and systemic lupus erythematosus. J. Rheumatol. **31:** 419–421.
27. KRAMER, P.R., S.F. KRAMER & G. GUAN. 2004. 17 beta-estradiol regulates cytokine release through modulation of CD16 expression in monocytes and monocyte-derived macrophages. Arthritis. Rheum. **50:** 1967–1975.
28. CUTOLO, M., S. CAPELLINO, P. MONTAGNA, et al. 2005. Sex hormone modulation of cell growth and apoptosis of the human monocytic/macrophage cell line. Arthritis. Res. Ther. **7:** R1124–R1132.
29. DORIA, A., M. CUTOLO, A. GHIRARDELLO, et al. 2002. Hormones and disease activity during pregnancy in systemic lupus erythematosus. Arthritis Rheum. **47:** 202–209.
30. DORIA, A., A. GHIRARDELLO, L. PUNZI, et al. 2004. Pregnancy, cytokines and disease activity in systemic lupus erythematosus. Arthritis Rheum. **51:** 989–995.
31. SANCHEZ-GUERRERO, J., A. VILLEGAS, A. MENDOZA, et al. 2001. Disease activity during the premenopausal and postmenopausal periods in women with systemic lupus erythematosus. Am. J. Med. **11:** 464–468.

32. CUTOLO, M., A. SULLI, K. OTSA, *et al.* 2006. Circadian rhythms: glucocorticoids and arthritis. Ann. N. Y. Acad. Sci. **1069:** 289–299.
33. KVIEN, T.K., T. UHLIG, S. ODEGARD, *et al.* 2006. Epidemiological aspects of rheumatoid arthritis: the sex ratio. Ann. N. Y. Acad. Sci. **1069:** 212–222.
34. STRAUB, R.H., P. HARLE, M. CUTOLO, *et al.* 2006. Tumor necrosis factor-neutralizing therapies improve altered hormone axes: an alternative mode of anti-inflammatory action. Arthritis Rheum. **54:** 2039–2046.

Index of Contributors